INTERNATIONAL SERIES OF MONOGRAPHS ON PURE AND APPLIED BIOLOGY

Division: **BIOCHEMISTRY**

VOLUME 3

PHYSICAL PROPERTIES OF THE STEROID HORMONES

OTHER TITLES IN THE SERIES ON PURE AND APPLIED BIOLOGY

BIOCHEMISTRY DIVISION

Vol. 1. PITT-RIVERS and TATA — *The Thyroid Hormones*
Vol. 2. BUSH — *The Chromatography of Steroids*

BOTANY DIVISION

Vol. 1. BOR — *Grasses of Burma, Ceylon, India and Pakistan*
Vol. 2. TURRILL (Ed.) — *Vistas in Botany*, Vol. 1
Vol. 3. SCHULTES — *Native Orchids of Trinidad and Tobago*
Vol. 4. COOKE — *Cork and the Cork Tree*
Vol. 5. TURRILL — *Vistas in Botany*, Vol. 2

MODERN TRENDS IN PHYSIOLOGICAL SCIENCES DIVISION

Vol. 1. FLORKIN — *Unity and Diversity in Biochemistry*
Vol. 2. BRACHET — *The Biochemistry of Development*
Vol. 3. GEREBTZOFF — *Cholinesterases*
Vol. 4. BROUHA — *Physiology in Industry*
Vol. 5. BACQ and ALEXANDER — *Fundamentals of Radiobiology*
Vol. 6. FLORKIN (Ed.) — *Aspects of the Origin of Life*
Vol. 7. HOLLAENDER (Ed.) — *Radiation Protection and Recovery*
Vol. 8. KAYSER — *The Physiology of Natural Hibernation*
Vol. 9. FRANÇON — *Progress in Microscopy*
Vol. 10. CHARLIER — *Coronary Vasodilators*
Vol. 11. GROSS — *Oncogenic Viruses*
Vol. 12. MERCER — *Keratin and Keratinization*
Vol. 13. HEATH — *Organophosphorus Poisons*
Vol. 14. CHANTRENNE — *The Biosynthesis of Proteins*
Vol. 15. RIVERA — *Cilia, Ciliated Epithelium and Ciliary Activity*
Vol. 16. ENSELME — *Unsaturated Fatty Acids in Atherosclerosis*

PLANT PHYSIOLOGY DIVISION

Vol. 1. SUTCLIFFE — *Mineral Salts Absorption in Plants*
Vol. 2. SIEGEL — *The Plant Cell Wall*
Vol. 3. MAYER and POLJAKOFF-MAYBER — *The Germination of Seeds*

PHYSICAL PROPERTIES OF THE STEROID HORMONES

Edited by
LEWIS L. ENGEL
ASSOCIATE PROFESSOR OF BIOLOGICAL CHEMISTRY
HARVARD UNIVERSITY MEDICAL SCHOOL

THE MACMILLAN COMPANY
NEW YORK
1963

THE MACMILLAN COMPANY
60 Fifth Avenue, New York 11, N.Y.

COLLIER-MACMILLAN CANADA LTD.
Galt, Ontario, Canada

PERGAMON PRESS LTD.
Headington Hill Hall, Oxford
4 & 5 Fitzroy Square, London, W.1

Library of Congress Card Number 61–12440

Set in Monotype Times New Roman 10 on 12 point and printed in Great Britain by Fisher, Knight & Co., Ltd., St. Albans.

CONTENTS

FOREWORD

THIS is an important volume written by an outstanding group of investigators who have given generously of their time so that the research efforts of their colleagues may be aided. It is important that this work has been done by practising scientists so that the information has been assured an efficient presentation. The individual contributors are congratulated on the excellency of their efforts.

The creation of a volume such as this is a task far beyond the abilities and energies of any single individual. It was imperative, therefore, to have an initiator, an inducer, a persuader, and a correlator. These four functions have been executed successfully and cheerfully by the Editor, Dr. Lewis Engel, who performed his duties in his usual scholarly manner. I can report that the co-authors still refer to the Editor with affection and respect.

This volume clearly illustrates the efficiency of modern methodology for the solution of problems of isolation, identification and quantitative determination of steroids. We have not only entered the era of " machine " chemistry but automation is essentially with us. I have not heard of an instrument which analyzes a mixture of steroids in a few milliseconds and presents the operator with a printed record of their structures and their quantitative abundance. The data so orderly presented in this volume will aid in the designing and executing of such valuable tools for the steroid chemist.

Steroid chemistry and all its subdivisions and interrelated fields have been enriched because this book was written. All who so profitably will use this volume will be grateful to those who labored so well.

RALPH I. DORFMAN.

EDITORIAL NOTE

It has not been found possible, without delaying publication and expanding editorial labor beyond reasonable limits, to eliminate from this book individual variation in some details of nomenclature and symbols. In the absence of agreed — and universally *accepted* — international conventions it is hoped that, although complete consistency has not been attained, any ambiguity has been avoided.

Examples of the variation in question are the use of the equivalent names allopregnane or 5α-pregnane, and of Δ^5-pregnene or 5-pregnene. Again, in the presentation of absorption data there are used the abbreviation "O.D." for optical density and "m." for mole, as in concentrations expressed in the form 2.1 mg (7.0×10^{-6} m.)/100 ml.

This volume is not an exhaustive compilation of physical data. Attention is directed to *Pouvoir Rotatoire Naturel*. I. *Steroides* by J.-P. Mathieu and A. Petit, Pergamon Press, as well as *Infrared Absorption Spectra of Steroids* by K. Dobriner, E. R. Katzenellenbogen and R. Norman Jones, Interscience Publishers, New York, 1953, and Volume II of the same work by G. Roberts, B. S. Gallagher and R. Norman Jones, Interscience Publishers, New York, 1958. Important data are also presented in *The Chromatography of Steroids* by I. E. Bush, Pergamon Press, Oxford, 1961, and in *Optical Rotatory Dispersion* by C. Djerassi, McGraw-Hill Book Company, Inc., New York, 1960.

PARTITION COEFFICIENTS*

LEWIS L. ENGEL† AND PRISCILLA CARTER

From the John Collins Warren Laboratories of the Collis P. Huntington Memorial Hospital of Harvard University at the Massachusetts General Hospital, and the Department of Biological Chemistry, Harvard Medical School, Boston, Massachusetts

IN the processing of tissues and body fluids for the isolation and identification of steroid hormones and their metabolites, partitions between two liquid phases play a predominant role. They are employed in the preliminary separation of these substances from other classes of compounds and also in the more delicate procedures involved in the resolution of mixtures of closely related substances by countercurrent distribution and liquid–liquid partition chromatography. For these reasons, increasing attention has been given to the measurement of partition coefficients of steroid hormones and their derivatives and metabolites in varous two-phase liquid–liquid systems. With the aid of these physical constants, it is possible to establish

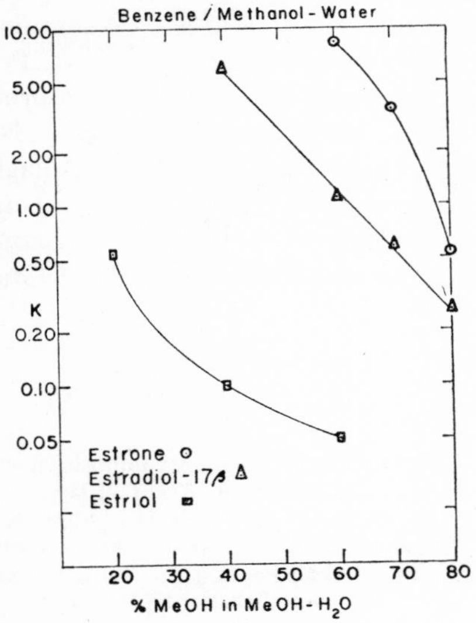

FIG. 1

Relation between phase composition and partition coefficient, K, for Estrone, Estradiol-17β and Estriol in the system Benzene/Methanol : Water

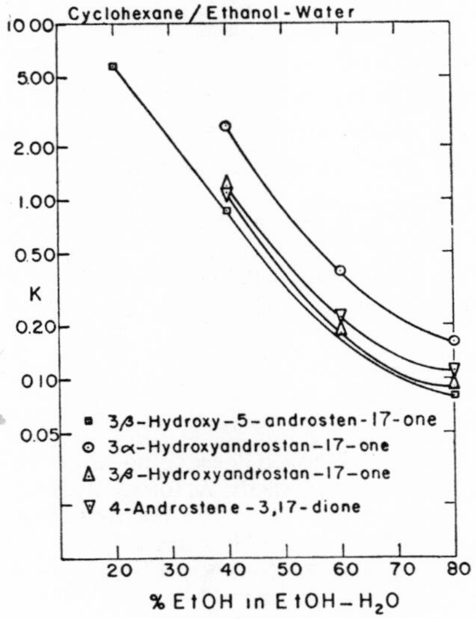

FIG. 2

Relation between phase composition and partition coefficient, K, for 3β-Hydroxy-5-androsten-17-one, 3α-Hydroxyandrostan-17-one, 3β-Hydroxyandrostan-17-one, and 4-Androstene-3,17-dione in the system Cyclohexane/Ethanol : Water

* This work was supported by grants from the National Cancer Institute, United States Public Health Service, a grant from the American Cancer Society, Inc., and a grant from the Jane Coffin Childs Memorial Fund for Medical Research.

This is publication Number 1056 of the Cancer Commission of Harvard University.

† Permanent Faculty Fellow of the American Cancer Society.

more rational methods of procedure for isolation and identification. Apparatus, some solvent systems and mathematical treatment of three-phase countercurrent distribution have been described,[34] but this procedure has not yet been applied to the separation of mixtures of steroids.

A knowledge of the value of the partition coefficient can be extremely useful in determining the type of process required to achieve a given separation. It can, for example, help to decide whether the best procedure in a given instance is continuous extraction in one of the many types of apparatus available for this purpose,[14] hand extraction or a short countercurrent distribution. In order to make these choices it is also necessary to know something of the properties of the substances which accompany the material whose isolation is sought. In these preliminary processes,

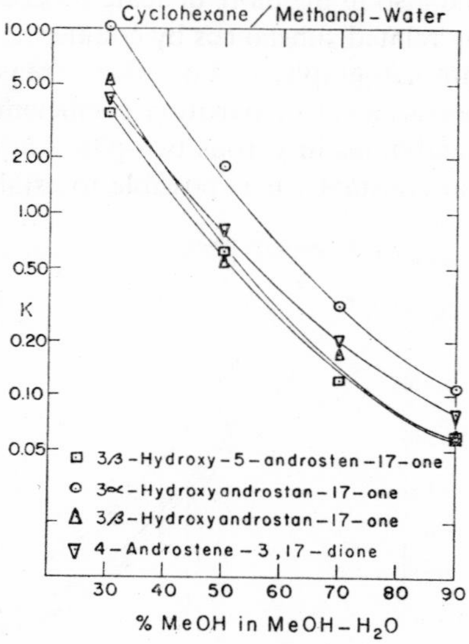

FIG. 3

Relation between phase composition and partition coefficient, K, for 3β-Hydroxy-5-androsten-17-one, 3α-Hydroxyandrostan-17-one, 3β-Hydroxyandrostan-17-one, and 4-Androstene-3,17-dione in the system Cyclohexane/Methanol : Water

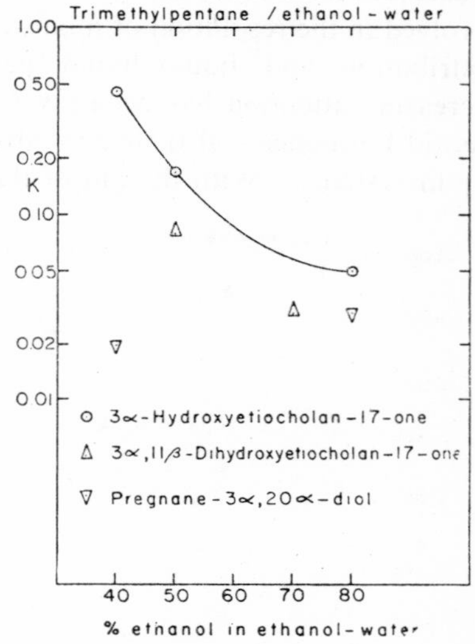

FIG. 4

Relation between phase composition and partition coefficient, K, for 3α-Hydroxy-etiocholan-17-one, 3α-11β-Dihydroxy-etiocholan-17-one, and Pregnane-3α,20α-diol in the system 2,2,4-Trimethylpentane/Ethanol : Water

employed for the concentration of the desired component, it is important to use partition coefficients that are either very large or very small; hopefully the corresponding constants for the contaminants are such that they will not be concentrated in the same phase as the steroids. These ends are only approximately possible, and for this reason finer fractionation becomes necessary.

A knowledge of the values of the partition coefficients of at least some of the components of a mixture is required in the application of countercurrent distribution. This technique has been discussed at length in numerous reviews,[14, 43] and it is only necessary to comment here that it is applicable for the separation of mixtures, for the characterization and quantitative estimation of individual components of such mixtures, and for the study of radiochemical purity.[4, 39a, 39b]

I. THE MEASUREMENT OF PARTITION COEFFICIENTS

The partition coefficient in this chapter is defined as follows:

$$K = \frac{C_u}{C_l} = \frac{W_u}{W_l} \cdot \frac{V_l}{V_u} \qquad \text{(A)}$$

where C, W and V are concentration of solute, weight of solute, and volumes of phases. u and l refer to the upper, less dense phase and lower, denser phase respectively. In principle, this constant can be determined by measurement of solute concentrations in the two phases at equilibrium after a single equilibration or after multiple equilibrations as in countercurrent distribution. In the latter case the calculation can be made from the analysis of the distribution.[14, 43] Such values are known with greater precision than those obtained by simple equilibration. They are, however, subject to certain errors inherent in the distribution process and the apparatus employed.

When the constant is measured by simple equilibration, the operation is carried out as follows:

Measured portions of a solution of the substance to be examined are transferred to glass stoppered tubes using a suitable solvent which is then removed under conditions which will not cause decomposition of the solute. Then measured volumes (usually equal) of the two mutually saturated phases are added, and the tubes are inverted gently twenty to thirty times to establish equilibrium. After the layers have separated, samples of the two phases are withdrawn from each tube and

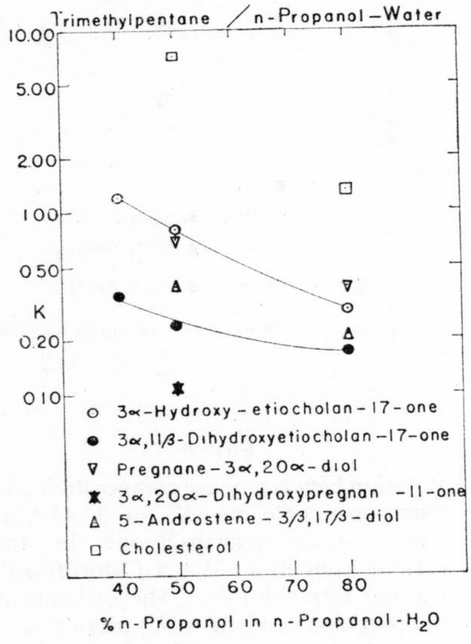

FIG. 5

Relation between phase composition and partition coefficient, K, for 3α-Hydroxyetiocholan-17-one, 3α,11β-Dihydroxyetiocholan-17-one, Pregnane-3α,20α-diol, 3α,20α-Dihydroxypregnan-11-one, 5-Androstene-3β,17β-diol, and Cholesterol in the system 2,2,4-Trimethylpentane/n-Propanol : Water

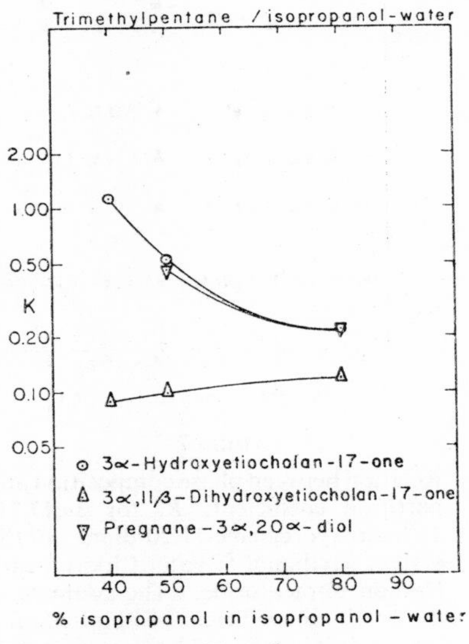

FIG. 6

Relation between phase composition and partition coefficient, K, for 3α-Hydroxyetiocholan-17-one, 3α,11β-Dihydroxyetiocholan-17-one, and Pregnane-3α,20α-diol in the system 2,2,4-Trimethylpentane/iso-Propanol : Water

the amount of solute in each phase measured by an appropriate method. The partition coefficient is then calculated using Equation (A). It is important that analyses be performed on both phases and the recovery calculated, since this provides the only means of knowing whether the solute has been completely dissolved. Analysis of both phases also increases the accuracy and precision in situations where the value of the partition coefficient differs greatly from unity. In such cases it is the ratio of a large to a small number (or the reciprocal) and a small error in the value of the small number produces a large effect upon the value of the ratio. If the partition coefficient in these situations is calculated from analysis of one phase only, a large error may be introduced.

It is difficult to assign limits of errors to the measurement of this constant, since they depend upon both the analytical procedure employed and the numerical value of the partition coefficient. As pointed out above, values differing greatly from one may be subject to quite considerable error.

The partition coefficient may also be estimated from countercurrent distribution curves. In this situation, both the precision and the accuracy of the value obtained

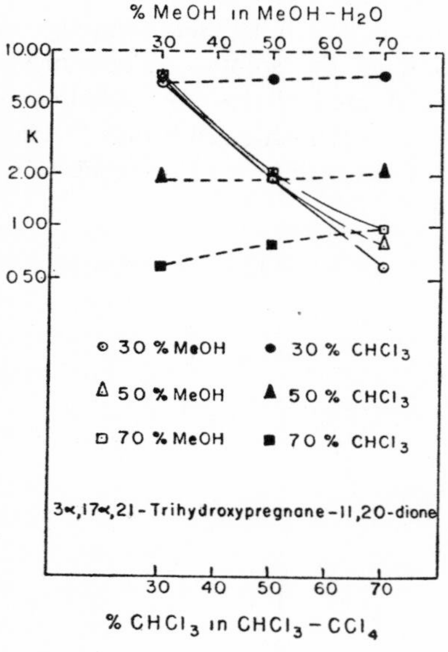

FIG. 7

Relation between phase composition and partition coefficient, *K*, for 3α,17,21-Trihydroxypregnane-11,20-dione in the system Methanol : Water/Chloroform : Carbon tetrachloride. The ordinate is the partition coefficient (*K*) plotted on a logarithmic scale. The lower (solid) abscissa gives the composition of the lower phase and the upper (dashed) abscissa gives the composition of the upper phase. —— Variation in *K* with changing lower phase composition at three fixed upper phase compositions. ------ Variation in *K* with changing upper phase composition at three fixed lower phase compositions

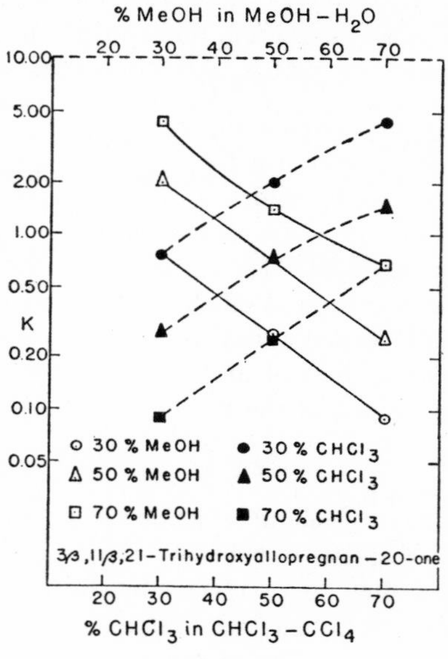

FIG. 8

Relation between phase composition and partition coefficient, *K*, for 3β,11β,21-Trihydroxyallopregnan-20-one in the system Methanol : Water/Chloroform : Carbon tetrachloride. The ordinate is the partition coefficient (*K*) plotted on a logarithmic scale. The lower (solid) abscissa gives the composition of the lower phase and the upper (dashed) abscissa gives the composition of the upper phase. —— Variation in *K* with changing lower phase composition at three fixed upper phase compositions. ------ Variation in *K* with changing upper phase composition at three fixed lower phase compositions

depend upon the variations in the exact phase compositions of the mixtures used in different runs and the variations in ambient temperature. However, since such a partition coefficient is calculated from essentially replicate determinations, it is generally a more reliable value that that determined by single equilibration procedures.

II. FACTORS WHICH INFLUENCE THE PARTITION COEFFICIENT

Although the partition coefficient is temperature dependent, in most of the systems with which experience has been obtained in this laboratory, where a constant temperature room is not available, this factor has not been disturbing in countercurrent distributions which last as long as three or four days. However, it can be expected that in multi-component systems, the compositions of which are such that the two phases are approaching miscibility, the temperature dependence would be great. Even in two component systems in which there is great mutual solubility marked temperature dependence of partition coefficients may be encountered.

Secondly, variations in the composition of the two phases may result in different values for partition coefficients, particularly in multi-component systems.

III. PREPARATION OF SOLVENT SYSTEMS

At any given temperature and pressure the composition of a two-component, two-phase system is fixed.[30] When more components are added, additional degrees of freedom are added and it becomes necessary to specify precisely how the system is made up. Common practice is to indicate the volumes of the individual components that are mixed and allowed to equilibrate. Finally, for measurement of the partition coefficient, equal volumes of the two phases are transferred into glass stoppered tubes as described above. This procedure has been employed in the preparation of all systems employed in this laboratory. The final equilibrium compositions of the two phases cannot be determined readily.*

IV. SOLVENT SYSTEMS

Certain general considerations dictate the choice of solvent systems for the countercurrent distribution of steroids. A primary consideration is that the solvents must neither react irreversibly with the substances present as solutes, nor must they interfere with any analytical procedure to be employed for the analysis of the distribution. The stability of the solvents is important. Since water is almost inevitably one component of a solvent system, care must be taken to employ substances which are not attacked rapidly by water. Esters, for example, present a risk in acidic or basic media, since hydrolysis of the ester with liberation of acid and alcohol would produce a changing phase composition, pH of the aqueous phase, and partition coefficient during the course of the distribution. Under some conditions, too, solvolysis of a solute may be a disturbing factor.[7]

It is generally true that the maximum resolution of two substances is achieved if the two phases in a countercurrent distribution have widely differing dielectric constants. Thus, a system consisting of an aliphatic hydrocarbon and water would be expected to give efficient separations. However, limitations of solubility may make such systems impractical. The addition of solvents in which the steroids

* Vapor phase chromatography may provide a solution to this analytical problem.

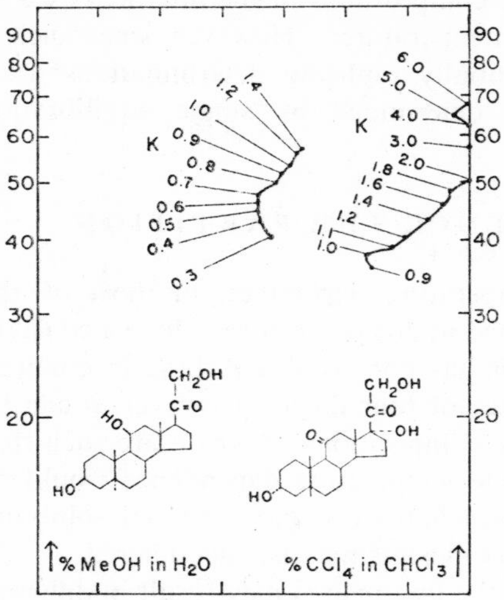

FIG. 9

Nomogram for the determination of the partition coefficients, *K*, of 3β,11β,21-Trihydroxyallopregnan-20-one and 3α,-17α,21-Trihydroxypregnane-11,20-dione in the system Methanol : Water/Chloroform : Carbon tetrachloride

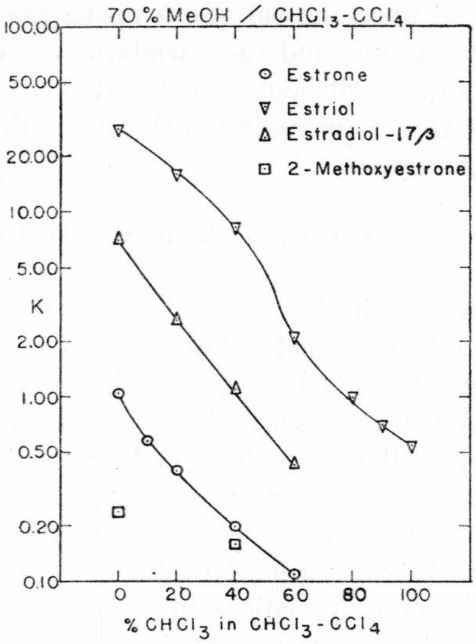

FIG. 10

Relation between phase composition and partition coefficient, *K*, for Estrone, Estradiol-17β, Estriol and 2-Methoxyestrone in the system 70% Methanol/Chloroform : Carbon tetrachloride

have more favorable solubilities will improve the capacity of the system at the expense of resolution. With increasing addition of the second type of solvent, capacity is increased, but resolution diminishes as the compositions of the two phases approach one another. In the limiting case, i.e. miscibility, when the phase compositions approach identity, all partition coefficients approach the same limiting value.[25]

Since the solvents are employed in relatively large volumes for countercurrent distributions, substances should be chosen which can be purified readily. The importance of trace contaminants in solvents should not be underestimated, since the solutes in low concentrations are exposed to them for relatively long periods of time. The role of traces of copper in the destruction of corticosteroids has been noted.[33] Furthermore, if infrared spectroscopy of residues from the tubes of the distribution is contemplated, the presence of residues from unpurified solvents often makes it impossible to obtain satisfactory spectra. A compendium of information concerning properties and purification of organic solvents has been published.[44]

Another factor which may contribute to the successful selection of solvent systems for countercurrent distribution is relative densities of the two phases. Solvents should be chosen which give the maximum difference in density so as to accelerate separation of the phases. This point should be borne in mind particularly when three- and four-component solvent systems are designed.

High boiling, essentially non-volatile liquids such as the glycols, which are employed so effectively in paper chromatography, are not convenient for countercurrent distribution because of the difficulty in removing them for analysis of the solute. Similarly, ether, pentane and similar low boiling solvents are unsatisfactory, since their rapid volatilization leads to changes in phase composition even during the course of a relatively short countercurrent distribution.

The toxicity of the solvent should also be considered and adequate ventilation provided and precautions taken when benzene, chlorinated hydrocarbons, or other toxic agents are employed.

A further factor is the tendency of the system to form emulsions, which not only slow down the distribution but also may lead to asymmetry of countercurrent distribution curves. In our experience benzene, toluene and cyclohexane are offenders, particularly in the presence of lipids derived from tissue and urinary extracts.

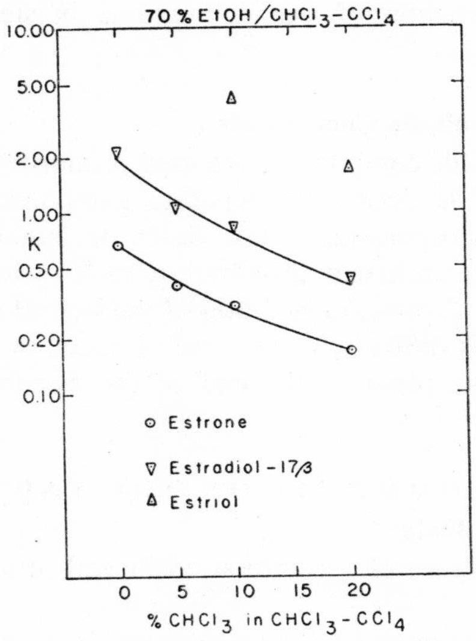

FIG. 11

Relation between phase composition and partition coefficient, *K*, for Estrone, Estradiol-17β, and Estriol in the system 70% Ethanol / Chloroform : Carbon tetrachloride

V. TYPES OF SOLVENT SYSTEMS

Two-Component Systems

Two-component, two-phase systems offer a wide choice and variety but in general have not provided very useful systems for countercurrent distribution, although preliminary separations into groups of compounds of similar polarity may be accomplished effectively with such systems.

Three-Component Systems

Systems composed of two organic solvents in addition to water have been extremely useful in countercurrent distributions. The possibilities of variation in phase composition over a relatively wide range make it possible to have a large choice of partition coefficients in related systems.[24, 31] In addition, this procedure has the advantage that the determination of partition coefficient in several related solvent systems is a more precise means of characterizing a solute than the determination of partition coefficient in a single system.

Four-Component Systems

Even greater latitude is permitted when four components are employed and a nomographic approach to systems of this type has already been reported.[25]

Simplifications of the nomographic technique have recently been made which avoid some of the laborious computations required in the earlier method. If, in the initial graphs, phase composition is plotted against partition coefficient on three cycle semilogarithmic paper, transformation of the measured partition coefficient values to the logarithms is avoided. If now the vertical axes of the solvent composition ratios of the two phases are plotted on the logarithmic scale of single cycle semilogarithmic paper, a second transformation to logarithms is avoided. The remainder of the construction of the nomograms is similar to that originally described.

Systems Containing Non-volatile Components

Systems with non-volatile components are used primarily for initial fractionations and separations when it is desired to separate compounds into groups. Such systems include those incorporating acids, bases or buffers. Their applications are numerous. For countercurrent distribution such systems are less convenient because of the difficulties involved in isolation of the steroid solutes. It is sometimes possible to circumvent this difficulty in the case of acidic or basic solutes by driving the solute into the organic phase at the end of the distribution by adjustment of pH of the aqueous phase.

VI. COMMENTS ON THE TABLES

Criteria for Acceptance of Data

The criteria for acceptance of a partition coefficient of a substance in the tables which follow are:

(1) that the constant must have been measured either on the pure crystalline compound by a single equilibration or by countercurrent distribution,

(2) that if it were measured by countercurrent distribution, only those cases in which a Gaussian curve is obtained are acceptable, and

(3) that the constant be measured by chemical and physical (including radio-chemical) methods. Partition coefficients measured by biological assay have not been included.

Tabulation of Compounds

Compounds are listed in the order of their empirical formulae. Alphabetical order prevails within groups of compounds having the same empirical formulae.

Systematic names are used except for those trivial names listed in Table I.

VII. INDEX OF SYSTEMS

Table No.	
I	Steroid index: structural name, and name used in tables
II	Ether / Acidic, Neutral, Basic Lower Phases
III	Ethyl acetate / Acidic, Basic Lower Phases
IV	Toluene / Acidic, Basic Lower Phases
V	Benzene / Acidic, Basic, Neutral Lower Phases

Acknowledgements — The authors wish to acknowledge their thanks to the following for making available to us unpublished measurements of partition coefficients: Drs. B. Baggett. R. H. Purdy, R. Walker and I. Weliky ; Misses I. Bjerkedal, A. Dimoline, L. L. Fielding, M. Halla, O. Klein, G. Lanman, M. Witkos and M. Zalkans ; and Mrs. N. Trofimow and Mr. A. Mahoney.

TABLE I. KEY TO NOMENCLATURE

Systematic Name	Trivial Name
C_{18}	
3-Hydroxy-1,3,5(10),6,8-estrapentaen-17-one	Equilenin
1,3,5(10),6,8,-Estrapentaene-3,17β-diol	Dihydroequilenin
3-Hydroxy-1,3,5(10),7-estratetraen-17-one	Equilin
3-Hydroxy-1,3,5(10)-estratriene-6-17-dione	6-Ketoestrone
3-Hydroxy-1,3,5(10)-estratriene-7,17-dione	7-Ketoestrone
3-Hydroxy-1,3,5(10)-estratriene-16-17-dione	16-Ketoestrone
3-Hydroxy-1,3,5(10)-estratrien-17-one	Estrone
3,17β-Dihydroxy-1,3,5(10)-estratrien-6-one	6-Ketoestradiol
3,17β-Dihydroxy-1,3,5(10)-estratrien-16-one	16-Ketoestradiol
1,3,5(10)-Estratrien-3-ol	Deoxyestrone
1,3,5(10)-Estratriene-3,17α-diol	Estradiol-17α
1,3,5(10)-Estratriene-3,17β-diol	Estradiol-17β
1,3,5(10)-Estratriene-3,16β,17β-triol	Epiestriol
1,3,5(10)-Estratriene-3,16α,17β-triol	Estriol
C_{19}	
3-Hydroxy,1-3,5(10)-Estratrien-17-one 2-methyl ether	2-Methoxyestrone
3-Hydroxy-1,3,5(10)-Estratrien-17-one 3-methyl ether	Estrone methyl ether
1,3,5(10)-Estratriene-3,17β-diol 3-methyl ether	Estradiol methyl ether
1,3,5(10)-Estratriene-2,3,17β-triol 2-methyl ether	2-Methoxyestradiol
1,3,5(10)-Estratriene-3,16α,17β-triol 3-methyl ether	Estriol methyl ether
1,3,5(10)-Estratriene-2,3,16α,17β-tetrol 2-methyl ether...	2-Methoxyestriol
3β-Hydroxy-5-androsten-17-one	Dehydroepiandrosterone
17β-Hydroxy-4-androsten-3-one	Testosterone
3α-Hydroxy-5α-androstan-17-one	Androsterone
C_{20}	
17α-Ethinyl-1,3,5(10)-estratriene-3,17β-diol	Ethinyl estradiol
1,3,5(10)-Estratriene-2,3,17β-triol 2,3-dimethyl ether	2-Methoxyestradiol methyl ether
$C_{21}H_{28}$	
1,3,5(10)-Estratriene-3,17β-diol 3-methyl ether 17-acetate	Estradiol methyl ether acetate
21-Hydroxy 4-pregnene-3,11,20-trione	Dehydrocorticosterone
11,21-Dihydroxy-18-aldo-4-pregnene-3,20-dione	Aldosterone
17,21-Dihydroxy-4-pregnene-3,11,20-trione	Cortisone
$C_{21}H_{30}$	
4-Pregnene-3,20-dione	Progesterone
21-Hydroxy-4-pregnene-3,20-dione	Cortexone
11β,21-Dihydroxy-4-pregnene-3,20-dione	Corticosterone
17,21-Dihydroxy-4-pregnene-3,20-dione	Cortexolone
11β,17,21-Trihydroxy-4-pregnene-3,20-dione	Cortisol
$C_{21}H_{34}$	
3α,17,21-Trihydroxy-5β-pregnane-11,20-dione	Tetrahydrocortisone
$C_{21}H_{36}$	
3α,11β,17,21-Tetrahydroxy-5β-pregnan-20-one	Tetrahydrocortisol

TABLE I—*continued* KEY TO NOMENCLATURE

Systematic Name	Trivial Name
C_{22}	
1,3,5(10)-Estratriene-2,3,17β-triol 2,3-dimethyl ether 17-acetate	2-Methoxyestradiol methyl ether acetate
C_{24}	
3-Hydroxy-1,3,5(10)-estratrien-17-one 3-(β-glucopyranosid)-uronic acid	Estrone glucosiduronic acid
C_{25}	
1,3,5(10)-Estratriene-3,16α,17β-triol 3-methyl ether 16,17-diacetate	Estriol methyl ether diacetate
3α-Hydroxy-5α-androstan-17-one 3-(β-glucopyranosid)-uronic acid	Androsterone glucosiduronic acid
3β-Hydroxy-5-androsten-17-one 3-(β-glucopyranosid)-uronic acid	Dehydroepiandrosterone glucosiduronic acid
C_{27}	
5-Cholesten-3β-ol	Cholesterol
3α,17,20β,21-Tetrahydroxy-5β-pregnan-11-one 3-(β-glucopyranosid)-uronic acid	β-Cortolone glucosiduronic acid
3α,17,21-Trihydroxy-5β-pregnane-11,20-dione 3-(β-glucopyranosid)-uronic acid	Tetrahydrocortisone glucosiduronic acid

TABLE II. SYSTEM – ETHER / ACIDIC, NEUTRAL, AND BASIC SOLUTIONS* †

	Compound			
	Estrone	Estradiol-17β	Estriol	16-Epiestriol
Lower phase				
15% HCl (v/v) (16)	70	50	80	
1.5 N H_2SO_4 (23)	100	80	50	
pH 4.0	∞		75	
H_2O (23)	∞	55	24	
H_2O (3)	90	75	55	
pH 8, Carbonate buffer	∞		60	
pH 9, Carbonate buffer (23)	∞	∞	22	
pH 9.3, Carbonate buffer (23)	∞	∞	13	
pH 10.5, Carbonate buffer (35)	∞	∞	13	
pH 10.9 Carbonate buffer (23)	28	34	0.1	
pH 11.9, Carbonate buffer (23)	2.7	3.8	0	
pH 12, Phosphate buffer ‡			0.49	3.4
1.0 N NaOH	0.4	0.7	0.03	
1.0 N NaOH (3) (13)	0.5–0.6	0.6	0	
0.10 N NaOH (3) (13)	2–4	2.0	0.03	
0.02 N NaOH (3)	10			
0.10 N NaOH in 20% NaCl (3)	19			
0.85 M Na_2CO_3 (3)	49	49	49	
1.07 M $NaHCO_3$ (3)	∞	∞	∞	

* Numerical values tabulated in this and subsequent tables are the partition coefficients as defined in Equation (A).
† Unless otherwise noted the partition coefficients tabulated in this and subsequent tables were measured in this laboratory and are either unpublished or may be found in references (4, 22, 23, 24, 25, 26, 27, 40).
‡ Diczfalusy, E. Private Communication, 1956.

TABLE III.—SYSTEM – ETHYL ACETATE / SALTS AND BUFFERS

	Compound		
	Estrone	Estradiol-17β	Estriol
Lower phase			
pH 4*	∞		∞
pH 8*	∞		∞
Saturated $NaHCO_3$ pH 7.9	∞	∞	∞
1 N NaOH†	∞	∞	∞
1 M $KHCO_3$ pH 8.1	1.17	1.27	1.27
3 M $KHCO_3$	0.19	0.47	0.35
0.25 M Na_2CO_3	0.39	0.72	0.43
1.0 M Na_2CO_3	0.61	0.92	0.92

* Dried estrogen dissolved in 25 ml. 1 N NaOH. pH adjusted with 6 N HCl.
† Hydrolysis occurred during extraction, final pH about 8.

TABLE IV. SYSTEM–TOLUENE / AQUEOUS ACIDS AND BASES

	Compound			
	Estrone	Estradiol-17β	Estriol	2-Methoxyestrone
Lower phase				
2.2 N HCl (35)			0.26	
1.5 N HCl (35)	24	19		
0.1 N NaOH (13)	1.47			
1.0 N NaOH (13)	0.27			
1.0 N NaOH (23, 26)	0.14	0.05	0	1.20
2.5 N NaOH	0.25	0.05	0	

TABLE V. SYSTEM – BENZENE / ACID, NEUTRAL, BASIC SOLUTIONS (3)

	Compound		
	Estrone	Estradiol-17β	Estriol
Lower phase			
80% H_2SO_4 — 20% H_2O	0		
67% H_2SO_4 — 33% H_2O	1.5		
50% H_2SO_4 — 50% H_2O	15.6	3.3	
40% H_2SO_4 — 60% H_2O		9.0	
33% H_2SO_4 — 67% H_2O	49	11.5	
10 N HCl	10	2.33	0.02
6.5 N HCl	∞	49	0.11
4 N HCl	∞	49	0.14
2.8 N HCl (35)			0.37
1.54 N HCl (35)	∞	∞	0.37
0.50 N HCl in 20% NaCl			2.03
0.34 M NaCl			2.03
1.1 M $NaHCO_3$			0.67
0.11 M $NaHCO_3$			0.20
0.11 M $NaHCO_3$ in 0.085 M Na_2CO_3			0.14
0.0085 M Na_2CO_3			0.02
0.85 M Na_2CO_3	∞	49	0.02
0.3 M Na_2CO_3	40	12	0.025
0.05 N NaOH in 20% NaCl	24	32	
0.10 N NaOH in 20% NaCl	24	4.6	
0.10 N NH_4OH	24	4.3	0
1.0 N NH_4OH	13.3	4.3	0
2.0 N NH_4OH		2.45	0
0.1 N NaOH	1.22	0.23	0
1.0 N NaOH	0.22	0.04	0
H_2O	∞	∞	0.28

TABLE VI. SYSTEM – BENZENE / METHANOL : WATER*

Compound	% Methanol in Methanol : Water						
	0	20	40	50(9)	60	70	80
C_{18}							
Estrone					8.3	3.5	0.54
Estradiol-17β			6.1		1.1	0.58	0.26
Estriol	0.19 (21)	0.54	0.10		0.05		
Epiestriol	3.4 (21)						
1,3,5(10)-Estratriene-3,16α, 17α-triol	3.8 (21)						
2-Methoxyestradiol	1.2 (28)						
2-Methoxyestriol	1.1 (28)						
C_{21}							
Cortisone	0.97 (9, 11)†			0.26			
Dehydrocorticosterone				2.6			
Cortexone	∞			16			
Corticosterone	10.1 (9, 11)			1.57			
Cortexolone	9.6 (9, 11)			1.22			
Cortisol	0.36 (9, 11)			0.14			

* Some of the data here can be found in graphical form in Figure 1.
† Values taken from references 9–12 may be averages of several values given.

TABLE VII. SYSTEM – 50-BENZENE : 50-PETROLEUM ETHER†/ETHANOL : WATER

Compound	% Ethanol in Ethanol : Water		
	0	2 (21)	30 (3)
Estrone			49
Estradiol-17β	24 (5)		3.16
Estriol	0 (3)		0.05
Epiestriol		0.41	
1,3,5(10)-Estratriene-3,16α, 17α,triol		0.57	

† INVESTIGATORS	Boiling point of petroleum ether used
Bachman & Petitt (3)	35–60° C
Brown, J. B. (5)	40–60° C
Diczfalusy, E. (15, 16, 21)	30–60° C (see Tables IX, X)
Pearlman & Cerceo (36, 37)	35–45° C (see Table IX)

TABLE VIII. SYSTEM – BENZENE : n-HEXANE/ETHANOL : WATER

Compound	% Benzene in Benzene: n-Hexane	0+0.05 % NaCl	% Ethanol in Ethanol : Water													
			0	2	3	5	10	20	47.5*	48.4*	50	52.5*	58*	61*	70	75
C_{18}																
Estriol (3)	100						0.15	0.19								
C_{19}																
4-Androstene-3,11,17-trione	0		1.22													
4-Androstene-3,17-dione (11)	0		6					2.4			0.17					0.08
Dehydroepiandrosterone (12)	0				14											
$C_{21}H_{28}$																
4,11-Pregnadiene-3,20-dione (15)	0									1.13						
Dehydrocorticosterone (9,11)	0		0.04													
Dehydrocorticosterone (9)	40					1.33										
Dehydrocorticosterone (11)	50		3.1													
Dehydrocorticosterone (9,11)	100										2.2				1.0	
Cortisone (11)	75		0.28													
Cortisone (9,11)	100	0.81					0.79				0.64					
$C_{21}H_{30}$																
Progesterone (11)	0								1.21	1.03	0.76	0.76	0.52	0.44		
Cortexone (9,11)	0		2.55					1.08			0.09					
Cortexone (11)	50		16													
Cortexone (9,11)	100						24				7.5					
Corticosterone (11)	38		0.64													
Corticosterone (9)	40					1.08										
Corticosterone (11)	50		1.06													
Corticosterone (11)	75		3.33													
Corticosterone (9,11)	100	9									1.31					

TABLE VIII—*continued*.

Compound	% Benzene in Benzene: n-Hexane	0+0.05 % NaCl	% Ethanol in Ethanol : Water													
			0	2	3	5	10	20	47.5*	48.4*	50	52.5*	58*	61*	70	75
Cortexolone (11)	38		1.08													
Cortexolone (9)	40					1.13										
Cortexolone (11)	50		2.24													
Cortexolone (9,11)	100	13									1.67					
Cortisol (11)	75		0.19													
Cortisol (9,11)	100	0.35									0.31					
$C_{21}H_{32}$																
3β-Hydroxy-5-pregnen-20-one (11,12)	0			18	38						0.54					
3β,17-Dihydroxy-5-pregnen-20-one (12)	0			1.3				0.76								
17-Hydroxy-4-pregnene-3,20-dione (11)	0		1.33					0.82			0.05					
$C_{21}H_{34}$																
Tetrahydrocortisol (11)	100	0.1														

* Figures estimated from graph (15).

TABLE IX. SYSTEM – PETROLEUM ETHER* / METHANOL : WATER

Compound	% Methanol in Methanol : Water		
	0	50	70
Estrone	3.34 (3)	0.06 (3)	
Estradiol-17β	0.79 (3)	0 (3)	
Estriol	0 (3)	0 (16)	
4-Androstene-3,17-dione			0.07 (36)
Testosterone			0.05 (37)
Progesterone			0.33 (36)
Cortexone			0.03 (37)
4-Cholesten-3-one			3.07 (36)
7-Ketocholesterol			1.8 (37)

* See footnote to Table VII.

TABLE X. SYSTEM – PETROLEUM ETHER* / ETHANOL : WATER

Compound	% Ethanol in Ethanol : Water			
	30 (3)	34.5 (15)	40 (3)	50 (3)
Estrone	0.56	0.24	0.14	0.08
Estradiol-17β	0.09	< 0.06	0.03	0
Estriol	0	< 0.01	0	0
Testosterone		0.28		
4,11-Pregnadiene-3,20-dione		5.15		
Cortisone		< 0.02		
Progesterone		3.55		
Cortexone		0.21		
Cortisol		< 0.02		

* See footnote to Table VII.

TABLE XI. SYSTEM – n-HEXANE / METHANOL : WATER

Compound	% Methanol in Methanol : Water				
	0	30	50	70	90
Estrone	6.8				
Estradiol-17β	1.07				
Estriol	0.06				
3α-Hydroxy-5α-estran-17-one			0.67 (27)		
3α-Hydroxy-5β-estran-17-one			0.32 (27)		
Dehydroepiandrosterone			0.26		
Dehydrocorticosterone	0.05 (11)				
Cortexone	2.65 (11)				
Progesterone			1.82		
3β-Hydroxy-5-pregnen-20-one			1.1		
Testosterone		0.48	0.12	0.06	0.03

TABLE XII. SYSTEM – sec-BUTANOL : n-HEXANE / WATER*

Compound	% sec-Butanol in sec-Butanol : n-Hexane					
	15	25	35	50	65	75
4-Androstene-3,11,17-trione		1.22				
4-Androstene-3,17-dione		12.5				
11β-Hydroxy-4-androstene-3,17-dione		2.23				
Aldosterone				1.44	3.5	
Cortisone		0.32	1.04	2.93	6.7	
Dehydrocorticosterone		0.51			8	
Cortexolone		2.85				
Corticosterone	0.25	0.96		7		
Cortisol		0.24	0.84			
Tetrahydrocortisone				3.6		10
Tetrahydrocortisol				5.3		9

* All values in this Table from (10, 11).

TABLE XIII. SYSTEM – ETHYL ACETATE : n-HEXANE / ETHANOL : WATER

Compound	% Ethyl Acetate in Ethyl Acetate : n-Hexane	% Ethanol in Ethanol : Water		
		0 (11)	20.5 (17)	50 (23)
Estrone	40			2.2
Estradiol-17β	40		15.4	0.9
Estriol	40		0.75	0.27
Cortisone	25	0.16		
Cortisone	50	1.38		
Cortexolone	50	6.1		
Corticosterone	25	0.72		
Corticosterone	50	4.3		
Cortisol	25	0.09		
Cortisol	50	1.00		
Tetrahydrocortisol	65	2.45		

TABLE XIV A. SYSTEM – ETHYL ACETATE : CYCLOHEXANE / ETHANOL : WATER

Compound	% Ethyl Acetate in Ethyl Acetate : Cyclohexane	% Ethanol in Ethanol : Water					
		0	33	40	50	60	70
C_{18}							
Equilenin (40)	50		20		4.2		1.0
Dihydroequilenin (40)	50		9		2.5		0.71
Equilin (40)	50		39		3.6		0.74
6-Ketoestrone (40)	50		4.6		3.3		0.59
7-Ketoestrone (40)	50		>10		6.3		1.0
16-Ketoestrone (40)	50		12		1.9		
Estrone (23)	10			1.8			
Estrone (23)	30				2.1		
Estrone (23)	40			10	2.6	0.78	
Estrone (40)	50	24	39		4.2		0.73
Estrone	100	37					
3-Hydroxy-1,3,5(10)-estratrien-16-one (40)	50		17		3.0		
6-Ketoestradiol (40)	50		3.6		2.4		0.42
16-Ketoestradiol	50		5.5 (40)		0.94		
Deoxyestrone (40)	50		33		26		3.1
Estradiol-17α (40)	50		>10		2.5		0.74
Estradiol-17β (23)	10			0.65			
Estradiol-17β (23)	30				0.92		
Estradiol-17β (23)	40			5.2	1.3	0.55	
Estradiol-17β (40)	50	7.6	16		2.9		0.64
Estradiol-17β	100	28					
1,3,5-Estratriene-3,16α, 17α-triol (21)	40			1.3			
16-Epiestriol (21)	40			1.6			
Estriol (23)	10			0.05			
Estriol (23)	30				0.15		
Estriol (23)	40			0.35	0.17	0.17	
Estriol (40)	50	2.9	1.3		0.35		0.35
C_{19}							
2-Methoxyestradiol (29)	50				2.64		
2-Methoxyestriol (28)	50				0.38		

TABLE XIV B. SYSTEM – ETHYL ACETATE : CYCLOHEXANE / ETHANOL : WATER*

Compound	% Ethyl Acetate in Ethyl Acetate : Cyclohexane	% Ethanol in Ethanol : Water						
		20	40	50	55	60	70	80
4-Androstene-3,11,17-trione	30			0.34				
4-Androstene-3,11,17-trione	40			0.67				
Δ^1-5α-Androstene-3,17-dione (25)	20		1.9			0.54	0.28	0.25
Δ^1-5α-Androstene-3,17-dione (25)	40		3.4			0.92	0.51	0.46
Δ^1-5α-Androstene-3,17-dione (25)	60		8.3			1.3	0.89	
4-Androstene-3,17-dione	0	6.5	0.84			0.22		0.11
11β-Hydroxy-4-androstene-3,17-dione	30			0.36				
11β-Hydroxy-4-androstene-3,17-dione	50			1.09				
Androstane-3,17-dione (25)	20		5.8			1.2	0.84	
Androstane-3,17-dione (25)	40		8.4			1.8	0.60	
Androstane-3,17-dione (25)	60		17	6.4		2.5	0.88	
Dehydroepiandrosterone	0	5.8	0.87			0.33		0.08
Dehydroepiandrosterone (25)	20		2.7			0.45		0.21
Dehydroepiandrosterone	30				1.04			
Dehydroepiandrosterone (25)	40		6.1			0.92		0.41
Dehydroepiandrosterone (25)	60		13			1.7	0.84	
Testosterone	30			0.68				
Androsterone	0	26	2.6			0.39		0.16
Androsterone (25)	20		7.3			0.89		0.29
Androsterone (25)	40		12.2			1.6		0.54
Androsterone (25)	60		24			2.4	1.1	
11β,17β-Dihydroxy-4-androsten-3-one	30			0.15				

TABLE XIV B—*continued.**

Compound	% Ethyl Acetate in Ethyl Acetate : Cyclohexane	% Ethanol in Ethanol : Water						
		20	40	50	55	60	70	80
3α-Hydroxy-5β-androstan-17-one (25)	20		2.8			0.52	0.28	
3α-Hydroxy-5β-androstan-17-one (25)	40		5.2			1.0	0.51	
3α-Hydroxy-5β-androstan-17-one (25)	60		12.3			2.0	1.2	
3β-Hydroxy-5α-androstan-17-one	0	22	1.2			0.18		0.09
3β-Hydroxy-5α-androstan-17-one (25)	20		2.9			0.56	0.31	
3β-Hydroxy-5α-androstan-17-one (25)	40		4.1			0.97	0.52	
3β-Hydroxy-5α-androstan-17-one (25)	60		10			1.9	0.95	

* Some of the data above can be found, in graphical form, in Figure 2.

TABLE XIV C. SYSTEM – ETHYL ACETATE : CYLCLOHEXANE/ETHANOL : WATER

Compound	% Ethyl Acetate in Ethyl Acetate : Cyclohexane	% Ethanol in Ethanol : Water					
		0	30	47.5	50	60	70
Progesterone	20					1.01	
Progesterone	30				2.8		
Cortexone	30		4.4	0.73	0.67		0.21
Cortexone	50		8		1.8		0.47
Cortexone	60		8		2.4		0.82
Cortexone	70		8		3.2		
6β-Hydroxy-4-pregnene-3,20-dione	30				0.57		
11β-Hydroxy-4-pregnene-3,20-dione	30				0.70		
16α-Hydroxy-4 pregnene-3,20-dione	30				0.20		
16α-Hydroxy-4 pregnene-3,20-dione	60				1.22		
17-Hydroxy-4-pregnene-3,20-dione	30				0.90		
3β-Hydroxy-5-pregnen-20-one	30				2.56		
3β,17-Dihydroxy-5-pregnen-20-one	30				0.90		
3α,20α-Dihydroxy-5β-pregnan-11-one	50		6.7				
Pregnane-3α,20α-diol	100	41					

TABLE XIV D. SYSTEM – ETHYL ACETATE : CYCLOHEXANE/ETHANOL : WATER

Compound	% Ethyl Acetate in Ethyl Acetate : Cyclohexane	% Ethanol in Ethanol : Water						
		0(6)	10	20	25	30	50	70
11-Dehydrocorticosterone	50					1.8		
Cortisone	50					1.2		
11β,17,21-Trihydroxy-4,6-pregnadiene-3,20-dione	100	12.6						
6β,17,21-Trihydroxy-4-pregnene-3,11,20-trione	100	2.2						
Cortexolone	10		0.66	0.43				
Cortexolone	30					1.33	0.48	
Cortexolone	50					3.8	0.96	
Corticosterone	10		0.25	0.14				
Corticosterone	30					0.91	0.28	
Corticosterone	50					2.3	0.65	
Cortisol	30					0.31	0.08	0.04
Cortisol	50					0.96	0.39	0.16
Cortisol	60					1.83	0.60	0.31
Cortisol	70					2.7	1.2	0.02
Cortisol	100	12.2						
9α,11β,17,21-Tetrahydroxy-4-pregnene-3,20-dione	100	2.0						
11β,17,20α,21-Tetra-hydroxy-4-pregnen-3-one	100	1.7						
Tetrahydrocortisone	30				0.43			
Tetrahydrocortisone	50					1.4		
11β,17,20β,21-Tetra-hydroxy-4-pregnen-3-one	100	1.6						
Tetrahydrocortisol	30				0.30			
Tetrahydrocortisol	100	11.0						

TABLE XV. SYSTEM – CYCLOHEXANE/METHANOL : WATER*

Compound	% Methanol in Methanol : Water			
	30	50	70	90
4-Androstene-3,17-dione	4.2	0.80	0.20	0.08
3β-Hydroxy-5-androsten-17-one	3.5	0.62	0.12	0.06
3α-Hydroxy-5α-androstan-17-one	10.7	1.8	0.33	0.11
3β-Hydroxy-5α-androstan-17-one	5.2	0.55	0.17	0.06
6β-Hydroxy-3,5-cycloandrostan-17-one (42)		1.7		

* Some of these data can be found in graphical form in Figure 3.

TABLE XVI. SYSTEM – 2,2,4-TRIMETHYLPENTANE/ETHANOL : WATER*

Compound	% Ethanol in Ethanol : Water			
	40	50	70	80
3α-Hydroxy-5β-androstan-17-one	0.46	0.17		0.05
3α,11β-Dihydroxy-5β-androstan-17-one	0.02			0.03
Pregnane-3α,20α-diol		0.08	0.03	

* These data are presented in graphical form in Figure 4.

TABLE XVII. SYSTEM – 2,2,4-TRIMETHYLPENTANE/n-PROPANOL : WATER†

Compound	% n-Propanol in n-Propanol : Water		
	40	50	80
5-Androstene-3β,17β-diol		0.39	0.21
3α-Hydroxy-5β-androstan-17-one	1.2	0.8	0.29
3α,11β-Dihydroxy-5β-androstan-17-one	0.35	0.24	0.17
3α,20α-Dihydroxy-5β-pregnan-11-one		0.11	
Pregnane-3α,20α-diol		0.71	0.39
Cholesterol		7.2	1.3

† These data are presented in graphical form in Figure 5.

TABLE XVIII. SYSTEM – 2,2,4-TRIMETHYLPENTANE/ISO-PROPANOL : WATER‡

Compound	% iso-Propanol in iso-Propanol : Water		
	40	50	80
3α-Hydroxy-5β-androstan-17-one	1.13	0.53	0.22
3α,11β-Dihydroxy-5β-androstan-17-one	0.09	0.10	0.12
Pregnane-3α,20α-diol			0.22

‡ These data are presented in graphical form in Figure 6.

TABLE XIX. SYSTEM – 2,2,4-TRIMETHYLPENTANE/ACETONE : WATER

Compound	% Acetone in Acetone : Water	
	50	80
Pregnane-3α,20α-diol	1.5	0.35

TABLE XX. SYSTEM – METHANOL : WATER/CHLOROFORM : CARBON TETRACHLORIDE

Compound	% Methanol in Methanol: Water	% Chloroform in Chloroform : Carbon Tetrachloride											
		0	5	10	20	30	40	50	60	70	80	90	100
C_{18}													
Equilenin (40)	50	0.55											
Dihydroequilenin (40)	50	2.9											
Equilin (40)	50	0.25											
6-Ketoestrone (40)	50	1.05											
7-Ketoestrone (40)	50	0.44											
16-Ketoestrone (40)	50	1.71											
Estrone (23)	0	0.0											
Estrone (23)	10	0.01											
Estrone (23)	20	0.04											
Estrone (23)	30	0.07											
Estrone (23)	40	0.15											
Estrone (40)	50	0.33											
Estrone	60	0.73											
Estrone	65	0.86											
Estrone‡	70	1.3(23)		0.58	0.42(24)		0.21(24)		0.11(24)				
Estrone	80	2.60											
Estrone	90	2.80											
3-Hydroxy-1,3,5(10)-estratrien-16-one (40)	50	0.37											
6-Ketoestradiol (40)	50	9.3											
16-Ketoestradiol (40)	50	5.9											
Deoxyestrone (40)	50	0.23											
Estradiol-17α (40)	50	1.64											
Estradiol-17β (23)	0	0.08											
Estradiol-17β (23)	10	0.15											
Estradiol-17β (23)	20	0.29											
Estradiol-17β (23)	30	0.64											
Estradiol-17β (23)	40	1.00											
Estradiol-17β (40)	50	2.10											
Estradiol-17β	60	4.70											
Estradiol-17β‡	70	7.0			2.31(24)		1.05(24)		0.43(24)				

TABLE XX—*continued.*

Compound	% Methanol in Methanol : Water	% Chloroform in Chloroform : Carbon Tetrachloride											
		0	5	10	20	30	40	50	60	70	80	90	100
Epiestriol	70								1.13				
Estriol (23)	10–60	10–20											
Estriol‡ (23,24)	70	20			16		8.2		2.1				
Estriol (24)	70										1.04	0.71	0.55
C_{19}													
4-Androstene-3,11,17-trione	70			0.76									
2-Methoxyestrone‡	70	0.3(32)					0.12(26)						
2-Methoxyestrone	80	0.74											
4-Androstene-3,17-dione	80	0.72		0.44									
11β-Hydroxy-4-androstene-3,17-dione	70			2.6	0.86	0.66							
Dehydroepiandrosterone	80	1.25		0.83									
Testosterone	70				0.46		0.25				0.09		
Testosterone	80			1.2									
C_{21}													
Cortisone	50	0.53											
Cortisone	70					2.6							
6β,17,21-Trihydroxy-4-pregnene-3,11,20-trione	0												3.311(6)
Progesterone	80	0.37											
Progesterone	85	0.57											
Progesterone	90	0.74											0.06
Cortexone	0												
Cortexone	80			0.92									
6β-Hydroxy-4-pregnene-3,20-dione	80			1.41									
11β-Hydroxy-4-pregnene-3,20-dione	70			0.96	0.41								
17-Hydroxy-4-pregnene-3,20-dione	70		0.96	0.49	0.34	0.23							

TABLE XX—*continued.*

Compound	% Methanol in Methanol : Water	% Chloroform in Chloroform : Carbon Tetrachloride											
		0	5	10	20	30	40	50	60	70	80	90	100
17-Hydroxy-4-pregnene-3,20-dione	80	2.0											
Cortexolone	10		0.42										
Cortexolone	20		0.61										
Cortexolone	30			0.74	0.40								
Cortexolone	50	3.2					0.29	0.13					
Cortexolone	60	4.7											
Cortexolone	70			3.4		0.83							
Corticosterone	10		0.77										
Corticosterone	20		1.27										
Corticosterone	30			1.05	0.50								
Corticosterone	50	4.2						0.18					
Corticosterone	60	5.6											
Corticosterone	70					1.1							
Cortisol	0												0.16‖(6)
Cortisol	30									0.70			
Cortisol	50						3.6	2.6					
Cortisol	70					5.9							
11β,17,21-Trihydroxy-1,4-pregnadiene-3,20-dione	0												0.28‖(6)
11β,17,21-Trihydroxy-4,6-pregnadiene-3,20-dione	0												0.21‖(6)
9α,11β,17,21-Tetrahydroxy-4-pregnene-3,20-dione	0												10‖ (6)
3β,17-Dihydroxy-5-pregnen-20-one	70			1.86	1.29								
17,21-Dihydroxy-5β-pregnane-3,20-dione	30									0.21			
3β,11β,21-Trihydroxy-5α-pregnan-20-one†	30					0.76		0.27		0.09			

TABLE XX—*continued.*

Compound	% Methanol in Methanol : Water	% Chloroform in Chloroform : Carbon Tetrachloride											
		0	5	10	20	30	40	50	60	70	80	90	100
3β,11β,21-Trihydroxy-5α-pregnan-20-one	50					2.01		0.72		0.25			
3β,11β,21-Trihydroxy-5α-pregnan-20-one	70					4.44		1.37		0.68			
3α,17,21-Trihydroxy-5β-pregnan-20-one	30									0.04			
3α,17,21-Trihydroxy-5β-pregnan-20-one	50							0.31					
Tetrahydrocortisone*	30					6.5		1.9		0.59			
Tetrahydrocortisone	50					6.9		1.9		0.79			
Tetrahydrocortisone	70					7.3		2.1		0.98			
11β,17,20α,21-Tetrahydroxy-4-pregnen-3-one	0												1.11‖(6)
11β,17,20β,21-Tetrahydroxy-4-pregnen-3-one	0												0.91‖(6)
Tetrahydrocortisol	0												0.42‖(6)
Tetrahydrocortisol	30									2.3			
Tetrahydrocortisol	50							5.8		2.4			
Tetrahydrocortisol	70									1.8			
11β,17β-Dihydroxy-4-androsten-3-one	70				4.2								
3β-Hydroxy-5-pregnen-20-one	80	0.80											
16α-Hydroxy-4-pregnene-3,20-dione	70			2.33									
20α-Hydroxy-4-pregnen-3-one	70	0.63											

* These values represented graphically in Figure 7 and Figure 9.
† These values represented graphically in Figure 8 and Figure 9.
‡ These values represented graphically in Figure 10.
‖ The values tabulated are the reciprocals of those published (6).

TABLE XXI. SYSTEM – ETHANOL : WATER / CHLOROFORM : CARBON TETRACHLORIDE*

Compound	% Ethanol in Ethanol : Water	% Chloroform in Chloroform : Carbon Tetrachloride				
		0	5	10	20	100
Estrone	70	0.67	0.40	0.31	0.17	
Estradiol-17β	70	2.2	1.1	0.86	0.44	
Estriol	70 + .05% NaCl			4.1	1.7	
Dehydrocorticosterone (11)	20	0.75				
Cortisone (11)	20			3.5		
Cortexolone (11)	10		0.46	0.31		
Cortexolone (9,11)	20	0.84				
Corticosterone (11)	10		1.08			
Corticosterone (9,11)	20	1.9		0.82		
Cortisol (11)	30					0.06

* Some of these data are represented graphically in Figure 11.

TABLE XXII. SYSTEMS – (A) ETHANOL : 0.05% NaCl IN WATER / n-HEXANE : CHLOROFORM
(B) ETHANOL : 0.05% NaCl IN WATER / n-HEXANE : CARBON TETRACHLORIDE

Compound	% Ethanol in Ethanol : 0.05% NaCl in Water	(A) % n-Hexane in n-Hexane : Chloroform		(B) % n-Hexane in n-Hexane : Carbon Tetrachloride	
		0	50	30	50
Aldosterone (10)	20		0.59		
Cortisone (11)	0		0.79		
Cortisone (9)	20		0.54		
Cortisone (11)	50		0.33		
Dehydrocorticosterone (11)	0			0.89	
Dehydrocorticosterone (11)	10			1.50	
Dehydrocorticosterone (11)	20				4.0
Cortexone (11)	60				3.6
Cortexolone (11)	0			1.00	
Cortexolone (11)	10			1.86	
Cortexolone (9,11)	20			1.94	3.6
Corticosterone (11)	0			2.23	
Corticosterone (9)	20			4.3	
Cortisol (11)	0		2.57		
Cortisol (9)	20		2.57		
Cortisol (11)	30	0.06	1.63		
Cortisol (11)	50		0.61		
3β,17-Dihydroxy-5-pregnen-20-one (12)	47.5†			1.29	2.7
17-Hydroxy-4-pregnene-3,20-dione (12)	47.5†			0.72	1.44

† No NaCl in aqueous phase.

TABLE XXIII A. SYSTEM – 2,2,4-TRIMETHYLPENTANE : sec-BUTANOL : WATER*

Compound	K	Compound	K
4-Androstene-3,17-dione	4.95	Cortexone	17.8
Testosterone	11.0	Progesterone	6.4
Cortisone	1.55	Corticosterone	3.73
Dehydrocorticosterone	2.0	Cortisol	1.35

* The system was made up using 400 ml. of water, 300 ml. of 2,2,4-Trimethylpentane and 200 ml. of sec-Butanol. Equal volumes of the two phases were used. (41)

TABLE XXIII B. SYSTEM – 2,2,4-TRIMETHYLPENTANE / AQUEOUS ALCOHOLS STEROID ACETATES

Compound	% Ethanol in Ethanol : Water				
	50	70	80	85	90
Pregnane-3α,20α-diol diacetate			2.7	1.7	1.2
Cholesteryl acetate	21	21		9.2	6.3
	% n-Propanol in n-Propanol : Water				
	50	60	70	75	80
Pregnane-3α,20α-diol diacetate	10.7	5.5	2.1	1.1	1.3
Cholesteryl acetate	87	10	5.6		2.7
	% iso-Propanol in iso-Propanol : Water				
	50	70	75	80	
Pregnane-3α,20α-diol diacetate	16	3.4	3.0	1.4	
Cholesteryl acetate	31	14		4.6	

TABLE XXIV. SYSTEM – METHANOL : WATER / CHLOROFORM : CARBON TETRACHLORIDE STEROID DERIVATIVES

Compound	% Methanol in Methanol : Water	% Chloroform in Chloroform : Carbon Tetrachloride					
		0	10	30	40	50	70
4-Androstene-3,17-dione 3-oxime	70	3.3	1.9	0.8		0.4	
4-Androstene-3,17-dione 3-oxime	80	4.5					
4-Androstene-3,17-dione 3-oxime	90	4.2					
6β Fluorotestosterone	90	2.8					
6β Fluorotestosterone propionate	90	0.4					
Methyl 11β,17-dihydroxy-3-oxo-4-etienate	70					0.41	0.22
17-Hydroxyprogesterone oxime	70				1.9		

TABLE XXV. MISCELLANEOUS SYSTEMS

Compound	Upper Phase	Lower Phase	K
Cortexone	Water	Methylene chloride	0.07
Cortisol	Water	Methylene chloride	0.13
5α-Pregnane-3β,11β,17,20β,21-pentol	Water	Methylene chloride	5.4
5α-Pregnane-3β,11β,17,20β,21-pentol	0.1 N Acetate buffer pH 5.1	Methylene chloride	4.6
Cortisol	0.1 N Acetate buffer pH 5.1	Methylene chloride	0.12
Cortisone (11)	20% Methanol: 80% Water +.05%NaCl w/v	50% n-Hexane 50% Chloroform	1.17
Cortisol (11)	20% Methanol: 80% Water +.05%NaCl w/v	50% n-Hexane 50% Chloroform	4.0
Cholesterol (1)	n-Heptane	80% Ethanol 20% Water	3.77*
Cortisol	80% Methanol: 20% Water	1,2-Dichloroethane	1.26
Progesterone	80% Methanol: 20% Water	1,2-Dichloroethane	0.26

* Figure corrected for equal volumes of upper and lower phases

TABLE XXVI. MISCELLANEOUS SYSTEMS, STEROID ACETATES

Compound	Upper Phase	Lower Phase	K
Testosterone acetate	10% Ethylacetate : 90% Cyclohexane	70% Ethanol : 30% Water	0.77
Testosterone acetate	90% Methanol : 10% Water	Carbon tetrachloride	0.56
Cortexone acetate	90% Methanol : 10% Water	Carbon tetrachloride	0.18
Cortisol 21-acetate (11)	n-Hexane	Water	0.01
Cortisol 21-acetate (11)	60% n-Hexane : 40% Benzene	5% Ethanol : 95% Water	0.43
16α-Hydroxyprogesterone acetate	80% Methanol: 20% Water	10% Chloroform 90% Carbon tetrachloride	0.58
16α-Hydroxyprogesterone acetate	90% Methanol: 10% Water	Carbon tetrachloride	1.40
16α-Hydroxyprogesterone acetate	30% Ethylacetate 70% Cyclohexane	50% Ethanol 50% Water	0.81

TABLE XXVII. MISCELLANEOUS SYSTEMS – ESTROGENS

Upper Phase	Lower Phase	Equilenin	Equilin	Estrone	Estra-diol-17β	Estriol	2-Methoxy-estrone	2-Methoxy-estradiol
n-Butanol	Water			5.3	9.4	5.1		
sec-Butanol	Water			19.	18.	6.		
2-Butanone	Water				26.	5.9		
70% Ethanol : 30% Water	Benzene (45)	0.17	0.40	0.33	1.0			
70% Methanol : 30% Water	10% Ethylacetate : 90% Carbon tetra-chloride (29)			0.37	1.59		0.19	0.85
50% Benzene : 50% Petroleum ether B.P. 40-60° C	0.4 N Sodium hydroxide (5)			0.11	0.04	0		

TABLE XXVIII A. MISCELLANEOUS SYSTEMS—ESTROGEN DERIVATIVES

Compound	Upper Phase	Lower Phase	*K*
Estrone 3-methyl ether (17)	n-Hexane	70% Methanol : 30% Water	4.9
Estrone 3-methyl ether	n-Hexane	90% Methanol : 10% Water	0.85 (17) 0.98 (38)
Estrone 3-methyl ether (17)	Petroleum ether B.P. 30–60° C	90% Methanol : 10% Water	0.85
Estrone 3-methyl ether (17)	90% Methanol : 10% Water	Toluene	0.29
Estrone 17-methoxime	90% Methanol: 10% Water	Carbon tetrachloride	1.15*
Estrone 3-methyl ether 17-thiosemicarbazone (17)	n-Hexane	55% Methanol : 45% Water	0.56
Estrone 3-methyl ether 17-thiosemicarbazone (17)	n-Hexane	70% Methanol : 30% Water	0.15
Estradiol-17β 3-methyl ether (17)	Petroleum ether B.P. 30–60° C	70% Methanol : 30% Water	1.0
Estradiol-17β 3-methyl ether (17)	n-Hexane	90% Methanol : 10% Water	0.27
Estradiol-17β 3-methyl ether (17)	70% n-Hexane : 30% Benzene	75% Methanol : 25% Water	1.95

* R. H. Purdy, Private Communication.

TABLE XXVIII B. MISCELLANEOUS SYSTEMS – ESTROGEN DERIVATIVES

Compound	Upper Phase	Lower Phase	*K*
Estriol 3-methyl ether (19)	10% Methanol : 90% Water	Carbon tetrachloride	0.20
Estriol 3-methyl ether (19)	40% Methanol : 60% Water	Carbon tetrachloride	0.85
Estriol 3-methyl ether (19)	70% Methanol : 30% Water	Carbon tetrachloride	2.5
17α-Ethinylestradiol (40)	50% Methanol : 50% Water	Carbon tetrachloride	1.04
17α-Ethinylestradiol (40)	50% Ethylacetate : 50% Cyclohexane	33% Ethanol : 67% Water	>10
17α-Ethinylestradiol (40)	50% Ethylacetate : 50% Cyclohexane	50% Ethanol : 50% Water	3.8
17α-Ethinylestradiol (40)	50% Ethylacetate : 50% Cyclohexane	70% Ethanol : 30% Water	0.68
2-Methoxyestradiol-17β 3-methyl ether (29)	90% Methanol : 10% Water	Carbon tetrachloride	1.25
2-Methoxyestradiol-17β 3-methyl ether (29)	70% n-Hexane : 30% Benzene	75% Methanol : 25% Water	0.52
Epiestriol monomethyl ether (21)	n-Hexane	50% Methanol : 50% Water	0.34
Epiestriol monomethyl ether (21)	n-Hexane	80% Methanol : 20% Water	0.08
1,3,5(10)-Estratriene-3,16α, 17α-triol 3-methyl ether (21)	n-Hexane	50% Methanol : 50% Water	0.39
Epiestriol acetonide (21)	Petroleum ether B.P. 30–60° C	50% Methanol : 50% Water	0.94
1,3,5,(10)-Estratriene-3,16α 17α-triol acetonide (21)	Petroleum ether B.P. 30–60° C	50% Methanol : 50% Water	1.1

TABLE XXVIII C. MISCELLANEOUS SYSTEMS – ESTROGEN DERIVATIVES

Compound	Upper Phase	Lower Phase	*K*
Estradiol-17β 3-methyl ether 17β-acetate (19)	n-Hexane	90% Methanol : 10% Water	3.5
Estradiol-17β 3-methyl ether 17β-acetate (19)	90% Methanol : 10% Water	Toluene	0.19
Estriol 3-methyl ether monoacetate (19)	n-Hexane	90% Methanol : 10% Water	0.20
2-Methoxyestradiol 3-methyl ether 17β-acetate (29)	90% Methanol : 10% Water	Carbon tetrachloride	0.28
2-Methoxyestradiol 3-methyl ether 17β-acetate (29)	70% n-Hexane : 30% Benzene	75% Methanol : 25% Water	14.5
Estriol 3-methyl ether, 16,17-diacetate (19)	n-Hexane	90% Methanol : 10% Water	0.96
Estriol 3-methyl ether, 16,17-diacetate (19)	n-Hexane	75% Methanol : 25% Water	3.8
Epiestriol 3-methyl ether, 16,17-acetonide (21)	n-Hexane	90% Methanol : 10% Water	5.7
1,3,5(10)-Estratriene-3-methoxy-16α,17α acetonide (21)	n-Hexane	90% Methanol : 10% Water	6.1
1,3,5(10)-Estratriene-16α, 17α-dimethoxy-3-acetate (21)	n-Hexane	80% Methanol : 20% Water	4.3

TABLE XXIX. MISCELLANEOUS SYSTEMS – ESTROGEN SULFATES (38)

Compound	Upper Phase	Lower Phase	*K**
Estrone sulfate	33% Benzene : 67% n-Butanol	0.1 N NH_4OH	0.92
Estrone sulfate	85% sec-Butanol : 15% 2,2,4-Trimethylpentane	0.1 N NH_4OH	2.70
Estrone sulfate	50% n-Butyl acetate : 50% n-Butanol	5% Pyridine : 95% Water	1.80
Estrone sulfate	60% n-Butyl acetate : 40% n-Butanol	0.1 N NH_4OH	4.3
Estrone sulfate	60% n-Butyl acetate : 40% n-Butanol	0.01 N NH_4OH	1.1
Estrone sulfate methoxime	60% n-Butyl acetate : 40% n-Butanol	0.01 N NH_4OH	8.7
Estrone sulfate methoxime	80% n-Butyl acetate : 20% n-Butanol	0.1 N NH_4OH	0.41

* These values are concentration dependent.

TABLE XXX. MISCELLANEOUS SYSTEMS – GLUCOSIDURONATES*

Compound	Upper Phase	Lower Phase	*K*
Estrone	sec-Butanol	0.1 N NH_4OH	1.3 (38)
Dehydroepiandrosterone	70% Toluene : 30% tert-Butanol	10% Acetic acid : 90% Water	0.90
Androsterone	71% Ethyl acetate : 29% n-Hexane	10% Acetic acid : 90% Water	1.21
3α-Hydroxy-5β-androstan-17-one	71% Ethyl acetate : 29% n-Hexane	10% Acetic acid : 90% Water	0.67
3α-Hydroxy-5β-androstan-17-one	70% Toluene : 30% tert-Butanol	10% Acetic acid : 90% Water	1.65
β-Cortolone	75% Ethyl acetate : 25% n-Butanol	0.01 N HCl	0.83
Tetrahydrocortisone	90% Ethyl acetate : 10% n-Butanol	0.01 N HCl	1.02

* All values from (39) except estrone glucosiduronate (38).

TABLE XXXI. MISCELLANEOUS SYSTEMS – BILE ACIDS (2)

Compound	n-Heptane†	75% iso-Propyl Ether : 25% n-Heptane	85% iso-Propyl Ether : 15% n-Heptane
	97.5% Acetic Acid : 2.5% Water	60% Acetic Acid : 40% Water	60% Acetic Acid : 40% Water
3,7,12-Triketocholanic acid		0.075	0.16
3,6-Diketo-5α-cholanic acid			1.06
3,6-Diketocholanic acid			1.05
3,12-Diketocholanic acid		0.49	1.05
3α-Hydroxy-7,12-diketocholanic acid			0.20
3-Ketocholanic acid		7.4	
3α-Hydroxy-12-ketocholanic acid			1.24
3α,7α-Dihydroxy-12-ketocholanic acid			0.20
3α,12α-Dihydroxy-7-ketocholanic acid			0.18
3α-Hydroxycholanic acid	0.24	7.7	12.4
3α,6α-Dihydroxycholanic acid			0.88
3α,12α-Dihydroxycholanic acid	0.06	1.14	2.14
3α,7α,12α-Trihydroxycholanic acid	0.017	0.14	0.31

† or 2,2,4-Trimethylpentane.

TABLE XXXII. MISCELLANEOUS SYSTEMS – CONJUGATED BILE ACIDS (2)

Upper Phase	Lower Phase	Compound		
		Glycocholic Acid	Glycodeoxy-cholic Acid	Taurocholic Acid Na Salt
n-Heptane	97.5% Acetic acid : 2.5% Water	0.004		
75% iso-Propyl ether : 25% n-Heptane	60% Acetic acid : 40% Water	0.024		
85% iso-Propyl ether : 15% n-Heptane	60% Acetic acid : 40% Water	0.06	0.25	
30% n-Butanol : 70% n-Heptane	10% Acetic acid : 90% Water	2.25	0.013	
sec-Butanol	3% Acetic acid : 97% Water	6.2	12.8	0.94

VIII. REFERENCES

[1] ABELL, L. L., LEVY, B. B., BRODIE, B. B. and KENDALL, F. E., *J. Biol. Chem.* **195**, 357–366 (1952).
[2] AHRENS, E. H., Jr. and CRAIG, L. C., *J. Biol. Chem.* **195**, 763–778 (1952).
[3] BACHMAN, C. and PETTIT, D. S., *J. Biol. Chem.* **138**, 689–704 (1941).
[4] BAGGETT, B. and ENGEL, L. L., *J. Biol. Chem.* **229**, 443–450 (1957).
[5] BAULD, W. S. and GREENWAY, R. M., in D. Glick, *Methods of Biochemical Analysis* Vol. 5, pp. 337–406 (1957).
[6] BURSTEIN, S., *Science* **124**, 1030 (1956).
[7] BURSTEIN, S. and LIEBERMAN, S., *J. Amer. Chem. Soc.* **80**, 5235–5239 (1958).
[8] BURSTEIN, S. and LIEBERMAN, S., *J. Biol. Chem.* **233**, 331–335 (1958).
[9] CARSTENSEN, H., *Acta Chem. Scand.* **9**, 1026–1027 (1955).
[10] CARSTENSEN, H., *Arkiv för Kemi* **10**, 235–238 (1956).
[11] CARSTENSEN, H., *Acta Soc. Med. Upsaliensis* **61**, 26–46 (1956).
[12] CARSTENSEN, H., OERTEL, G. W., and EIK-NES, K. B., *J. Biol. Chem.* **234**, 2570–2577 (1959).
[13] COHEN, S. L. and MARRIAN, G. F., *Biochem. J.* **28**, 1603–1614 (1934).
[14] CRAIG, L. C. and CRAIG, D. in Weissberger, *Technique of Organic Chemistry* Vol. 3, pp. 149–393. Interscience, New York (1956).
[15] DICZFALUSY, E., *Acta Endocr.* **10**, 373–389 (1952).
[16] DICZFALUSY, E., *Acta Endocr.* **12**, Suppl. 12 (1953).
[17] DICZFALUSY, E., *Acta Endocr.* **15**, 317–324 (1954).
[18] DICZFALUSY, E., *Acta Endocr.* **20**, 216–229 (1955).
[19] DICZFALUSY, E. and LINDKVIST, P., *Acta Endocr.* **22**, 203–223 (1956).
[20] DICZFALUSY, E. *Acta Endocr.* Suppl. 31, 11–26 (1957).
[21] DICZFALUSY, E. and HALLA, M., *Acta Endocr.* **27**, 303–313 (1958).
[22] ENGEL, L. L., *Recent Progr. Hormone Res.* **5**, 335–372 (1950).
[23] ENGEL, L. L., SLAUNWHITE, W. R., Jr., CARTER, P. and NATHANSON, I. T., *J. Biol. Chem.* **185**, 255–263 (1950).
[24] ENGEL, L. L., SLAUNWHITE, W. R., Jr., CARTER, P. and OLMSTED, P. C., *J. Biol. Chem.* **191**, 621–625 (1951).
[25] ENGEL, L. L., ALEXANDER, J., CARTER, P., ELLIOTT, J. and WEBSTER, M., *Analyt. Chem.* **26**, 639–641 (1954).
[26] ENGEL, L. L., BAGGETT, B. and CARTER, P., *Endocrinology* **61**, 113–114 (1957).
[27] ENGEL, L. L., ALEXANDER, J. and WHEELER, M., *J. Biol. Chem.* **231**, 159–164 (1958).
[28] FISHMAN, J. and GALLAGHER, T. F., *Arch. Biochem. Biophys.* **77**, 511–512 (1958).
[29] FRANDSEN, V. Aa., *Acta Endocr.* **31**, 603–607 (1959).
[30] GIBBS, J. W., *Trans. Conn. Acad.* **3**, 108–248 (1876) ; **3**, 343–524 (1878).
[31] HOLLINGSWORTH, C. A., TABER, J. J. and DAUBERT, B. F., *Science* **120**, 306–307 (1954).
[32] KRAYCHY, S. and GALLAGHER, T. F., *J. Amer. Chem. Soc.* **79**, 754 (1957).
[33] LEWBART, M. L. and MATTOX, V. R., *Nature, Lond.* **183**, 820–821 (1959).

[34] MELTZER, H. L., *J. Biol. Chem.* **233**, 1327–1336 (1958).
[35] NAPP, J-H. and KERSTEN, I., *Arch. f. Gynäkol.* **188**, 279–298 (1957).
[36] PEARLMAN, W. H. and CERCEO, E., *J. Biol. Chem.* **176**, 847–856 (1948).
[37] PEARLMAN, W. H., *Recent Progr. Hormone Res.* **9**, 27–44 (1954).
[38] PURDY, R. H., ENGEL, L. L. and ONCLEY, J. L., *J. Biol. Chem.* **236**, 1043–1050 (1961).
[39] SCHNEIDER, J. J. and LEWBART, M. L., *Recent Progr. Hormone Res.* **15**, 201–230 (1959).
[39a] SHEPS, M. C., PURDY, R. H., ENGEL, L. L. and ONCLEY, J. L., *J. Biol. Chem.* **235**, 3033–3041 (1960).
[39b] SHEPS, M. C., PURDY, R. H., ENGEL, L. L. and ONCLEY, J. L., *J. Biol. Chem.* **235**, 3042–3048 (1960).
[40] SLAUNWHITE, W. R., Jr., ENGEL, L. L., OLMSTED, P. C. and CARTER, P., *J. Biol. Chem.* **191**, 627–631 (1951).
[41] TALBOT, N. B., ULICK, S., KOUPREIANOW, A. and ZYGMUNTOWICZ, A., *J. Clin. Endocrin. and Metab.* **15**, 301–316 (1955).
[42] TEICH, S., ROGERS, J., LIEBERMAN, S., ENGEL, L. L. and DAVIS, J. W., *J. Amer. Chem. Soc.* **75**, 2523–2524 (1953).
[43] WEISIGER, J. R. in Mitchell, Kolthoff, Proskauer and Weissberger, *Organic Analysis* Vol. 2, pp. 277–326. Interscience, New York (1954).
[44] WEISSBERGER, A., PROSKAUER, E. S., RIDDICK, J. A. and TOOPS, E., Jr., *Technique of Organic Chemistry* (2nd edition) Vol. 7. Interscience, New York (1955).
[45] WESTERFELD, W. W., THAYER, S. A., MACCORQUODALE, D. W. and DOISY, E. A., *J. Biol. Chem.* **126**, 181–193 (1938).

CHROMATOGRAPHIC MOBILITIES

R. NEHER

From the Laboratories of CIBA Ltd., Basle

I. INTRODUCTION

THE chief purpose of the present compilation of chromatographic mobilities of steroids is to assist in identifying individual steroids, as well as more or less complicated mixtures of steroids. This task appears to be most difficult of all where natural extracts are concerned, since here one does not know at the start exactly what type of steroids one is dealing with. The number of known steroids is so vast that for the moment we are compelled to confine ourselves to a selection, and have therefore chosen approximately 250 compounds, i.e. C_{18}, C_{19} and C_{21} steroid hormones known to occur naturally in the animal world, their metabolites and closely related isomers and analogs. Steroids and steroid esters which can only be obtained by synthesis or by microbiological methods have not been listed ; hence, for example, most of the 11α-, 12α-, 14α-, or 15α-oxygenated derivatives have been excluded — an omission which, if anything, facilitates reference to this compilation for purposes of identification. An exception has been made in the case of certain artefacts or synthetic analogs of natural steroid hormones, which today are frequently encountered in clinical specimens subjected to chromatographic analysis. Only a few metabolites of such synthetic hormonal analogs have been included, however, as many of them have not yet been systematically investigated.

The present compilation is based partly on the detailed reviews of Savard,[30] Reineke[29] and Neher[24] and partly on other relevant papers,[1, 3, 5, 11, 12, 14, 16, 17, 18, 19, 22, 24a–c, 35] from which the values quoted have been converted to a common denominator. The data assembled here have been supplemented by many new values obtained from our laboratories and from personal communications.

Those who have had experience of paper chromatography will know that, even where the methods employed are strictly standardized, the problem of reproducibility involves certain difficulties which recur again and again and which tend, of course, to be magnified when attempts are made in one laboratory to reproduce results obtained in another. This is a point to be borne in mind when using the present compilation.

II. GENERAL METHODS

The general procedure employed for the paper chromatography of steroids, as broadly elaborated by Zaffaroni[36] and Bush[6, 7] and as described in various other published monographs,[4, 10, 24, 32] cannot be dealt with in detail here. For the most part, the mean values quoted in the tables have been based on 3 to 12 determinations carried out according to the method already described elsewhere[24] (Whatman paper No. 1, UV print, color reactions BT*, DNB*, H_3PO_4, $SbCl_3$, DNPH*, etc., descending). As a rule, the temperature was 22 ± 2° in the case of Zaffaroni-type systems, and

* BT = blue tetrazolium ; DNB = *m*-dinitrobenzene ; DNPH = 2,4-dinitrophenyl hydrazine.

$22 \pm 2°$ or $38 \pm 1°$, as indicated, in the case of Bush-type systems. The chromatoplate technique[13, 33] on silicic acid was carried out at $22 \pm 2°$ in jars saturated with the ascending solvent, the arrangement described by Stahl[33] yielding good results here. The detecting agent used was a spray of concentrated sulfuric acid.

The fact that all the mobilities derived from various sources have had to be incorporated into a uniform and serviceable pattern is the reason why as a rule no R_f values have been quoted, but instead R_S values,[24] which relate not to the solvent front but to the following four standard steroids (S), which are readily accessible, easily detectable, and of varying polar strength: Δ^4-pregnene-3,20-dione (progesterone), 21-hydroxy-Δ^4-pregnene-3,20-dione (cortexone), 11β,21-dihydroxy-Δ^4-pregnene-3,20-dione (corticosterone), and 11β,17α,21-trihydroxy-Δ^4-pregnene-3, 20-dione (cortisol). Since, for practical purposes, all that matters is the relative sequence of the steroids in each individual system, any steroid can if necessary be taken as a standard and the new R_S values immediately obtained by simple conversion. For this reason, it is also advisable always to chromatograph standard substances at the same time.

To give some practical idea of the actual distance travelled on paper, Table I quotes the R_f values of the four standard substances in each of the systems employed, as obtained in our laboratories under normal conditions and with a simple descending run (mean values based on several determinations). In this way, the R_f values of all the steroids listed can if necessary be directly calculated ; this may prove useful, for example, in selecting the correct solvent systems.

In practice, allowance must be made for a margin of error of about ± 5 per cent in the R_S values of pure or fairly pure steroids. The discrepancy may be even greater where abundant impurities are present (effect on solubility) or where several steroids with similar flow rates are involved (displacement effect). (For a preliminary approach of calculating the running properties of steroids using a generalized R_M function cf. Ref. 18a.)

III. NOTES ON THE USE OF THE TABLES AND FIGURES*

The chromatographic mobilities shown in the tables and figures have been so listed that they can be consulted for various purposes, e.g. to find the values for individual steroids or to identify steroids by comparing the experimental values with those listed within a certain group.

For this reason the steroids have been broadly divided into three groups, viz. C_{18}, C_{19} and C_{21} steroids. The tables themselves have been grouped by reference to the method by which the steroids can be detected (UV, BT, etc.), i.e. either on the basis of their structural formula or on the basis of the reactions they yielded. These same steroids have been further subdivided into separate tables according to their degree of polarity as compared with that of the four standard steroids. Finally, in each table the steroids have been arranged according to their molecular formulae, listed in order of progression ; where the molecular formula is the same, they have been listed in alphabetical order by reference to their systematic names.

* Since the completion of the manuscript in November 1959 many new values and further compounds have been inserted in or added to the tables, but this was not possible in the case of the figures. Furthermore, a full account on the execution and application of the new methods of thin layer and gas chromatography developed since then to as useful techniques as paper chromatography is given by the author in a most recent monograph.[38]

Excluding the 17 phenolic steroids (" C_{18} steroids"), which are compiled separately in Table XXII and which can easily be identified using ferric chloride–potassium ferricyanide[2] as a reagent, the 227 neutral steroids listed here can be readily classified using the absorption at 240 mμ (UV), the reducing power for blue tetrazolium (BT) and the color reaction with *m*-dinitrobenzene (DNB). According to their positive or negative behavior against these three indicators the following 6 groups can be established:

1. UV+ BT+ DNB− 34 C_{21} and C_{22} steroids
2. UV+ BT− DNB+ 15 C_{19} steroids
3. UV+ BT− DNB− 56 C_{19}, C_{20} and C_{21} steroids
4. UV− BT+ DNB− 28 C_{21} steroids
5. UV− BT− DNB+ 26 C_{19} steroids
6. UV− BT− DNB− 68 C_{19} and C_{21} steroids

Further subdivision or characterization of these steroids — which is particularly necessary in the case of the 6th group — is possible with, for example, antimony trichloride ($SbCl_3$), phosphoric acid (H_3PO_4), and dinitrophenylhydrazine (DNPH); within the groups with UV+, soda fluorescence also renders excellent service. (Attention should be paid to the specificity of color reactions referred to in section 5.)

To simplify matters, the C_{19} and C_{21} steroids have been grouped separately throughout the tables; only two indicators have been quoted in each instance (UV and BT, or UV and DNB), as these would appear sufficient for differentiation, particularly since the BT+ and DNB+ properties are more or less mutually exclusive. But this means, for example, that for purposes of identification the experimentally ascertained R_S values of spots which have been differentiated as UV+, BT−, and DNB− have to be compared with those listed in the tables (in the sub-group having the appropriate polarity) under UV+ and BT−, as well as under UV+ and DNB−. Furthermore, the mobilities of a number of steroids have been related to more than one of the four standard steroids, and hence are to be found in more than one table.

It has been found in practice that, when identifying steroids or mixtures of steroids by the chromatographic technique, the simultaneous use of several systems — if possible both of the Bush *and* Zaffaroni type — as well as of several color reactions offers great advantages and largely eliminates the risks of misinterpretation. Accordingly, in the tables the R_S values are also always quoted for a number of solvent systems, the choice of which has for practical reasons been confined to those listed in Table I, since these have been widely used with satisfactory results.

Some tables are rather large, however, and contain so many values that checking the R_S values found against those listed in the tables often becomes a rather difficult and uncertain procedure. In order to make the task easier in such cases, the chromatographic sequence of the steroids in the various solvent systems has been presented in diagrammatic form in Figs. 1–11. To afford a clearer overall picture, the names have been replaced by numbers referring to the steroids listed in the respective tables, and the standard steroid appears as a horizontal line (S) above all the systems; the distance between this line and the other steroids is true to scale. This form of presentation proved a satisfactory method of enabling one to see at a glance the chromatographic pattern of each steroid, to note changes in

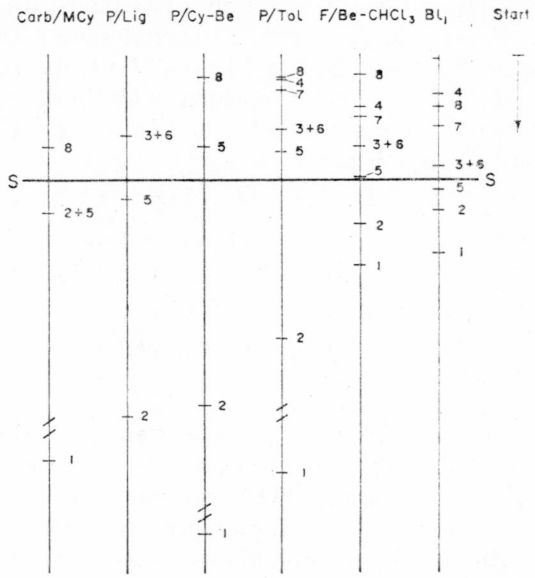

FIG. 1

C_{21}-Steroids UV+BT+ (Table II)
R_S-values (S = corticosterone)

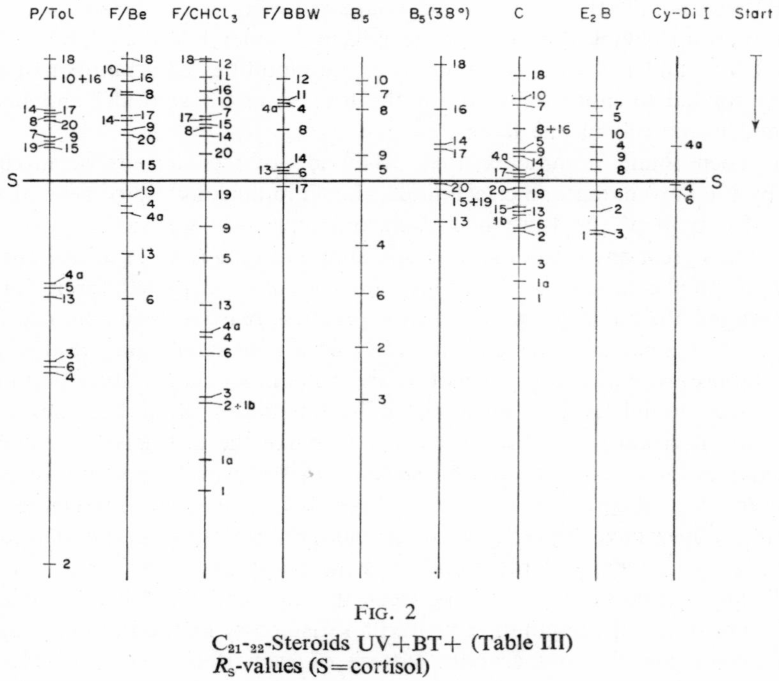

FIG. 2

C_{21}-$_{22}$-Steroids UV+BT+ (Table III)
R_S-values (S = cortisol)

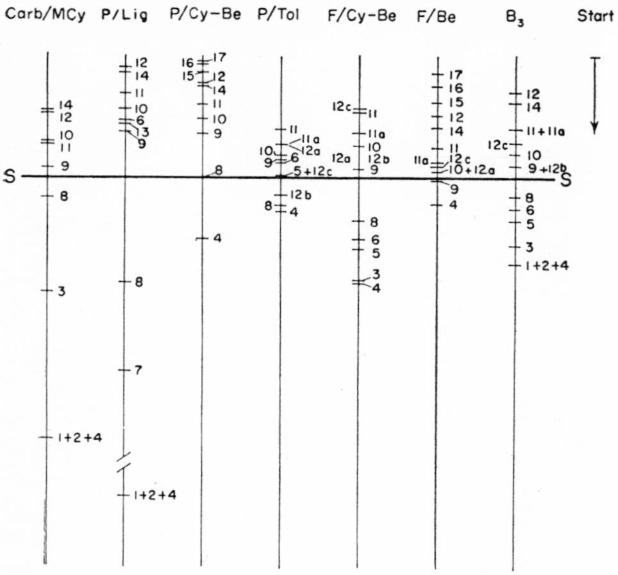

FIG. 3

C_{21}-Steroids UV+BT− (Table V)
R_S-values (S=cortexone)

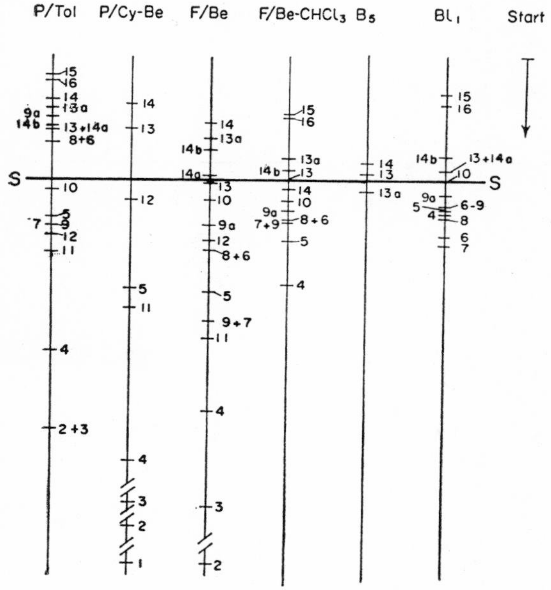

FIG. 4

C_{21}-Steroids UV+BT− (Table VI)
R_S-values (S=corticosterone)

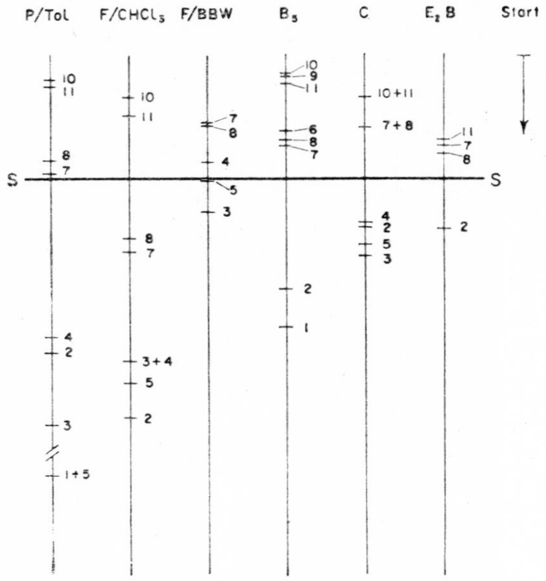

FIG. 5

C_{21}-Steroids UV+BT− (Table VII)
R_S-values (S=cortisol)

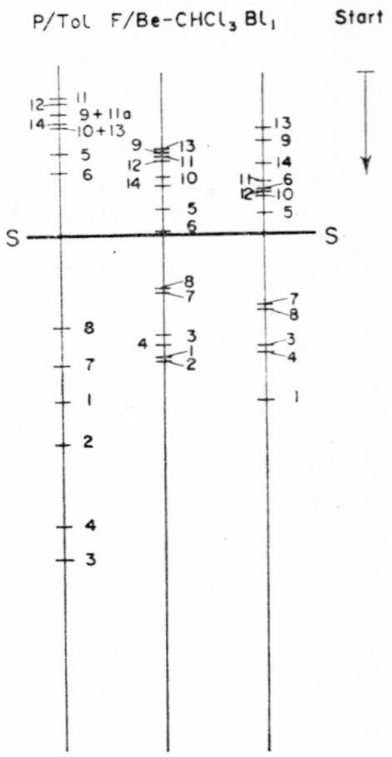

FIG. 6

C_{21}-Steroids UV−BT+ (Table IX)
R_S-values (S=corticosterone)

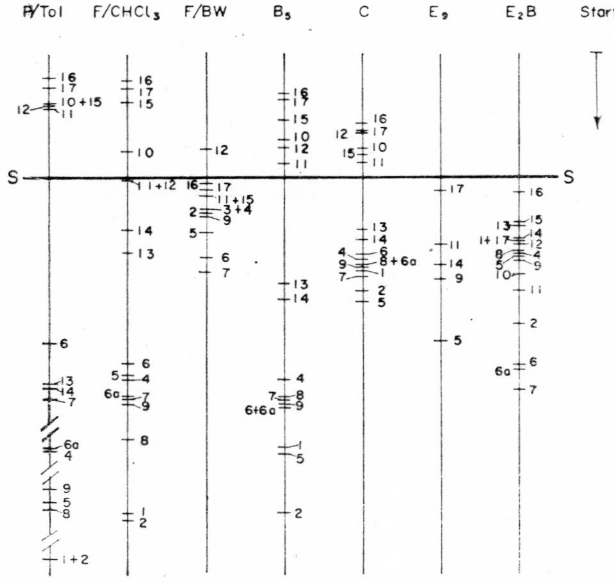

FIG. 7

C_{21}-Steroids UV−BT+ (Table X)
R_S-values (S=cortisol)

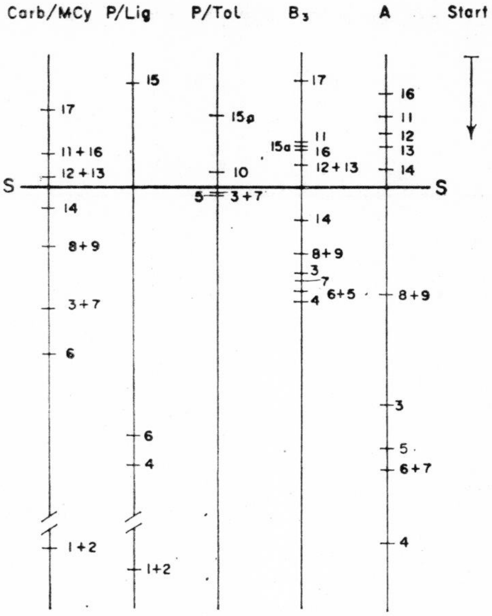

FIG. 8

C_{21}-Steroids UV−BT− (Table XIII)
R_S-values (S=cortexone)

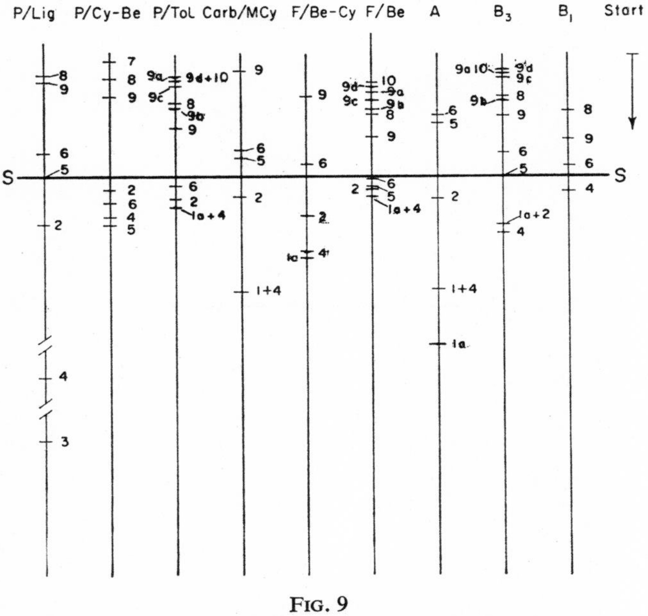

FIG. 9

C_{19}-Steroids (17-Ketosteroids) UV+DNB+ (Table XVI)
R_S-values (S=cortexone)

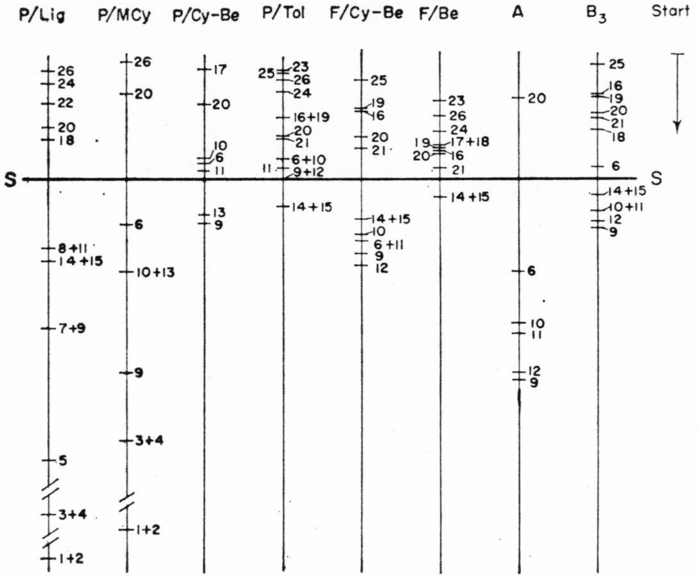

FIG. 10

C_{19}-Steroids (17-Ketosteroids) UV−DNB+ (Table XVIII)
R_S-values (S=cortexone)

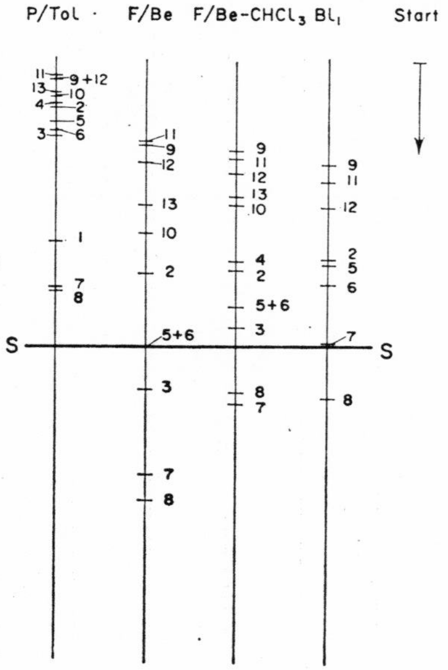

FIG. 11

C_{19}-Steroids UV−DNB− (Table XXI)
R_S-values (S=corticosterone)

sequence, and to select the system affording the best separation. Patterns of this kind are extremely useful for the characterization and identification of steroids by paper chromatography, which should finally be rounded off by alternating parallel chromatograms using authentic material.

A few published mobilities that have not been incorporated into Tables II–XXII are referred to in each instance at the end of the appropriate table. In this connection, attention is drawn to several further studies dealing with the paper chromatography of steroid sulfates[31] and steroid glucuronides.[8, 20, 26, 27]

Table XXII is reserved for the 17 C_{18} steroids, which represent most of the known natural oestrogens and their metabolites.[21] The R_S values listed in this table were either actually determined by us or converted from values quoted in various publications[1, 5, 11, 19, 29, 32] and personal communications. A few further values[5a, 8b, 23, 28, 34] obtained using other solvent systems have also been published.

IV. CHROMATOPLATE TECHNIQUE

This technique of adsorption chromatography on thin layers of silicic acid, which is a counterpart to filter-paper chromatography, has only recently been applied to steroids. It involves less expenditure of time and material than conventional paper chromatography, and it also affords far better possibilities of detection by means of fluorescence with strong acids such as concentrated sulfuric acid. On the other hand, it greatly restricts the use of relatively specific detection reactions such as UV, BT, and soda fluorescence. For this reason the chromatoplate technique is chiefly suited for checking degrees of purity and tracing chemical reactions. Nevertheless, the very fact that the chromatographic sequence often differs from that seen in paper chromatography is sufficient justification for resorting to the

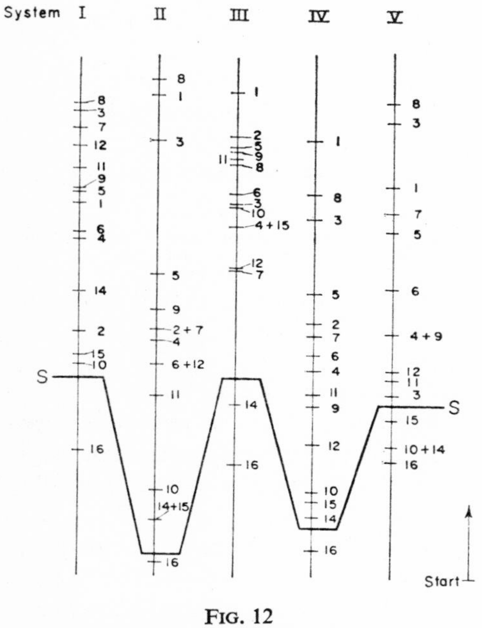

FIG. 12

Steroids of lower polarity (Table XXIII)
R_S-values (S=corticosterone) on chromatoplates

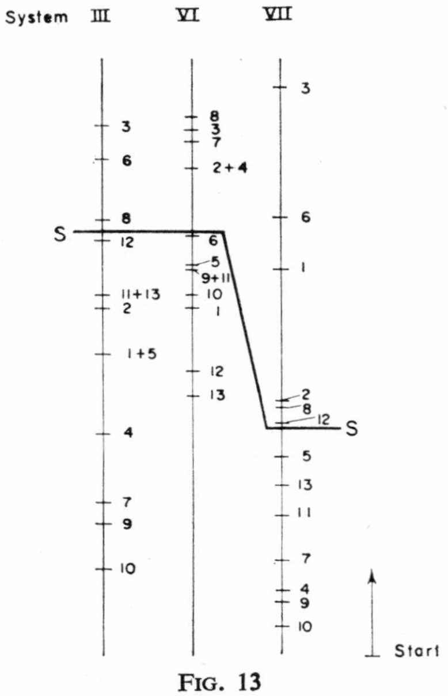

FIG. 13

Steroids of higher polarity (Table XXIV)
R_S-values (S=cortisol) on chromatoplates

chromatoplate technique for purposes of identification as well, particularly as a supplement to paper chromatography. This is evident from Tables XXIII and XXIV as well as from Figs. 12 and 13, where the restricted selection of steroids and solvent systems listed is designed merely as a suggestion. It is therefore unnecessary here to subdivide the steroids on the basis of their physicochemical properties ; instead, they have simply been divided into two groups according to their polarity. Figures 12 and 13, in particular, when compared with the paper-chromatographic patterns, are intended to give some idea as to the cases in which it may be useful to resort to the chromatoplate technique in addition.

Other solvent systems offering advantages in some special cases include: benzene–acetone (9:1, 1:1), benzene–ether (6:4), benzene–methanol (95:5), benzene–ethyl acetate (8:2, 1:1, 3:7), ether, ether–dimethylformamide (99:1), chloroform–ether (6:4), chloroform–acetone (7:3), ethyl acetate, and ethyl acetate–methanol (99:1). Alumina or Celite with 5 per cent gypsum added may be used as adsorbing material instead of silicic acid. Further examples for the application of thin layer chromatography of etianic acid esters and weakly polar steroids were recently presented by Barbier *et al.*[1a] and van Dam and co-workers.[35a] Since the completion of the manuscript in 1959 this technique has fully developed and is thoroughly reviewed by the author in a recent monograph.[38]

V. SPECIFICITY OF COLOR REACTIONS

In paper-chromatographic analysis, the detection reactions are just as important as the mobilities themselves. In fact, only when both are combined does paper chromatography afford a rational method of identification. Hence, it is necessary to know as far as possible the precise degree of specificity of the color reactions. Attention is therefore drawn to the reviews already mentioned,[7, 24, 29, 36] and the essentials — including points which have emerged from recent experiences — briefly summarized below:

(a) Blue tetrazolium (BT): Reducing groups, such as α-ketols in the side chains or in rings, immediately produce bright blue spots. It is important to note that α-ketols, which readily form cyclohemiketals with a neighboring hydroxyl group, as e.g. in some 18-hydroxy-compounds (cf. Table III A), show an extremely slow and faint color formation.

Ketol esters produce spots more slowly, depending on their acid residue. Occasionally, glycol side chains and Δ^4-3-ketones show a greyish-blue to bluish-violet reaction, although only slowly and very faintly, e.g., progesterone, testosterone, and a few of their oxygenated derivatives. Less suitable for the chromatoplate technique.

(b) Soda fluorescence ; yellow with Δ^4-3-ketosteroids ; Δ^1-3-ketones and α,β-unsaturated ketones in positions other than position 3 do not react. Exceptions reacting positively: certain triterpenes and cyclic compounds containing a group comparable to that of the Δ^4-3-ketosteroids ; 3,6-diketones ; even in normal light, Δ^4-3,6-diketones give a yellow color reaction.

Exceptions reacting negatively: progesterone and certain progesterone derivatives, such as 17α, 20α, and 20β-dihydroxy-Δ^4-pregnen-3-one, 6β, 11β, 14α-, 17α- or 18-hydroxyprogesterone, 11β,17α-dihydroxy-Δ^4-pregnene-3,20-dione, or 17αhydroxy-Δ^4-androsten-3-one show a much fainter, somewhat reddish fluorescence ; the reaction of 19-norsteroids and 2αhydroxysteroids is also fainter.

No reaction is shown by polyconjugated Δ^4-3-ketones, or 7-hydroxy-Δ^4-3-ketones; a more or less pronounced shift towards green or bluish-green occurs with 19-hydroxy-Δ^4-3-ketones. Soda fluorescence is unsuitable for the chromatoplate technique.

(c) *m*-Dinitrobenzene (DNB): cardenolides and 17-ketones, including particularly 17-ketones with a Δ^4-3-keto group, yield a strong violet reaction; color reactions far weaker and of much briefer duration are observed with 3-ketones (blue to bluish-violet) and 16-ketones (yellowish-brown), whereas Δ^4-3,6-diketones show an intense orange-yellow to bluish-green reaction. Exceptions: 14α-, 15α- and 18-hydroxyl groups largely suppress the color reaction of 17-ketones. Suitable for the chromatoplate technique.

(d) Dinitrophenylhydrazine (DNPH): reactive keto groups; sequence in descending order of sensitivity: Δ^4-3-ketones>3-ketones>20-ketones>17-ketones $\Delta^{1,4}$-3-ketones; α-ketols of the side chain react very poorly, and the same applies to certain Δ^4-3-ketosteroids specially substituted in rings C and D; 11-ketones do not react at all. Suitable for the chromatoplate technique.

(e) Antimony trichloride ($SbCl_3$), particularly suitable for Δ^5-3β-hydroxysteroids, which yield an orange to red color reaction even in normal light; the same applies to the C_{19}-17α-hydroxycompounds[24a]! The fluorescence reactions (UV light), though very unspecific, are often extremely useful because they permit marked color differentiation (also in the case of phosphoric acid, etc.); blue color reaction with 3β,7-dihydroxy-Δ^5-steroids[1b,31a]; very suitable for the chromatoplate technique.

(f) Ferric chloride–potassium ferricyanide: phenols and enols. Suitable for the chromatoplate technique.

For details of further color reactions and additional methods of identification in connection with chromatography, readers are referred to our recent review[38] and to other chapters in this book.

Where the *R* values obtained in experiments fail to tally satisfactorily with those listed in the present compilation, even allowing for normal margins of error, the closest of the divergent mobilities may suggest a certain structure or an isomeric steroid not included in the tables if the relationships between chemical structure and chromatographic mobilities are taken into account. These relationships have already been described in detail elsewhere[24] and, since no new aspects have emerged meanwhile, they need not be dealt with again here. It is interesting to note, however, that the mobilities are to a certain degree reversed in the case of steroid esters (see e.g. Bush and Mahesh[8a]).

Acknowledgements — I should like to express my sincerest thanks to Drs. I. E. Bush, C. Djerassi, T. F. Gallagher, K. Heusler, O. Jeger, W. Klyne, G. F. Marrian, C. Meystre, T. Reichstein, L. H. Sarett, J. Schmidlin, St. Ulick, J. Urech, and P. Wieland for placing substances at my disposal or supplying me with chromatographic data. I should also like to thank Dr. A. Wettstein for the encouragement he has given me in this work, as well as Mr. E. von Arx and Miss J. Vogt for their technical assistance and Mr. H. D. Philps, M.A., for his help with the translation.

TABLE I. MEAN R_f-VALUES OF 4 STANDARD STEROIDS IN ZAFFARONI- AND BUSH-TYPE SOLVENT SYSTEMS

Zaffaroni-type* Systems, 22° C	% stat. phase†	Progesterone	Cortexone	Corticosterone	Cortisol
P/Lig	50	0.17	0.03	0.02	—
P/Cy-Be (1 : 1)	50	0.45	0.07	0.01	—
F/Cy	20	0.58	0.08	—	—
P/MCy	25	0.55	0.21	0.03	—
Carb/MCy	100	0.73	0.16	0.01	—
F/Cy-Be (1 : 1)	20	0.91	0.52	0.05	—
P/Tol	20	0.92	0.73	0.23	0.01
F/Be	20	—	0.85	0.33	0.02
F/Be-$CHCl_3$ (1 : 1)	20	—	0.92	0.54	0.05
F/$CHCl_3$	20	—	—	0.77	0.24
F/EBW	20	—	—	0.65	0.40
F/BW	20	—	—	—	0.42
F/BBW	20	—	—	—	0.60
Bush-type Systems‡	**Temp. °C**				
A	22	0.67	0.15	—	—
	38	0.71	0.19	—	—
B_3	22	—	0.52	0.09	—
	38	—	0.52	0.11	—
B_1	38	—	0.75	0.25	—
BL_1	22	—	0.91	0.58	—
	38	—	0.91	0.60	—
E_9	38	—	—	—	0.19
Cy-Di I	38	—	—	0.45	0.25
B_5	22	—	—	0.77	0.25
	38	—	—	0.78	0.32
C	22	—	—	0.80	0.37
	38	—	—	0.78	0.38
E_2B	38	—	—	—	0.48

* P = Propylenglycol
Carb = Carbitol
Di = Dioxane
EBW = Ethyl acetate-butyl acetate-water (15: 85:5)
F = Formamide
BW = Butylacetate-water (100:5)[22]
BBW = n-Butanol-butyl acetate-water (15: 85: 5)
Lig = Ligroin
Cy = Cyclohexane
Be = Benzene
MCy = Methylcyclohexane
Tol = Toluene

† Concentration of stationary phase in impregnating solution

‡ A : Petroleum ether-methanol-water (100: 80: 20)
B_3 : Petroleum ether-benzene-methanol-water (33: 17: 40: 10)
B_1 : Petroleum ether-toluene-methanol-water (25: 25: 35: 15)
BL_1 : Petroleum ether-benzene-methanol-water (30: 70: 50: 50)
E_9 : Hexane-tert. butanol-methanol-water (50: 22.5: 22.5: 20)[14]
B_5 : Benzene-methanol-water (100: 50: 50)
C : Toluene-ethylacetate-methanol-water (90: 10: 50: 50)
E_2B : iso-Octane-tert. butanol-water (10: 5: 9)[14]
Cy-Di I: Cyclohexane-dioxane-methanol-water (4: 4: 2: 1)[9]

TABLE II. C_{21} STEROIDS UV+ BT+ (FIG. 1). R_s values (S = corticosterone)

	Carb/MCy	P/Lig	P/Cy-Be	P/Tol	F/Be-CHCl$_3$	BL$_1$/38°
1 21-Hydroxy-Δ^4-pregnene-3,20-dione	3.91		8.15	4.00	1.70	1.60
2 21-Hydroxy-Δ^4-pregnene-3,11,20-trione	1.27	2.96	2.86	2.30	1.36	1.25
3 6β,21-Dihydroxy-Δ^4-pregnene-3,20-dione		0.64		0.59	0.73	0.89
4 16α,21-Dihydroxy-Δ^4-pregnene-3,20-dione				0.19	0.41	0.31
5 17α,21-Dihydroxy-Δ^4-pregnene-3,20-dione	1.27	1.16	0.73	0.77	0.98	1.08
6 18,21-Dihydroxy-Δ^4-pregnene-3,20-dione		0.64		0.59	0.73	0.89
7 19,21-Dihydroxy-Δ^4-pregnene-3,20-dione				0.28	0.49	0.57
8 17α,21-Dihydroxy-Δ^4-pregnene-3,11,20-trione	0.73		0.17	0.17	0.15	0.41

TABLE III : C_{21-22} STEROIDS UV+ BT+ (FIG. 2). R_s values (S = cortisol)

No.	Compound	F/EBW 38°	P/Tol	F/Be	F/ $CHCl_3$	F/ BBW	B_5 22°	C 38°	E_2B 38°	CyDi I 38°
1a	6β,21-Dihydroxy-Δ^4-pregnene-3,20-dione				3.24			1.80		
1	11β,21-Dihydroxy-Δ-pregnene-3,20-dione	1.35			3.51			1.95	1.43	
1b	16α,21-Dihydroxy-Δ^4-pregnene-3,20-dione				2.75			1.28		
2	19,21-Dihydroxy-Δ^4-pregnene-3,20-dione		4.11		2.79		2.34	1.40	1.24	
3	20,20,21-Trihydroxy-Δ^4-pregnen-3-one-18-acid-lactone (18→20)		2.46		2.75		2.76	1.67	1.39	
4	11β,21-Dihydroxy-Δ^4-pregnen-18-al-3,20-dione (aldosterone)	0.41	2.55	1.20	2.25	0.40	1.52	0.97	0.75	1.03
4a	11β,21-Dihydroxy-Δ^4-17-iso-pregnen-18-al-3,20-dione (17-isoaldosterone)		1.83	1.26	2.22	0.41		0.92		0.73
5	6β,21-Dihydroxy-Δ^4-pregnene-3,11,20-trione	0.51	1.87		1.62		0.91	0.75	0.49	1.08
6	17α,21-Dihydroxy-Δ^4-pregnene-3,11,20-trione	1.05	2.51	1.95	2.39	0.95	1.91	1.38	1.09	
7	6β,11β,21-Trihydroxy-Δ^4-pregnene-3,20-dione	0.39	0.66	0.30	0.50		0.31	0.40	0.41	
8	6β,17α,21-Trihydroxy-Δ^4-pregnene-3,20-dione	0.66	0.49	0.31	0.58	0.60	0.44	0.59	0.85	
9	11β,19,21-Trihydroxy-Δ^4-pregnene-3,20-dione	0.44	0.69	0.60	1.37		0.80	0.77	0.79	
10	17α,19,21-Trihydroxy-Δ^4-pregnene-3,20-dione	0.44	0.19	0.13	0.36		0.20	0.35	0.53	
11	2α,11β,17α,21-Tetrahydroxy-Δ^4-pregnene-3,20-dione				0.17	0.36				
12	6β,11β,17α,21-Tetrahydroxy-Δ^4-pregnene-3,20-dione				0.04	0.19				
							38°			
13	17α,21-Dihydroxy-$\Delta^{1,4}$-pregnadiene-3,11,20-trione		1.94	1.59	2.00	0.93	1.33	1.24		
14	11β,17α,21-Trihydroxy-$\Delta^{1,4}$-pregnadiene-3,20-dione		0.46	0.53	0.65	0.90	0.71	0.80		
15	6α-Chloro-17α,21-dihydroxy-$\Delta^{1,4}$-pregnadiene-3,11,20-trione		0.73	0.88	0.56		1.09	1.21		
16	9α-Fluoro-11β,17α,21-trihydroxy-$\Delta^{1,4}$-pregnadiene-3,20-dione		0.19	0.21	0.28		0.43	0.59		
17	9α-Fluoro-11β,17α,21-trihydroxy-Δ^4-pregnene-3,20-dione		0.47	0.48	0.51	1.05	0.75	0.96		
18	9α-Fluoro-11β,16α,17α,21-tetrahydroxy-$\Delta^{1,4}$-pregnadiene-3,20-dione*		0.03	0.02	0.03		0.07	0.16		
19	6α-Methyl-11β,17α,21-trihydroxy-$\Delta^{1,4}$-pregnadiene-3,20-dione		0.71	1.13	1.11		1.09	1.10		
20	9α-Fluoro-16α-methyl-11β,17α,21-trihydroxy-$\Delta^{1,4}$-pregnadiene-3,20 dione		0.52	0.64	0.79		1.01	1.05		

* The mobilities of this compound and its derivatives in other systems were recently described by Florini and Buyske[15] and Smith *et al.*[32a,b]

† Relative mobilities of 19-norcorticosteroid hormones have been published by Zaffaroni *et al.*[37]

TABLE III A: C_{21} STEROIDS UV+ BT+24C
Chromatographic differentiation of aldosterone from closely related steroids
$R_{cortisol}$-values (mean values of spot center)

	P/Tol	F/Be	F/CHCl₃	F/BBW	C 38°†	E_2B 38°	Cy-Di I 38°†	B^5 38°†	BT	NaOH	H_3PO_4	SbC_3
1 18-HO-corticosterone	0.57	0.36	0.88	0.70	0.54		0.76		+‡	yellow	–	–
2 aldosterone	2.55	1.20	2.25	0.40	0.97	0.77	1.03	1.22	++	yellow	–	–
3 17iso-aldosterone	1.83	1.26	2.22	0.41	0.92	0.73	0.73	1.09	++	yellow	–	–
4 18-HO-comp.A	2.95	1.82	2.20	0.74	1.08	0.74	0.91	1.20	+‡	pale yellow	light pink	light violet
5 18-Oxo-comp.A* (11-dehydro-aldosterone)	~4.50	2.65	2.78	0.77	1.18	0.64	0.94	1.39	++	yellow	–	–
6 cortisone	2.51	1.95	2.39	0.95	1.38	1.13	1.08	1.43	++	yellow	blue	–

Systematic names:
1 11β,18,21-Trihydroxy-Δ⁴-pregnene-3,20-dione.
2 11β,21-Dihydroxy-Δ⁴-pregnen-18-al-3,20-dione.
3 11β,21-Dihydroxy-Δ⁴-17-iso-pregnen-18-al-3,20-dione.
4 18,21-Dihydroxy-Δ⁴-pregnene-3,11,20-trione.
5 21-Hydroxy-Δ⁴-pregnen-18-al-3,11,20-trione.
6 17α,21-Dihydroxy-Δ⁴-pregnene-3,11,20-trione.

* Tailing spots in all solvent systems, possibly caused by tautomerism.
† Bush type solvent systems are well suited for the sensitive 18-HO-compounds if the paper is *pre*-equilibrated and the substance brought on to the paper shortly before the run: otherwise these compounds decompose partly.
‡ Only weak and particularly slow color formation [20(18)-cyclohemiketal-grouping].

TABLE IV: C_{21} STEROIDS UV+ BT−. R_s values (S = progesterone)

		Carb/ McCy	P/Lig	A 38°
1	$\Delta^{4,16}$-Pregnadiene-3,20-dione	1.00	1.00	1.00(22°)
2	$\Delta^{4,9(11)}$-Pregnadiene-3,20-dione	1.00		0.90(22°)
3	$\Delta^{1,4}$-Pregnadiene-3,20-dione	0.62		0.60(22°)
4	20β-Hydroxy-Δ^{4}-pregnen-3-one			0.68
5	20α-Hydroxy-Δ^{4}-pregnen-3-one		0.10	0.50
6	Δ^{4}-Pregnene-3,6,20-trione		0.50	
7	Δ^{4}-Pregnene-3,11,20-trione	0.37 :	0.37	0.29
8	17α-Hydroxy-Δ^{4}-pregnene-3,20-dione	0.29	0.12	0.17
9	11β-Hydroxy-Δ^{4}-pregnene-3,20-dione	0.22		0.13
10	6β-Hydroxy-Δ^{4}-pregnene-3,20-dione	0.23		0.12
11	16α-Hydroxy-Δ^{4}-pregnene-3,20-dione	0.15		0.03
11a	21-Hydroxy-Δ^{4}-pregnene-3,20-dione	0.32	0.20	0.27
12	17α-Hydroxy-Δ^{4}-pregnene-3,11,20-trione	0.15		

TABLE V: C_{20-21} STEROIDS UV+ BT− (FIG. 3). R_s values (S = cortexone)

	Carb/MCy	P/Lig	P/Cy-Be	P/Tol	F/Cy-Be	F/Be	B_3 38°
1 $\Delta^{4,16}$-Pregnadiene-3,20-dione	3.14	5.10					1.70
2 $\Delta^{4,9(11)}$-Pregnadiene-3,20-dione	3.14	5.10					1.70
3 $\Delta^{1,4}$-Pregnadiene-3,20-dione	1.94				1.84		1.55
4 Δ^{4}-Pregnene-3,20-dione	3.14	5.10	1.50	1.28	1.86	1.21	1.70
5 20β-Hydroxy-Δ^{4}-pregnen-3-one				0.99	1.59		1.35
6 20α-Hydroxy-Δ^{4}-pregnen-3-one		0.53		0.88	1.50		1.25
7 Δ^{4}-Pregnene-3,6,20-trione		2.58					
8 Δ^{4}-Pregnene-3,11,20-trione	1.16	1.86	1.00	1.22	1.35		1.15
9 17α-Hydroxy-Δ^{4}-pregnene-3,20-dione	0.92	0.62	0.64	0.86	0.95	1.01	0.93
10 11β-Hydroxy-Δ^{4}-pregnene-3,20-dione	0.70	0.44	0.52	0.81	0.74	0.95	0.80
11 6β-Hydroxy-Δ^{4}-pregnene-3,20-dione	0.73	0.31	0.40	0.59	0.48	0.75	0.60
11a 14α-Hydroxy-Δ^{4}-pregnene-3,20-dione				0.71	0.64	0.87	0.60
12 16α-Hydroxy-Δ^{4}-pregnene-3,20-dione	0.47	0.10	0.23			0.49	0.30
12a 18-Hydroxy-Δ^{4}-pregnene-3,20-dione				0.73	0.90	0.95	1.78
12b 18-Hydroxy-Δ^{4}-etienic acid lactone (20→18) 3-one (C_{20}-steroid)				1.14	0.91		0.90
12c 11β,18-Oxido-18-hydroxy-Δ^{4}-etienic acid-lactone (20→18)-3-one (C_{20}-steroid) = aldosterone lactone				0.99	0.44	0.91	0.52
13 Δ^{4}-Pregnene-3,6,11,20-tetrone		0.56					
14 17α-Hydroxy-Δ^{4}-pregnene-3,11,20-trione	0.46	0.14	0.25			0.59	0.38
15 6β-Hydroxy-Δ^{4}-pregnene-3,11,20-trione			0.14			0.39	
16 11β,17α-Dihydroxy-Δ^{4}-pregnene-3,20-dione			0.07			0.26	
17 6β,17α-Dihydroxy-Δ^{4}-pregnene-3,20-dione			0.05			0.14	

TABLE VI : C_{20-21} STEROIDS UV+ BT− (FIG. 4). R_s values (S = corticosterone)

		P/Tol	P/Cy-Be	F/Be	F/Be-$CHCl_3$	B_5 22°	BL_1 38°
1	Δ^4-Pregnene-3,11,20-trione		8.16				
2	17α-Hydroxy-Δ^4-pregnene-3,20-dione	3.00	5.20	6.54			
3	11β-Hydroxy-Δ^4-pregnene-3,20-dione	3.00	4.28	3.64			
4	6β-Hydroxy-Δ^4-pregnene-3,20-dione	2.38	3.27	2.87	1.85		1.27
5	16α-Hydroxy-Δ^4-pregnene-3,20-dione	1.30	1.88	1.90	1.49		1.25
6	17α,20α-Dihydroxy-Δ^4-pregnen-3-one	0.70		1.58	1.32		1.20
7	17α,20β-Dihydroxy-Δ^4-pregnen-3-one	1.37		2.15	1.34		1.20
8	11β,20α-Dihydroxy-Δ^4-pregnen-3-one	0.70		1.58	1.32		1.20
9	11β,20β-Dihydroxy-Δ^4-pregnen-3-one	1.37		2.15	1.34		1.20
9a	20β,21-Dihydroxy-Δ^4-pregnen-3-one	*ca.*0.50*		1.37	1.25		1.13
10	11β,18-Dihydroxy-Δ^4-etienic acid lactone (20→18)-3-one (C_{20}-steroid)	1.08		1.17	1.17		1.01
11	17α-Hydroxy-Δ^4-pregnene-3,11,20-trione	1.59	2.04	2.28			
12	6β-Hydroxy-Δ^4-pregnene-3,11,20-trione	1.45	1.16	1.49			
13	11β,17α-Dihydroxy-Δ^4-pregnene-3,20-dione	0.60	0.59	1.04	0.99	0.95	0.92
13a	11β,18-Dihydroxy-Δ^4-pregnene-3,20-dione	0.43		0.66	0.83	1.10	1.46†
14	6β,17α-Dihydroxy-Δ^4-pregnene-3,20-dione	0.35	0.39	0.54		0.86	
14a	17α,20β-Dihydroxy-Δ^4-pregnene-3,11-dione	0.62		0.97	1.07		0.93
14b	17α,20α-Dihydroxy-Δ^4-pregnene-3,11-dione	0.58		0.75	0.92		0.81
15	20β,21-Dihydroxy-Δ^4-pregnene-3,11-dione	0.16			0.47		0.31
16	17α,20β,21-Trihydroxy-Δ^4-pregnen-3-one	0.20			0.50		0.39

* Tailing. † Decomposition product?

TABLE VII : C_{21} STEROIDS UV+ BT− (FIG. 5). R_s values (S = cortisol)

		P/Tol	F/$CHCl_3$	F/BBW	B_5 22°	C 38°	E_2B 38°	F/Be
1	11β,17α-Dihydroxy-Δ^4-pregnene-3,20-dione	6.60			2.20			
1a	11β,18-Dihydroxy-Δ^4-pregnene-3,20-dione	5.50			2.65			7.30
2	20β,21-Dihydroxy-Δ^4-pregnene-3,11-dione	2.41	2.94		1.89	1.39	1.40	
3	11β,17α,20β-Trihydroxy-Δ^4-pregnen-3-one	*ca.*3.06*	2.48	1.26		1.62		*ca.*5.05*
4	17α,20α,21-Trihydroxy-Δ^4-pregnen-3-one	*ca.*2.30*	2.48	0.88		1.35		2.34
5	17α,20β,21-Trihydroxy-Δ^4-pregnen-3-one	*ca.*3.10*	2.66	1.02		1.53		3.33
6	17α,20β,21-Trihydroxy-$\Delta^{1,4}$-pregnadiene-3,11-dione				0.60			
7	17α,20α,21-Trihydroxy-Δ^4-pregnene-3,11-dione	0.95	1.59	0.54	0.72	0.58	0.72	0.48
8	17α,20β,21-Trihydroxy-Δ^4-pregnene-3,11-dione	0.84	1.48	0.55	0.67	0.58	0.79	0.51
9	11β,17α,20β,21-Tetrahydroxy-$\Delta^{1,4}$-pregnadiene-3-one				0.16			
10	11β,17α,20α,21-Tetrahydroxy-Δ^4-pregnen-3-one	0.20	0.33		0.15	0.32		
11	11β,17α,20β,21-Tetrahydroxy-Δ^4-pregnen-3-one	0.25	0.48		0.22	0.32	0.68	

* Tailing.

TABLE VIII: C_{21} STEROIDS UV− BT+
R_S values (S = cortexone)

		P/Lig	P/Tol	F/Cy-Be	B_3 22°
1	21-Hydroxyallopregnane-3,20-dione	2.36			
2	3β,21-Dihydroxy-Δ^5-pregnen-20-one		0.47	0.77	0.68
3	3β,21-Dihydroxyallopregnan-20-one		0.48	0.87	0.79
4	3α,21-Dihydroxypregnan-20-one		0.64	0.87	0.85
5	21-Hydroxypregnane-3,6,20-trione		0.81	0.12	
6	21-Hydroxyallopregnane-3,11,20-trione		0.80	0.33	0.37
7	21-Hydroxypregnane-3,11,20-trione		0.75	0.32	0.35
8	11β,21-Dihydroxyallopregnane-3,20-dione		0.49		0.24
9	3α,17α,21-Trihydroxypregnan-20-one		0.36	0.21	0.33

TABLE IX: C_{21} STEROIDS UV− BT+ (FIG. 6)
R_S values (S = corticosterone)

		P/Tol	F/Be-$CHCl_3$	BL_1 22°
1	3β,21-Dihydroxyallopregnan-20-one	2.03	1.76	2.03
2	3α,21-Dihydroxypregnan-20-one	2.21	1.80	
3	21-Hydroxyallopregnane-3,11,20-trione	3.02	1.62	1.69
4	21-Hydroxypregnane-3,11,20-trione	2.81	1.68	1.73
5	3β,21-Dihydroxyallopregnane-11,20-dione	0.48	0.83	0.86
6	3α,21-Dihydroxypregnane-11,20-dione	0.60	0.97	0.71
7	11β,21-Dihydroxyallopregnane-3,20-dione	1.81	1.35	1.43
8	17α,21-Dihydroxypregnane-3,20-dione	1.57	1.34	1.46
9	3β,11β,21-Trihydroxyallopregnan-20-one	0.24	0.48	0.41
10	3α,11β,21-Trihydroxypregnan-20-one*	0.32	0.63	0.73
11	3β,17α,21-Trihydroxyallopregnan-20-one	0.14	0.50	0.66
11a	3α,17α,21-Trihydroxyallopregnan-20-one	0.24		
12	3α,17α,21-Trihydroxypregnan-20-one	0.18	0.53	0.72
13	17α,21-Dihydroxyallopregnane-3,11,20-trione	0.32	0.46	0.33
14	17α,21-Dihydroxypregnane-3,11,20-trione	0.30	0.68	0.55

* The corresponding allopregnane isomer ("allo-TH-corticosterone") was not available; it is supposed to run slightly faster than No. 10.

Table X: C_{21} Steroids UV− BT+ (Fig. 7). R_s values (S = cortisol)

		P/Tol	F/$CHCl_3$	F/BW	B_5 22°	C 38°	E_9 38°	E_2B 38°	F/EBW
1	3β,21-Dihydroxyallopregnane-11,20-dione	>6.0	3.71		3.19	1.74		1.52	
2	3α,21-Dihydroxypregnane-11,20-dione	>6.0	3.75	1.29	3.71	1.92		2.18	
3	3β,17α,21-Trihydroxy-Δ^5-pregnen-20-one			1.26					
4	3β,11β,21-Trihydroxyallopregnan-20-one	4.00	2.63	1.26	2.64	1.67		1.61	
5	3α,11β,21-Trihydroxypregnan-20-one*	5.43	2.60	1.45	3.24	2.01	2.32	1.62	
6	3β,17α,21-Trihydroxyallopregnan-20-one	2.34	2.50	1.64	2.87	1.63		2.51	
6a	3α,17α,21-Trihydroxyallopregnan-20-one	3.98	2.78		2.87	1.70		2.56	
7	3α,17α,21-Trihydroxypregnan-20-one	2.80	2.79	1.76	2.81	1.81		2.71	
8	17α,21-Dihydroxyallopregnane-3,11,20-trione	5.47	3.11		2.80	1.71		1.60	
9	17α,21-Dihydroxypregnane-3,11,20-trione	5.31	2.84	1.31	2.83	1.73	1.83	1.66	
10	3β,17α,21-Trihydroxyallopregnane-11,20-dione	0.40	0.79		0.70	0.77		1.78	
11	3α,17α,21-Trihydroxypregnane-11,20-dione	0.42	1.01	1.14	0.89	0.88	1.55	1.92	1.14
12	3α,11β,21-Trihydroxypregnan-18-al-20-one	0.41	1.01	0.78°	0.76	0.66		1.54	0.48
13	11β,17α,21-Trihydroxyallopregnane-3,20-dione	2.67	1.61		1.86	1.43		1.40	
14	11β,17α,21-Trihydroxypregnane-3,20-dione	2.70	1.43		1.99	1.51	1.71	1.49	
15	3α,11β,17α,21-Tetrahydroxyallopregnan-20-one	0.40	0.40	1.14°	0.55	0.82		1.37	
16	3β,11β,17α,21-Tetrahydroxyallopregnan-20-one	0.20	0.22	1.05°	0.33	0.57		1.12	0.96
17	3α,11β,17α,21-Tetrahydroxypregnan-20-one	0.29	0.28	1.08°	0.38	0.63	1.11	1.51	1.07

* The corresponding allopregnane isomer ("allo-TH-corticosterone") was not available; it is supposed to run slightly faster than No. 5.

† Other $R_{cortisol}$-values: B_5 (38°), 0.63; Cy-Di I (38°) 1.01; F/CH_2Cl_2 0.73; Ethylene glycol/$C_2H_4Cl_2$-Tol (1 : 1) 0.48.

° in F/BBW—system which is somewhat more polar than F/BW and runs with a sharper solvent front; the *relative* mobilities are, however, nearly identical in both systems.

TABLE XI: C_{21} STEROIDS UV− BT−
R_f values from ref. [3,12]

		P/Tol	B_4 22°	X 22°
1	Allopregnane-3,20-dione	0.91		
2	3β-Hydroxy-Δ5-pregnen-20-one	0.78	0.88	
3	3β-Hydroxyallopregnan-20-one	0.86	0.89	
4	3α-Hydroxypregnan-20-one	0.85		
5	Allopregnane-3α,20α-diol	0.35	0.71	
6	Allopregnane-3β,20α-diol	0.31	0.77	
7	Allopregnane-3β,20β-diol	0.41	0.78	
8	Pregnane-3α,20α-diol	0.32	0.73	
9	Δ5-Pregnene-3β,17α,20α-triol			0.26
10	Δ5-Pregnene-3β,17α,20β-triol			0.33
11	Allopregnane-3α,17α,20α-triol			0.38
12	Allopregnane-3α,17α,20β-triol			0.48
13	Pregnane-3α,17α,20α-triol	0.08		0.33
14	Pregnane-3α,17α,20β-triol			0.42

X = iso-Octane-toluene-methanol-water (5 : 15 : 16 : 4)[12].

TABLE XII: C_{21} STEROIDS UV− BT−
R_S values (S = progesterone)

		A 38°	B_3 38°	F/Cy	P/MCy
1	3β-Hydroxy-Δ5-pregnen-20-one	0.79	0.89	0.93	0.55
2	3α-Hydroxyallopregnan-20-one	1.08	0.99	1.19	
3	3β-Hydroxyallopregnan-20-one	0.90	0.95	1.02	0.62
4	3α-Hydroxypregnan-20-one	0.95	0.95	1.08	

TABLE XIII : C_{21} STEROIDS UV− BT− (FIG. 8)
R_S values (S = cortexone)

		Carb/MCy	P/Lig	P/Tol	B_3 22°	A 22°
1	Allopregnane-3,20-dione	4.07	6.7			
2	Pregnane-3,20-dione	4.07	6.7			
3	3β-Hydroxy-Δ^5-pregnen-20-one	1.92	2.80	1.04	1.65	2.65
4	3α-Hydroxy-allopregnan-20-one		3.11		1.87	3.57
5	3β-Hydroxy-allopregnan-20-one			1.05	1.79	2.98
6	3α-Hydroxy-pregnan-20-one	2.27	2.89		1.79	3.14
7	3β-Hydroxy-pregnan-20-one	1.92		1.04	1.71	3.14
8	Allopregnane-3,11,20-trione	1.45			1.50	1.81
9	Pregnane-3,11,20-trione	1.45			1.50	1.81
10	3α-Hydroxyallopregnane-11,20-dione			0.88		
11	3β-Hydroxyallopregnane-11,20-dione	0.74			0.65	0.46
12	3α-Hydroxypregnane-11-20-dione	0.92			0.83	0.59
13	3β-Hydroxypregnane-11,20-dione	0.92			0.83	0.69
14	11β-Hydroxypregnane-3,20-dione	1.16			1.25	0.86
15	3α,17α-Dihydroxypregnan-20-one		0.20			
15a	3β,21-Dihydroxy-Δ^5-pregnen-20-one			0.47	0.68	
16	17α-Hydroxypregnane-3,11,20-trione	0.74			0.71	0.29
17	3α,17α-Dihydroxypregnane-11,20-dione	0.41			0.19	

TABLE XIV : C_{21} STEROIDS UV− BT−
R_S values (S = corticosterone)

		P/Tol	F/Be-$CHCl_3$	BL_1 22°
1	3β,17α-Dihydroxyallopregnan-20-one	1.12	1.68	2.13
2	Allopregnane-3β,17α-20α-triol	0.30	1.06	1.11
3	Allopregnane-3β,17α,20β-triol	0.42	1.28	1.15
4	Pregnane-3α,17α,20α-triol	0.40	1.07	1.08

TABLE XIV A: C_{21} STEROIDS UV— BT— (DNPH+)[24a]. R_S values (S = corticosterone)

		P/Tol	F/Be	F/Be-$CHCl_3$	B_3 38°	BL_1 38°	E_4 38°
1	3β,16α-Dihydroxy-Δ^5-pregnen-20-one	0.26	1.10		0.64		1.52
2	3β,16β-Dihydroxy-Δ^5-pregnen-20-one	0.26	1.06		0.60		1.36
3	3β,17α-Dihydroxy-Δ^5-pregnen-20-one	1.12	2.75	1.54	2.68	1.30	
4	3β,21-Dihydroxy-Δ^5-pregnen-20-one	2.00	3.06	1.63	4.10	1.40	
5	3α,16α-Dihydroxyallopregnan-20-one	0.46	1.57		1.19		2.26
6	3β,16α-Dihydroxyallopregnan-20-one	0.29	1.15	1.08	0.71	0.94	1.63
7	3β,16β-Dihydroxyallopregnan-20-one	0.29	1.13		0.70		1.43
8	3α,16α-Dihydroxypregnan-20-one	0.33	1.27		0.98		2.26
9	3β,16α-Dihydroxypregnan-20-one	0.49	1.77		1.08		2.13

TABLE XV: C_{21} STEROIDS UV— BT—. R_S values (S = cortisol)

		P/Tol	F/$CHCl_3$	B_5 22°	C 38°	E_2B 38°	Trivial Names
1	Allopregnane-3β,17α,20β,21-tetrol	0.47	0.46		1.12	1.88	Reichstein's K
2	3α,17α,20α,21-Tetrahydroxypregnan-11-one		0.37	0.10			Cortolone
3	3α,17α,20β,21-Tetrahydroxypregnan-11-one		0.37	0.10			β-Cortolone
4	Allopregnane-3β,11β,17α,20β,21-pentol	0.04	0.04		0.13	0.67	Reichstein's A
5	Pregnane-3α,11β,17α,20α,21-pentol		0.11	0.04			Cortol
6	Pregnane-3α,11β,17α,20β,21-pentol		0.14	0.05			β-Cortol

TABLE XVI : C_{19} STEROIDS (17-KETOSTEROIDS) UV+ DNB+ (FIG. 9). R_s values (S = cortexone)

		P/Lig	P/Cy-Be	P/Tol	Carb/MCy	F/Cy-Be	F/Be	A 38°	B_3 22°	B_1 22°
1	$\Delta^{4,9(11)}$-Androstadiene-3,17-dione				1.92			1.90		
1a	$\Delta^{4,11}$-Androstadiene-3,17-dione			1.25		1.66	1.15	2.37	1.40	
2	$\Delta^{1,4}$-Androstadiene-3-17-dione	1.38	1.10	1.18	1.16	1.33	1.10	1.17	1.45	
3	Δ^{1}-Androstene-3,17-dione	4.40								
4	Δ^{4}-Androstene-3,17-dione	3.80	1.32	1.26	1.92	1.62	1.17	1.90	1.45	1.11
5	Δ^{4}-Androstene-3,6,17-trione	1.00	1.38		0.84		1.07	0.56	1.00	
6	Δ^{4}-Androstene-3,11,17-trione	0.80	1.20	1.07	0.79	0.89	1.01	0.50	0.80	0.90
7	6α-Hydroxy-Δ^{4}-androstene-3,17-dione		0.06							
8	6β-Hydroxy-Δ^{4}-androstene-3,17-dione	0.18	0.20	0.36			0.49		0.35	0.46
9	11β-Hydroxy-Δ^{4}-androstene-3-17-dione	0.22	0.35	0.56	0.14	0.35	0.68		0.51	0.69
9a	11α-Hydroxy-Δ^{4}-androstene-3,17-dione			0.22			0.32		0.18	
9b	12α-Hydroxy-Δ^{4}-androstene-3,17-dione			0.44			0.46		0.39	
9c	14α-Hydroxy-Δ^{4}-androstene-3,17-dione			0.27			0.39		0.21	
9d	15α-Hydroxy-Δ^{4}-androstene-3,17-dione			0.19			0.28		0.14	
10	19-Hydroxy-Δ^{4}-androstene-3,17-dione			0.18			0.25		0.17	

TABLE XVI A: C_{19} STEROIDS (17-KETOSTEROIDS) UV+ DNB+. R_S values

	S = corticosterone					S = cortisol	
	P/Tol	F/Be	F/Be-$CHCl_3$	B_3 38°	BL_1 38°	F/$CHCl_3$	C 38°
1 6β-Hydroxy-Δ^4-androstene-3,17-dione	1.57	1.92	1.35	2.00	1.15		
2 11β-Hydroxy-Δ^4-androstene-3,17-dione	2.40	2.65	1.58	2.98	1.36		
3 11α-Hydroxy-Δ^4-androstene-3,17-dione	1.04	1.24	1.21	0.99	0.92		
4 12α-Hydroxy-Δ^4-androstene-3,17-dione	2.09	1.76	1.44	2.13	1.21		
5 14α-Hydroxy-Δ^4-androstene-3,17-dione	1.29	1.51	1.26	1.21	1.05	3.46	1.91
6 15α-Hydroxy-Δ^4-androstene-3,17-dione	0.90	1.10	1.10	0.79	0.80	3.28	1.86
7 19-Hydroxy-Δ^4-androstene-3,17-dione	0.83	1.03	1.06	0.98	0.86		

TABLE XVII: C_{19-20} STEROIDS UV+ DNB−. R_S values (S = cortexone)

	P/Lig	P/Cy-Be	P/Tol	Carb/MCy	F/Cy-Be	F/Be	A 38°	B_3 22°	P/MCy
1 17β-Hydroxy-$\Delta^{1,4}$-androstadien-3-one	0.27	0.34	0.40	0.60	0.69	0.83	0.48	0.65	0.96
1a 17α-Hydroxy-Δ^4-androsten-3-one			0.81		1.13		1.27	1.07	
2 17β-Hydroxy-Δ^4-androsten-3-one	0.73	0.50	0.70	1.03	1.01	0.96	1.05	0.95	0.58
2a 1-Dehydrotestololactone			0.60		0.25	0.69	0.11	0.28	
2b Testololactone			0.84		0.44	0.81	0.24	0.50	
3 17β-Hydroxy-Δ^4-androstene-3,11-dione		0.15	0.35	0.10	0.21	0.43		0.25	
3a 17α-Hydroxy-Δ^4-androstene-3,11-dione			0.41		0.33			0.43	
4 6β,17β-Dihydroxy-Δ^4-androsten-3-one		0.03	0.07			0.11			
5 11β,17β-Dihydroxy-Δ^4-androsten-3-one	0.05	0.05	0.11	0.07	0.09	0.19			
6 17α-Methyl-17β-hydroxy-Δ^4-androsten-3-one		0.80	0.77	1.34		1.10	1.44	1.23	
7 17α-Methyl-17β-hydroxy-Δ^4-androstene-3,11-dione		0.33	0.45			0.67		0.40	

TABLE XVII A: C_{19} STEROIDS UV+ DNB−. R_S values

		S = Corticosterone				S = Cortisol				
		P/Tol	F/Be	F/Be-$CHCl_3$	BL_1 38°	P/Tol	F/Be	F/$CHCl_3$	C 38°	Cy-Di I 38°
1	17β,Hydroxy-Δ4-androstene-3,15-dione	0.94	1.31	1.24	0.92					
2	2α,17β-Dihydroxy-Δ4-androsten-3-one	1.05	1.42	1.16	1.17					
3	2β,17β-Dihydroxy-Δ4-androsten-3-one	1.46		1.38	1.32					
4	6β,17β-Dihydroxy-Δ4-androsten-3-one	0.21	0.37	0.56	0.58	2.55	5.15	2.38	1.54	
5	11β,17β-Dihydroxy-Δ4-androsten-3-one	0.37	0.73	0.83	0.73	6.0	10.0	2.83	1.83	
6	11β,17α-Dihydroxy-Δ4-androsten-3-one	0.47	1.14	1.04	0.89					
7	15α,17β-Dihydroxy-Δ4-androsten-3-one			0.34		1.05	2.22	1.98	0.83	0.77
8	16α,17β-Dihydroxy-Δ4-androsten-3-one			0.31		1.22	1.80	2.14	1.10	

TABLE XVIII: C_{19} STEROIDS (17-KETOSTEROIDS) UV− DNB+ (FIG. 10). R_s values (S = cortexone)

		P/Lig	P/MCy	P/Cy-Be	P/Tol	F/Cy-Be	F/Be	A 38°	B_3 38°
1	Δ^2-Androsten-17-one	20.4	6.45						
2	3β-Chlor-Δ^5-androsten-17-one	20.4	6.45						
3	Androstane-3,17-dione	5.5	3.14						
4	Etiocholane-3,17-dione	5.5	3.14						
5	6-Hydroxy-i-androsten-17-one	3.3							
6	3β-Hydroxy-Δ^5-androsten-17-one		1.37	0.87	0.84	1.50		1.75	1.18
7	3α-Hydroxy-Δ^9-androsten-17-one	2.22							
8	3α-Hydroxy-Δ^9-etiocholen-17-one	1.56							
9	3α-Hydroxyandrostan-17-one	2.22	2.58	1.36	1.00	1.60		2.63	1.40
10	3β-Hydroxyandrostan-17-one		1.76	0.83	0.84	1.45		2.20	1.26
11	3α-Hydroxyetiocholan-17-one	1.56		0.93	0.90	1.50		2.28	1.26
12	3β-Hydroxyetiocholan-17-one				1.00	1.70		2.58	1.35
13	Androstane-3,7,17-trione		1.76	1.29					
14	Androstane-3,11,17-trione	1.67			1.22	1.32	1.14		1.13
15	Etiocholane-3,11,17-trione	1.67			1.22	1.32	1.14		1.13
16	3β-Hydroxy-Δ^5-androstene-11,17-dione				0.50	0.45	0.76		0.32
17	3β-Hydroxyandrostane-6,17-dione			0.11			0.74		
18	3α-Hydroxyandrostane-11,17-dione	0.67					0.74		0.60
19	3β,Hydroxyandrostane-11,17-dione				0.50	0.44	0.75		0.34
20	3α-Hydroxyetiocholane-11,17-dione	0.58	0.31	0.38	0.65	0.66	0.77	0.35	0.47
21	3β-Hydroxyetiocholane-11,17-dione				0.67	0.75	0.90		0.50
22	11β-Hydroxyandrostane-3,17-dione	0.38							
23	3β,11β-Dihydroxy-Δ^5-androsten-17-one				0.12		0.36		
24	3α,11β-Dihydroxyandrostan-17-one	0.22			0.29		0.61		
25	3β,11β-Dihydroxyandrostan-17-one				0.14	0.20			0.08
26	3α,11β-Dihydroxyetiocholan-17-one*	0.11	0.05		0.20		0.49		

* The chromatographic mobilities of a few more polar 17-Ketosteroids are given by Okeda *et al.*[25]

TABLE XIX: C_{19} STEROIDS (17-KETOSTEROIDS) UV− DNB+
R_S values (S = corticosterone)

		P/Lig	P/Tol	F/Be	F/Be-$CHCl_3$	BL_1 38°
1	3β-Hydroxy-Δ5-androstene-11,17-dione		2.34	3.20	1.67	1.40
2	3α-Hydroxyandrostane-11,17-dione			3.20	1.68	
3	3β-Hydroxyandrostane-11,17-dione		2.39	3.23	1.69	1.40
4	3α-Hydroxyetiocholane-11,17-dione		2.30	3.30	1.79	
5	3β-Hydroxyetiocholane-11,17-dione		3.06	3.80	1.80	1.48
6	11β-Hydroxyandrostane-3,17-dione	6.80				
7	3β,11β-Dihydroxy-Δ5-androsten-17-one		0.60	1.50	1.16	1.06
8	3α,11β-Dihydroxyandrostan-17-one	4.0	1.02	2.12	1.40	1.28
9	3β,11β-Dihydroxyandrostan-17-one		0.68	1.43	0.98	1.20
10	3α,11β-Dihydroxyetiocholan-17-one	1.92	0.76	1.69	1.19	1.26

TABLE XX: C_{19} STEROIDS UV− DNB−
R_S values (S = cortexone)

		P/Cy-Be	P/Tol
1	17β-Hydroxyandrostan-3-one*	1.04	1.56
2	17β-Hydroxyetiocholan-3-one	1.02	1.56
3	Δ5-Androstene-3β,17α-diol	0.16	
4	Δ5-Androstene-3β,17β-diol	0.10	0.20
5	Androstane-3α,17β-diol	0.23	
6	Androstane-3β,17β-diol	0.17	
7	Androstane-3β,17α-diol	0.21	
8	Etiocholane-3α,17β-diol	0.18	
9	Etiocholane-3α,17α-diol	0.22	
10	17β-Hydroxyetiocholane-3,11-dione	0.24	
11	3β,17β-Dihydroxy-Δ5-androsten-16-one	0–0.08	
12	3α,17β-Dihydroxyandrostan-16-one	0.16	

* Additional values
$R_{cortexone}$ P/MCy 1.75; F/Cy 5.93; A(38°) 3.45.
$R_{progesterone}$ 0.23; 0.50; 0.93.

TABLE XXI: C_{19} STEROIDS UV− DNB− (FIG. 11)
R_S values (S = corticosterone)

		P/Tol	F/Be	F/Be-$CHCl_3$	BL_1 38°
1	Δ5-Androstene-3β,17β-diol	0.63		1.41	
2	3β,17β-Dihydroxy-Δ5-androsten-11-one	0.16	0.74	0.73	0.69
3	3α,17β-Dihydroxyandrostan-11-one	0.26	1.15	0.93	
4	3β,17β-Dihydroxyandrostan-11-one	0.15		0.70	
5	3α,17β-Dihydroxyetiocholan-11-one	0.21	1.00	0.86	0.71
6	3β,17β-Dihydroxyetiocholan-11-one	0.24	1.00	0.86	0.78
7	11β,17β-Dihydroxyandrostan-3-one	0.79	1.45	1.20	0.99
8	11β,17β-Dihydroxyetiocholan-3-one	0.80	1.54	1.16	1.18
9	Δ5-Androstene-3β,11β,17β-triol	0.06	0.29	0.31	0.36
10	Androstane-3α,11β,17β-triol	0.12	0.60	0.50	
11	Androstane-3β,11β,17β-triol	0.05	0.28	0.34	0.42
12	Etiocholane-3α,11β,17β-triol	0.06	0.35	0.39	0.51
13	Etiocholane-3β,11β,17β-triol	0.11	0.50	0.47	

TABLE XXII: "C_{18} STEROIDS" (ESTROGENS, TRIVIAL NAMES)

Blue color reaction with ferric chloride-potassium ferricyanide[2] — R_S values; R_f values of standard estrogens in brackets

	a	b		c	d	e	f	g	h	i	k	l
1 Equilin	0.88	0.91		0.95		2.13	2.32	1.68				
2 Equilenin	0.62	0.72		0.77		1.96	2.09	1.61				
3 Dihydroequilin-17α	0.27	0.14		0.39		1.07	1.04	0.94				
4 Dihydroequilenin-17α	0.15	0.09		0.26		0.81	0.81	0.72				
5 4-Methoxyestrone	1.97	1.84		1.46		2.74	2.74	1.90				
6 2-Methoxyestrone	1.43	1.87		0.92	4.95	2.26	2.48	1.72				
7 Estrone	1.00 (0.35)	1.00 (0.38)	8.34	1.00 (0.45)	2.50	2.25	2.24	1.73	1.35	1.22	4.02	2.22
8 2-Methoxyestradiol				0.92*	~2.0*	2.20*	2.45*					
9 Estradiol-17β	0.28	0.12	1.00 (0.06)	0.39	1.00 (0.20)	1.00 (0.35)	1.00 (0.35)	1.00 (0.50)	1.00 (0.71)	1.00 (0.75)	3.91	2.06
10 Estradiol-17α	0.41	0.16	0.36	0.52		1.28	1.26	1.18	1.08	1.05	4.16	2.12
11 16-Oxo-estrone		0.11	0.94	0.24		0.26				0.88	3.83	
12 16α-Hydroxyestrone	0.05	0.07	0.62	0.11		0.27	0.24	0.39	0.70	0.60	3.35	1.90
13 16β-Hydroxyestrone			0.82			0.26		0.33	0.59	0.59	3.40	1.92
14 18-Hydroxyestrone									0.62*			
15 16-Oxo-estradiol-17β			0.81			0.27		0.34	0.59	0.62	3.45	1.89
16 16-Epiestriol			0.19			0.11		0.18	0.33	0.37	2.86	1.68
17 Estriol			< 0.01			< 0.01	0.01	< 0.01	0.07	0.05	1.00 (0.24)	1.00 (0.43)

a Formamide/cyclohexane-benzene (1 : 1)

b Propyleneglycol/toluene

c Bush B_3, 38°C

d Dao's System, 38°C: n-heptane-CH_3OH 1 : 1[11]

e Formamide/benzene

f Formamide/dichlorbenzene[1] (Formamide/monochlorbenzene cf. 5)

g Formamide/benzene-chloroform (1 : 1)

h Formamide/Chloroform

i BL_1, 38°C

k Bush C, 38°C

l Marrian's System, 38°C: chloroform-benzene-methanol-water (36 : 64 : 66 : 33)[19]

TABLE XXIII : STEROIDS OF LOWER POLARITY (FIG. 12)
R_S values (S = corticosterone) on *chromatoplates* (thin layer chromatography)

		I	II	III	IV	V
1	Estrone	1.89	21.6	2.45	8.82	2.26
2	Estradiol-17β	1.24	11.2	2.23	5.12	1.05
3	Δ^4-Androstene-3,17-dione	2.35	19.6	1.89	7.25	2.63
4	17β-Hydroxy-Δ^4-androsten-3-one	1.71	10.6	1.77	4.19	1.41
5	3α-Hydroxyandrostan-17-one	1.95	13.6	2.17	5.75	2.00
6	3α-Hydroxyetiocholan-17-one	1.74	9.6	1.94	4.50	1.67
7	Δ^4-Androstene-3,11,17-trione	2.26	11.2	1.55	4.87	2.11
8	Δ^4-Pregnene-3,20-dione	2.39	22.8	2.09	7.75	2.74
9	3β-Hydroxy-Δ^5-pregnen-20-one	1.96	12.0	2.15	3.45	1.41
10	Pregnane-3α,20α-diol	1.07	4.14	1.87	1.73	0.76
11	17α-Hydroxy-Δ^4-pregnene-3,20-dione	2.06	8.15	2.11	3.20	1.14
12	21-Hydroxy-Δ^4-pregnene-3,20-dione	2.18	9.59	1.56	2.69	1.19
14	21-Hydroxy-Δ^4-pregnane-3,11,20-trione	1.44	2.57	0.87	1.24	0.76
15	17α,21-Dihydroxy-Δ^4-pregnene-3,20-dione	1.12	2.57	1.77	1.55	0.91
16	3α,21-Dihydroxypregnane-11,20-dione	0.64	0.71	0.57	0.55	0.67
S = Corticosterone	R_f values	0.37	0.04	0.32	0.15	0.30

I CHCl₃-MeOH 95 : 5
II $CHCl_3$-Ether 80:20
III Butylacetate-MeOH 99 : 1
IV Benzene-Acetone 80 : 20
V Benzene-MeOH 90 : 10

TABLE XXIV : STEROIDS OF HIGHER POLARITY (FIG. 13)
R_S values (S = cortisol) on *chromatoplates* (thin layer chromatography)

		III	VI	VII
1	3α,21-Dihydroxypregnan-20-one	0.71	0.82	1.71
2	11β,21-Dihydroxy-Δ^4-pregnene-3,20-dione	0.82	1.15	1.12
3	17α,21-Dihydroxy-Δ^4-pregnene-3,20-dione	1.25	1.24	2.53
4	3α,21-Dihydroxypregnane-11,20-dione	0.52	1.15	0.29
5	3α,11β,21-Trihydroxypregnan-20-one	0.71	0.92	0.88
6	3α,17α,21-Trihydroxypregnan-20-one	1.17	0.99	1.94
7	11β,21-Dihydroxy-Δ^4-pregnen-18-al-3,20-dione	0.36	1.20	0.38
8	17α,21-Dihydroxy-Δ^4-pregnene-3,11,20-trione	1.03	1.27	1.10
9	17α,20α,21-Trihydroxy-Δ^4-pregnene-3,11-dione	0.31	0.91	0.24
10	17α,20β,21-Trihydroxy-Δ^4-pregnene-3,11-dione	0.27	0.85	0.14
11	3α,17α,21-Trihydroxypregnane-11,20-dione	0.85	0.91	0.62
12	3α,11β,17α,21-Tetrahydroxyallopregnan-20-one	0.98	0.68	1.05
13	3α,11β,17α,21-Tetrahydroxypregnan-20-one	0.85	0.61	0.76
S = Cortisol	R_f values	0.48	0.42	0.19

III Butylacetate-MeOH 99 : 1 VI $CHCl_3$-MeOH 90 : 10 VII Ether-MeOH 99 : 1

VI. REFERENCES

[1] AXELROD, L. R., *Recent Progr. Hormone Res.* **9**, 69–89 (1954); *J. Biol. Chem.* **201**, 59–69 (1953).

[1a] BARBIER, M., JÄGER, H., TOBIAS, H. and WYSS, E., *Helv. Chim. Acta* **42**, 2440–2446 (1959).

[1b] BARR, T., HEILBRON, I. M., PARRY, E. G. and SPRING, F. S., *J. Chem. Soc.* 1437 (1936).

[2] BARTON, G. M., EVANS, R. S. and GARDNER, J. A. F., *Nature, Lond.* **170**, 249 (1952).

[3] BLOCH, H. S., ZIMMERMANN, B. and COHEN, S. L., *J. Clin. Endocrin. and Metab.* **13**, 1206–1212 (1953).

[4] BLOCK, R. J., DURRUM, E. L. and ZWEIG, G., *A manual of paper chromatography and paper electrophoresis* (2nd Ed.) Academic Press (1958).

[5] BREUER, H. and NOCKE, L., *Acta Endocr.* **29**, 489–498 (1958).

[5a] BREUER, H., KNUPPEN, R. and PANGELS, G., *Hoppe-Seyl. Z.* **317**, 248–256 (1959).

[6] BUSH, I. E., *Biochem. J.* **50**, 370–378 (1952).

[7] BUSH, I. E., *Recent Progr. Hormone Res.* **9**, 321–335 (1954); *Brit. Med. Bull.* **10**, 229–236 (1954).

[8] BUSH, I. E., *Biochem. J.* **67**, 23P (1957).

[8a] BUSH, I. E. and MAHESH, V. B., *Biochem. J.* **71**, 705–717; 718–742 (1959).

[8b] BUSH, I. E., KLYNE, W. and SHORT, R. V., *J. Endocrin.* **20**, i–ii (1960).

[9] CHEN, P. S., SCHEDL, H. P., ROSENFELD, G. and BARTTER, F. C., *Proc. Soc. Exp. Biol. Med.* **97**, 683–685 (1958), this solvent system was developed originally by Ralph E. Peterson.

[10] CRAMER, F., *Paperchromatography* (4th Ed.) Verlag Chemie, Weinheim (1958).

[11] DAO, TH. L., *Endocrinology* **61**, 242–255 (1957).

[12] DECOURCEY, C., *J. Endocrin.* **14**, 164–170 (1956).

[13] DEMOLE, E., *J. Chromatogr.* **1**, 24–34 (1958).

[14] EBERLEIN, W. R. and BONGIOVANNI, A. M., *Arch. Biochem. Biophys.* **59**, 90–96 (1955).

[15] FLORINI, J. R. and BUYSKE, D. A., *Arch. Biochem. Biophys.* **79**, 8–12 (1959).

[16] GÖBEL, P., HENI, F. and D'ADDABBO, A., *Hoppe-Seyl. Z.* **311**, 201–212 (1958).

[17] GRAY, C. H., GREEN, M. A. S., HOLNESS, N. J. and LUNNON, J. B., *J. Endocrin.* **14**, 146–154 (1956).

[18] HUBENER, H. J., FUKUSHIMA, D. K. and GALLAGHER, T. F., *J. Biol. Chem.* **220**, 501–511 (1956).

[18a] KABASAKALIAN, P. and BASCH, A., *Analyt. Chem.* **32**, 458–460 (1960).

[19] LAYNE, D. S. and MARRIAN, G. F., *Biochem. J.* **70**, 244–248 (1958).

[20] LEWBART, M. L. and SCHNEIDER, J. J., *Nature, Lond.* **176**, 1175 (1955).

[21] MARRIAN, G. F., *Proc. IVth Internat. Congress of Biochemistry* Vol. 4, pp. 208–222. Pergamon (1959).

[22] MATTOX, V. R. and LEWBART, M. L., *Arch. Biochem. Biophys.* **76**, 362–366 (1958).

[23] MITCHELL, F. L. and DAVIES, R. E., *Biochem. J.* **56**, 690–698 (1954).

[24] NEHER, R., *J. Chromatogr.* **1**, 205–258 (1958) (in German); in M. LEDERER, *Chromatographic Reviews* Vol. 1, 99–192. Elsevier (1959) (in English).

[24a] NEHER, R., MEYSTRE, CH. and WETTSTEIN, A., *Helv. Chim. Acta* **42**, 132–152 (1959).

[24b] NEHER, R. and WETTSTEIN, A., *Helv. Chim. Acta* **43** 1171–1191 (1960).

[24c] NEHER, R. and WETTSTEIN, A., *Helv. Chim. Acta* **43**, 1628–1639 (1960).

[25] OKADA, M., FUKUSHIMA, D. K. and GALLAGHER, T. F., *J. Biol. Chem.* **234**, 1688–1692 (1959).

[26] PELZER, H., *Hoppe-Seyl. Z.* **314**, 234–239 (1959).

[27] PELZER, H., STAIB, W. and OTT., D., *Hoppe-Seyl. Z.* **312**, 15–21 (1958).

[28] PUCK, A., *Klin. Wochschr.* **33**, 865–867 (1955).

[29] REINEKE, L. M., *Analyt. Chem.* **28**, 1853–1858 (1956).

[30] SAVARD, K., *Recent Progr. Hormone Res.* **9**, 185–208 (1954).

[31] SCHNEIDER, J. J. and LEWBART, M. L., *J. Biol. Chem.* **222**, 787–794 (1956).

[31a] SCHNEIDER, J. J. and LEWBART, M. L., *Recent Progr. Hormone Res.* **15**, 201–225 (1959).

[32] SIBLIKOVA, O., in HAIS, I. M. and MACEK, K., *Handbuch der Papierchromatographie* Vol. 1, 342–385; G. Fischer, Jena (1958).

[32a] SMITH, L. L. and FOELL, T., *J. Chromatogr.* **3**, 321–388 (1960).

[32b] SMITH, L. L., FOELL, T., MAIO, R. DE and HALWEN, M., *J. Amer. Pharm. Ass.* (Sc. Ed.) **48**, 528–532 (1959).

[33] STAHL, E., *Chemikerztg* **82**, 323–329 (1958).

[34] STRUCK, H., *Naturwissenschaften*, **45**, 41–42 (1958).

[35] ULICK, ST. and LIEBERMAN, S., *J. Amer. Chem. Soc.* **79**, 6567–6568 (1957).

[35a] VAN DAM, M. J. D., DE KLEUVER, G. J. and DE HEUS, J. G., *J. Chromatogr.* **4**, 26–33 (1960).

[36] ZAFFARONI, A., *Recent Progr. Hormone Res.* **8**, 51–83 (1953).

[37] ZAFFARONI, A., RINGOLD, H. J., ROSENKRANZ, G., SONDHEIMER, F., THOMAS, G. H. and DJERASSI, C., *J. Amer. Chem. Soc.* **80**, 6110–6114 (1958).

[38] NEHER, R., *Steroid Chromatography*, Elsevier (1963).

ULTRAVIOLET ABSORPTION

JOHN P. DUSZA, MILTON HELLER AND SEYMOUR BERNSTEIN

From the Organic Chemical Research Section, Lederle Laboratories, a Division of American Cyanamid Co., Pearl River, N.Y.

I. INTRODUCTION AND SCOPE

THE application of ultraviolet absorption spectroscopy in the field of steroid chemistry and biochemistry has been extensive and its utility has been well established.

Dannenberg in 1939[93] wrote the first comprehensive review on the correlation of structure of steroids with their ultraviolet absorption properties. Subsequently a large number of publications have appeared which deal with structural correlations and methods for calculating the absorption band for certain chromophores (*inter alios*: Koch,[241] Turner and Voitle,[410] Woodward,[440–442] Fieser and Fieser[148] and Dorfman[116]).

The Dorfman review[116] which appeared in 1953 is an outstanding and comprehensive contribution, and covered steroids generally through 1951 with a few selected references in 1952. In the present review the literature has been surveyed from 1952 through 1959. However, in the latter year, only the " principal " journals have been covered. Moreover, this survey has been restricted to include only steroid hormones and related compounds. It does not include sterols, bile acids, sapogenins, butenolides and the like. Where necessary for the sake of completion some of the Dorfman data on such compounds as, e.g., testosterone, have been included in the present survey.

II. TECHNIQUE

The types of instrumentation used most commonly at the present time for ultraviolet absorption spectroscopy are based upon the absorption of specific radiation by a medium (in this case *usually* the steroid in solution) which is interposed between a source of continuous radiation and a spectroscope. The modern photo-electric spectrophotometer incorporates a device for reading intensities directly so that a monochromator is incorporated to isolate rays of a selected, very narrow, wave length range. In this way a complete absorption curve may be mapped out by taking successive intensity readings at different wave length settings until the whole range is covered. The modern photo-electric instruments, which are easy and rapid to use, are claimed to be accurate to within ± 0.2 per cent[160] (in terms of intensities).

Both the *Beckman DU quartz spectrophotometer* and the *Unicam photo-electric quartz spectrophotometer SP* 500 are now the most popular of this type. It is not possible to distinguish any difference in capabilities of these two instruments, the main difference being the use of the Beckman instrument in America, and the use of the Unicam instrument in Europe. The use of the quartz optics in air restricts the use of either instrument below 200 mμ, although some attempts have been made with the Unicam instrument to determine intensities in this range. In either case, concentration of 10–20 μg steroid/ml are necessary for most accurate determinations for the stronger types of absorption (α,β-unsaturated ketones, etc.). For accurate determinations of aromatic types of absorption concentrations of ten to a hundred times that mentioned above are necessary.

The most common solvents used in the steroid field as shown in the tables are methanol, ethanol, ether and chloroform.

More recently, the commercial introduction of a continuously recording spectrophotometer — the *Cary Recording Spectrophotometer* (Model 11MS or Model 14M) — has enabled the user to observe a complete absorption curve in a very rapid time interval. This is done by allowing the output from the radiation receiver, a photomultiplier tube, to activate a pen-and-ink recorder. There is a possibility in this case of some small lag in the instrument, and also more difficulty in interpreting the exact reading due to the spacing of the lines on the recording paper and the thickness of the tracing of the spectrum so that readings of the wave length and intensity may not be quite so precise as in the instruments mentioned above. In general, almost all the absorption values recorded in the tables have been taken with one of these three instruments. Since even the authors very often no longer mention the particular type of instrument used, it would be of no value to attempt any distinction of these instruments. They all meet a very high demand of accuracy.

III. STRUCTURAL CORRELATIONS

1. Scope

The cited review article by Dorfman[116] contains an extensive treatment of the structural correlations of steroids with their ultraviolet absorption properties. As stated, the present review has been restricted to the compilation of the absorption properties of steroid hormones and related compounds from 1952 through 1959. As a consequence of this narrowing of the scope and the lack of additional data it was found that in a few cases little of significance could be added to the already established correlations. However, we wish to present and review here a number of structural correlations with steroids containing certain chromophores which we feel will be of principal interest to the steroid hormone chemists and biochemists.

2. Ultraviolet Absorption of Steroids Containing Isolated Double Bonds*

An isolated double bond shows selective absorption in the ultraviolet between 160–206 mμ with a strong maximum (ε *ca.* 3,980–12,600). Also the position and intensity of maximal absorption is dependent on the degree of substitution of the double bond, increasing substitution resulting in bathochromic shifts to longer wave lengths. These measurements below 200 mμ were obtained by vacuum spectroscopic techniques which unfortunately do not lend themselves readily to the routine procedure desired by steroid investigators.

Bladon *et al.* found that with a quartz spectrophotometer (Unicam SP 500) and a hydrogen light source absorption values down to about 205 mμ may be obtained. The solvents employed were cyclohexane, absolute and 95 per cent ethanol. Ethanol

* The discussion in this section is based principally on the publications of Bladon, P., Henbest, H. B. and Wood, G. W., *J. Chem. Soc.* 2737 (1952); Stich, K., Rotzler, G. and Reichstein, T., ref. 562, and Ellington, P. S. and Meakins, G. D., *J. Chem. Soc.* 697 (1960). The Swiss reference contains an extensive bibliography on double bond spectroscopy.

was preferred due to the increased solubilities of steroids in this solvent. It is important to note that in this work the maxima observed for the double bonds concerned were only " apparent maxima " and were not located at the true positions. This is ascribable to false energy (scattered light) which causes decreases in absorption intensities in the shorter wave lengths. It was established that by this technique the presence of a double bond in a steroid molecule could be detected. Also it was concluded that the absorption due to a steroid double bond appears to be dependent on (1) the degree of substitution, (2) whether it is in an exocyclic position, (3) the absorption of (potential) adjacent olefinic centers, and (4) the influence of neighboring substituents or groups.

With the current development of recording spectrophotometers steroid double bond spectroscopy will probably become a routine procedure and its usefulness fully exploited. Stich *et al.* have reported on a study of the absorption properties of 44 compounds (34 steroids are included) employing the Beckman recording spectrophotometer model DK 2 with a hydrogen light source. The analyses were carried out in a nitrogen atmosphere and the solvents employed were cyclohexane (absorption possible down to about 190 mμ) and alcohol (absorption possible down to about 195 mμ). Also the observed maxima and extinction coefficients were corrected for scattered light. Some of the Reichstein data are recorded in the tables of data.

More recently Ellington and Meakins examined 47 steroids and triterpenoids containing an isolated double bond in the region 192–250 mμ. The instrument employed was the Cary recording spectrophotometer model 14 M, and the determinations were carried out in a nitrogen atmosphere. Generally their findings were in agreement with those of the Reichstein group. With one exception these compounds in alcohol solution showed selective absorption between 193–205 mμ. These bands, it was concluded, are true absorption maxima and are not due to instrumental factors.

Ellington and Meakins concluded that structural diagnosis by this method requires examination of band widths and intensities as well as the wave length of maximal absorption. In some cases the type of double bond present may be determined but in others a clear distinction between two or more possibilities is not possible. Their results are summarized in Table I.

As pointed out by Henbest *et al.* and Reichstein *et al.*, Ellington and Meakins also found that the degree of substitution is not the only factor influencing double bond absorption. This is shown by a comparison of Δ^4- and Δ^5-steroids and Δ^{12}-triterpenes which give fairly consistent absorption bands for exocyclic trisubstituted double bonds with the formally similar Δ^7-steroids which have much broader bands with lower $\varepsilon_{\overline{max}}$ and higher ε_{210} values. It is also shown that the proximity of certain substituents to a double bond can also cause marked changes. For example, the allylic acetoxyl group in 3β-acetoxy-4-cholestene leads to an unusually high extinction value, λ_{max} 197 mμ (ε12,400), in contrast to the normal values for the free steroid 4-cholesten-3β-ol, λ_{max} 197 mμ (9000). Although no compound with only a 1,2-disubstituted-*trans*-double bond center was studied, the results with 4 compounds containing such a double bond show that such a grouping has a λ_{max} ~ 196 mμ, ε_{max} ~6000.

Unfortunately the Ellington–Meakins publication appeared too late for inclusion of their compound data in the tables of data.

TABLE I. DOUBLE BOND ABSORPTIONS IN ALCOHOL SOLUTIONS
(According to Ellington and Meakins, *loc. cit.*)

Type of Double Bond	λ_{max}(mμ)	$\Delta\lambda_{\frac{1}{2}}$ [a]	ε_{max}	ε_{210} [b]
—HC=CH— (*cis*)	<196	12–18	6200– 7500	200– 1900
CH_2=C<	195–196	20–22	8700– 9300	2200– 2500
—HC=C< (exocyclic)	195–196	18–25	8100– 9700	1400– 3200
Δ^7 steroids	196–197	32–34	5700– 7500	4300– 4700
>C=C<(not exocyclic)	196–198	24–30	7300– 9000	3400– 4700
>C=C< (doubly exocyclic)	204	29–30	11,300–12,200	10,000–10,700

[a] $\Delta\lambda_{\frac{1}{2}}$ is a measure of the band width and is defined as twice the difference between λ_{max} and the wave length (on the higher wave length side of the band) at which $\varepsilon = \frac{1}{2}\varepsilon_{max}$.
[b] The ε_{210} values appear to be as useful as the ε_{max} values in distinguishing between different types of double bonds. While ε_{210} values are generally in line with those of the corresponding ε_{max} change in band shape (as in the Δ^7-steroids) can upset this relationship.

3. Ultraviolet Absorption of Conjugated Dienes and Polyene Steroids

Two double bonds in conjugation with each other constitute a chromophore whose principal absorption band has shifted 30–40 mμ toward longer wave lengths (bathochromic effect) and whose extinction coefficient has increased (hyperchromic effect) compared to that of an isolated double bond. Linearly conjugated steroid trienes and tetraenes can be viewed as dienes in which the additional double bonds extend the conjugation. Each additional double bond results in a bathochromic shift of *ca.* 30 mμ.

Annular dienic steroids may be classified according to the relative locations of the double bonds; homoannular (located in same ring) and heteroannular (distributed between two adjoining rings).

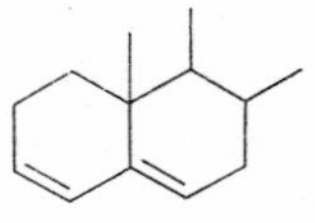

Heteroannular diene
Transoid

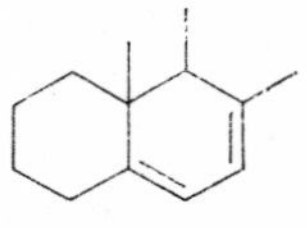

Homoannular diene
Cisoid

The homoannular (*cisoid*) dienes generally possess an absorption band between 260–285 mμ with a ε_{max} of 5000–15,000; whereas the heteroannular (*transoid*) dienes absorb at 220–250 mμ with a ε_{max} 14,000–28,000. It is to be noted that the ε_{max} of the latter (*transoid* dienes) are higher than those of the *cisoid* dienes.*

Dorfman[116] has noted that many dienes exhibit three absorption bands with one on each side of the principal band and almost equidistant from it. The band at the longest wave length has the lowest extinction coefficient. The two secondary bands are approximately −7 and +8 mμ away from the principal band in the case of the heteroannular dienes, −10 and +12 mμ apart for the homoannular dienes, and −13 and +15 mμ apart in the trienes.

The dienic and polyenic chromophores are listed in the following tables.

* In this connection, see MULLIKEN, R. S., *J. Chem. Phys.* **7**, 121 (1939); *Rev. Modern Phys.* **14**, 265 (1942); and KOCH, H. P., *Chem. & Ind.* **61**, 273 (1942).

TABLE II. ULTRAVIOLET ABSORPTION OF CONJUGATED STEROID DIENES

Chromophore	Range		Comments
	λ_{max}(mμ)	ε_{max}	
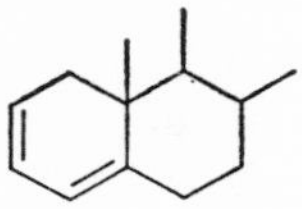 $\Delta^{2,4}$	~ 266 275 ~ 287	6300–15,000 6300–20,000 13,500	Ref. 116
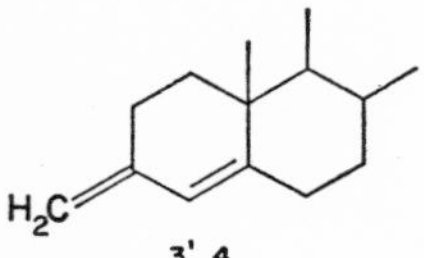 $\Delta^{3',4}$	233 239	16,200 17,300	Ref. 116 and present work
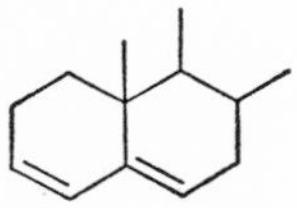 $\Delta^{3,5}$	226–228 233–235 241–243	16,500–20,900 17,100–21,900 12,000–14,500	Ref. 116 and present work. A 11-carbonyl group exerts *ca.* a 2 mμ hypsochromic effect.
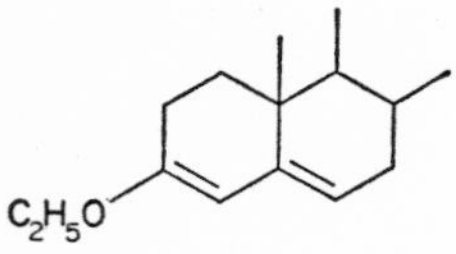	240–242	12,600–23,450	Ref. 116 and present work. A 11-carbonyl group appears not to exert a hypsochromic effect on this chromophore. A 6-methyl group exerts *ca.* a 6 mμ bathochromic effect, i.e., λ_{max} 247 mμ. A 6-chlorine atom exerts *ca.* a 10 mμ bathochromic effect.
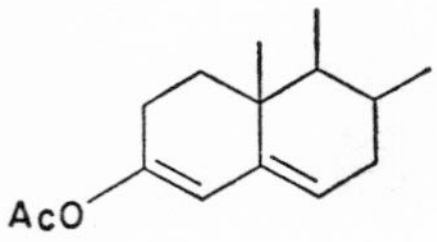	234–236	15,900–21,000	A 6-methyl group exerts *ca.* a 8–10 mμ bathochromic effect. A 6-cyano group exerts *ca.* a 28 mμ bathochromic effect.
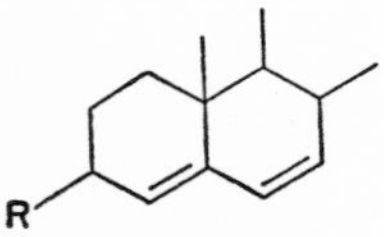 $\Delta^{4,6}$ (R = OH, CH_3COO)	232 238–240 248	17,800–24,000 20,100–28,200 12,700–19,500	Ref. 116

TABLE II (*continued*)

Chromophore	Range		Comments
	λ_{max}(mμ)	ε_{max}	
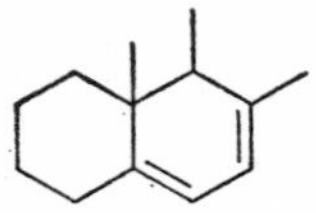 $\Delta^{5,7}$	262(*i*) 270–273 280–283 292–296	7400–8000 9500–15,500 10,000–15,900 5700–9780	Ref. 116 and present work (13 examples)
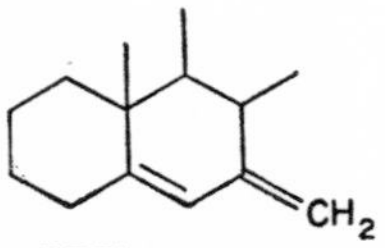 $\Delta^{5,7(7')}$	236 237(I)	20,000 22,400	Ref. 116 1 example in present work
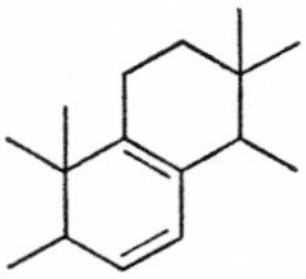 $\Delta^{6,8(9)}$	275	4700–5300	Ref. 116
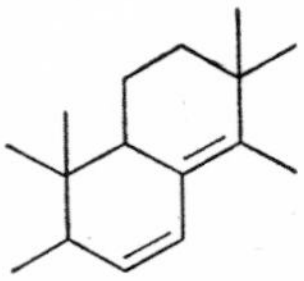 $\Delta^{6,8(14)}$	252–253	17,000–21,800	Ref. 116 and HUNZIKER, F. *et al.*, *Helv. Chim. Acta* **38**, 1316 (1955)
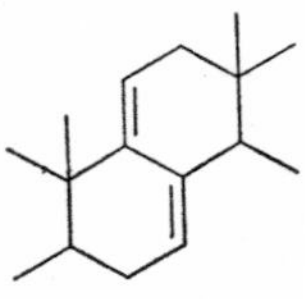 $\Delta^{7,9(11)}$	234–236 242–245 250–252	10,000–15,900 10,700–17,400 9000–12,600	Ref. 116 See ZÜRCHER, A. *et al.*, *Helv. Chim. Acta* **37**, 1562 (1954): 6β-hydroxy: 246 mμ (ε14,800) 6β-acetoxy: 246 mμ (ε18,600) 6β-ethoxy: 246 mμ (ε15,100) 5α-hydroxy: 244 mμ (ε16,600)
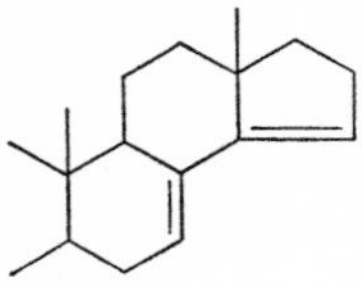 $\Delta^{7,14}$	242–250	9900–15,000	Ref. 116

TABLE II (*continued*)

Chromophore	Range		Comments
	λ_{max}(mμ)	ε_{max}	
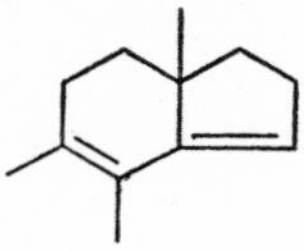 $\Delta^{8,14}$	245–250	16,100–21,500	Ref. 116 and present work (3 examples)
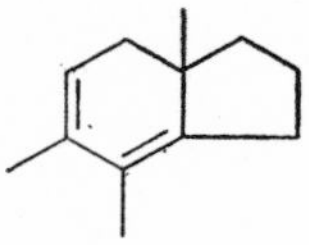 $\Delta^{8(14),9(11)}$	271	4600	Correlation based on 1 example in present work
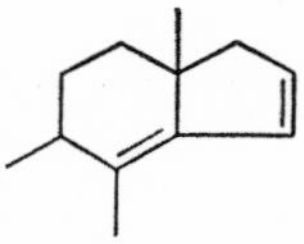 $\Delta^{8(14),15}$	247	2500	Correlation based on 1 example in present work
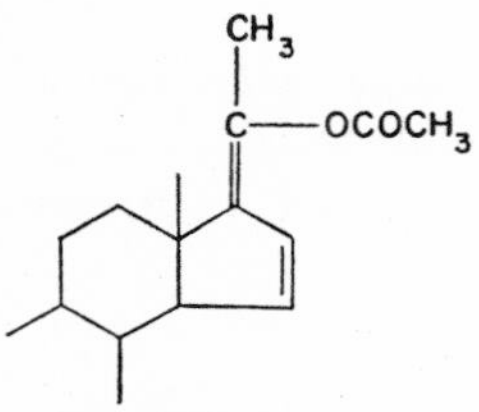 $\Delta^{15,17(20)}$	242	13,700	Correlation based on 1 example in present work
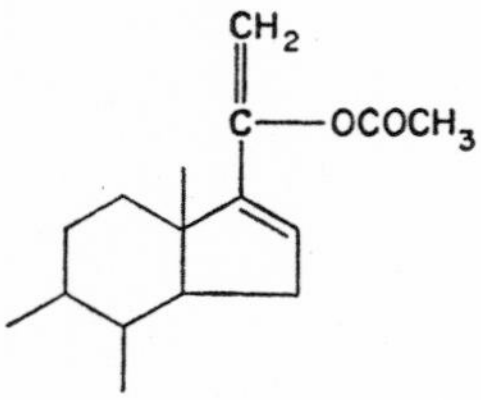 $\Delta^{16,20}$	238	14,100–15,900	Ref. 116 and present work (5 examples)
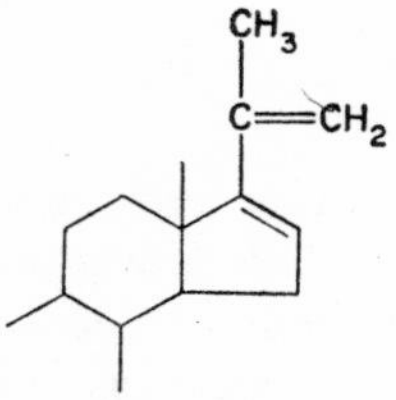 $\Delta^{16,20(22)}$	239 (inflection)	16,200	Correlation based on 1 example in present work

TABLE III. ULTRAVIOLET ABSORPTION OF CONJUGATED STEROID TRIENES

Chromophore	Range		Comments
	λ_{max}(mμ)	ε_{max}	
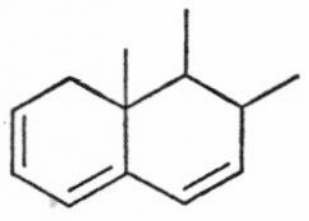 $\Delta^{2,4,6}$	296 304–307 320	12,600–16,600	Ref. 116
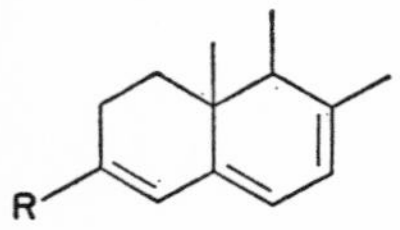 $\Delta^{3,5,7}$ (R=H, CH_3COO)	301–305 314–317 320–332	12,500–20,000 15,700–23,400 11,100–17,400	Ref. 116
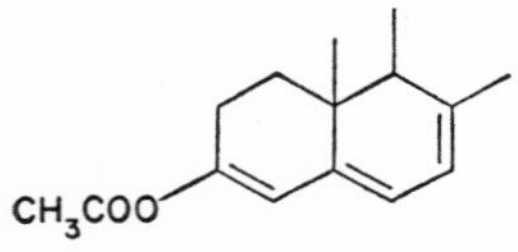	300–302 313–314 327.5–329	18,000–18,200 22,000–22,350 15,500–16,200	Values according to present work (2 examples, including 1–19 nor-compound)
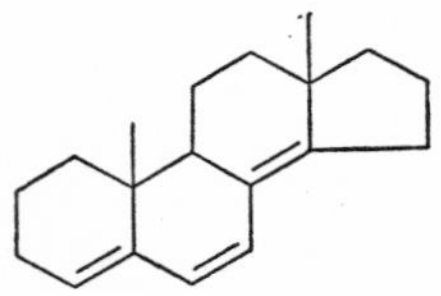 $\Delta^{4,6,8(14)}$	283	33,000	Ref. 116
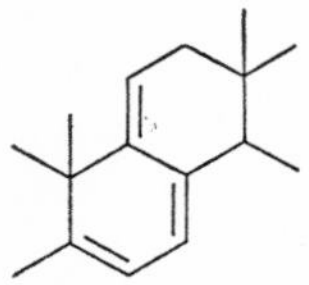 $\Delta^{5,7,9(11)}$	310–313 322–325 338–340	8100–11,600 9200–14,500 5800–8200	Ref. 116 and present work (6 examples). Sometimes secondary bands appear as inflections.

TABLE III (*continued*)

Chromophore	Range		Comments
	$\lambda_{max}(m\mu)$	ε_{max}	
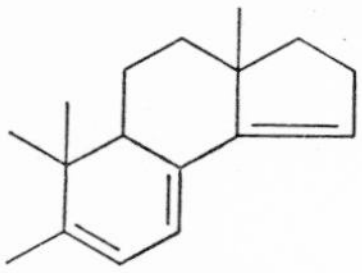 $\Delta^{5,7,14}$	319	15,000–17,500	Ref. 116
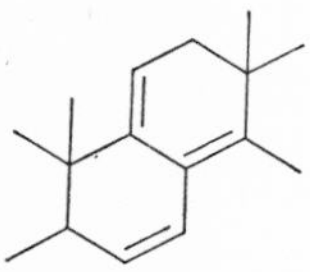 $\Delta^{6,8(14),9(11)}$	~ 243 285	~ 12,100 9100	Ref. 116
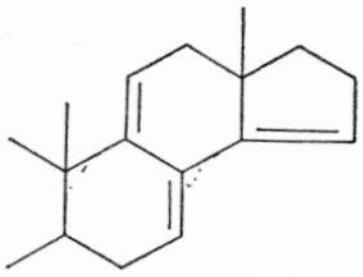 $\Delta^{7,9(11),14}$	227 235 268	11,000 9300 9100	See LAUBACH, G. D. *et al.*, *J. Amer. Chem. Soc.* **78**, 4743 (1956).

TABLE IV. ULTRAVIOLET ABSORPTION OF CONJUGATED STEROID TETRAENES

Chromophore	Range		Comments
	$\lambda_{max}(m\mu)$	ε_{max}	
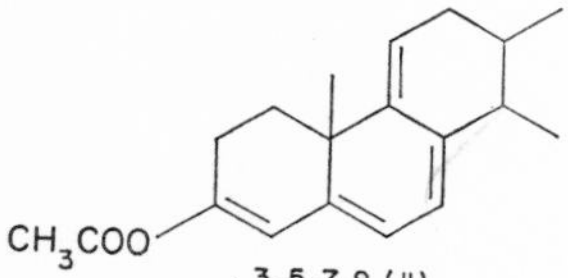 $\Delta^{3,5,7,9(11)}$	336–339 354–356 372–375	15,000–17,800 17,400–21,900 13,000–16,200	Ref. 116
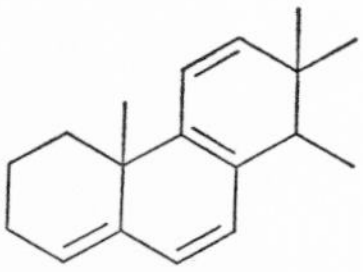 $\Delta^{4,6,8(9),11}$	355	13,500	Ref. 116

TABLE IVA

Chromophore	Range		Comments
	$\lambda_{max}(m\mu)$	ε_{max}	
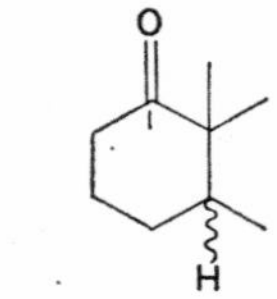	292–298	25–50	
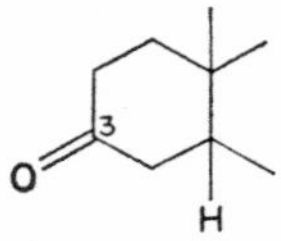	275–285	17–155	This overlaps the range reported by Dorfman
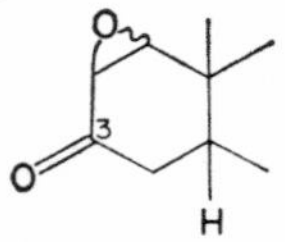	295–300	21–23	2 examples
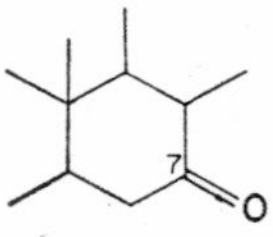	288	26	1 example
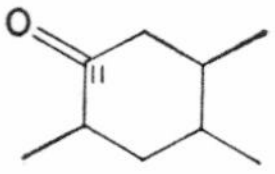	288–298	32–316	Same comment as for 3-ketones
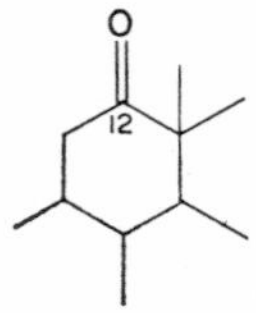	285–298	46–160	Same comment as for 3-ketones
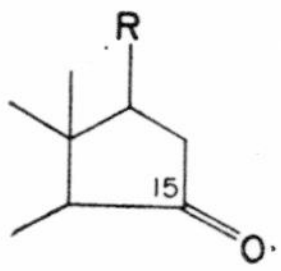	285–295	25	
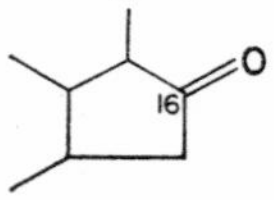	280	50	1 example

TABLE IVA (*continued*)

Chromophore	Range		Comments
	λ_{max}(mμ)	ε_{max}	
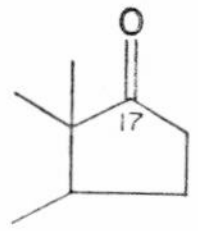	292–294	40–50	Same comment as for 3-ketones
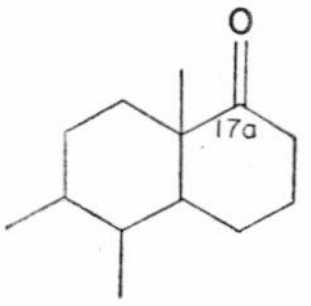	290–292	32–40	
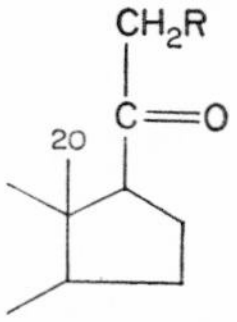	270–295	32–80	Same comment as for 3-ketones

4. Ultraviolet Absorption of Steroids Containing Isolated Carbonyl Groups

It is well known that the isolated carbonyl group has an intense ultraviolet absorption at 170–210 mμ.[562] However, except for the case of specialized equipment used by Stich *et al.*, [562] the ordinary spectrophotometers have a limited value in this area. An investigation by Bird *et al.** using a Unicam S.P. 500 spectrophotometer showed that these end-absorption intensities vary within a wide range from ε200–3500 at 205 mμ and from ε80–2400 at 210 mμ for a large number of steroids. These absorptions overlap the end absorptions of isolated double bonds, of course, and caution must be exercised.

It is, moreover, emphasized in this paper that due to deviations from Beer's law, sensitivity of the particular instrument used and other inherent difficulties, this region is not yet too useful. Ellington and Meakins (*loc. cit.*) have indicated similar results may be obtained with the use of a Cary spectrophotometer (model 14 M).

The absorptions of simple ketones listed in this report have to do with the bond at approximately 280 mμ which is also well defined, but unfortunately of much less intensity. It may be noticed in Table IVA that isolated carbonyl groups show the same type of absorption peaks (270–300 mμ) of low intensity (ε16–316). It is difficult in view of the small number of examples to verify Dorfman's suggestion[116] that an ethylene bond in the vicinity of the carbonyl group exerts a hypsochromic effect. However, it is interesting to note the bathochromic effect of the 1,2-epoxy function on the absorption of a 3-keto group (10–15 mμ) which is in line with Dorfman's comment of the bathochromic effect of an epoxy function on a carbonyl group.

* BIRD, C. W., NORYMBERSKI, J. K. and WOODS, G. F., *J. Chem. Soc.* 4149 (1957).

TABLE V

Chromophore	Range		Comments
	$\lambda_{max}(m\mu)$	ε_{max}	
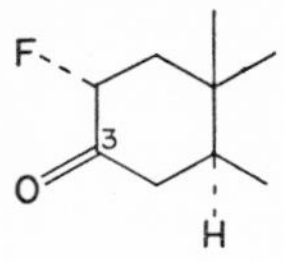	283	27–35	
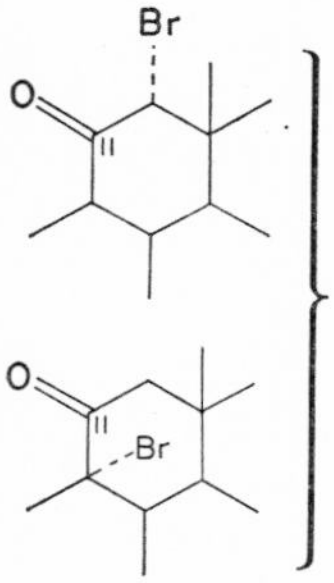	319–320	100–150	
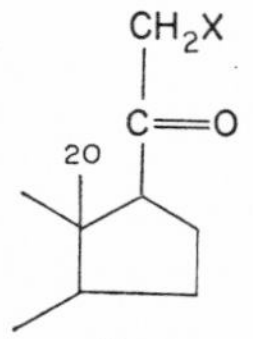 X=F, Cl	282–284	69–76	
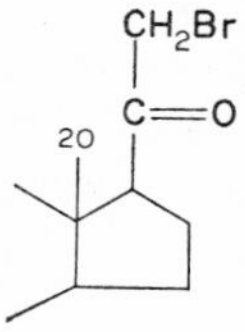	292–294	89	
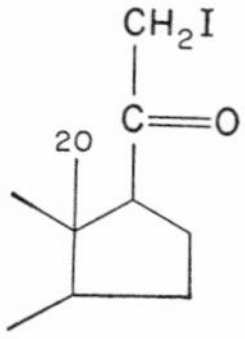	268–270	41	
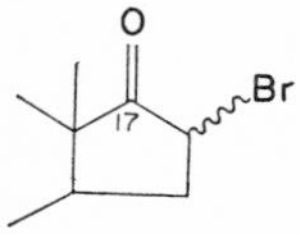	310–314	80–160	
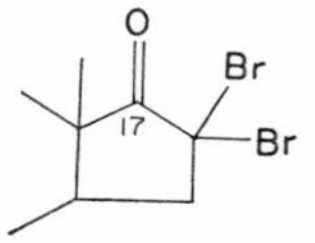	320	81	

Cookson* has shown the effect of halogen substituents alpha to a six-membered ring carbonyl function. In general, equatorial halogen substituents have very little influence while axial substituents give a bathochromic shift (*ca.* 28 mμ). This principle may be observed in Table V wherein a 2α-fluoro (equatorial)-3-one has very little effect on the 3-one absorption while a 9α- or 12α-bromo (axial)-11-one affords a bathochromic effect of *ca.* 25 mμ.

In cases in which the above steric effects are non-existent other electronic or bulk steric factors assume importance, which at the present time are not easily explained. It may be noticed that a 21-fluoro or chloro substituent *alpha* to a 20-ketone exerts little effect on the ketone absorption while a 21-bromo compound gives a considerable bathochromic effect which might be expected due to a greater overlap of π orbitals with the larger bromine atom. However, a 21-iodo substituent actually exerts a hypsochromic effect so that this sort of explanation is not useful. Again it is to be noted that a 16α- or β-(or both) bromo-17-ketone exerts a considerable bathochromic effect on the 17-ketone absorption.

5. Ultraviolet Absorption of Steroids Containing Double Bond Conjugated Carbonyl Groups

Enones

The ultraviolet absorption maximum arising from the conjugative interaction of a carbonyl grouping and a double bond has been studied at great length. This intensive investigation has shown that there exists a predictable relationship between maximal absorption and its intensity and the structure of the chromophore. As more information was gathered, subtle structural variations about the chromophore could be distinguished, thereby increasing the importance of this analytical technique. Application of ultraviolet spectroscopy in the field of steroid chemistry has been widespread and proven to be highly useful. This review concerns itself chiefly with recent developments correlating spectra and structural variations.

The chromophoric system resulting from the conjugation of a carbonyl group and a double bond (enone) is characterized by a strong absorption maximum in the range 225–265 mμ and a weak band at 300–340 mμ. The latter, arising from the displacement of the normal carbonyl maximum, is of weak intensity and is

TABLE VI. CALCULATION OF ABSORPTION MAXIMA OF ENONES

$-\overset{\overset{\displaystyle O}{\|}}{C}-\underset{\alpha}{C}=\underset{\beta}{C}-$		Wave length
Standard value		215 mμ
Increments for alkyl substituents	α	+10 mμ
	β	+12 mμ
Increment for each exocyclic double bond		+ 5 mμ

* COOKSON, R. C., *J. Chem. Soc.* 282 (1954).

seldom reported. The ranges may be broadened considerably by substituents exhibiting either hypsochromic or bathochromic effects on the enone.

There exist a wide variety of possible enone structures within the steroid ring system and most of these have been reported. All such enones may be generalized into the equivalent representation, $-\overset{\overset{\displaystyle O}{\|}}{C}-\underset{\alpha}{C}=\underset{\beta}{C}-$. Through the application of standard increments originally suggested by Woodward[440, 442] and further expanded by Fieser[148] and Dorfman,[116] an approximate value for the absorption maximum of any chromophore may be derived. For most systems this approximation can be quite precise. An abbreviated table for enone systems is summarized in Table VI.

As more compounds are studied, the number of applicable corrections is increased. This procedure can be somewhat self-defeating in this respect. As the discussion of particular chromophores is expanded substituent effects will be evaluated. A detailed discussion of the Δ^4-3-ones has been included after the general comments listed below.

TABLE VII

	Range		Comments
	λ_{max}(mμ)	ε_{max}	
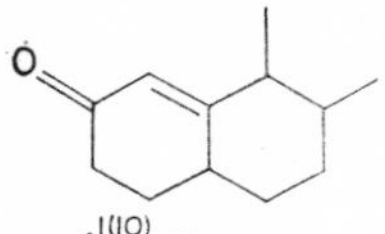 $\Delta^{1(10)}$-2-ones	240	15,900	Only one member of this class has been reported.
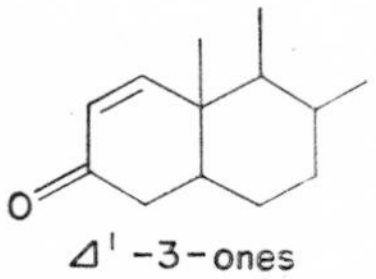 Δ^{1}-3-ones	224–233	9000–15,000	The absorption maximum of this chromophore may vary considerably and is influenced by (1) substituents on the chromophore at C-1 and C-2, (2) substituents at C-4, (3) configuration at C-5, (4) and other long-range effects in the molecule.
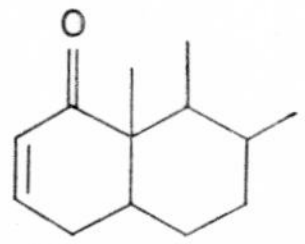 Δ^{2}-1-ones	224–226 330–340	7200–8500 47–90	A limited number of representatives of this chromophore have been reported.

TABLE VII (*continued*)

	Range		Comments
	λ_{max}(mμ)	ε_{max}	
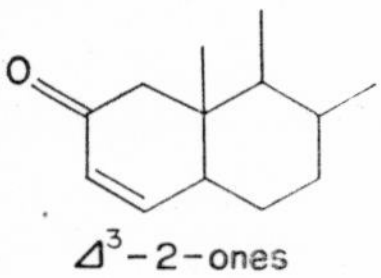 Δ^3-2-ones			No representatives for the simple chromophore are known. The 5α-hydroxylcholesterol derivative [CONCA, R. J. and BERGMANN, W., *J. Org. Chem.* **18**, 1104 (1953)] has a maximum at 223 mμ. Dorfman reports a value 238 mμ (ε7,400) for the 3-acetoxy system.
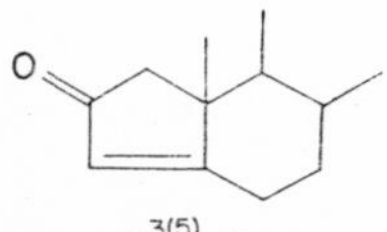 A-nor-$\Delta^{3(5)}$-2-ones	229–234	14,000–16,000	These A-nor derivatives exhibit the hypsochromic effect encountered in confining the chromophore in a five-membered ring. The absorption maximum is influenced by an oxygen function at the 11-position in the typical manner to be elaborated in the expanded discussion of the Δ^4-3-one chromophore.
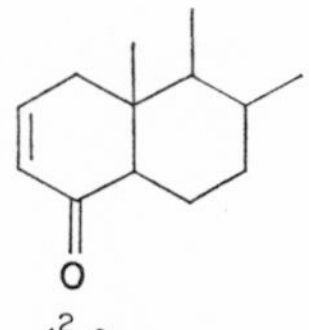 Δ^2-4-ones			No representatives of this or the 19-nor$\Delta^{5(10)}$-4-ones have been reported.
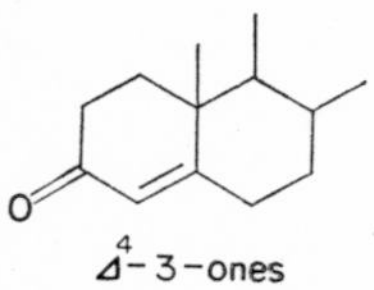 Δ^4-3-ones	232–244	10,000–20,000	Discussion of this chromophore can be found as a separate section following these general comments.

TABLE VII (*continued*)

	Range		Comments
	λ_{max}(mμ)	ε_{max}	
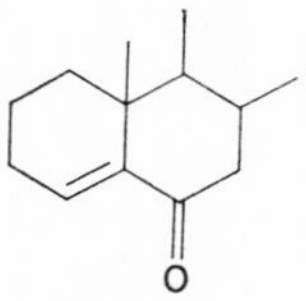 Δ^4-6-ones	236–244 300–320	6300–6400 85–120	No representatives of this system are included in the tables. Dorfman[116] reports several examples in the ranges cited.
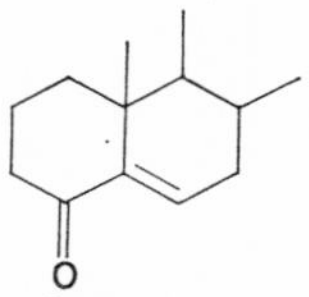 Δ^6-4-ones	240–241	3200–7200	See above.
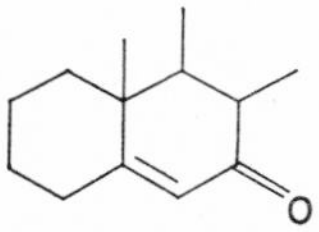 Δ^5-7-ones	235–241	11,000–13,500	Acetylation of the 3β-hydroxyl group (equatorial) produces a hypsochromic shift (−3 mμ). A limited number of examples for the chromophore are reported.
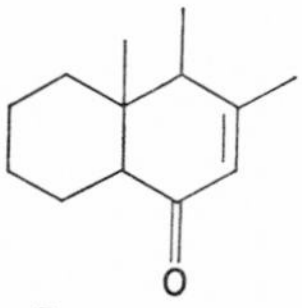 Δ^7-6-ones	241	15,800	The tables cite only two examples of this chromophore.
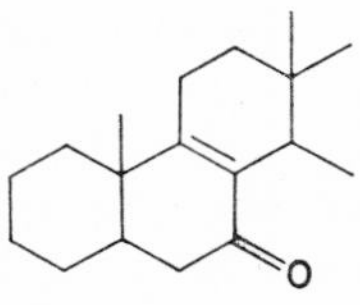 Δ^8-7-ones	252–253	7900–13,000	The maximum is shifted to 268 mμ when a carbonyl group is present at C-11.

TABLE VII (*continued*)

	Range		Comments
	λ_{max}(mμ)	ε_{max}	
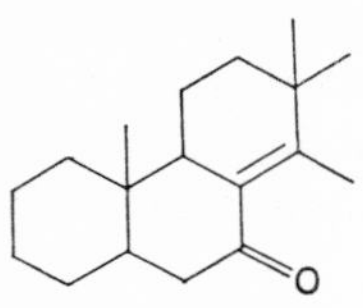 $\Delta^{8(14)}$-7-ones	260–263	7800–10,800	No representatives of this class are included in this chapter. Dorfman[116] cites four examples.
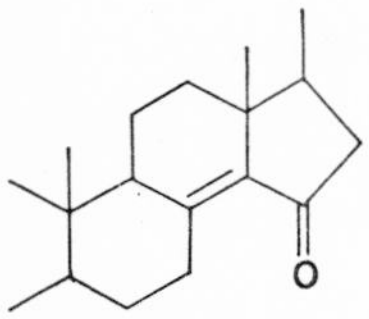 $\Delta^{8(14)}$-15-ones	259	12,700–13,300	See above.
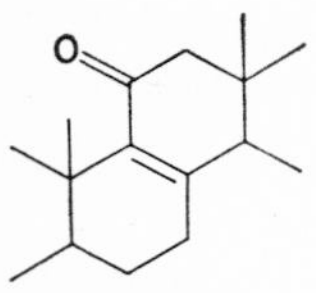 Δ^{8}-11-ones	248–256	8000–9100	The normal range for compounds with this chromophore is 252–254 mμ. A carbonyl group at C-7 produces the expected bathochromic effect (+16 to + 20 mμ).
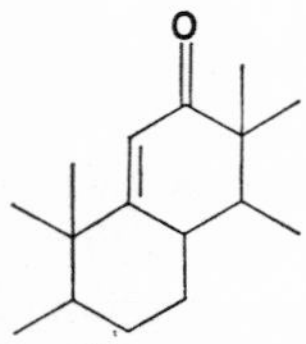 $\Delta^{9(11)}$-12-ones	238–242 320–322	12,300–16,600 70–190	A limited number of examples are included in the tables. A review of the sapogenin field would produce more examples of the system. A 7α-acetoxyl group shows a slight hypsochromic effect.
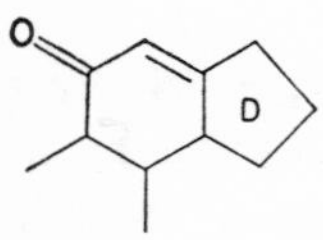 13-nor-Δ^{12}-11-ones	240	17,200	Only one compound of this system is included in the tables. Several examples of 13,17-seco steroids are known (234–239 mμ). Representative compounds where ring-D is six-membered can be found in the triterpenoid field.

TABLE VII (*continued*)

	Range		Comments
	λ_{max}(mμ)	ε_{max}	
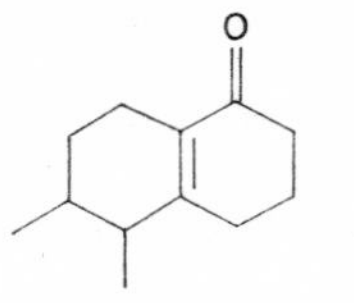 13-nor-Δ^{13}-17a-ones	246–248.5	12,600–15,600	Members of this group are encountered in papers dealing with the total synthesis of steroids.
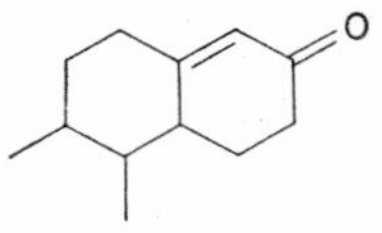 13-nor-$\Delta^{13(17a)}$-17-ones	238–244	13,000–17,000	See above.
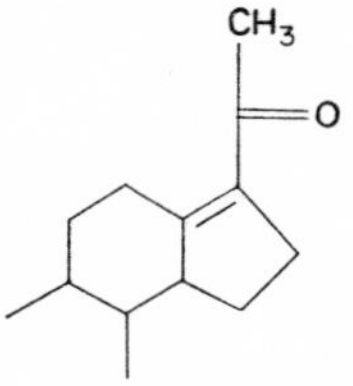 13-nor-$\Delta^{13(17)}$-20-ones	256	11,200	1 example of this system has been reported.
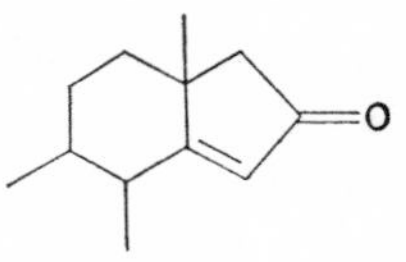 Δ^{14}-16-ones	221–249	9800–17,000	Examples of this system are in general limited to synthetic compounds involving 11 and 18 oxygenated systems.
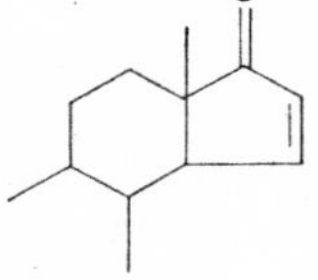 Δ^{15}-17-ones	230–233	7200–13,500	When the 14α-hydrogen is substituted by a 14β-hydroxyl group, a hypsochromic shift to 213 mμ has been observed. A 16-bromo group gives the expected large bathochromic effect (+20 mμ).

TABLE VII (*continued*)

	Range		Comments
	λ_{max}(mμ)	ε_{max}	
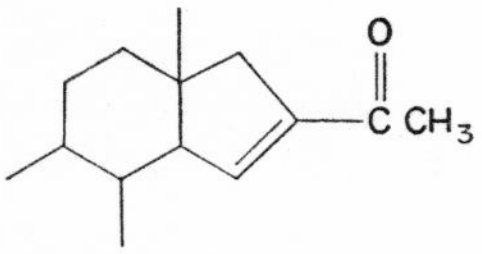 Δ^{15}-16'-ones	244	12,300	This system is limited to 1 example.
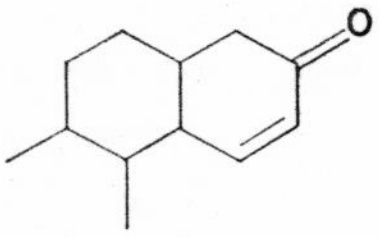 D-homo-Δ^{15}-17-ones	233–234	6000	The introduction of an acetoxyl group at C-16 shows no effect. Hydrolysis of the acetate gives rise to the α-diketone (272 mμ).
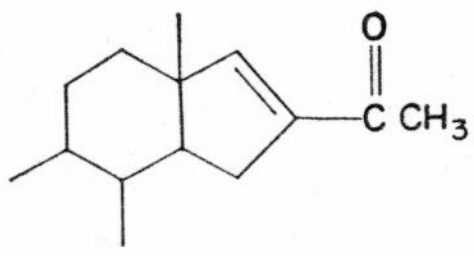 Δ^{16}-16'-ones	237–242	9800–12,300	A methyl group at C-17 gives a chromophore with a maximum at 251 mμ. An amino group at C-17 gives a compound having a peak at 314 mμ.
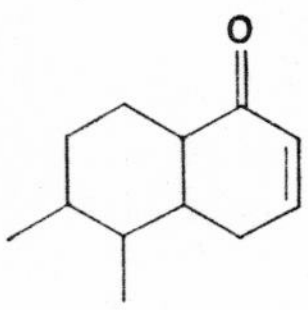 D-homo-Δ^{16}-17a-ones	224.7–225	8200–8700	Only a few examples of this chromophore have been reported.
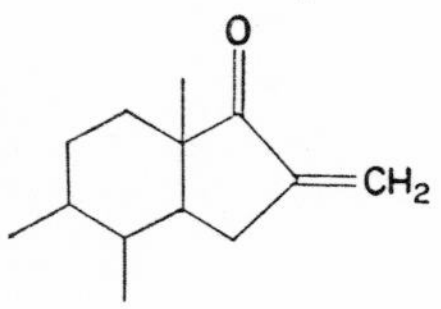 $\Delta^{16'}$-17-ones	228	8000–8800	See above.

TABLE VII (*continued*)

	Range		Comments
	λ_{max}(mμ)	ε_{max}	
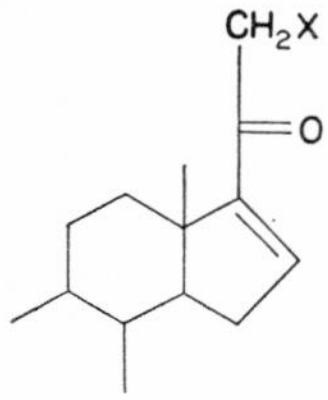 Δ^{16}-20-ones	225–250	6500–9900	A typical value for the system would be 238–240 mμ. Surrounding substituents have a pronounced effect on the chromophore. A 12-carbonyl shows a hypsochromic effect (−11 mμ). Another group showing a small hypsochromic effect is the 15β-hydroxyl. The absorption maximum of a 21-iodo group is 250 mμ. A methyl group at C-16 gives a value of 248–252 mμ to the chromophore.
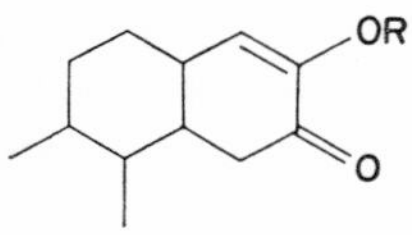 D-homo-Δ^{17}-16-ones			No representatives of the simple system are known. When the chromophore arises from the enolization of the α-diketone (R=H) the compound exhibits absorption at 277–279 mμ, the acetate 241–245 mμ (R=$COCH_3$).
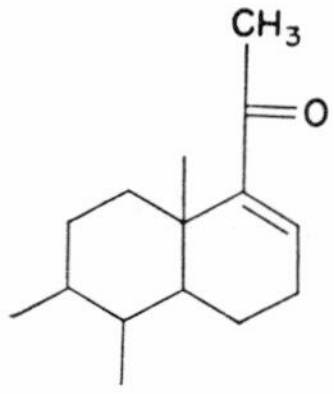 D-homo-$\Delta^{17(17a)}$-20-ones	230	10,100	Only one example of this chromophore is listed in the tables.

TABLE VII (*continued*)

	Range		Comments
	$\lambda_{max}(m\mu)$	ε_{max}	
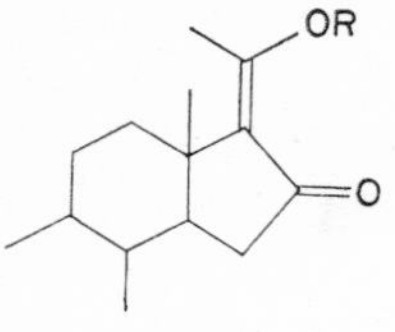 $\Delta^{17(20)}$-16-ones			Two compounds with this chromophore appear in the tables. R = isopropyl (281 mμ) and R = acetyl (246 mμ).
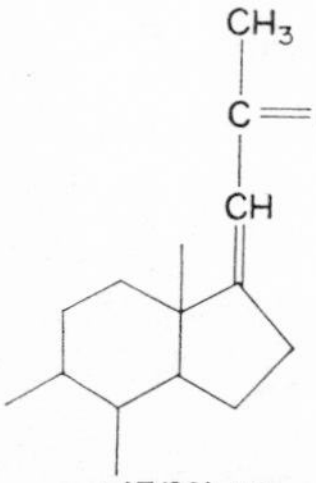 $\Delta^{17(20)}$-21-ones	242	17,800	Only one example of this chromophore is listed in the tables.

The Δ^4*-3-ones*

Comprising approximately one third of the table entries, the Δ^4-3-ones represent the single largest group of compounds studied. In addition, they provide the most variation in structure and thus lend themselves to a close study of structure–absorption correlations. The search for compounds possessing interesting physiological properties has stimulated interest in such modifications. These modifications can be broadly separated into two classes (1) those that are made on the molecule at a site removed from the chromophore and (2) those that alter the hydrogen atom distribution of the system or on immediately adjacent carbon atoms.

A representative absorption range for the Δ^4-3-ones would be difficult to define. However, the range 240–242 mμ (in alcohol), adequately describes the absorption maximum of simple systems. The calculated value for the Δ^4-3-ones is 244 mμ. A molecular extinction coefficient of 16,000 represents an approximation which is also quite variable. A second absorption maximum is noted near 310 mμ. Being of such low intensity (max ~100), this broad peak is seldom reported.

The influence exerted by substituents located on carbon atoms removed from the chromophore may result in bathochromic or hypsochromic effects on the absorption maximum of the Δ^4-3-one. The greatest number of substituents have been introduced at the 9-position replacing the 9α-hydrogen atom. Table VIII summarizes compounds in the 9α-substituted hydrocortisone and cortisone series.

The introduction of a 11β-hydroxyl group or its 11α-epimer has no influence on the absorption maximum of the Δ^4-3-ones. Oxidation to the 11-carbonyl compounds has the reported hypsochromic effect (−3 to −5 mμ) commonly used to establish the presence of a 11-oxygenated grouping. The presence of a methyl group at the 9-position may have a bathochromic effect but few examples of this

TABLE VIII

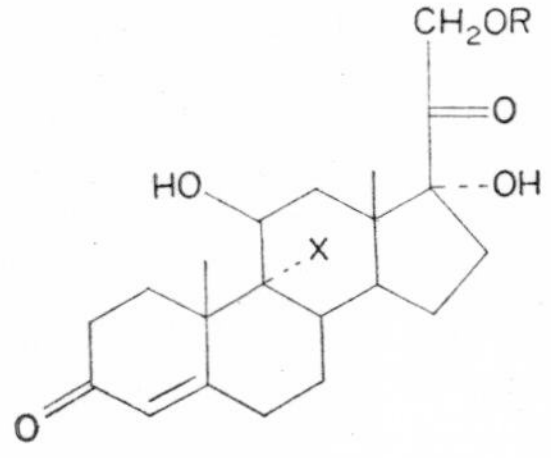

X	λ_{max}(mμ)(11-OH)	λ_{max}(mμ)(11-CO)
H	241	238
CH_3	244	—
OH	242	237
OCH_3	243	238
F	238	234
Cl	241	236
Br	243	237
I	243	—
SCN	243	238

substitution are known. The influence of the halogen atom appears to be related to its electronegativity with fluorine, the most electronegative having the greatest hypsochromic effect (−3 mμ). The bathochromic shift in proceeding from fluorine to chlorine to bromine is not confined to the series mentioned above but is observed in a number of 9α-halo series. The influence of other groups mentioned in the table cannot be properly evaluated since differences from the reference compounds are slight and represent insufficient numbers of examples to warrant detailed study.

A variety of substituents in rings C and D also influence the Δ^4-3-one chromophore by some type of long range interaction. Bathochromic effects have been observed for the 9β, 11β-epoxides (+2 to +3 mμ) and 11α-methyl compounds (+2 mμ). Hypsochromic effects are noted with a greater number of substituents such as the Δ^7, Δ^8, $\Delta^{8(14)}$, $\Delta^{9(11)}$, Δ^{11} and Δ^{14} olefins (−2 to −3 mμ). Other hypsochromic shifts of −2 to −3 mμ are observed for the 9α, 11α-epoxides, 11β, 12β-epoxides, 14α, 15α-epoxides, the 12-carbonyl derivatives and the 11β⟶18 lactone and hemiacetal groupings. Comparison of compounds in the androstane series indicates that a hypsochromic effect (−2 mμ) is associated with the transformation of a 17β-hydroxyl to a 17-carbonyl grouping in a great many cases.

Substitutions at C-1 and C-7 are not common and are restricted to a hydroxyl, acetoxyl, methyl and esterified thiol groups. Each carbon atom possesses a β-equatorial conformation, and in the acetylation of the 1β-hydroxyl, the hypsochromic effect (-2 mμ) in forming the acetate is observed. This shift takes place with the 7α-hydroxyl epimer thereby questioning its configurational assignment. A shift to longer wave length is observed for the 7β-methyl group and what may be a smaller bathochromic effect for the 7α-methyl series.

The influence of various groups at C-2 has been studied in the α-series since this represents the stable conformation at the 2-position. The 2α-equatorial hydroxyl group upon acetylation shows the expected hypsochromic effect (-2 mμ) while the epimeric 2β-hydroxyl group (axial) does not. Alkyl substituents may exhibit small bathochromic effects ($+1$ to $+2$ mμ) in studying particular series. The 2α-halo compounds do not show any dramatic effects but appear to follow the same electronegativity relationship shown at C-9. The ranges of fluorine (241–242 mμ), chlorine (242–243 mμ) and bromine (244 mμ) are based on a limited number of examples.

Replacement of the hydrogen atom at the 4-position markedly changes the Δ^4-3-one chromophore and this is shown in considering Table IX.

TABLE IX

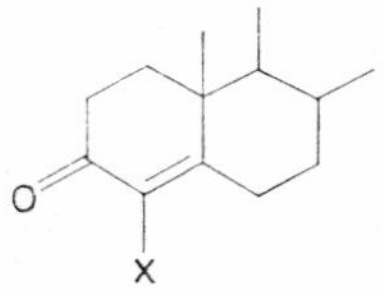

X	λ_{max}(mμ)
H	241
CH_3 (Alkyl)	249–251
C_6H_5	240–241
OH	277
$OCOCH_3$	246
F	241
Cl	254–256
Br	260–262

The addition of a 4-alkyl group imparts the predicted bathochromic effect ($+8$ to $+10$ mμ) to the chromophore associated with the addition of an "α"-substituent to an α,β-unsaturated ketone. The 4-phenyl group, showing no influence on the chromophore, must assume an orientation out-of-the-plane of the chromophore to minimize the orbital overlap. The 4-halo-substituents exhibit an influence on the chromophore which is probably related to overlap of the oxygen-halogen orbitals. The rigidity of this planar system can be contrasted to the 2α-equatorial conformation assumed by the 2-halo derivatives. The largest halogen atom studied, bromine, exhibits the strongest bathochromic effect ($+19$ to $+22$ mμ) on the chromophore. The acetylation of the 4-hydroxyl gives the large hypsochromic effect (-30 mμ) associated with enol acetylation.

A summary of the various groups introduced at the 6-position is presented in Table X. Both conformations for each substituent, except the 6-cyano, have been reported. The 6β-axial group can be isomerized to the 6α-equatorial conformation and the resulting change in the absorption maximum is quite unpredictable.

TABLE X

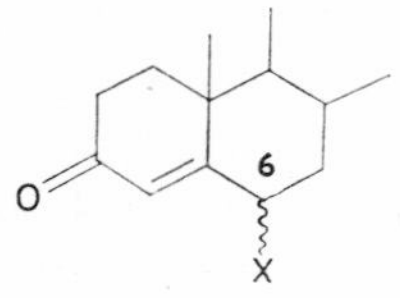

X	λ_{max}(mμ) α	β
H	241	
F	236–237	232–234
Cl	236–237	239–240
Br	236	246
OH	239–240	235–236
$OCOCH_3$	235–237	235–237
CH_3 (Alkyl)	240–242	241–242
C_6H_5	244–246	242
NO_2	232–234	234–236
CN	230; 288–290	—

Review of the 6β-substituents does not reveal any unexpected values with the possible exception of the 6β-hydroxyl and acetoxyl. Anomalous results are encountered in the epimerization to the 6α-series. The fluoro, hydroxyl and phenyl groups show a bathochromic effect, while hypsochromic effects are noted with the bromo, alkyl and nitro groups. The acetylation of the 6α-equatorial hydroxyl group gives the hypsochromic effect (-3 to -4 mμ) associated with such a transformation. An interesting situation arises with 6-cyano derivatives in that they exhibit two maxima, the one at longer wave length (288–290 mμ) being of much stronger intensity. An explanation of this may rest in consideration of the tautomeric equilibrium possible with the enolic component absorbing at the longer wave length.

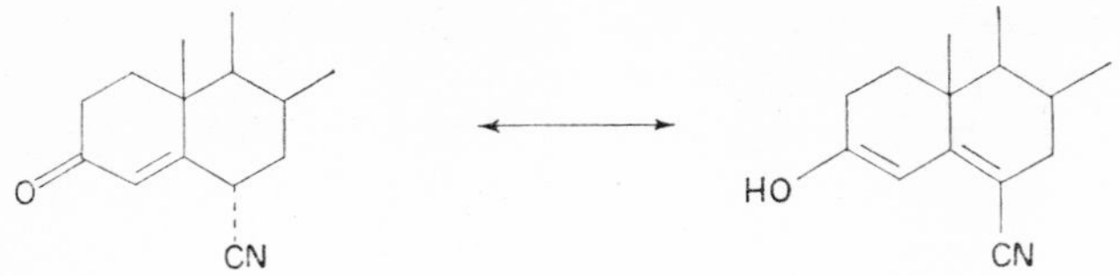

If the 6α-configuration is the more stable, and all evidence seems to indicate this in other series studied, the equilibrium precludes the isolation of the 6β-cyano-Δ^4-3-one system.

A limited number of 10-substituted steroids have been reported and for those compounds whose exact stereochemistry is known, only the 10β-conformation has been assigned. The absorption maximum of the 10β-hydroxy- and 10β-cyano-compounds are approximately the same as the 6-substituted products with the qualification that the 10β-cyano-compound displays only one peak as compared to two cited in the 6α-cyano series. The 10-cyano group cannot participate in an equivalent tautomeric system as suggested for the 6-cyano compound and thus would not be expected to exhibit the long wave length peak of the latter. Whether this observation questions the assignment of the 6α-configuration in the 6-cyano-Δ^4-3-one is difficult to determine. Other 10β-substituents include the formyl and hydroxymethyl groups. Acetylation of the latter is accompanied by a hypsochromic effect (-4 to -5 mμ) observed in previous cases. Table XI summarizes the 10β-substituents.

TABLE XI

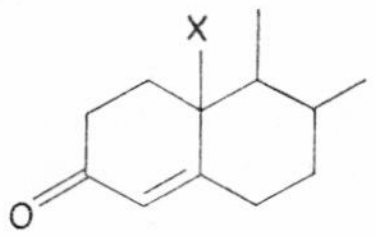

X (β-configuration)	λ_{max}(mμ)
H	241
CH_3	241
OH	234–237
CN	229–230
CHO	241–245
CH_2OH	242–243
CH_2OCOCH_3	238–239

Dienones

The coupling of a second double bond to an α,β-unsaturated ketone system may give rise to one of two generalized chromophoric systems. The added double bond may extend the conjugation if it is incorporated so as to occupy the γ,δ-positions in respect to the α,β-unsaturated ketone. This can be illustrated in the case of the $\Delta^{4,6}$-3-ones (X) and is referred to as a conjugated dienone. A second alternative is that

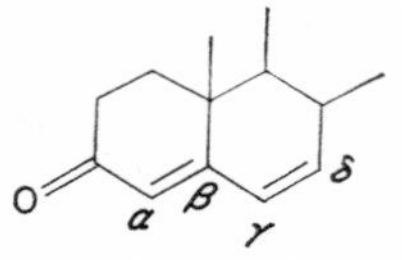

(X)

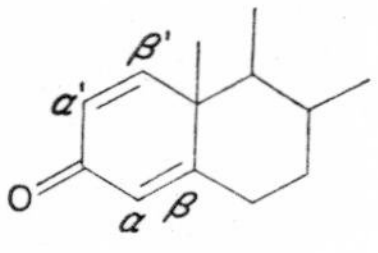

(Y)

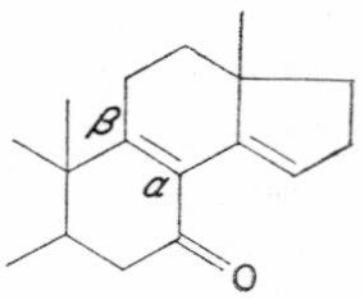

(Z)

the newly introduced double bond may be placed at either the α',β'-positions, giving rise to a chromophore best illustrated by consideration of the $\Delta^{1,4}$-3-one (Y) or be attached to the α-position as in a $\Delta^{8,14}$-7-one (Z). The latter two examples can be broadly termed cross-conjugated systems due to the branching of the chromophore.

When a new double bond is added to an existing chromophore a change in absorption maximum and extinction coefficient is observed. In the case of the conjugated dienones a shift to longer wave length is noted. The change in extinction coefficient is less predictable. In a number of dienones a second short wave length peak is present which may be more intense than the longer wave length maximum. The cross-conjugated dienones of the α',β'-type exhibit a single maximum and the added double bond imparts a slight bathochromic effect to the maximum. The lone example of the α-type cross-conjugated system gives an anomalous spectrum containing a short wave length maximum (224–226 mμ) of high intensity and also a maximum of lower extinction found in the region of conjugated dienones (298 mμ).

For calculation of the approximate absorption maxima of conjugated dienones, several values must be added to the simplified table listed under the general discussion of enones.

TABLE XII

Increment for each alkyl substituent at γ-position or higher	+38 mμ
Increment for each double bond extending conjugation	+18 mμ
Increment for the presence of a homoannular diene component	+30 mμ

The various types of dienones usually encountered in the steroid field are tabulated and presented with an approximate maximal absorption range and extinction values for each system. Comments are included as a guide. A detailed discussion of the $\Delta^{1,4}$-3-ones and the $\Delta^{4,6}$-3-ones can be found as separate sections following the general comments on dienones.

TABLE XIII
ULTRAVIOLET ABSORPTION OF DIENONE CHROMOPHORES

	Range		Comments
	$\lambda_{max}(m\mu)$	ε_{max}	
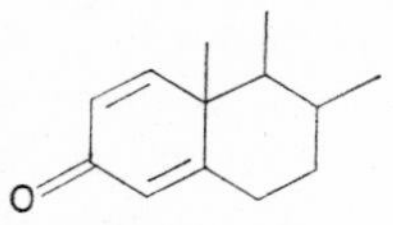 $\Delta^{1,4}$-3-ones	235–250	9700–19,000	The discussion of this chromophoric system has been treated separately and appears as a supplement to the general comments.
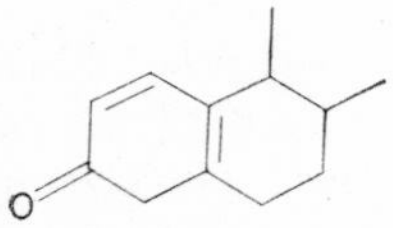 19-nor-$\Delta^{1,5(10)}$-3-ones	335	3500	The lone representative of this system, 4,4-diacetoxy-1,5(10)-estra-diene-3,17-dione, is of questionable purity.
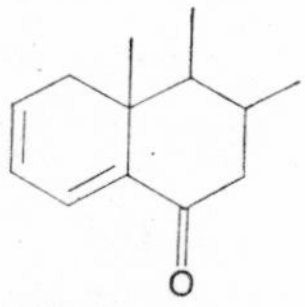 $\Delta^{2,4}$-6-ones	314–317	6300–7600	No representatives of this chromophore are included in the tables. Dorfman[116] cites a limited number of examples.
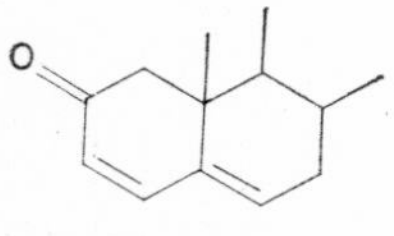 $\Delta^{3,5}$-2-ones	290	12,600	See above.
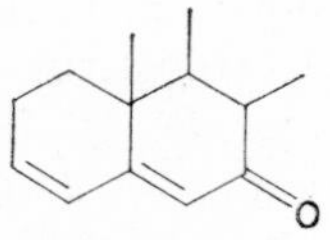 $\Delta^{3,5}$-7-ones	278–284	26,000–31,000	Compounds having a hydroxyl or alkoxyl substituent at C-3 show the expected bathochromic shift. Values for a hydroxyl substituent at C-3 fall in the range 320–322 mμ and in alkaline solution a shift to 390–392 mμ is observed with a high extinction coefficient. Alkoxyl groups fall in the range 309–311 mμ.

TABLE XIII (*continued*)

	Range		Comments
	λ_{max}(mμ)	ε_{max}	
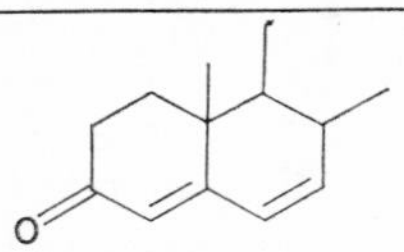 $\Delta^{4,6}$-3-ones	280–286	20,000–32,000	The range cited is for the unsubstituted chromophore. A discussion of this system is treated separately and appears as the second supplement to these comments.
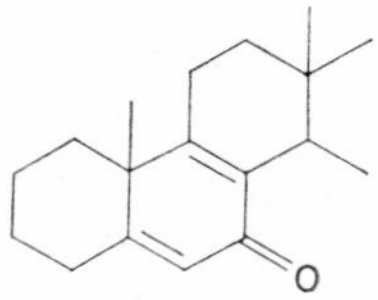 $\Delta^{5,8}$-7-ones	244–248	11,600–12,800	The range is based on a limited number of examples. The compounds in the cholesterol and ergosterol series have been reported [INHOFFEN, H. H. and MENGEL, W., *Chem. Ber.* **87**, 146 (1954)].
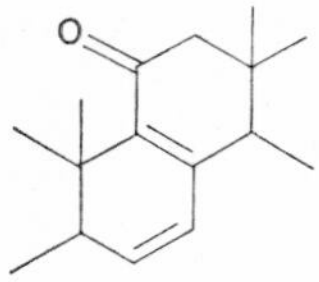 $\Delta^{6,8}$-11-ones	308	6900	One example of this chromophore is reported by Dorfman.[116]
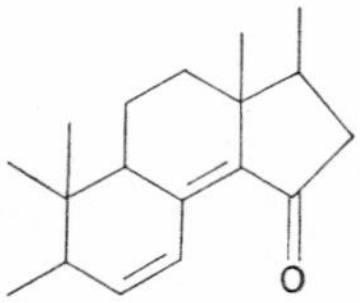 $\Delta^{6,8(14)}$-15-ones	297	20,400	One example of this chromophore is known in the ergosterol series [BARTON, D. H. R. and LAWS, G. F., *J. Chem. Soc.* 52 (1954)].
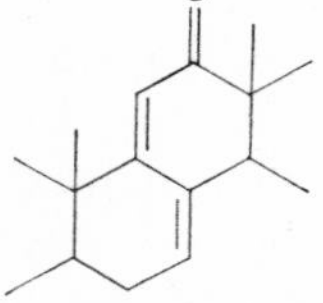 $\Delta^{7,9(11)}$-12-ones	238–240 290–293	3000–3800 12,000–14,500	The range is based on a limited number of examples.

TABLE XIII (*continued*)

	Range		Comments
	λ_{max}(mμ)	ε_{max}	
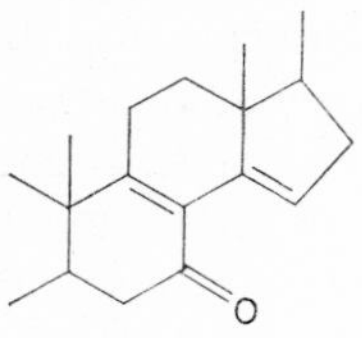 $\Delta^{8,14}$-7-ones	224–226 298	15,600–18,000 5000–6500	Several examples of this chromophore are known. Structures once postulated as $\Delta^{8,11}$-7-ones and $\Delta^{8(14),15}$-7-ones are most likely $\Delta^{8,14}$-7-ones.
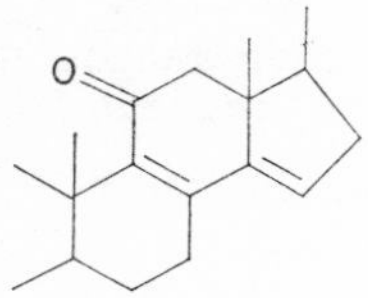 $\Delta^{8,14}$-11-ones	210–214 292–294	8900–11,700 12,000–13,700	This chromophore has been reported in the ergosterol series [GRIGOR, J., NEWBOLD, G. T. and SPRING, F. S., *J. Chem. Soc.*, 1170 (1955)].
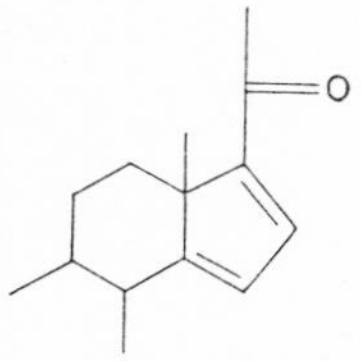 $\Delta^{14,16}$-20-ones	305–307	9000–17,000	The range is based on a very limited number of examples.
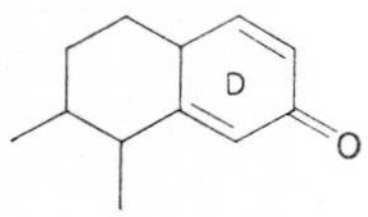	246.5	17,600	Only one representative of this class has been reported.

The $\Delta^{1,4}$*-3-ones*

The biological importance achieved by certain 1-dehydro-Δ^4-3-ones has resulted in the synthesis in recent years of a great number of compounds having this structural feature. As a result, this system probably ranks second only to the parent Δ^4-3-ones in the number of representatives listed in the tables. With such interest currently centered on these compounds, extensive structural modifications have been reported.

The ultraviolet absorption spectrum of the $\Delta^{1,4}$-3-ones is represented by a single intense band which is characteristic of homoannular cross-conjugated dienones. In simple unsubstituted compounds, the maximum falls in the short range of 243–244 mμ with molecular extinction values of the order of 15,000–17,000. The introduction of substituents into the molecule may change this range considerably.

Of the various substituents introduced at sites apart from the chromophore itself, only those at the C-9 and C-11 positions seem to have any effect and they are identical to the situation encountered in the discussion of the Δ^4-3-ones.

The introduction of a 11β-hydroxyl group appears to have little or no effect on the chromophore. Maximum absorption falls in the range 242–244 mμ. Considering a large number of these derivatives, significantly more show absorption at the lower end of the range. The epimeric 11α-hydroxyl group shows a bathochromic effect (+3 mμ) in this series. The typical hypsochromic effect (−6 mμ) encountered in the 11-carbonyl derivative is noted in this system. The absorption maximum for Δ^1-dehydrocortisone is 238 mμ. A strong hypsochromic effect is also noted for the $\Delta^{9(11)}$ olefin (−6 mμ) while the 9β,11β-epoxide function shows a strong bathochromic effect (+3 to +5 mμ).

When the 9α-hydrogen is replaced by a group of stronger electronegativity, a hypsochromic effect is always noted in the $\Delta^{1,4}$-3-ones. In this series the 9α-bromo, -chloro and -fluoro derivatives are known and the respective ranges for the compounds also possessing a 11β-hydroxyl group are 240–242, 238–239 and 237–239 mμ. The additional hypsochromic effect of the 11-carbonyl is also superimposed. A few 9α,11β-dihalo-$\Delta^{1,4}$-3-ones have been reported. On the basis of a limited number of compounds, the 11β-halogen approximates the effect produced by the 11-carbonyl grouping. A summary of the effects of substituents at the 9α- and 11-positions is presented in Table XIV.

TABLE XIV

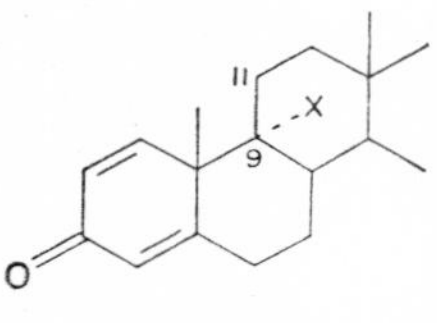

X λ_{max}	11β-Hydroxy λ_{max}(mμ)	11-Carbonyl λ_{max}(mμ)	11α-Hydroxy λ_{max}(mμ)
H	242–244	238–239	247–248
Br	240–242	238–240	
Cl	238–239	236–237	
F	237–239	235	

Considering substituents that are placed on or immediately adjacent to the $\Delta^{1,4}$-3-one system, carbon positions 1, 2, 4, 6, and 10 are possibilities. All may possibly influence the electron distribution about the chromophore and thereby alter its absorption maximum. In the period covered in this survey, no 1-substituted $\Delta^{1,4}$-3-ones have been reported with the exception of 1,2-dichloro-17β-hydroxy-1,4-androstadien-3-one propionate (λ_{max} 257.5 mμ).

Substitution at the C-2 position has been confined to chlorine, methyl and oxygenated derivatives each of which produces the expected bathochromic effect associated with the addition of a grouping to the α-position on an α,β-unsaturated ketone. A range of 247–254 mμ would include all such substituents with the 2-hydroxy compounds being confined in the range 252–254 mμ, and the 2-methyl compounds at 247–248 mμ, the effects of ring-C substituents not being considered.

A limited number of 4-substituted compounds have been reported but these seem to indicate that neither methyl nor halogen substitution at this position exhibits any marked effects on the absorption maximum. This is in marked contrast to the Δ^4-3-ones. A larger number of 6-substituted derivatives are known. However, these are confined to the 6α- rather than 6β-substituent since these possess the more marked physiological activities. The introduction of a 6-methyl group has no apparent influence on the chromophore similarly observed in the Δ^4-3-ones. The halogen derivatives (bromo, chloro and fluoro) follow the same pattern previously noted. The 6α-fluoro derivatives show a slight hypsochromic effect (−2 to −4 mμ). A single 6β-bromo compound (250 mμ) demonstrates a bathochromic effect over the α-epimer (244 mμ) and the parent compound (243 mμ). The 6α-chloro compounds show little change in absorption from the parent compounds. The hypsochromic effects of the 9α-halo and 11-carbonyl groupings are superimposed on any effect exhibited by the 6-substituted compounds.

Substitution of various groups at the C-10 position, replacing the normal 10-methyl group, has provided a limited number of interesting compounds. The configuration has not been established for all such substitutions. However, certain derivatives follow the pattern established by the 6-substituted compounds. Of the halo derivatives a 10β-chloro compound gives the expected bathochromic shift (+4 mμ) while the 10β-fluoro derivative shows a small hypsochromic effect (−3 to −4 mμ). The configuration of the 10-hydroxyl group reported in compounds of the 1,4-androstadien-3-one series is unestablished; they apparently are β-substituents and show selective absorption in the range of 235–242 mμ. This indicates a

TABLE XV

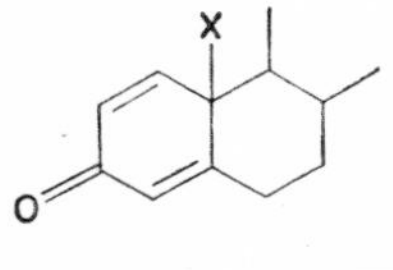

X	λ_{max}(mμ)
β-F	240–241
β-Cl	250
ξ-OH	235–242
ξ-$OCOCH_3$	248–250
β-CH_2OH	245–246 (11-carbonyl correction applied)
β-CH_2OCOCH_3	243

hypsochromic effect for this grouping. A strong bathochromic effect (+4 to +6 mμ) is noted with a 10-acetoxyl substituent suggesting a strong interaction with the dienone system. A lone compound having a 10β-hydroxymethyl grouping has been reported. Compensating for the effect of the 11-carbonyl group, the hydroxymethyl probably has a slight bathochromic effect. This has also been observed in the Δ^4-3-one series. The 10β-acetoxymethyl shows little or no effect. The 10-substituted compounds are given in Table XV.

The $\Delta^{4,6}$-3-ones

Extending the conjugation of the Δ^4-3-ones by the addition of another double bond to give the $\Delta^{4,6}$-3-one system, brings about both the displacement of the maximum to longer wave length and an intensification of the extinction value. In general the range of 283–284 mμ can be assigned to the simple chromophore with molecular extinction values ranging from 25,000–30,000. These particular values are subject to considerable variance depending on the arrangement of neighboring functional groups in the molecule and by the substitution of various groups onto the chromophore, replacing the hydrogen atoms.

In considering the functional groups not attached directly to the conjugated system, it can be seen that they may produce either hypsochromic or bathochromic effects on the system or have no influence on the 283–284 mμ value assigned to the chromophore. Substituents producing hypsochromic effects in this series are essentially those encountered in the discussions of the Δ^4-3-ones and the $\Delta^{1,4}$-3-ones. The presence of a 9α-fluorine lowers the maximum to 281 mμ while the 11-carbonyl group shifts the value of the chromophore to 280 mμ with the effects being additive. Bathochromic effects produced by neighboring groups are also observed. The introduction of a 11α-hydroxyl group produces a shift to 286 mμ but the 11α-acetoxyl group has no influence on the system. It has also been observed

TABLE XVI

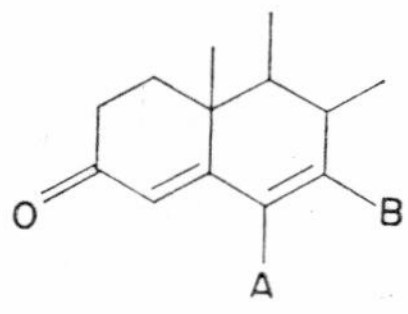

A	B	λ_{max}(mμ)	ε_{max} (approx)
H	H	284	25,000
CH_3	H	288–289	24,000
H	CH_3	294–298	25,000
F	H	282–284	24,500
Cl	H	285	20,000
OCH_3	H	304	16,100

that a 1α-thioacetate grouping has a bathochromic effect (+3 mμ) on the chromophore. A lone compound having a 1α,2β-dichloro grouping (λ_{max} 296.5 mμ) shows a strong bathochromic effect.

The absorption maximum of a chromophoric system may be most easily altered by the introduction of various substituents directly on the system. In such cases bathochromic effects are observed. Current interest in the chemistry of the $\Delta^{4,6}$-3-ones has centered about substituents at the 6- and 7-positions. These are summarized in Table XVI.

The introduction of methyl groups at positions 6 and 7 produces a bathochromic effect but not in the expected magnitude. The 6-methyl group exhibits a bathochromic effect of +4 to +5 mμ, a value slightly lower than predicted from the generalized expressions derived for extended chromophores. The bathochromic effect of the 7-methyl group (+10 to +14 mμ) is more in conformity. The large bathochromic effect seen in the 4-halo-Δ^4-3-ones may be ascribed primarily to orbital overlap between the halogen atom and the oxygen as stated. The absence of this bathochromic effect in the 6-halo-$\Delta^{4,6}$-3-ones may be attributed to the increased distance between the halogen and oxygen atoms. As expected the introduction of an oxygenated function (methoxyl group, +20 mμ) imparts a strong bathochromic effect to the chromophore.

The hypsochromic effect of the 11-carbonyl group is also observed in the 7-methyl-$\Delta^{4,6}$-3-one system. The value of 294 mμ for 7-methyl-6-dehydrocortisone is contrasted by the maximum of 296–298 mμ for 7-methyl-6-dehydro-hydrocortisone which is representative for the system in general.

Trienones

The addition of a double bond to a dienone system can give rise to a variety of trienones whose spectral properties will be expected to differ from the original dienone chromophore. Covering seven carbon atoms, the new trienones may possess a homoannular diene component as in the $\Delta^{4,6,8}$-3-ones (A), or may be heteroannular as in the $\Delta^{4,6,8(14)}$-3-one (B) or $\Delta^{6,8,14}$-11-one (C) types. The

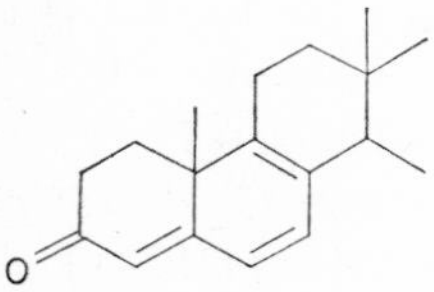

(a)

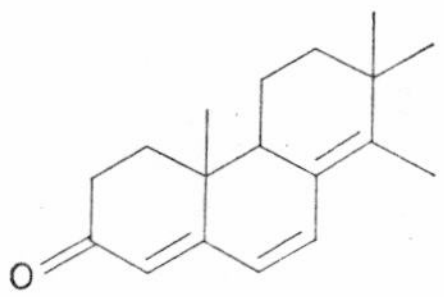

(b)

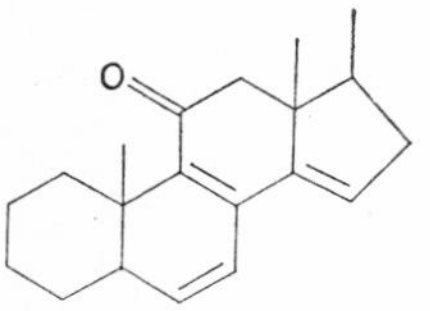

(c)

classification of conjugated and cross-conjugated systems can also be imposed to further specify a particular chromophore. The number of representatives for each system is in general quite limited and in some cases only one member is known. Furthermore, controversy concerning several of the proposed structures has not been resolved, further complicating a general review of these systems.

As expected, the trienones exhibit an absorption band at long wave length but this maximum may appear over a considerable range (296–390 mμ) depending on the chromophore in question. In addition, the spectrum contains at least one additional peak at lower wave length, the most common systems having three absorption bands. A considerable variation is noted in the relative intensities of these bands. The pattern in the molecular extension values is characteristic of the chromophore but may be varied by individual substituents of the system.

The various trienone systems have been tabulated to provide a summary of the tables and examples quoted in the Dorfman review.[116] A detailed discussion of the $\Delta^{1,4,6}$-3-one system has been included to discuss the effects of various substituents on the chromophore.

TABLE XVII. THE ULTRAVIOLET ABSORPTION OF TRIENONE CHROMOPHORES

	Range		Comments
	λ_{max} (mμ)	ε_{max}	
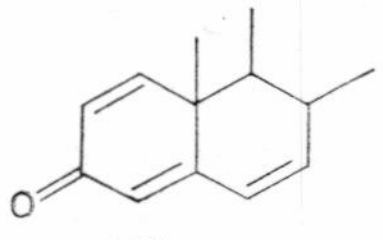 $\Delta^{1,4,6}$-3-one	221–224 255–256 295–301	10,000–13,400 9100–16,700 10,200–13,700	A detailed discussion of this chromophore can be found as a supplement to these general comments.
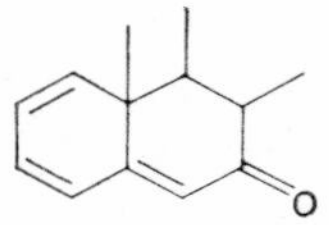 $\Delta^{1,3,5}$-7-one	230 278–281 348–350	14,400–18,600 2600–3700 8700–11,000	This system has been reported only in the cholesterol series. [HENBEST, H. B. and WILSON, R. A. L., *Chem. & Ind.* 86 (1956).]
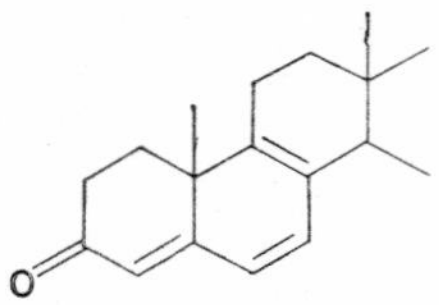 $\Delta^{4,6,8}$-3-one	244–245.5 285–300 390	14,300–16,700 3100 3900–6700	A very limited number of examples of this chromophore are known. [ELKS, J., EVANS, R. M., OUGHTON, J. F. and THOMAS, G. H., *J. Chem. Soc.* 463 (1954).] The tables list a representative of this system in the pregnane series.
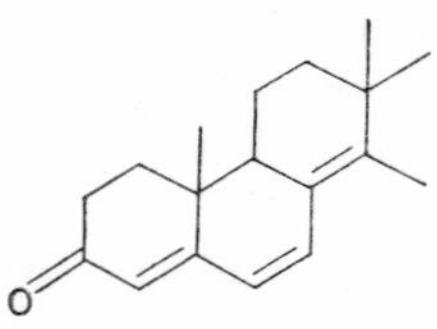 $\Delta^{4,6,8(14)}$-3-one	237 282 334–350	4700 7100 25,800–27,500	See above. In some cases a lone maximum in the range 334–348 mμ has been reported for this system.

TABLE XVII (*continued*)

	Range		Comments
	$\lambda_{max}(m\mu)$	ε_{max}	
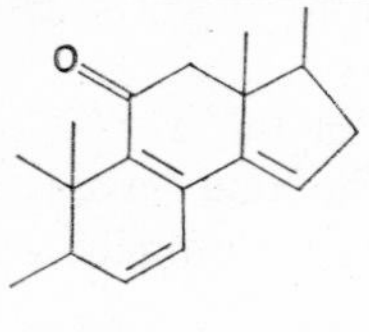 $\Delta^{6,8,14}$-11-one	237 341	11,000 11,500	A lone representative of this chromophore appears in the ergosterol series. [LAUBACH, G. D., SCHREIBER, E. C., AGNELLO, E. J., LIGHTFOOT, E. N. and BRUNINGS, K. J., *J. Amer. Chem. Soc.* **75**, 1514 (1953).]
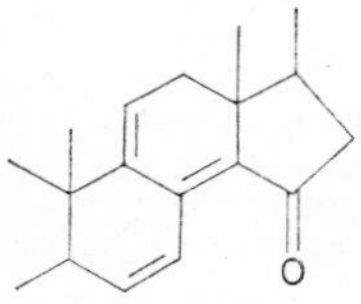 $\Delta^{6,8(14),9(11)}$-15-one	233 326	15,000 8910	A lone representative of this chromophore appears in the ergosterol series. [AGNELLO, E. J., PINSON, R., JR. and LAUBACH, G. D., *J. Amer. Chem. Soc.* **78**, 4756 (1956).]
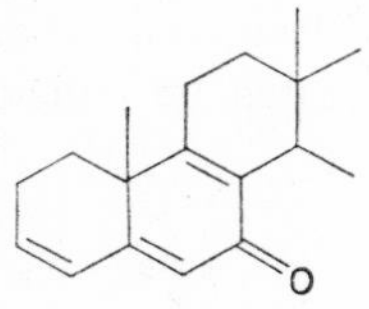 $\Delta^{3,5,8}$-7-one	215–217 272	19,000 14,600	A compound in the ergosterol series of doubtful purity has been suggested to possess this structure. See reference cited in the $\Delta^{4,6,8}$-3-ones.

The $\Delta^{1,4,6}$*-3-ones*

Thus far, the $\Delta^{1,4,6}$-3-ones are the only class of trienones that contains a sufficient number of representatives to warrant a detailed discussion concerning the influence of various substituents on the basic chromophore. As in the case of the $\Delta^{1,4}$-3-ones, the increased biological interest in dehydro-Δ^{4}-3-ones has stimulated interest in the $\Delta^{1,4,6}$-3-ones and substituted derivatives.

The chromophore can be classified as a cross-conjugated trienone. As we have seen, the $\Delta^{1,4}$-3-ones exhibit a single absorption maximum. With the addition of the 6,7-double bond, the resulting $\Delta^{1,4,6}$-3-one system exhibits a spectrum that contains two or three maxima depending on the substitution pattern. Systems of this general type appear at first glance to be composites of the individual chromophores comprising the system, i.e. Δ^{1}-3-ones, $\Delta^{1,4}$-3-ones and $\Delta^{4,6}$-3-ones.

The spectrum of 1,4,6-androstadien-3,17-dione has bands at 222, 256 and 298 mμ. The addition of a 2-methyl substituent should therefore eliminate the maximum at 222 mμ. This has been observed for 2-methyl-1,4,6-androstatrien-3,17-dione which has only two maxima at 266 and 301 mμ with the peak at lower wave length becoming the more intense. An extension of this argument to other trienone systems is not as obvious.

The substitution of methyl groups at the 4- and 6-positions of the $\Delta^{1,4,6}$-3-ones has a slight bathochromic effect on the 222 mμ peak and also on the long wave length peak. The influence of a methyl group at the various positions is summarized in Table XVIII.

TABLE XVIII

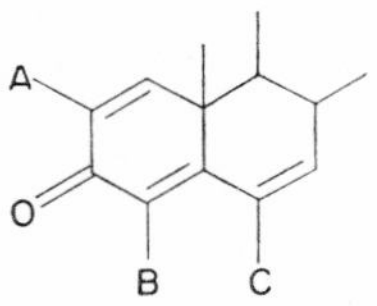

A	B	C	λ_{max}(mμ)		
H	H	H	222–223	254–256	294–297
CH_3	H	H	—	265.5–266	300–301
H	CH_3	H	226	255	306
H	H	CH_3	228	253	304

The substitution of a halogen atom at the 2-, 4-, and 6-positions on the chromophore has a similar effect and this can be best demonstrated by considering Table XIX.

TABLE XIX

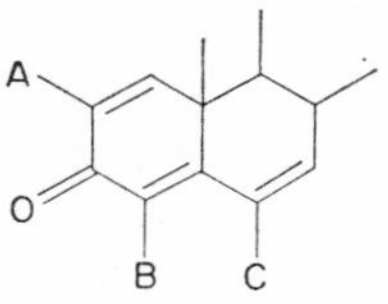

A	B	C	λ_{max}(mμ)		
H	H	H	222–223	254–256	294–297
Cl	H	H	—	267.5	305
H	Cl	H	229	255	310.5
H	H	Cl	228–229	258–260	295–297
H	H	F	225	254	298

1,4,6-Androstatrien-3,11,17-trione (λ_{max} 222, 255 and 296 mμ), the lone 11-carbonyl representative, does not show the hypsochromic effect of the 11-carbonyl group as is manifested in the Δ^1-3-ones, Δ^4-3-ones, $\Delta^{1,4}$-3-ones and $\Delta^{4,6}$-3-ones.

6. Ultraviolet Absorption of Steroids Containing Aromatic Rings

The general types of absorption typical of an aromatic system have been well outlined by both Gillam and Stern[160] and Dorfman.[116] There are some additions to the information previously reported, which have come about either through closer examination of the absorption spectra or through previously unreported types of substitution affecting the chromophoric system.

The absorption spectra of the C-3 oxygenated aromatic A ring generally fit the limits set by Dorfman[116] subject to the refinements mentioned in Table XX. Dorfman[116] listed very few compounds alkylated in ring A and none of more than one oxygen function on ring A. Compounds with amino or nitro substituent groups have not been previously listed.

Compounds which have a double bond conjugated with an aromatic A ring show the same types of absorption previously elaborated by Dorfman.[116] These absorptions are also given in Table XX.

A large number of synthetic D-homo steroids containing an aromatic D ring have been prepared by W. S. Johnson and collaborators.[212–214, 219–223] It may be

TABLE XX

Chromophore	Range		Comments
	λ_{max}(mμ)	ε_{max}	
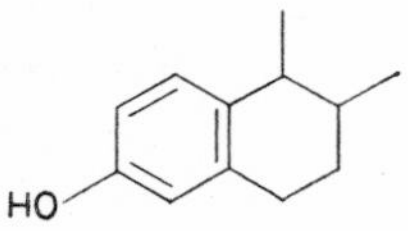	279–284 287	1600–6900 1950	The maximum at 287 mμ has been only occasionally reported. The earlier maximum at 279–289 mμ is the basic peak for this type of compound as mentioned in ref. 116.
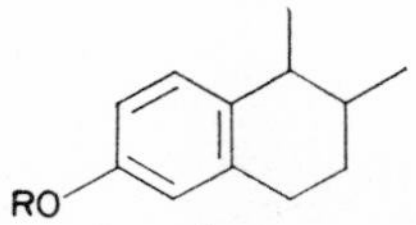	266–269 273–276	480–2140 480–1600	The hypsochromic and hyperchromic effect of 3-acylation is again noticed. The second peak at 273–276 mμ has not been mentioned in ref. 116.
R=CH_3CO =CH_2CH_3CO R=C_6H_5CO	226–230	17,800–27,500	
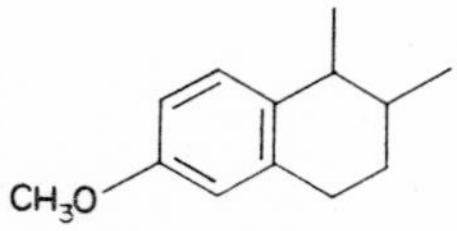	276–279 285–287	2000–3160	The 285–287 mμ peak had not previously been mentioned.

TABLE XX (*continued*)

Chromophore	Range		Comments
	$\lambda_{max}(m\mu)$	ε_{max}	
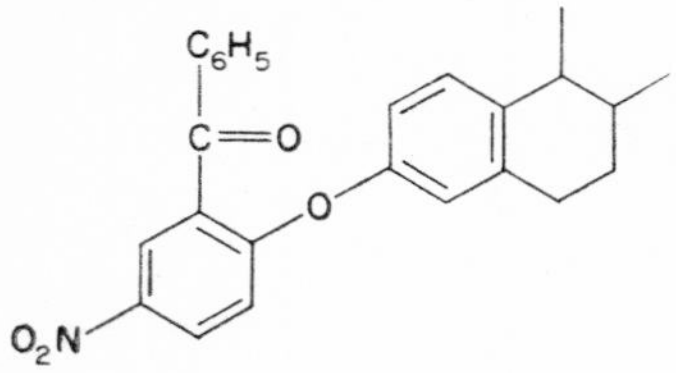	254 296	17,000 12,000	There are only a limited number of these compounds.
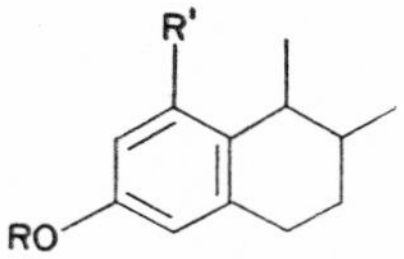 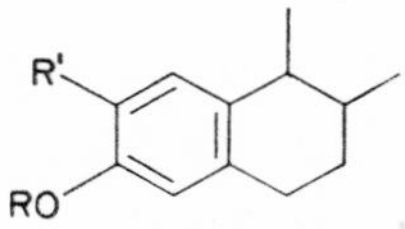 R=H or CH_3 R'=CH_3	280–287	1600–2500	A slight bathochromic effect seems to exist due to alkylation at C-1 or C-2. This is not observed with alkylation at C-4.
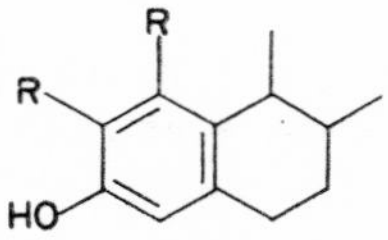 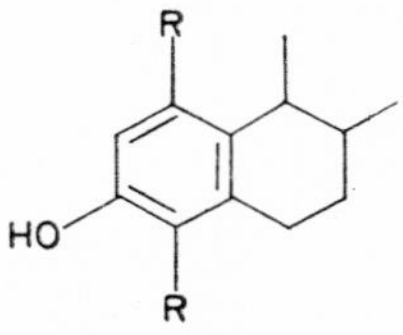 R=CH_3	288	1780	A bathochromic effect is again observed. Very few examples are available.

TABLE XX (*continued*)

Chromophore	Range		Comments
	λ_{max}(mμ)	ε_{max}	
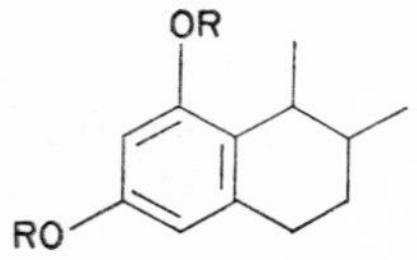 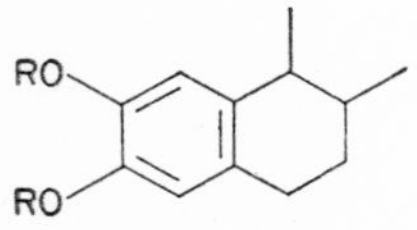 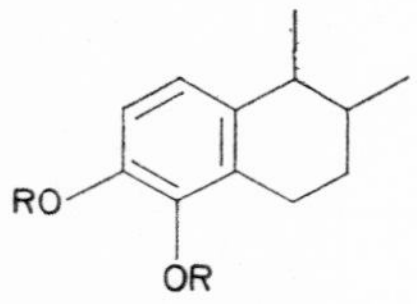 R=H or CH_3	277–287	2000–4000	A slight bathochromic effect exists on substitution of a second oxygen function.
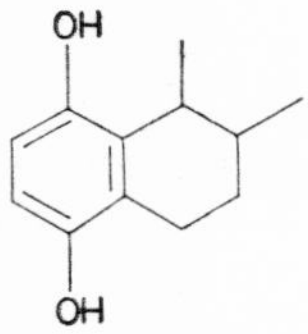	295 265	3600 340	1 example is available.
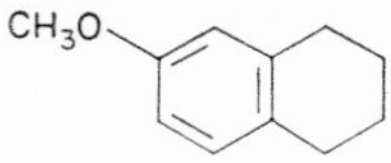	286	3700	A very limited number of examples is available.
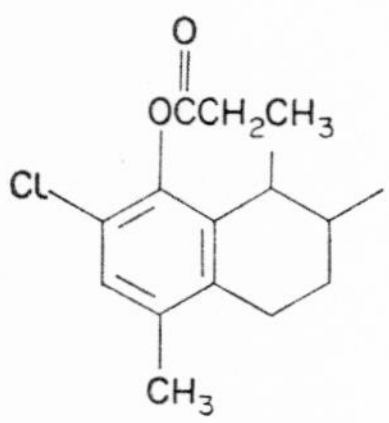	274	485	1 example is available.
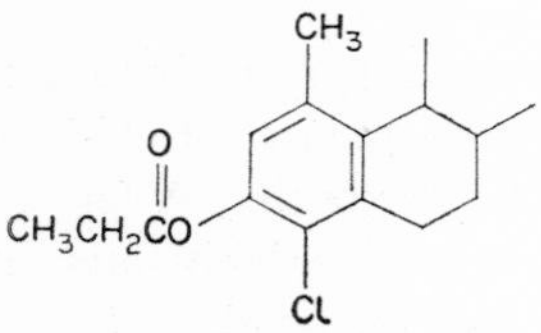	285(inf.) 290	1875 1940	1 example is available.

TABLE XX (*continued*)

Chromophore	Range		Comments
	$\lambda_{max}(m\mu)$	ε_{max}	
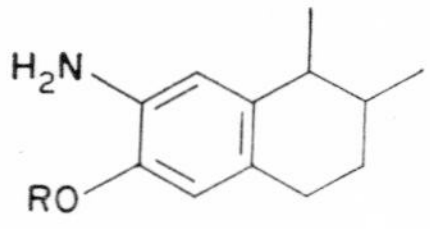 R=H or CH_3	295–297	4000	2 examples are available.
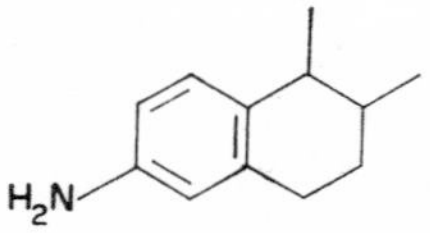	237–9	8000–9000	Only limited number of examples are available.
N-Acetyl	247–9	15–16,000	
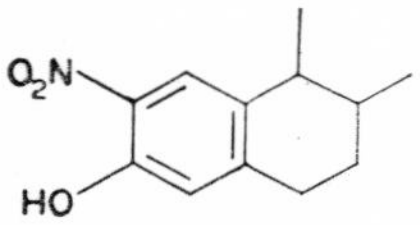	293 364–366	8100 3690	1 example only is available.
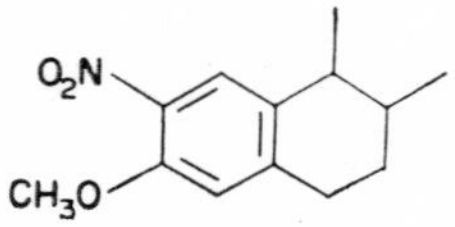	272.5 336	4510 3130	1 example is available.
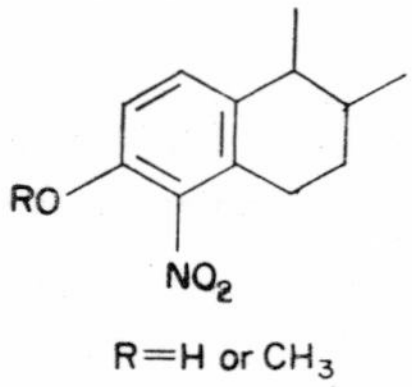 R=H or CH_3	275–278	1500–1800	2 examples
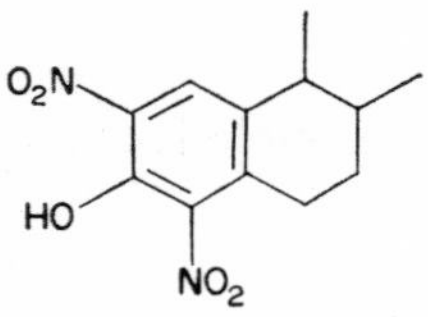	277–279 352–354	6500 3500	2 examples
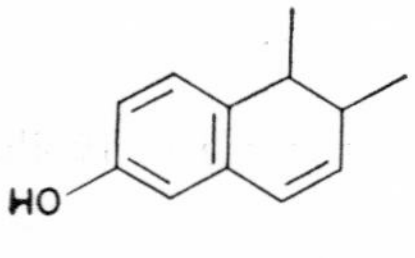	262–272 302–306	7950–10,000 2250–2500	These may include alkyl substituents at C-1 or C-2 or both. A few C-6 methyl substituents are also included.

TABLE XX (*continued*)

Chromophore	Range		Comments
	λ_{max}(mμ)	ε_{max}	
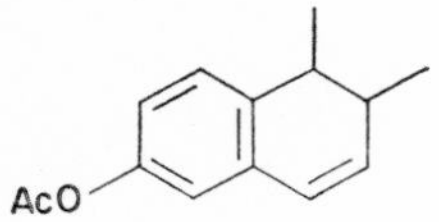	224–225 262–268	25,000–31,600 1260–7950	These may include alkyl substituents at C-1 or C-2 or both.
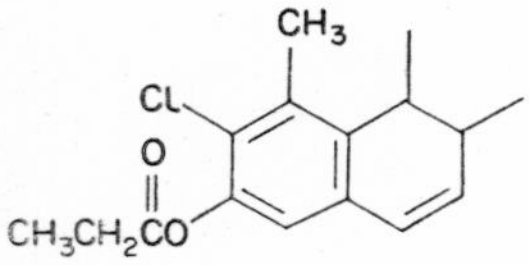	226 232 271	29,450 25,450 12,700	1 example
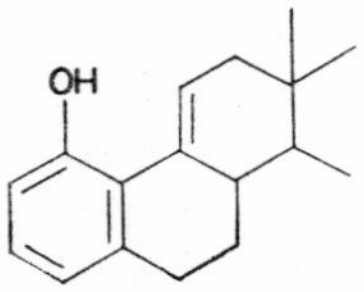	255.5 300	13,200 3830	1 example
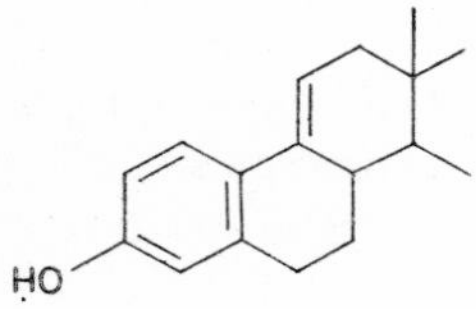	263 298	18,050 3125	1 example
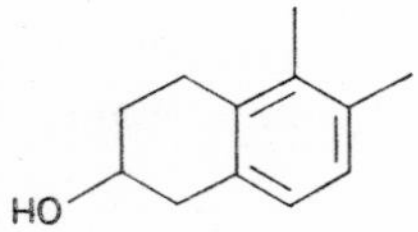	269	395	1 example in this work
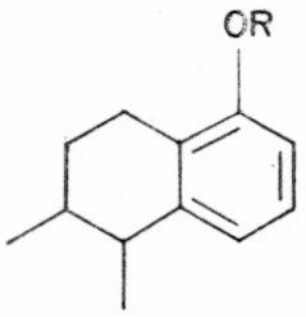 R=H or CH_3	271–275 277–282	1260 2500	
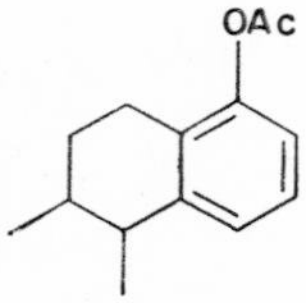	260–262	250–630	The acetate group again shows a hypsochromic and hyperchromic effect.

TABLE XX (*continued*)

Chromophore	Range		Comments
	λ_{max}(mμ)	ε_{max}	
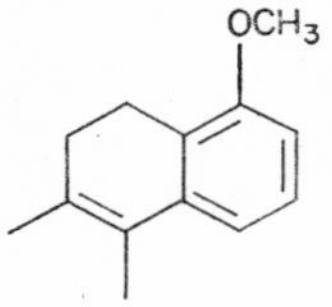	217–222 265–272	27,500–31,000 9000–13,800	
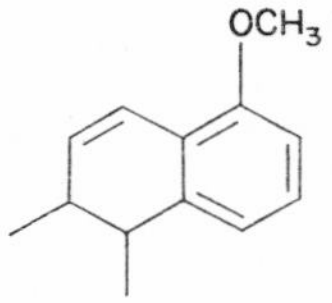	268–271 298–300 308–312	6170–10,200 3470–5130 3160–5000	
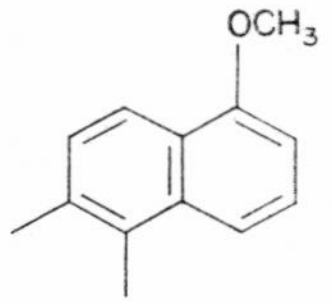	224–227 285–287 295–298 310–312 323–325	50,000 5000–6300 6920–7410 4680–5500 2340–2890	2 examples
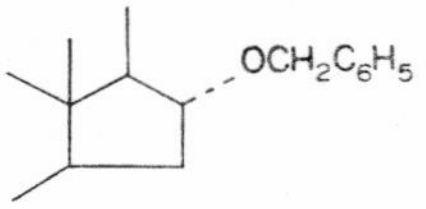	247–8 252 258 264	130 156–198 196–227 149–184	Only limited number of compounds; a typical benzene absorption curve
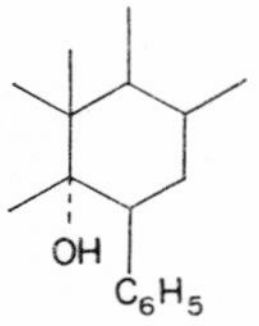	254 260 266	174–220 205–240 148–195	A typical benzene absorption curve
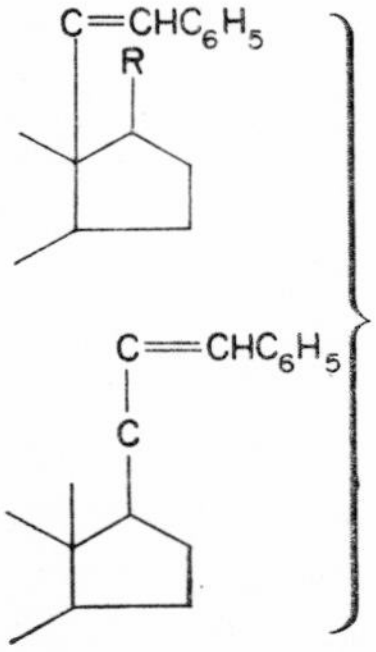	254–255	18,900–20,900	A typical "styrene" absorption

TABLE XX (*continued*)

Chromophore	Range		Comments
	$\lambda_{max}(m\mu)$	ε_{max}	
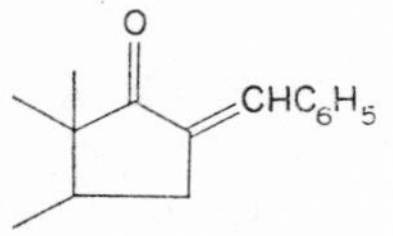 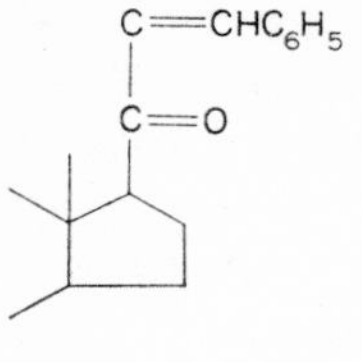 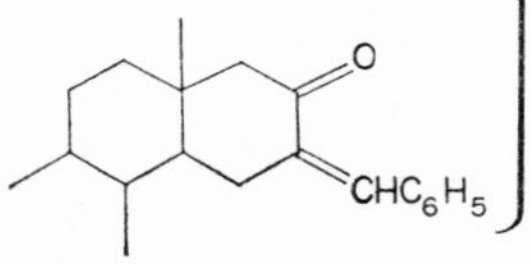	220–225 285–295	8000–16,000 21,000–27,000	Ultraviolet data of this type of compound have not been recorded to a large extent.
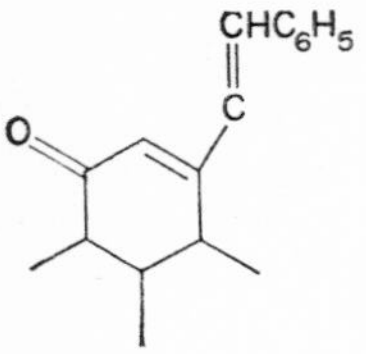	238–240 325	10,600–14,000 35,000	2 examples
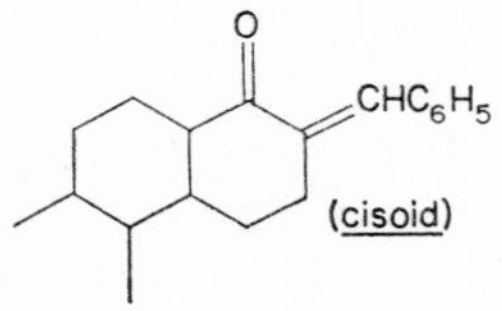 (cisoid)	219–221 269–278	11,500–13,200 8130–8910	The differentiation between these compounds and the *transoid* isomer (see below) may be made on the basis of the lower range of maxima of the *cisoid* compounds.
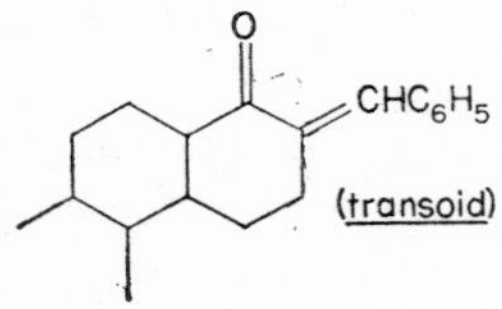 (transoid)	222 286.5–292	5890–7950 15,800	See above.

TABLE XX (*continued*)

Chromophore	Range		Comments
	λ_{max}(mμ)	ε_{max}	
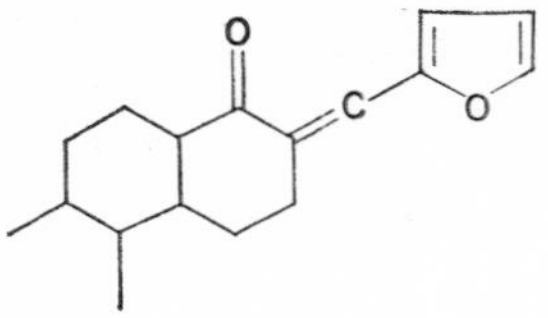	320–329	20,000–25,000	The furfurylidenes exhibit maxima at longer wave lengths than the benzylidenes (see above) and this approximates the relative K-band displacement in furfuraldehyde compared to benzaldehyde.
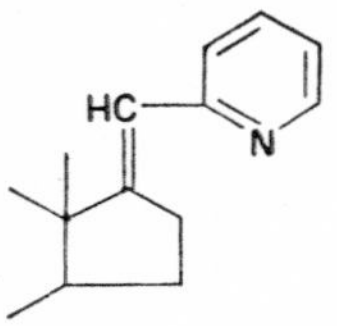	250	19,100	1 example
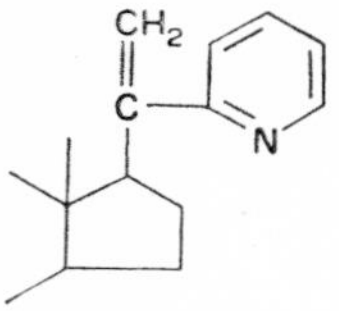	230	7350	1 example

seen in Table XX that these compounds, both conjugated with a double bond and non-conjugated, have absorptions similar to the aromatic A ring compound.

The naphthalene type compounds, both AB aromatic and CD-homo aromatic have complex absorptions typical of these structures.

Steroids with a substituent phenyl group give typical benzene absorptions while conjugation gives the expected enhancement of intensity and bathochromic effects. The large peaks noticed in conjugated benzene compounds are probably the double bond peak which in an unconjugated compound is below the limit (<200 mμ) at which these instruments are effective.

It may be noticed in Table XX that compounds in which the stereochemistry of the aryl substituents about a conjugated double bond is known (*cisoid* or *transoid*), a characteristic difference in absorption maxima and intensity of the extinction coefficient appears.

IV. TABLES OF ULTRAVIOLET ABSORPTION DATA

1. Introduction to the Tables

The compilation of the vast amount of data presented in the following tables makes it essential that the user of the tables be familiar with the basic rules, arbitrarily selected by the authors, for the presentation of the data. The usefulness of the tables will be directly related to the facility with which the information can be gleaned from the text. Consequently this short presentation describing the extent, composition and cataloguing of the material abstracted from the literature has been included.

In an attempt to conform to the general tenets of the volume and to restrict the number of table entries, primary emphasis has been confined to steroid hormones and related compounds. The literature has been reviewed from 1952 to 1958 and it is presumed that the tables are complete in this respect. After completion of the 1952–1958 tables and references, it was deemed advisable to include data from the 1959 literature. This material appears separately and represents only a survey of the primary journals. The patent literature has not been included in this survey.

The compounds have been grouped into tables based on their ultraviolet absorption chromophores. Within each table the entries have been further subdivided and arranged systematically according to their empirical formulae. Simple derivatives of these compounds (i.e. acetates, benzoates, acid esters, etc.) are included under the parent compound and are so indicated. However, derivatives that result in a change of the chromophoric system are listed separately under the particular system in question. In a number of cases spectral data have not been reported for the parent compound and this results in blank entries in the tables. A great many compounds possessing chromophores are recorded in the literature without complete spectral characterization and accordingly are not listed in the tables. Therefore, caution is advised if the tables are to be used as a literature searching device.

Attempted standardization of nomenclature has resulted in changes in compound names from those found in the original references. The compounds have been named as derivatives of the androstane, etiocholane, 5α-pregnane, pregnane and estrane ring systems with the various substituents listed alphabetically. D-Homo-, nor- and seco-steroids are named using the intact ring systems stated.

The absorption maxima (λ_{max}) are reported in millimicrons (mμ) and the extinction coefficients (as ε, $\log\varepsilon$ or $E^{1\%}_{1\,cm}$) are reported in the convention appearing in the original text. A separate column has been provided for the solvent employed. Blank spaces appearing in any of the first three columns indicate that the data have not been provided. The reference column has been indexed in the bibliography. Authors are listed alphabetically in the periods 1952–1958 and 1959. No attempt has been made to review the data critically; hence all references to a specific compound are included in the tables. On occasion, this allows an evaluation of solvent effect and an alternate expression of the molecular extinction value. The term "chart" appears in the tables. This term is used to indicate that the authors have interpreted or have hesitated to interpret a published curve for which the actual values have not been stated. In any event the curve may be found in the original text and should be consulted.

The following solvent abbreviations are employed in the tables:

A	Ethanol
C	Cyclohexane
Ch	Chloroform
D	Dioxane
E	Ether
H	Hexane
I	iso-Octane
IP	iso-Propanol
M	Methanol
W	Water

In addition, Ac refers to an acidic solution of the solvent specified while B indicates a basic solution.

2. Index to the Tables

3. Tables

TABLE I. ISOLATED DOUBLE BONDS

Formula	Compound	λ_{max}	Ext.	Sol.	Ref.
$C_{19}H_{26}O$	2,9(11)-Androstadien-17-one	200	6012		240
		205	4202		240
		210	1748		240
		215	480		240
		220	166		240
$C_{19}H_{28}O$	9(11)-Androsten-17-one	200	5340		240
		205	3410		240
		210	1233		240
		215	86		240
$C_{20}H_{30}O_4$	17β-Carboxy-8(14)-etiocholene-3β,11α-diol Diacetate, methyl ester	204	3.98	Ch	245
$C_{21}H_{28}O_2$	4,9(11)-Pregnadiene-3,20-dione	206	3.67	A	360

TABLE II. DIENES

Formula	Compound	λ_{max}	Ext.	Sol.	Ref.
3,5-Dienes					
$C_{20}H_{26}O_3$	17β-Carboxy-3,5,14-androstatrien-19-ol				
	Ethyl ester	234	17,130	A	119
	Acetate, ethyl ester	234	20,240	A	119
$C_{20}H_{28}O_2$	3,5-Androstadiene-17β-carboxylic acid				
	Methyl ester	234	4.3	A	446
$C_{20}H_{30}O$	3-Methyl-3,5-androstadien-17β-ol	233	4.28	E	387
$C_{21}H_{29}O_2Cl$	21-Chloro-3,5-pregnadien-19-ol	234	22,800	A	181
	Acetate	234	17,400	A	181
$C_{21}H_{30}O_2$	19-Hydroxy-3,5-pregnadien-20-one				
	Acetate	234	19,800	A	119
$C_{21}H_{32}O$	3,5-Pregnadien-20β-ol	235	30,000		64
$C_{21}H_{32}O_2$	3,5-Pregnadiene-20β,21-diol	228	16,500	A	74
		235	17,000	A	74
		243	12,700	A	74
3,5-Dienol Acetates					
$C_{20}H_{28}O_3$	3-Acetoxy-19-nor-3,5-androstadien-17β-ol				
	Acetate	235	18,950	A	412
		234	21,000	A	173
	Benzoate	231	18,390	A	173
$C_{21}H_{30}O_3$	3-Acetoxy-3,5-androstadien-17β-ol				
	Acetate	234	4.22	A	347
$C_{23}H_{28}O_5$	3-Acetoxy-3,5-pregnadien-21-al-11,20-dione				
	21, 21-Diacetoxyacetal	231	$E^{1\%}_{1\,cm}$ 385		163
$C_{23}H_{30}O_5$	3-Acetoxy-16α,17α-epoxy-21-hydroxy-3,5-pregnadien-20-one				
	Acetate	234	4.26	A	351
$C_{23}H_{31}O_4Br$	3-Acetoxy-16β-bromo-17α-hydroxy-3,5-pregnadien-20-one	234	4.30	A	351
$C_{23}H_{32}O_3$	3-Acetoxy-3,5-pregnadien-20-one	234	4.21	A	347
$C_{23}H_{32}O_4$	3-Acetoxy-17α-hydroxy-3,5-pregnadien-20-one				
	Acetate	234.5	21,000	A	281

TABLE II—*continued*

Formula	Compound	λ_{max}	Ext.	Sol.	Ref.
3,5-Dienol Acetates (cont.)					
$C_{23}H_{32}O_5$	3-Acetoxy-16α,17α-dihydroxy-3,5-pregnadien-20-one 16-Acetate	234	4.31	A	351
$C_{23}H_{32}O_6$	3-Acetoxy-16α,17α,21-trihydroxy-3,5-pregnadien-20-one 16,21-Diacetate	234	4.29	A	351
$C_{24}H_{34}O_5$	3-Acetoxy-21-hydroxy-16α-methoxy-3,5-pregnadien-20-one Acetate	235	19,700	IP	90
$C_{25}H_{34}O_4$	3,5,17(20)-Pregnatriene-3,20-diol-diacetate	235	4.23	A	98
	3,5,20-Pregnatriene-3,20-diol-diacetate	235	4.29	A	283
3,5-Dienol Ethers					
$C_{20}H_{28}O_2$	3-Ethoxy-19-nor-3,5-androstadien-17-one	242	4.26	A	393
		242	4.26	A	106
		242	4.2	A	95
$C_{21}H_{28}O_3$	3-Ethoxy-3,5-androstadiene-11,17-dione	241	19,400	A	43
		240	19,400	M	261
$C_{21}H_{29}O_2N$	17ξ-Cyano-3-ethoxy-19-nor-3,5-androstadien-17ξ-ol	242	4.2	A	95
$C_{22}H_{28}O_2$	*d,l*-3-Ethoxy-17a-methoxy-D-homo-18-nor-9β-3,5,13(17a),14,16-androstapentaene	241	4.37	A	212
$C_{22}H_{32}O_2$	3-Ethoxy-16β-methyl-3,5-androstadien-17-one	240	4.25	A	341
$C_{22}H_{32}O_3$	3-Ethoxy-17β-hydroxy-19-nor-17α-3,5-pregnadien-20-one Acetate	242	4.16	A	280
$C_{22}H_{34}O_2$	3-Ethoxy-16β-methyl-3,5-androstadien-17β-ol	240	4.28	A	341
$C_{23}H_{32}O_5$	3-Ethoxy-17α,21-dihydroxy-3,5-pregnadiene-11,20-dione 21-Acetate	242	4.27		305
$C_{23}H_{34}O_2$	3-Ethoxy-3,5,17(20)-pregnatrien-21-ol	241	4.3	A	318
$C_{23}H_{34}O_3$	17β-Carboxy-3-ethoxy-17α-methyl-3,5-androstadiene Methyl ester	241	4.1	A	131
$C_{26}H_{30}O_3$	3-Benzyloxy-3,5-androstadiene-11,17-dione	240–241.5	21,000	A	43
$C_{26}H_{34}O_3$	3-Benzyloxy-3,5-androstadiene-11β,17β-diol	240.5–241	22,300	A	43
$C_{26}H_{36}O_6F$	3-Ethoxy-9α-fluoro-11β,21-dihydroxy-16α,17α-isopropylidenedioxy-3,5-pregnadien-20-one 21-Acetate	241	4.31	A	334

TABLE II—*continued*

Formula	Compound	λ_{max}	Ext.	Sol.	Ref.
3,5-Dienol Ethers					
$C_{28}H_{34}O_2S$	3-Benzylthio-17α-methyl-3,5-androstadiene-17β-carboxylic acid				
	Methyl ester	269	4.06	A	131
3,5-Dienes-3-halo					
$C_{19}H_{27}OCl$	3-Chloro-3,5-androstadien-17β-ol	Chart			158
$C_{19}H_{27}OBr$	3-Bromo-3,5-andostadien-17β-ol	Chart			158
$C_{20}H_{27}OCl$	3-Chloro-19-nor-10ξ,14β,17α-3,5-pregnadien-20-one	243	19,000	A	29
3,5-Dienes-3-enamines					
$C_{23}H_{32}O_3N$	3-Morpholinyl-3,5-androstadiene-11,17-dione	269	21,300	E	194
$C_{23}H_{33}ON$	3-(1-Pyrrolidinyl)-3,5-androstadien-17-one	281		E	193
$C_{23}H_{35}ON$	3-(1-Pyrrolidinyl)-3,5-androstadien-17β-ol	280		E	193
$C_{24}H_{31}ON$	3-(2-Pyridinyl)-3,5-androstadien-17β-ol				
	Acetate	304	19,300		174
$C_{24}H_{34}ON$	3-(1-Pyrrolidinyl)-6-methyl-3,5-androstadien-17-one	281	17,900	M	72
		284	23,150	E	72
$C_{24}H_{35}O_2N$	11β-Hydroxy-11α-methyl-3-(1-pyrrolidinyl)-3,5-androstadien-17-one	281	4.35	E	333
$C_{24}H_{37}ON$	17α-methyl-3-(1-pyrrolidinyl)-3,5-androstadien-17β-ol	281		E	193
$C_{25}H_{33}O_3N$	3-(1-Pyrrolidinyl)-3,5,17(20)-*cis*-pregnatrien-11-one-21-oic-acid				
	Methyl ester	274	21,825	M	204
		225	14,550	AcM	204
$C_{25}H_{35}O_2N$	3-(1-Pyrrolidinyl)-3,5-pregnadiene-11,20-dione	282		E	193
$C_{25}H_{37}ON$	3-(1-Pyrrolidinyl)-3,5-pregnadien-20-one	281		E	193
$C_{25}H_{37}O_2N$	11α-Hydroxy-3-(1-pyrrolidinyl)-3,5-pregnadien-20-one	281		E	193
$C_{26}H_{35}O_3N$	3-(1-Pyrrolidinyl)-6-methyl-3,5,17(20)-pregnatrien-11-one-21-oic acid				
	Methyl ester	224	16,650	AcM	396
		272	21,450	M	396
		360	1200	M	396

TABLE II—*continued*

Formula	Compound	λ_{max}	Ext.	Sol.	Ref.
5,7-Dienes					
$C_{18}H_{26}O_2$	19-Nor-5,7-androstadiene-3β,17β-diol	272	4.05	A	445
		282–284	4.06	A	445
		296	3.80	A	445
		272	11,170	A	412
		283	11,650	A	412
		295	6580	A	412
$C_{19}H_{26}O_2$	3β-Hydroxy-5,7-androstadien-17-one iso-Caproate	270	10,330	A	293
		281	10,800	A	293
		293	6270	A	293
$C_{19}H_{28}O_2$	5,7-Androstadiene-3β,17β-diol 3-iso-Caproate,17-benzoate	229	14,800	A	295
		271	12,100	A	295
		281	12,300	A	295
		293	6500	A	295
$C_{21}H_{30}O_3$	3-Ethylenedioxy-5,7-androstadien-17β-ol	271	9850	A	17
		281	10,500	A	17
		293	6000	A	17
	Acetate	271	10,100	A	17
		281–281.5	10,600	A	17
		293	6100	A	17
	Benzoate	229	15,100	A	17
		271	12,800	A	17
		281	13,300	A	17
		293	7100	A	17
$C_{21}H_{30}O_2$	3β-Hydroxy-5,7-pregnadien-20-one	271	11,200	A	294
		282	12,000	A	294
		294	7000	A	294
	iso-Caproate	271.5	11,250	A	294
		282.5	12,000	A	294
		294.7	7000	A	294

TABLE II—*continued*

Formula	Compound	λ_{max}	Ext.	Sol.	Ref.
5,7-Dienes (cont.)					
$C_{23}H_{32}O_4$	3-Ethylenedioxy-21-hydroxy-5,7-pregnadien-20-one				
	Acetate	272	11,700	A	16
		282	12,600	A	16
		294	7500	A	16
$C_{25}H_{36}O_4$	3,20-Bisethylenedioxy-5,7-pregnadiene	271	10,800	A	16
		282	11,300	A	16
		294	6500	A	16
$C_{25}H_{36}O_6$	3,20-Bisethylenedioxy-5,7-pregnadiene-17α,21-diol	271	10,600		15
		281.5	11,200		15
		293	6500		15
	21-Acetate	271	9500		15
		281.5	10,100		15
		293	5900		15
7,9(11)-Dienes					
$C_{19}H_{28}O_2$	7,9(11)-Androstadiene-3β,17β-diol	236	4.20		189
		242	4.24		189
		250	4.06		189
	Diacetate	235	4.14		189
		242	4.18		189
		250	4.00		189
$C_{21}H_{28}O_2$	3β-Hydroxy-5α-7,9(11)-pregnadien-20-one				
	Acetate	235	14,500	A	361
		242.5	16,000	A	361
		251	10,400	A	361
$C_{21}H_{30}O_3$	3β,17α-Dihydroxy-5α-7,9(11)-pregnadien-20-one				
	3-Acetate	234	4.05	A	317
		242	4.11	A	317

TABLE II—*continued*

Formula	Compound	λ_{max}	Ext.	Sol.	Ref.
8(14),9(11)-Dienes					
$C_{21}H_{28}O_4$	17α,21-Dihydroxy-8(14),9(11)-pregnadiene-3,20-dione				
	21-Acetate	271	4600	M	423
		271	3800	A	156
	17α,21-Dihydroxy-5ξ-8(14),9(11)-pregnadiene-3,20-dione				
	21-Acetate	271	4600	M	167
8,14-Dienes					
$C_{21}H_{28}O_4$	17α,21-Dihydroxy-8,14-pregnadiene-3,20-dione				
	21-Acetate	246	21,500	M	423
	17α,21-Dihydroxy-5ξ-8,14-pregnadiene-3,20-dione				
	21-Acetate	246	21,500	M	167
8(14),15-Dienes					
$C_{20}H_{26}O_5$	17β-Carboxy-3β,11α-dihydroxy-8(14),15-etiocholadien-12-one				
	Diacetate, methyl ester	242	4.28	A	366
$C_{21}H_{32}O_3$	5α-8(14),15-Pregnadiene-3β,7ξ,20β-triol	247	3.90	A	249
15,17(20)-Dienes					
$C_{23}H_{32}O_3$	20-Acetoxy-5,15,17(20)-pregnatrien-3β-ol				
	Acetate	242	13,700	IP	90
16,20-Dienes-20-enol acetates					
$C_{22}H_{26}O_3$	20-Acetoxy-19-nor-1,3,5(10),16,20-pregnapentaen-3-ol				
	Acetate	238	4.15	A	101
		265(sh)			101
$C_{23}H_{32}O_3$	20-Acetoxy-5,16,20-pregnatrien-3β-ol				
	Formate	238	4.2	A	349
	Acetate	238	4.15	A	283
$C_{23}H_{34}O_3$	20-Acetoxy-5α-16,20-pregnadien-3β-ol				
	Acetate	238	4.19	A	283

TABLE II—*continued*

Formula	Compound	λ_{max}	Ext.	Sol.	Ref.
16,20-Dienes-20-enol acetates (cont.)					
$C_{23}H_{34}O_4$	20-Acetoxy-5α-16,20-pregnadiene-3β,6β-diol				
	Diacetate	238	4.18	A	348
Dienes-Cumulative					
$C_{22}H_{24}O_3$	*d,l*-3-Acetoxy-17a-methoxy-D-homo-18-nor-3,5,8,13(17a),14,16-androstahexaene	224	4.61	A	222
$C_{22}H_{26}O_2$	*d,l*-3-Ethoxy-17a-methoxy-D-homo-18-nor-3,5,8,13(17a),14,16-androstahexaene	227	4.58	A	222
Dienes–One double bond exocyclic					
$C_{20}H_{30}O$	3-Methylene-4-androsten-17β-ol	239	4.36	I	387
$C_{20}H_{30}O_2$	7-Methylene-5-androstene-3β,17β-diol				
	Diacetate	237	4.35	I	388
$C_{22}H_{32}O$	20-Methylene-5,16-pregnadien-3β-ol				
	Acetate	239	4.21	I	387

TABLE III. TRIENES

Formula	Compound	λ_{max}	Ext.	Sol.	Ref.
3,5,7-Trienes					
$C_{20}H_{26}O_3$	3-Acetoxy-19-nor-3,5,7-androstatrien-17β-ol				
	Acetate	300	4.32	A	445
		312	4.41	A	445
		328	4.27	A	445
		290	11,580	A	412
		300	18,000	A	412
		313	22,350	A	412
		327.5	16,200	A	412
	Benzoate	228	17,600	A	42
		302	18,200	A	42
		314	22,000	A	42
		329	15,500	A	42
5,7,9(11)-Trienes					
$C_{19}H_{24}O_2$	3β-Hydroxy-5,7,9(11)-androstatrien-17-one				
	iso-Caproate	321	9950	A	293
		311(inf)	11,250	A	293
		336	6950	A	293
$C_{19}H_{26}O_2$	5,7,9(11)-Androstatriene-3β,17β-diol	312	9500	A	293
		324	10,800	A	293
		338	6700	A	293
	17-Benzoate	227	16,900	A	295
		311(inf)	10,300	A	295
		323	10,700	A	295
		339(inf)	7400	A	295
	3-iso-Caproate	310	10,300	A	295
		324	11,600	A	295
		339	7200	A	295

TABLE III—*continued*

Formula	Compound	λ_{max}	Ext.	Sol.	Ref.
5,7,9(11)-Trienes (cont.)					
$C_{19}H_{26}O_2$	3-iso-Caproate,17-benzoate	227	17,100	A	295
		310	11,600	A	295
		324	12,100	A	295
		339	8200	A	295
$C_{21}H_{28}O_2$	3β-Hydroxy-5,7,9(11)-pregnatrien-20-one	313(inf)	9880	A	294
		324	11,000	A	294
		338(inf)	6900	A	294
$C_{25}H_{34}O_6$	3,20-Bisethylenedioxy-5,7,9(11)-pregnatriene-17α,21-diol				
	21-Acetate	312	8100	A	15
		325	9200	A	15
		340–341	5800	A	15
Misc.					
$C_{23}H_{32}O$	20-Ethinyl-5,20(21)-pregnadien-3β-ol				
	Acetate	223	10,500	A	379
$C_{40}H_{54}O_2$	Di-17-(5,16-androstadien-3β-ol)-acetylene	272	4.21	A	382
		285	4.14	A	382

TABLE IV. SIMPLE KETONES

Formula	Compound	λ_{max}	Ext.	Sol.	Ref.
1-Ones					
$C_{20}H_{30}O_3$	17β-Carboxy-etiocholan-1-one				
	Methyl ester	292–294	1.70	A	368
		220–240(sh)	2.4–2.0	A	368
	17β-Carboxy-androstan-1-one				
	Methyl ester	296	1.51		362
$C_{20}H_{30}O_4$	17β-Carboxy-14β-hydroxy-etiocholan-1-one				
	Methyl ester	293–294	1.66	A	368
		230–255(sh)	1.86–1.58	A	368
$C_{20}H_{32}O_2$	17β-Hydroxymethyl-androstan-1-one				
	Acetate	297	1.41	A	362
$C_{20}H_{32}O_3$	3β-Hydroxy-17β-hydroxymethyl-androstan-1-one				
	Diacetate	298	1.59	A	362
$C_{21}H_{34}O_3$	3β,20β-Dihydroxy-5α-pregnan-1-one				
	Diacetate	294	1.72	A	373
		294	1.72	A	374
	3β,20α-Dihydroxy-5α-pregnan-1-one				
	Diacetate	295	1.67	A	374
3-Ones					
$C_{18}H_{26}O_2$	17β-Hydroxy-5(10)-estren-3-one	282–289	36	A	437
$C_{20}H_{28}O_4$	17β-Carboxy-1α,2α-epoxy-androstan-3-one				
	Methyl ester	300	1.36	A	362
	17β-Carboxy-1ξ,2ξ-epoxy-etiocholan-3-one				
	Methyl ester	295	1.33	A	369
$C_{20}H_{30}O_3$	17β-Carboxy-etiocholan-3-one				
	Methyl ester	280–281	1.23	A	362
$C_{20}H_{30}O_4$	17β-Carboxy-1β-hydroxy-etiocholan-3-one				
	Methyl ester	276	1.27	A	369
	17β-Carboxy-7α-hydroxy-etiocholan-3-one				
	Acetate, methyl ester	275	1.45	A	231

TABLE IV—*continued*

Formula	Compound	λ_{max}	Ext.	Sol.	Ref.
7-Ones					
$C_{20}H_{30}O_4$	17β-Carboxy-3α-hydroxy-etiocholan-7-one				
	Acetate, methyl ester	288	1.42	A	231
11-Ones					
$C_{19}H_{28}O_3$	3β,17β-Dihydroxy-9β-7-androsten-11-one				
	Diacetate	295	1.98		190
$C_{20}H_{28}O_5$	17β-Carboxy-3β,12β-dihydroxy-14-etiocholan-11-one				
	Diacetate, methyl ester	211	3.32	A	244
		295	2.53	A	244
$C_{20}H_{30}O_5$	17β-Carboxy-3β,12β-dihydroxy-etiocholan-11-one				
	Methyl ester	288	1.60	A	367
	12-Acetate, methyl ester	288–290	1.61	A	367
	Diacetate, methyl ester	295	1.63	A	244
$C_{20}H_{30}O_6$	17β-Carboxy-3β,12β,14β-trihydroxy-etiocholan-11-one	292–293	1.62	A	367
	3,12-Diacetate, methyl ester	294	1.57	A	244
12-Ones					
$C_{20}H_{28}O_4$	17β-Carboxy-3β-hydroxy-14-etiocholen-12-one				
	Acetate, methyl ester	292	2.21		367
$C_{20}H_{28}O_6$	17β-Carboxy-3β,11α,15α-trihydroxy-8(14)-etiocholen-12-one				
	3,11-Diacetate, methyl ester	285	2.12		366
$C_{20}H_{30}O_4$	17β-Carboxy-3β-hydroxy-etiocholan-12-one				
	Acetate, methyl ester	288	1.70	A	367
$C_{20}H_{30}O_5$	17β-Carboxy-3α,7α-dihydroxy-etiocholan-12-one				
	Diacetate, methyl ester	288	1.70	A	231
	17β-Carboxy-3β,11β-dihydroxy-etiocholan-12-one				
	Diacetate, methyl ester	298	1.97	A	367
	17β-Carboxy-3β,14β-dihydroxy-etiocholan-12-one				
	3-Acetate, methyl ester	287–288	1.66	A	367

TABLE IV—*continued*

Formula	Compound	λ_{max}	Ext.	Sol.	Ref.
15-Ones					
$C_{22}H_{28}O_5$	*d,l*-18-Carboxy-3-ethylenedioxy-11β-hydroxy-14ξ-5-androsten-16-one-18′→ 11-lactone	285	20(approx.)	A	187
16-Ones					
$C_{21}H_{32}O_5$	3β-Hydroxy-5α-pregnan-16-one-21-oic acid				
	Hexahydrobenzoate, ethyl ester	280(chart)	1.7	A	76
17-Ones					
$C_{19}H_{26}O_2$	3-Methoxy-2,5(10)-estradien-17-one	278	76		86
$C_{19}H_{28}OBr_2$	16,16-Dibromo-androstan-17-one	320	1.91	A	376
$C_{19}H_{28}O_2$	3β-Hydroxy-5-androsten-17-one	292	45	A	116
	3β-Hydroxy-14-androsten-17-one	292	1.62	A	397
$C_{19}H_{28}O_3$	1ξ,3β-Dihydroxy-5-androsten-17-one				
	1-Acetate	294	34	A	62
	Diacetate	294	41	A	62
$C_{19}H_{29}OBr$	16α-Bromo-androstan-17-one	314	2.01	A	376
	16β-Bromo-androstan-17-one	312	1.90	A	376
$C_{19}H_{29}O_2Br$	16α-Bromo-3β-hydroxy-androstan-17-one	314	121	A	142
	Acetate	314	159	A	142
	16β-Bromo-3β-hydroxy-androstan-17-one	314	109	A	142
	Acetate	314	93	A	142
$C_{19}H_{30}O$	Androstan-17-one	292	1.72	A	376
$C_{19}H_{30}O_2$	3α-Hydroxy-androstan-17-one	294	48	A	116
	3β-Hydroxy-androstan-17-one				
	Acetate	294	48	A	142
$C_{19}H_{30}O_3$	3β,16α-Dihydroxy-androstan-17-one				
	Diacetate	302	80	A	217
	3β,16β-Dihydroxy-androstan-17-one				
	Diacetate	306	46	A	217
$C_{20}H_{31}O_3Br$	16β-Bromo-3β-hydroxy-15ξ-methoxy-androstan-17-one				
	Acetate	310	133	A	142

TABLE IV—*continued*

Formula	Compound	λ_{max}	Ext.	Sol.	Ref.
17a-Ones					
$C_{20}H_{30}O_2$	3β-Hydroxy-D-homo-5-androsten-17a-one				
	Acetate	292	1.55	A	362
$C_{20}H_{32}O_2$	3β-Hydroxy-D-homo-androstan-17a-one				
	Acetate	292	1.61	A	362
$C_{21}H_{34}O_2$	3β-Hydroxy-17α-methyl-D-homo-androstan-17a-one	290			362
20-Ones					
$C_{21}H_{30}O_3$	16α,17α-Epoxy-3β-hydroxy-5-pregnen-20-one	292	1.81	A	362
	Acetate	292	1.50	A	362
	3β,16α-Dihydroxy-17β-methyl-18-nor-17α-5,13-pregnadiene				
	3-Acetate, 16-formate	295	185	A	188
	Diacetate	295	180	A	188
$C_{21}H_{30}O_4$	16α,17α-Epoxy-3β,21-dihydroxy-5-pregnen-20-one				
	21-Acetate	292	1.73	A	362
	Diacetate	292	1.71	A	362
$C_{21}H_{32}O_2$	3β-Hydroxy-5-pregnen-20-one	284	1.79	M	365
	3α-Hydroxy-7-pregnen-20-one				
	Acetate	284	1.81	A	411
	3β-Hydroxy-8(14)-pregnen-20-one				
	Acetate	205	10,500	A	258
		282	60	A	258
$C_{21}H_{32}O_3$	16α,17α-Epoxy-3β-hydroxy-5α-pregnan-20-one				
	Acetate	299	1.6	A	66
		299	1.65		362
	1ξ,3β-Dihydroxy-5-pregnen-20-one				
	Diacetate	286	45	A	62
	3β,5α-Dihydroxy-6-pregnen-20-one	284	1.74	M	364
	3β,7α-Dihydroxy-5-pregnen-20-one	283	1.68		365

TABLE IV—*continued*

Formula	Compound	λ_{max}	Ext.	Sol.	Ref.
20-Ones (cont.)					
$C_{21}H_{32}O_3$	3β,21-Dihydroxy-5-pregnen-20-one				
	21-Acetate	284	1.82	A	362
	Diacetate	284	1.82	A	362
	3β,16α-Dihydroxy-17β-methyl-18-nor-17α-13-pregnen-20-one	295	150		188
$C_{21}H_{32}O_4$	3β-Hydroxy-5α-hydroperoxy-6-pregnen-20-one	282	1.79	M	364
	3β-Hydroxy-7α-hydroperoxy-5-pregnen-20-one	282	1.76	M	365
$C_{21}H_{32}O_5$	3β,16β,17α,21-Tetrahydroxy-5-pregnen-20-one				
	3,16,21-Triacetate	295	80		188
$C_{21}H_{34}O_2$	3β-Hydroxy-5α-pregnan-20-one	270	295	A	68
$C_{21}H_{34}O_3$	3β,5α-Dihydroxy-pregnan-20-one	284	1.82	M	368
	3β,16α-Dihydroxy-5α-pregnan-20-one	287	1.74	M-Ch (1 : 1)	290
	3β,21-Dihydroxy-pregnan-20-one				
	21-Acetate	283	1.88	A	362
	Diacetate	282.5	1.84	A	362
Misc.					
$C_{21}H_{28}O_6$	3β,12β,14β-Trihydroxy-pregnane-11,20-dione-21-oic acid-21 → 14-lactone, 3,12-Diacetate	358	1.54	A	244
$C_{21}H_{30}O_5$	1β,3β,14β-Trihydroxy-pregnan-20-one-21-oic acid-21 → 14-lactone, Diacetate	355	1.62	A	369
$C_{21}H_{30}O_8$	1β,3β,5β,11α,14β,19-Hexahydroxy-pregnan-20-one-21-oic acid-21 → 14-lactone, 1,3,11,19- Tetra-acetate	355	1.67	A	402
$C_{21}H_{32}O_2$	16α-Acetyl-5-androsten-3β-ol				
	Acetate	280	28	A	146
	16β-Acetyl-5-androsten-3β-ol				
	Acetate	280	40	A	146
$C_{21}H_{34}O_2$	16α-Acetyl-androstan-3β-ol				
	Acetate	280	50	A	146
	16β-Acetyl-androstan-3β-ol				
	Acetate	280	25	A	146

TABLE IV—*continued*

Formula	Compound	λ_{max}	Ext.	Sol.	Ref.
Cumulative Ketones					
1,20-Diones					
$C_{21}H_{32}O_2$	5α-Pregnane-1,20-dione	287	1.93	A	373
		287	1.93	A	374
3,17-Diones					
$C_{19}H_{28}O_2$	Androstane-3,17-dione	290	61	A	116
3,12-Diones					
$C_{20}H_{26}O_3$	17β-Carboxy-8(14)?-etiocholene-3,12-dione				
	Methyl ester	208	3.60	A	229
		285	1.83	A	229
3,20-Diones					
$C_{21}H_{30}O_3$	1α,2α-Epoxy-5α-pregnane-3,20-dione	290	1.87	A	373
$C_{21}H_{32}O_2S$	21-Thio-5α-pregnane-3,20-dione				
	Acetate	230.5	3.54	A	108
7,11-Diones					
$C_{19}H_{26}O_5$	8α,9α-Epoxy-3β,17β-dihydroxy-androstane-7,20-dione				
	Diacetate	280(sh)	1.80	A	192
		310	1.96	A	192
$C_{21}H_{32}O_4$	3β,20β-Dihydroxy-5α-pregnane-7,11-dione	294	1.90	A	350
11,20-Diones					
$C_{21}H_{32}O_4$	3β,12β-Dihydroxy-5α-pregnane-11,20-dione				
	Diacetate	288	1.94	A	287
$C_{23}H_{32}O_5$	3-Ethylenedioxy-17α-hydroxy-5-pregnene-11,20-dione	295	86	M	326

TABLE IV—*continued*

Formula	Compound	λ_{max}	Ext.	Sol.	Ref.
3,11,20-Triones					
$C_{21}H_{28}O_5Br_2$	2,2-Dibromo-17α,21-dihydroxy-5α-pregnane-3,11,20-trione				
	21-Acetate	206	3710	A	140
		292	422	A	140
	2ξ,4ξ-Dibromo-17α,21-dihydroxy-5α-pregnane-3,11,20-trione				
	21-Acetate	210	2580	A	140
		292	141	A	140
$C_{21}H_{29}O_5Br$	2ξ-Bromo-17α,21-dihydroxy-5α-pregnane-3,11,20-trione				
	21-Acetate	207	2320	A	140
		292	131	A	140
	4ξ-Bromo-17α,21-dihydroxy-5α-pregnane-3,11,20-trione				
	21-Acetate	292	122	A	140
$C_{21}H_{30}O_5$	17α,21-Dihydroxy-5α-pregnane-3,11,20-trione	295	249	A	140
3,7,11,20-Tetraones					
$C_{21}H_{28}O_4$	5α-Pregnane-3,7,11,20-tetraone	292	2.03	A	103

TABLE V. ENONES

Formula	Compound	λ_{max}	Ext.	Sol.	Ref.
1-en-3-Ones					
$C_{19}H_{24}O_3$	1-Androstene-3,11,17-trione	228	11,350	A	271
	1-Etiocholene-3,11,17-trione	224	9425	A	271
$C_{19}H_{27}O_2Br$	4β-Bromo-17β-hydroxy-1-etiocholen-3-one				
	Acetate	236	8480	A	224
$C_{19}H_{28}O_2$	17β-Hydroxy-1-androsten-3-one				
	Acetate	232	4.00		141
$C_{20}H_{26}O_7$	17β-Carboxy-5β,14β,19-trihydroxy-1-etiocholene-3,11-dione				
	Methyl ester	233	4.09	A	402
		305–310	1.75	A	402
$C_{20}H_{28}O_3$	17β-Carboxy-1-etiocholen-3-one				
	Methyl ester	231.5	4.12	A	369
		323	1.59	A	369
$C_{20}H_{28}O_7$	17β-Carboxy-5β,11α,14β,19-tetrahydroxy-1-etiocholen-3-one				
	11-Acetate, methyl ester	233	4.06	A	402
		315	1.55	A	402
$C_{21}H_{27}O_5Br$	2-Bromo-17α,21-dihydroxy-5α-1-pregnene-3,11,20-trione				
	21-Acetate	255	7500	A	140
	4β-Bromo-17α,21-dihydroxy-1-pregnene-3,11-20-trione				
	21-Acetate	229	7750	A	224
$C_{21}H_{28}O_5$	17α,21-Dihydroxy-1-pregnene-3,11,20-trione	224	8700	M	75
	17α,21-Dihydroxy-5α-1-pregnene-3,11,20-trione				
	21-Acetate	228	4.1	A	439
		228	4.24		305
		227	11,700	A	140
		225	9130	M	224
$C_{21}H_{28}O_5BrF$	2-Bromo-9α-fluoro-11β,17α,21-trihydroxy-5α-1-pregnene-3,20-dione				
	21-Acetate	250	8000	A	154
$C_{21}H_{29}O_5F$	9α-Fluoro-11β,17α,21-trihydroxy-5α-1-pregnene-3,20-dione				
	21-Acetate	222	4.03	M	201
		228	6100	A	154

TABLE V—*continued*

Formula	Compound	λ_{max}	Ext.	Sol.	Ref.
1-en-3-Ones (cont.)					
$C_{21}H_{30}O_2$	17β-Hydroxy-4,4-dimethyl-1,5-androstadien-3-one				
	Propionate	227	4.0	A	6
$C_{22}H_{32}O_2$	17β-Hydroxy-4,4,17α-trimethyl-1,5-androstadien-3-one	226–227	3.97	A	6
	Acetate	227	3.99	A	6
1(10)-en-2-Ones					
$C_{18}H_{26}O_2$	17β-Hydroxy-19-nor-1(10)-androsten-2-one	240	15,900		150
2-en-1-Ones					
$C_{20}H_{28}O_3$	17β-Carboxy-2-etiocholen-1-one				
	Methyl ester	225	3.93	A	368
		333	1.96	A	368
		225	3.93	A	362
		333	1.96	A	362
$C_{20}H_{30}O_2$	17β-Hydroxymethyl-2-androsten-1-one				
	Acetate	224	3.89	A	362
		333	1.74	A	362
		220	3.90	E	362
		340	1.68	E	362
$C_{21}H_{30}O_2$	5α-2-Pregnene-1,20-dione	226	3.89	A	373
		286	1.82	A	373
		335	1.75	A	373
		226	3.89	A	374
$C_{21}H_{32}O_2$	20β-Hydroxy-5α-2-pregnen-1-one				
	Acetate	224	3.91	A	373
		330	1.70	A	373
		225	3.98	A	374
		331	1.90	A	374

TABLE V—*continued*

Formula	Compound	λ_{max}	Ext.	Sol.	Ref.
2-en-1-Ones (cont.)					
$C_{21}H_{32}O_2$	20α-Hydroxy-5α-2-pregnen-1-one				
	Acetate	225	3.90	A	374
		333	1.79	A	374
4-en-3-Ones					
$C_{18}H_{22}O_2$	19-nor-4,7-androstadiene-3,17-dione	238	4.16	A	445
$C_{18}H_{22}O_3$	19-nor-4-androstene-3,6,17-trione	254	9550	A	320
	19-nor-4-androstene-3,11,17-trione	240	14,600	A	320
$C_{18}H_{24}O_2$	19-nor-4-androstene-3,17-dione	240	4.24	A	393
		239	16,900	A	437
		239	4.20		329
		240	4.24	A	106
$C_{18}H_{24}O_3$	10ξ-Hydroxy-19-nor-4-androstene-3,17-dione	235.5	14,025	A	320
$C_{18}H_{26}O_2$	17β-Hydroxy-19-nor-4-androsten-3-one	240.5	17,000	A	437
	Acetate	240	18,100	A	173
	Acetate, oxime	240	18,390	A	173
	Benzoate	235	29,450	A	173
	d,l-18,19-Bisnor-D-homo-4-androsten-3-one	240.5	17,000	A	216
$C_{18}H_{26}O_3$	6β,17β-Dihydroxy-19-nor-4-androsten-3-one	238	13,875	A	320
	Diacetate	236	13,550	A	320
	11α,17β-Dihydroxy-19-nor-4-androsten-3-one	242	15,475	A	320
	10β,17β-Dihydroxy-19-nor-4-androsten-3-one	234–236	4.12	A	359
	10ξ,17β-Dihydroxy-19-nor-4-androsten-3-one	237	15,025	A	320
$C_{19}H_{23}O_3F$	9α-Fluoro-4-androstene-3,11,17-trione	234	17,000	A	156
$C_{19}H_{24}O_2$	4,9(11)-Androstadiene-3,17-dione	238–239	14,800	A	46
		238	16,800	A	44
		240	16,925		194
$C_{19}H_{24}O_3$	4-Androstene-3,6,17-trione	250	10,600	A	13
	4-Androstene-3,11,17-trione	238	15,300	A	263
		238	15,100	A	184

TABLE V—*continued*

Formula	Compound	λ_{max}	Ext.	Sol.	Ref.
4-en-3-Ones (cont.)					
$C_{19}H_{24}O_3$	4-Androstene-3,15,17-trione	242	17,400	M	38
	9β,11β-Epoxy-4-androstene-3,17-dione	242.5–243	14,000	A	250
$C_{19}H_{24}O_4$	*d,l*-11β,18-Epoxy-18-hydroxy-4-androstene-3,16-dione	240	16,500	A	433
$C_{19}H_{25}O_2Br$	16α-Bromo-4-androstene-3,17-dione	239	4.179	A	147
		239.5	4.21	A	122
	16β-Bromo-4-androstene-3,17-dione	239	4.214	A	147
$C_{19}H_{25}O_2Br_2Cl$	2α,6β-Dibromo-4-chloro-17β-hydroxy-4-androsten-3-one	270	4.08	A	239
$C_{19}H_{25}O_2Cl$	4-Chloro-4-androstene-3,17-dione	254–255	4.19	IP	237
	16α-Chloro-4-androstene-3,17-dione	239.5	4.19	A	122
	16β-Chloro-4-androstene-3,17-dione	239.5	4.22	A	122
$C_{19}H_{25}O_2F$	6α-Fluoro-4-androstene-3,17-dione	234–236	4.19	A	58
	6β-Fluoro-4-androstene-3,17-dione	234	4.10	A	58
$C_{19}H_{25}O_2N$	17ξ-Cyano-17ξ-hydroxy-19-nor-4-androsten-3-one	240	4.2	A	95
$C_{19}H_{25}O_3Br$	9α-Bromo-11β-hydroxy-4-androstene-3,17-dione	242.5	16,200	A	250
$C_{19}H_{25}O_3Cl$	9α-Chloro-11β-hydroxy-4-androstene-3,17-dione	240	17,200	A	250
$C_{19}H_{25}O_3F$	9α-Fluoro-11β-hydroxy-4-androstene-3,17-dione	238	17,200	A	250
$C_{19}H_{26}O$	4,16-Androstadien-3-one	240	4.22	A	385
	17-Methyl-18-nor-4,17(18)-androstadien-3-one	240	4.23	A	385
$C_{19}H_{26}O_2$	18,19-Dinor-4-pregnene-3,20-dione	239.5	15,000	A	292
		240	17,900	M	211
		240	17,000	A	399
	1ξ-Methyl-19-nor-4-androstene-3,17-dione	242	4.16	A	339
	4-Androstene-3,17-dione	240	17,170	A	116
	8α-4-Androstene-3,17-dione	243	4.17	A	97
	13α-4-Androstene-3,17-dione	243	4.17	A	105
		240	17,250	A	56
	17β-Hydroxy-4,7-androstadien-3-one	238.5	15,100	A	17
	Benzoate	232–233	30,800	A	17
	16α,17α-Epoxy-4-androsten-3-one	240	4.22	A	385
	d,l,-18-Nor-D-homo-4-androstene-3,17a-dione	240	4.2	A	214
$C_{19}H_{26}O_2BrCl$	2ξ-Bromo-4-chloro-17β-hydroxy-4-androsten-3-one	260	4.08	A	239

TABLE V—*continued*

Formula	Compound	λ_{max}	Ext.	Sol.	Ref.
4-en-3-Ones (cont.)					
$C_{19}H_{26}O_2Cl_2$	1α,2β-Dichloro-17β-hydroxy-4-androsten-3-one	250	4.16	A	239
$C_{19}H_{26}O_3$	1α-Hydroxy-4-androstene-3,17-dione	240	15,000	M	112
	Acetate	239.5	16,500	M	112
	2α-Hydroxy-4-androstene-3,17-dione	241	4.21	A	353
	2β-Hydroxy-4-androstene-3,17-dione	242	14,200	M	112
	Acetate	243	15,300	M	112
	6α-Hydroxy-4-androstene-3,17-dione	239.5	16,170	A	23
		239	15,300	A	72
	Acetate	236	15,350	A	72
		235	15,520	A	23
	6β-Hydroxy-4-androstene-3,17-dione	235.5	13,550	A	23
		237	12,700	A	134
	Acetate	235	13,200	A	134
		235	12,480	A	23
	9α-Hydroxy-4-androstene-3,17-dione	242	14,400	A	135
		241	16,100	M	114
	11α-Hydroxy-4-androstene-3,17-dione	241	14,800	A	45
		242	14,600	A	134
	Acetate	238–239.5	15,500	A	44
	11β-Hydroxy-4-androstene-3,17-dione	240–241	15,300	A	43
	Acetate	239	16,000	M	301
	14α-Hydroxy-4-androstene-3,17-dione	241	16,100	A	135
	14ξ-Hydroxy-4-androstene-3,17-dione	240	4.18	A	397
	19-Hydroxy-4-androstene-3,17-dione	242	16,100	A	119
	Acetate	237.5		A	119
	17β-Hydroxy-4-androstene-3,6-dione	250	11,200	A	13
	17β-Hydroxy-4-androstene-3,11-dione	238	16,200	A	259
		238	14,400	A	184
		237.5	14,000	A	43
	Acetate	237–238	14,200	A	43
	17β-Hydroxy-4-androstene-3,16-dione	240.5	16,600	A	276

Table V—*continued*

K

Formula	Compound	λ_{max}	Ext.	Sol.	Ref.
4-en-3-Ones					
$C_{19}H_{26}O_3$	17α-Carboxy-19-nor-14β-4-androsten-3-one	240	18,360	A	25
	Methyl ester	239	14,900	A	25
	Ethyl ester	239	17,700	A	25
	17β-Carboxy-19-nor-4-androsten-3-one	240	4.23	A	394
	Methyl ester	240	4.24	A	394
	d,l-11β-Hydroxy-18-nor-D-homo-4-androstene,3,17a-dione	240	4.21	A	220
	Testololactone	237	17,900	A	157
$C_{19}H_{26}O_4$	6β,11β-Dihydroxy-4-androstene-3,17-dione	238	15,200	M	321
	9α,11β-Dihydroxy-4-androstene-3,17-dione	241–242	15,500	A	250
$C_{19}H_{26}O_5$	16 : 17-Seco-4-androsten-3-one-16,17-dioic acid				
	Dimethyl ester	239	4.24	IP	5
$C_{19}H_{27}O_2Br$	4-Bromo-17β-hydroxy-4-androsten-3-one	262	4.10	A	331
	Acetate	261	11,600		69
	Propionate	261	4.09	A	236
	16α-Bromo-17β-hydroxy-4-androsten-3-one	239	4.303	A	147
	Acetate	239	4.208	A	147
	16β-Bromo-17β-hydroxy-4-androsten-3-one	239	4.186	A	147
		240	4.22	A	122
	Acetate	239	4.190	A	147
$C_{19}H_{27}O_2Cl$	2α-Chloro-17β-hydroxy-4-androsten-3-one				
	Acetate	242	4.14	IP	123
	4-Chloro-17β-hydroxy-4-androsten-3-one	256	4.13	A	331
	Acetate	255	13,300		69
	Propionate	254	4.12	IP	237
	16α-Chloro-17β-hydroxy-4-androsten-3-one	240	4.2	A	122
	16β-Chloro-17β-hydroxy-4-androsten-3-one	240	4.2	A	122
$C_{19}H_{27}O_2F$	4-Fluoro-17β-hydroxy-4-androsten-3-one				
	Acetate	241	11,670		69
	6α-Fluoro-17β-hydroxy-4-androsten-3-one	236–238	4.16	A	58
	6β-Fluoro-17β-hydroxy-4-androsten-3-one	234	4.09	A	58

TABLE V—*continued*

Formula	Compound	λ_{max}	Ext.	Sol.	Ref.
4-en-3-Ones (cont.)					
$C_{19}H_{28}O_2$	17β-Hydroxy-4-methyl-19-nor-4-androsten-3-one	250	15,400	M	21
	Acetate	249.5	17,100	M	21
		249	15,300	A	173
	17β-Hydroxy-17α-methyl-19-nor-4-androsten-3-one	240	4.2	A	95
		240	4.23	A	106
	1ξ-Methyl-19-nor-4-androsten-3-one	242	4.15	A	339
	17β-Hydroxymethyl-19-nor-4-androsten-3-one	240	4.23	A	394
	17aβ-Hydroxy-19-nor-D-homo-4-androsten-3-one	241.5	17,000		51
	d,l-17aβ-Hydroxy-18-nor-D-homo-4-androsten-3-one				
	Acetate	241	4.22	A	214
	17β-Hydroxy-8α-4-androsten-3-one	242	4.18	A	97
		242	4.18	A	105
	17α-Hydroxy-13α-4-androsten-3-one	241	16,700	A	56
	17α-Hydroxy-4-androsten-3-one	240	4.23	A	385
	Acetate	240	4.22	A	385
	17β-Hydroxy-4-androsten-3-one	241	15,800	A	116
	Phosphate	240	16,900	A	159
	Dimethylphosphate	238	15,800	A	159
$C_{19}H_{28}O_3$	2α,17β-Dihydroxy-4-androsten-3-one	242	4.24	A	381
	17-Acetate	240	4.22	A	353
	Diacetate	240	4.24	A	381
	2β,17β-Dihydroxy-4-androsten-3-one				
	Diacetate	243	4.2	A	79
		242	4.23	A	381
	4,17β-Dihydroxy-4-androsten-3-one				
	17-Acetate	277	12,100		69
	Diacetate	246	15,500		69
	6β,17β-Dihydroxy-4-androsten-3-one	236	13,800	A	13
		238	13,700		134
	17-Acetate	236	4.14	A	347
	Diacetate	236	13,100	A	13

TABLE V—*continued*

Formula	Compound	λ_{max}	Ext.	Sol.	Ref.
4-en-3-Ones (cont.)					
$C_{19}H_{28}O_3$	11α,17β-Dihydroxy-4-androsten-3-one	243	14,275		134
	Diacetate	238–239	15,700	A	43
	11β,17β-Dihydroxy-4-androsten-3-one	242	16,600	A	259
		242	14,900	A	43
	17-Acetate	241	16,100	A	43
	Diacetate	237	15,900	M	301
	14α,17β-Dihydroxy-4-androsten-3-one	242	14,600	A	135
	17-Acetate	241	16,300	A	135
	16α,17β-Dihydroxy-4-androsten-3-one	240.5	4.2	IP	5
$C_{19}H_{28}O_4$	*d,l*-11β,17β,18-Trihydroxy-4-androsten-3-one	242	16,400	A	436
$C_{20}H_{24}O_2$	*d,l*-17a-Methoxy-D-homo-18-nor-4,13(17a),14,16-androstatetraen-3-one	232	4.32	A	222
		278(sh)	3.35	A	222
	d,l-17a-Methoxy-D-homo-18-nor-8α-4,13(17a),14,16-androstatetraen-3-one	231	4.21	A	222
		241	4.20	A	222
		278(sh)	3.28	A	222
	d,l-17a-Methoxy-D-homo-18-nor-9β-4,13(17a),14,16-androstatetraen-3-one	232	4.27	A	212
		240	4.26	A	212
		278(sh)	3.30	A	212
	d,l-17a-Methoxy-D-homo-18-nor-8α,9β-4,13(17a),14,16-androstatetraen-3-one	231	4.21	A	222
		243	4.21	A	222
		278(sh)	3.31	A	222
$C_{20}H_{24}O_4$	17β-Carboxy-11β, 18-epoxy-18-hydroxy-4-androsten-3-one-lactone	239		A	172
$C_{20}H_{24}O_5$	*d,l*-17α-Carboxy-11β-hydroxy-14β-4-androsten-3-one-18-oic acid-18 → 11-lactone				
	17-Methyl ester	238	17,400	A	434

TABLE V—*continued*

Formula	Compound	λ_{max}	Ext.	Sol.	Ref.
4-en-3-Ones (cont.)					
$C_{20}H_{24}O_5$	*d,l*-17β-Carboxy-11β-hydroxy-4-androsten-3-one-18-oic acid-18 → 11-lactone				
	17-Methyl ester	239	16,200	A	434
$C_{20}H_{26}O_2$	16-Methylene-4-androstene-3,17-dione	236	4.37	A	297
	17α-Ethinyl-17β-hydroxy-19-nor-4-androsten-3-one	240	4.24	A	393
		240	4.24	A	106
		240	4.2	A	95
$C_{20}H_{26}O_2Br_2$	2β,6β-Dibromo-2α-methyl-4-androstene-3,17-dione	251	4.11	A	209
$C_{20}H_{26}O_3$	19-Nor-4-pregnene-3,11,20-trione	240	4.20	A	57
	17α-Ethinyl-10β,17β-dihydroxy-19-nor-4-androsten-3-one	236	4.16	A	359
	17β-Carboxy-4, 9(11)-androstadien-3-one				
	Methyl ester	240	4.07	A	73
	17β-Carboxy-4,14-androstadien-3-one				
	Methyl ester	240	16,950	A	277
	17β-Carboxy-18-hydroxy-4-androsten-3-one-lactone	240			233
	D-Homo-4-androstene-3,11,17a-trione	239	15,400	A	80
$C_{20}H_{26}O_3Br_2$	17β-Carboxy-2ξ,6ξ-dibromo-4-androsten-3-one				
	Methyl ester	250	4.17	A	394
$C_{20}H_{26}O_4$	17β-Carboxy-19-formyl-19-nor-4-androsten-3-one				
	Ethyl ester	241	12,600	A	28
$C_{20}H_{26}O_5$	17α,21-Dihydroxy-19-nor-4-pregnene-3,11,20-trione	238	4.21	A	443
		238	4.21	A	444
$C_{20}H_{27}O_2N$	17β-Cyano-17α-hydroxy-4-androsten-3-one	240	4.20	A	136
$C_{20}H_{28}O$	19-Nor-4,17(20)-pregnadien-3-one	242	4.22		86
	17-Methylene-4-androsten-3-one	240	4.23	A	385
$C_{20}H_{28}O_2$	2α-Methyl-4-androstene-3,17-dione	242	4.22	A	209
	6α-Methyl-4-androstene-3,17-dione	242	15,650	A	72
		240	4.21	A	332
	6β-Methyl-4-androstene-3,17-dione	240	4.2	IP	1
		242	16,200	A	72
		242	4.19	A	332

TABLE V—*continued*

Formula	Compound	λ_{max}	Ext.	Sol.	Ref.
4-en-3-Ones (cont.)					
$C_{20}H_{28}O_2$	16β-Methyl-4-androstene-3,17-dione	240	4.22	A	341
		240	4.23	A	297
	16-Methylene-17β-hydroxy-4-androsten-3-one	240	4.22	A	297
	Acetate	240	4.24	A	297
	17α,20-Epoxy-21-nor-4-pregnen-3-one	240	4.24	A	385
	17β-Hydroxy-17α-vinyl-19-nor-4-androsten-3-one	240	4.25	A	393
		240	4.23	A	394
	19-Nor-4-pregnene-3,20-dione	240	4.24	A	107
	19-Nor-10ξ,14β,17α-4-pregnene-3,20-dione	240	16,000	A	29
$C_{20}H_{28}O_3$	16α-Carboxy-4-androsten-3-one	241	11,500	A	146
	16β-Carboxy-4-androsten-3-one	241	15,500	A	146
	11β-Hydroxy-11α-methyl-4-androstene-3,17-dione	243	4.19	A	333
	17β-Hydroxy-17α-methyl-4-androstene-3,6-dione	251	8,350	A	134
	17β-Hydroxy-17α-methyl-4-androstene-3,11-dione	239	13,300	A	134
	11α-Hydroxy-19-nor-4-pregnene-3,20-dione	242	4.22	A	57
	11β-Hydroxy-19-nor-4-pregnene-3,20-dione	242	4.20	A	57
	17α-Hydroxy-19-nor-4-pregnene-3,20-dione	240	4.23	A	443
		240	4.23	A	444
	21-Hydroxy-19-nor-4-pregnene-3,20-dione	240	4.24	A	393
		240	4.24	A	394
	Acetate	240	4.26	A	393
		240	4.24	A	394
	17β-Hydroxy-19-nor-17α-4-pregnene-3,20-dione				
	Acetate	240	4.23	A	280
	21-Hydroxy-19-nor-10ξ,14β,17α-4-pregnene-3,20-dione	240	15,600	A	29
	Acetate	240	17,000	A	29
	17aβ-Hydroxy-D-homo-4-androstene-3,11-dione	238	16,100	A	80
	Benzoate	232	27,700	A	80
	Propionate	239	15,400	A	80
$C_{20}H_{28}O_4$	17β-Carboxy-7α-hydroxy-4-androsten-3-one	243	15,100	A	277
	Acetate, methyl ester	238	15,900	A	277

TABLE V—*continued*

Formula	Compound	λ_{max}	Ext.	Sol.	Ref.
4-en-3-Ones (cont.)					
$C_{20}H_{28}O_4$	17β-Carboxy-15β-hydroxy-4-androsten-3-one				
	Methyl ester	241	16,900	A	277
	17α-Carboxy-19-hydroxy-14β-4-androsten-3-one	243	19,300	A	120
	Acetate	239	15,100	A	120
	Methyl ester	243	16,300	A	120
	Ethyl ester	243	19,100	A	120
	Acetate, methyl ester	239	16,900	A	120
	Acetate, ethyl ester	239	18,100	A	120
	17β-Carboxy-19-hydroxy-4-androsten-3-one	242	15,000	A	180
	Methyl ester	242	14,000	A	180
	Amide	242	13,300	A	26
	17β-Carboxy-11α-hydroxy-4-androsten-3-one				
	Acetate, methyl ester	240	4.23	A	330
	11β,21-Dihydroxy-19-nor-4-pregnene-3,20-dione	241	4.21	A	444
		241	4.21	A	443
	21-Acetate	240	4.23	A	444
		240	4.22	A	443
$C_{20}H_{28}O_5$	11β,17α,21-Trihydroxy-19-nor-4-pregnene-3,20-dione	241	4.23	A	443
		241	4.21	A	253
		242	4.21	A	256
		241	4.23	A	444
$C_{20}H_{29}O_2Br$	2α-Bromo-17β-hydroxy-17α-methyl-4-androsten-3-one	244	4.15	IP	123
	4-Bromo-17β-hydroxy-17α-methyl-4-androsten-3-one	262	4.06	A	331
$C_{20}H_{29}O_2Cl$	2α-Chloro-17β-hydroxy-17α-methyl-4-androsten-3-one	243	4.10	IP	123
	4-Chloro-17β-hydroxy-17α-methyl-4-androsten-3-one	255–256	4.14	IP	237
		256	4.12	A	331
$C_{20}H_{29}O_3F$	9α-Fluoro-11β,17β-Dihydroxy-17α-methyl-4-androsten-3-one	240	16,700	A	177
$C_{20}H_{30}O$	17β-Methyl-4-androsten-3-one	241	14,400	A	176
$C_{20}H_{30}O_2$	17β-Hydroxy-17α-ethyl-19-nor-4-androsten-3-one	240	4.22		86
	20ξ-Hydroxy-19-nor-4-pregnen-3-one	240	4.25	A	107
	17β-Hydroxy-2α-methyl-4-androsten-3-one	242	4.19	A	335

TABLE V—*continued*

Formula	Compound	λ_{max}	Ext.	Sol.	Ref.
4-en-3-Ones (cont.)					
$C_{20}H_{30}O_2$	17β-Hydroxy-4-methyl-4-androsten-3-one	250	4.21	A	336
		251	4.16	A	386
		250	14,200	M	21
	Acetate	251	4.17	A	386
	17β-Hydroxy-6α-methyl-4-androsten-3-one	242	15,150	A	72
		242	4.2	A	332
		241	4.2	IP	1
	17β-Hydroxy-6β-methyl-4-androsten-3-one	242	16,200	A	72
		242	4.19	A	332
		241–242	4.19	IP	1
	17α-Hydroxy-16β-methyl-4-androsten-3-one	240	4.35	A	341
	Acetate	240	4.32	A	341
	Propionate	240	4.30	A	341
	17β-Hydroxy-16β-methyl-4-androsten-3-one	240	4.23	A	297
		240	4.27	A	341
	17α-Hydroxy-17β-methyl-4-androsten-3-one	240	4.23	A	385
	20ξ-Hydroxy-19-nor-4-pregnen-3-one				
	Acetate	240	4.25	A	107
	17β(?)-Hydroxy-8β,14α-dimethyl-18-nor-4-androsten-3-one	242	19,300	A	91
$C_{20}H_{30}O_3$	2α,17β-Dihydroxy-17α-methyl-4-androsten-3-one				
	2-Acetate	241	15,600	M	24
	6β,17β-Dihydroxy-17α-methyl-4-androsten-3-one	238	13,600		134
	11β,17β-Dihydroxy-11α-methyl-4-androsten-3-one	244	4.18	A	333
	11α,17β-Dihydroxy-17α-methyl-4-androsten-3-one	243	14,700	A	134
	11β,17β-Dihydroxy-17α-methyl-4-androsten-3-one	243	15,575	A	177
	17α-Hydroxy-17β-hydroxymethyl-4-androsten-3-one	240	4.23	A	385
	11β,17β-Dihydroxy-1-(α-hydroxyethyl)-19-nor-4-androsten-3-one	247	15,000	A	253
$C_{21}H_{24}O_5$	*d,l*-16α,17α-Epoxy-11β-hydroxy-4-pregnene-3,20-dione-18-oic-acid-18 → 11-lactone	238	16,750	A	435
$C_{21}H_{26}O_3$	17β-Hydroxy-17α-ethinyl-4-androstene-3,11-dione	238	15,000	M	261
		238	15,300	A	413

TABLE V—*continued*

Formula	Compound	λ_{max}	Ext.	Sol.	Ref.
4-en-3-Ones (cont.)					
$C_{21}H_{26}O_3$	4,9(11)-Pregnadien-21-al-3,20-dione 21,21-Dimethylacetal	238	4.23	M	406
$C_{21}H_{26}O_4$	*d,l*-11β-Hydroxy-17α-4-pregnene-3,20-dione-18-oic-acid-18 → 11-lactone	238	17,200	A	371
	d,l-11β-Hydroxy-14β,17α-4-pregnene-3,20-dione-18-oic acid-18 → 11-lactone	239	16,200	A	370
	d,l-11β-Hydroxy-4-pregnene-3,20-dione-18-oic acid-18 → 11-lactone	238	14,300	A	370
	4,16-Pregnadiene-3,11-dione-21-oic acid Methyl ester	239	15,450	A	204
	4-Pregnen-21-al-3,11,20-trione	238	15,300	M	48
	Dimethylacetal	236	15,600	A	163
		238	15,100	M	265
	Dibenzylacetal	238	4.24	A	260
	16α,17α-Epoxy-4-pregnene-3,11,20-trione	239	15,600	A	323
		238	4.18		137
	16α,17α-Epoxy-4-pregnene-3,12,20-trione	238.5	16,190	M	358
	13α,21-Epoxy-17β-methyl-18-nor-17β-4-pregnene-3-20,dione	236	15,200	A	195
	4-Pregnene-3,6,11,20-tetraone	247	10,250	A	67
		257	12,120	BA	67
	4-Pregnene-3,11,15,20-tetraone	238	4.18	A	372
	4-Pregnene-3,12,15,20-tetraone	238	4.2	A	372
$C_{21}H_{26}O_5$	17α-Hydroxy-4-pregnen-21-al-3,11,20-trione	238	$E^{1\%}_{1cm.}$ 437	Ch	247
		450	$E^{1\%}_{1cm.}$ 107	Ch	247
	Hydrate	238	15,700	M	340
		238	$E^{1\%}_{1cm.}$ 418	M	247
	Dimethylacetal	240	$E^{1\%}_{1cm.}$ 387	M	247
	Diethylacetal	238	$E^{1\%}_{1cm.}$ 372	M	247
	Diacetylacetal	238	$E^{1\%}_{1cm.}$ 321	M	247
	Quinazolone	238	$E^{1\%}_{1cm.}$ 1045	M	247
		319	$E^{1\%}_{1cm.}$ 185	M	247
	Potassium bisulphite addition compound	245	$E^{1\%}_{1cm.}$ 349	W	247

TABLE V—*continued*

Formula	Compound	λ_{max}	Ext.	Sol.	Ref.
4-en-3-Ones (cont.)					
$C_{21}H_{26}O_5$	Sodium bisulphite addition compound	238	$E_{1cm.}^{1\%}$ 342	M	247
		245	$E_{1cm.}^{1\%}$ 354	W	247
	16α,17α-Epoxy-21-hydroxy-4-pregnene-3,11,20-trione				
	Acetate	238	15,500	M	228
		238	16,550	M	269
	16α,17α-Epoxy-21-hydroxy-4-pregnene-3,12,20-trione				
	Acetate	237	17,200	M	358
	17α,21-Dihydroxy-9ξ-4,8(14)-pregnadiene-3,11,20-trione				
	21-Acetate	239	15,650	M	420
	17α,21-Dihydroxy-4,8(14)-pregnadiene-3,11,20-trione				
	21-Acetate	239	15,650	M	423
	17,21-Diacetate	238	15,100	M	423
	11β,17α,21-Trihydroxy-4,14-pregnadiene-3,20-dione				
	21-Acetate	242	4.21	A	7
	d,l-11β,21-Dihydroxy-4-pregnene-3,20-dione-18-oic acid-18 → 11-lactone, 21-Acetate	238	17,400	A	371
	d,l-11β,21-Dihydroxy-14β,17α-4-pregnene-3,20-dione-18-oic acid-18 → 11-lactone	238	17,250	A	434
$C_{21}H_{26}O_5ClF$	6α-Chloro-9α-fluoro-17α,21-dihydroxy-4-pregnene-3,11,20-trione				
	21-Acetate	230	4.16	A	334
	6β-Chloro-9α-fluoro-17α,21-dihydroxy-4-pregnene-3,11,20-trione				
	21-Acetate	234	4.18	A	334
$C_{21}H_{26}O_6$	6α,7α-Epoxy-17α,21-dihydroxy-4-pregnene-3,11,20-trione				
	21-Acetate	238	13,000	M	302
	8ξ,14ξ-Epoxy-17α,21-dihydroxy-4-pregnene-3,11,20-trione	240	12,700	M	423
	21-Acetate	238	14,600	M	423
	Diacetate	238	16,600	M	423
	14α,15α-Epoxy-17α,21-dihydroxy-4-pregnene-3,11,20-trione				
	21-Acetate	237	4.22	A	7
	17α,21-Dihydroxy-4-pregnene-3,6,11,20-tetraone				
	21-Acetate	245	4.04	A	383

TABLE V—*continued*

Formula	Compound	λ_{max}	Ext.	Sol.	Ref.
4-en-3-Ones (cont.)					
$C_{21}H_{27}O_2Cl_3$	21,21,21-Trichloro-4-pregnene-3,20-dione	240	17,300		234
$C_{21}H_{27}O_3Br$	4-Bromo-4-pregnene-3,11,20-trione	258–259	4.00		236
	17α-Bromo-4-pregnene-3,11,20-trione	239	16,625	A	257
$C_{21}H_{27}O_3Cl$	4-Chloro-4-pregnene-3,11,20-trione	257	4.12	A	237
$C_{21}H_{27}O_3F$	12α-Fluoro-4-pregnene-3,11,20-trione	236	16,500	A	179
$C_{21}H_{27}O_4Cl$	9α-Chloro-11β-hydroxy-4-pregnen-21-al-3,20-dione				
	Dimethylacetal	240	17,800	A	156
$C_{21}H_{27}O_4Br$	16β-Bromo-17α-hydroxy-4-pregnene-3,12,20-trione	238.3	18,000	M	358
$C_{21}H_{27}O_4F$	13α,21-Epoxy-9α-fluoro-11β-hydroxy-17β-methyl-18-nor-17α-4-pregnene-3,20-dione	237	17,700	A	178
	17α,21-Epoxy-9α-fluoro-11β-hydroxy-4-pregnene-3,20-dione	237	18,300	A	178
	9α-Fluoro-11β-hydroxy-4-pregnen-21-al-3,20-dione				
	Dimethylacetal	237	16,800	A	156
	12α-Fluoro-21-hydroxy-4-pregnene-3,11,20-trione				
	21-Acetate	237	15,800	A	404
		237	15,800	M	405
$C_{21}H_{27}O_5Br$	6ξ-Bromo-17α,21-dihydroxy-4-pregnene-3,11,20-trione				
	21-Acetate	243	13,200	A	266
	9α-Bromo-17α,21-dihydroxy-4-pregnene-3,11,20-trione				
	21-Acetate	237	16,100	A	156
	16β-Bromo-17α,21-dihydroxy-4-pregnene-3,11,20-trione				
	21-Acetate	238	15,700	M	228
$C_{21}H_{27}O_5Cl$	4-Chloro-17α,21-dihydroxy-4-pregnene-3,11,20-trione	254	4.11	A	331
	21-Acetate	253	4.11	A	237
	6α-Chloro-17α,21-dihydroxy-4-pregnene-3,11,20-trione				
	21-Acetate	233	4.16	A	334
	6β-Chloro-17α,21-dihydroxy-4-pregnene-3,11,20-trione				
	21-Acetate	237	4.16	A	334
	9α-Chloro-17α,21-dihydroxy-4-pregnene-3,11,20-trione				
	21-Acetate	236	16,600	A	156

TABLE V—*continued*

Formula	Compound	λ_{max}	Ext.	Sol.	Ref.
4-en-3-Ones (cont.)					
$C_{21}H_{27}O_5Cl$	12α-Chloro-17α,21-dihydroxy-4-pregnene-3,11,20-trione	237	12,700	A	155
	21-Acetate	236	14,000	A	155
	16β-Chloro-17α,21-dihydroxy-4-pregnene-3,11,20-trione				
	21-Acetate	238	15,700	M	47
$C_{21}H_{27}O_5F$	6α-Fluoro-17α,21-dihydroxy-4-pregnene-3,11,20-trione				
	21-Acetate	233	4.21	A	60
	Diacetate	233	4.20	A	60
	6β-Fluoro-17α,21-dihydroxy-4-pregnene-3,11,20-trione				
	Diacetate	230	4.09	A	60
	9α-Fluoro-17α,21-dihydroxy-4-pregnene-3,11,20-trione	234	16,000	A	156
	21-Acetate	234	17,000	A	156
$C_{21}H_{27}O_6Br$	6β-Bromo-7α,17α,21-trihydroxy-4-pregnene-3,11,20-trione				
	21-Acetate	240	12,000	M	302
	15β-Bromo-14α,17α,21-trihydroxy-4-pregnene-3,11,20-trione				
	21-Acetate	237	4.21	A	7
$C_{21}H_{27}O_6Cl$	15β-Chloro-14α,17α,21-trihydroxy-4-pregnene-3,11,20-trione				
	21-Acetate	237	4.21	A	7
$C_{21}H_{27}O_6F$	9αFluoro-16α,17α,21-trihydroxy-4-pregnene-3,11,20 trione				
	16,21-Diacetate	235	15,100	A	407
$C_{21}H_{28}O_2$	17α-Ethinyl-17β-hydroxy-1ξ-methyl-19-nor-4-androsten-3-one	242	4.16	A	339
	17α-Ethinyl-17β-hydroxy-4-androsten-3-one	240	16,400	A	116
	4,7-Pregnadiene-3,20-dione	237	15,700	A	16
		238	4.28		109
	4,9(11)-Pregnadiene-3,20-dione	240	4.15	A	360
		240	4.22	A	352
	4,11-Pregnadiene-3,20-dione	239	4.2	A	232
$C_{21}H_{28}O_3$	17β-Carboxy-17α-methyl-4,11-androstadien-3-one				
	Methyl ester	239	4.27	A	130
	17α-Ethinyl-11β,17β-dihydroxy-4-androsten-3-one	242	16,000	M	261
		242	15,800	A	413
	17-Acetate	242	15,800	M	261

TABLE V—*continued*

Formula	Compound	λ_{max}	Ext.	Sol.	Ref.
4-en-3-Ones (cont.)					
$C_{21}H_{28}O_3$	17β-Hydroxy-17α-vinyl-4-androstene-3,11-dione	237.5	16,000	M	261
	17-Ethylenedioxy-4,9(11)-androstadien-3-one	239	16,500	A	44
	4-Pregnen-21-al-3,20-dione				
	21,21-Dibenzylacetal	240	4.23	A	260
	11β,12β-Epoxy-4-pregnene-3,20-dione	238	16,300	A	179
	19-Formyl-19-nor-4-pregnene-3,20-dione	241	11,250	A	28
	21-Hydroxy-4,7-pregnadiene-3,20-dione				
	Acetate	237–238	13,800	A	16
	4-Pregnene-3,6,20-trione	250	10,600	A	13
	4-Pregnene-3,16,20-trione	240	16,900	A	41
		285	5430	A	41
$C_{21}H_{28}O_3N_2$	21-Diazo-19-hydroxy-14β-4-pregnene-3,20-dione	243	14,800	A	120
$C_{21}H_{28}O_4$	16α,17α-Epoxy-11α-hydroxy-4-pregnene-3,20-dione	242	15,300	A	323
		242	4.15		137
	Acetate	240	4.18		137
	13α,21-Epoxy-11β-hydroxy-17β-methyl-18-nor-17α-4-pregnene-3,20-dione	240	16,800	A	178
	17α,21-Epoxy-11β-hydroxy-4-pregnene-3,20-dione	241	16,300	A	178
	11β-Hydroxy-4-pregnen-21-al-3,20-dione				
	21,21-Dimethylacetal	242	4.21	M	406
	21,21-Dibenzylacetal	240	4.24	A	260
	17α-hydroxy-4-pregnene-3,12,20-trione	238.5	16,190	M	358
	17α,21-Dihydroxy-4,7-pregnadiene-3,20-dione	238–239	14,800		15
	21-Acetate	238–239	14,000		15
	17α,21-Dihydroxy-4,9(11)-pregnadiene-3,20-dione	237.5–239	16,000	A	46
		239	17,600	A	156
	21-Acetate	238	16,500	A	156
		240	$E^{1\%}_{1cm.}$ 407	M	166
		238.5–240	16,600	A	132
	21-Acetate, 17-formate	238	16,400	A	156
	17α,21-Dihydroxy-4,14-pregnadiene-3,20-dione	240	4.21	A	55

TABLE V—*continued*

Formula	Compound	λ_{max}	Ext.	Sol.	Ref.
4-en-3-Ones (cont.)					
$C_{21}H_{28}O_4$	11β,12β-Epoxy-21-hydroxy-4-pregnene-3,20-dione				
	21-Acetate	238.5	17,400	A	404
		238.5	17,400	M	405
	17α-Hydroxy-4-pregnene-3,6,20-trione	248	9000	A	273
		312	1000	A	273
	21-Hydroxy-4-pregnene-3,6,20-trione				
	Acetate	250	10,800	A	13
	21-Hydroxy-19-formyl-19-nor-4-pregnene-3,20-dione	245	12,000	A	28
	Acetate	243	12,000	A	28
$C_{21}H_{28}O_4ClF$	21-Chloro-9α-fluoro-11β,17α-dihydroxy-4-pregnene-3,20-dione	238	17,700		178
$C_{21}H_{28}O_4F_2$	9α,21-Difluoro-11β,17α-dihydroxy-4-pregnene-3,20-dione	239	16,400	A	178
$C_{21}H_{28}O_4S$	17α-Hydroxy-21-thio-4-pregnene-3,11,20-trione				
	21-Acetate	236	4.39	A	108
$C_{21}H_{28}O_5$	Aldosterone				
	21-Acetate	240	16,400	A	172
	20,20,21-Trihydroxy-4-pregnen-3-one-18-oic acid-18 → 20 lactone	241	4.24		291
	11β,17α-Dihydroxy-4-pregnen-21-al-3,20-dione				
	Hydrate	242	16,000	M	340
		244	$E^{1\%}_{1cm.}$ 423	M	247
	Quinazolone	237	$E^{1\%}_{1cm.}$ 985	M	247
		318	$E^{1\%}_{1cm.}$ 185	M	247
	9α,11α-Epoxy-17α,21-dihydroxy-4-pregnene-3,20-dione				
	21-Acetate	238	16,000	A	156
	9β,11β-Epoxy-17α,21-dihydroxy-4-pregnene-3,20-dione	243	14,500	A	156
	21-Acetate	243	15,500	A	156
		244	4.17	A	55
		242	13,800	A	252
	14α,15α-Epoxy-17α,21-dihydroxy-4-pregnene-3,20-dione	239	4.24	A	55
	d,l-18,20-Epoxy-17α,20-dihydroxy-4-pregnene-3,11-dione	238	15,000	A	435

TABLE V—*continued*

Formula	Compound	λ_{max}	Ext.	Sol.	Ref.
4-en-3-Ones (cont.)					
$C_{21}H_{28}O_5$	11β,17α,21-Trihydroxy-4,8-pregnadiene-3,20-dione				
	21-Acetate	238	16,400	M	423
	11,21-Diacetate	237	16,000	M	423
	11β,17α,21-Trihydroxy-4,8(14)-pregnadiene-3,20-dione				
	21-Acetate	240	17,200	M	423
		239	20,000	M	156
		238	4.21	M	420
	11-Propionate, 21-Acetate	238	18,200	A	156
	11-Mesylate, 21-Acetate	237	17,800	A	156
	11β,17α,21-Trihydroxy-9ξ-4,8(14)-pregnadiene-3,20-dione				
	21-Acetate	240	17,200	M	420
	16β,21-Epoxy-11β,17α-dihydroxy-4-pregnene-3,20-dione	241	15,900	A	11
	17α,21-Dihydroxy-4-pregnene-3,6,20-trione				
	21-Acetate	250	4.05	A	383
	12α,21-Dihydroxy-4-pregnene-3,11,20-trione				
	Diacetate	238	16,000	M	405
	16α,21-Dihydroxy-4-pregnene-3,11,20-trione				
	21-Acetate	238	16,326	M	228
	17α,21-Dihydroxy-4-pregnene-3,11,20-trione	238	16,000	A	116
	21-Dibenzylphosphate	238	16,700	M	92
	21-Dihydrogenphosphate	244	15,900	W	327
		238	14,700	M	92
	21-Dimethylphosphate	238	15,600	M	327
	21-Disodiumphosphate	238	13,100	M	92
	17α,21-Dihydroxy-4-pregnene-3,12,20-trione	239	16,846	M	227
	21-Acetate	238	4.23		4
		238	16,773	M	227
$C_{21}H_{28}O_5BrF$	2ξ-Bromo-9α-fluoro-11β,17α,21-trihydroxy-4-pregnene-3,20-dione				
	21-Acetate	242	12,200	A	154
$C_{21}H_{28}O_5ClF$	6α-Chloro-9α-fluoro-11β,17α,21-trihydroxy-4-pregnene-3,20-dione				
	21-Acetate	234	4.11	A	334

TABLE V—*continued*

Formula	Compound	λ_{max}	Ext.	Sol.	Ref.
4-en-3-ones (cont.)					
$C_{21}H_{28}O_5ClF$	6β-Chloro-9α-fluoro-11β,17α,21-trihydroxy-4-pregnene-3,20-dione				
	21-Acetate	238	4.17	A	334
$C_{21}H_{28}O_6$	8ξ,14ξ-Epoxy-11β,17α,21-trihydroxy-4-pregnene-3,20-dione				
	21-Acetate	242	14,000	M	423
	14α,15α-Epoxy-11β,17α,21-trihydroxy-4-pregnene-3,20-dione	239	4.23	A	7
	21-Acetate	240	4.21	A	7
	2α,17α,21-Trihydroxy-4-pregnene-3,11,20-trione	237	4.21	A	353
	21-Trimethylacetate	237	12,600	M	24
	2-Acetate,21-trimethylacetate	238	15,400	M	24
	2,17,21-Triacetate	237	4.21	A	353
	6β,17α,21-Trihydroxy-4-pregnene-3,11,20-trione	232	4.14	A	383
	6,21-Diacetate	232	4.13	A	383
	7α,17α,21-Trihydroxy-4-pregnene-3,11,20-trione				
	21-Acetate	238	15,000	M	302
	9α,17α,21-Trihydroxy-4-pregnene-3,11,20-trione				
	21-Acetate	238	15,620	M	423
		238	16,500	A	156
	14α,17α,21-Trihydroxy-4-pregnene-3,11,20-trione	237	4.20	A	7
	21-Acetate	237	4.22	A	7
	16α,17α,21-Trihydroxy-4-pregnene-3,11,20-trione	237–238	16,500	A	10
	21-Acetate	238	15,900		121
	16,21-Diacetate	237–238	16,400	A	10
$C_{21}H_{29}O_2Br$	4-Bromo-4-pregnene-3,20-dione	261	4.07	A	236
		260	4.07	A	331
	6ξ-Bromo-4-pregnene-3,20-dione	248	4.22	A	381
	17α-Bromo-4-pregnene-3,20-dione	241	4.2	A	129
$C_{21}H_{29}O_2Cl$	4-Chloro-4-pregnene-3,20-dione	255	4.125	IP	237
		256	4.15	A	331
	21-Chloro-4-pregnene-3,20-dione	240	4.14	A	131
$C_{21}H_{29}O_2Cl_3$	21,21,21-Trichloro-20ξ-hydroxy-4-pregnen-3-one	240	16,500		234

TABLE V—*continued*

Formula	Compound	λ_{max}	Ext.	Sol.	Ref.
4-en-3-Ones (cont.)					
$C_{21}H_{29}O_2F$	6α-Fluoro-4-pregnene-3,20-dione	236	4.19	A	58
	6β-Fluoro-4-pregnene-3,20-dione	234-236	4.12	A	58
$C_{21}H_{29}O_3Br$	4-Bromo-17α-hydroxy-4-pregnene-3,20-dione	259	4.04	A	236
	Acetate	260	4.08	A	331
	12α-Bromo-11β-hydroxy-4-pregnene-3,20-dione	239	16,000	A	179
	16β-Bromo-17α-hydroxy-4-pregnene-3,20-dione	240–242	4.24	A	351
		300	2.07	A	351
	17α-Bromo-11α-hydroxy-4-pregnene-3,20-dione				
	Acetate	240	16,100	A	257
$C_{21}H_{29}O_3Cl$	4-Chloro-11α-hydroxy-4-pregnene-3,20-dione	256	4.12	IP	237
	4-Chloro-17α-hydroxy-4-pregnene-3,20-dione	255	4.12	IP	237
	4-Chloro-21-hydroxy-4-pregnene-3,20-dione				
	Acetate	256	4.12	A	331
		255	4.12	A	237
	12α-Chloro-11β-hydroxy-4-pregnene-3,20-dione	239	17,000	A	179
$C_{21}H_{29}O_3F$	6α-Fluoro-17α-hydroxy-4-pregnene-3,20-dione	236	4.21	A	60
	12α-Fluoro-11β-hydroxy-4-pregnene-3,20-dione	239	18,000	A	179
$C_{21}H_{29}O_4Br$	6ξ-Bromo-17α,21-dihydroxy-4-pregnene-3,20-dione				
	21-Acetate	242	4.25	A	378a
	12α-Bromo-11β,21-dihydroxy-4-pregnene-3,20-dione	240	16,300	M	404
		240	16,300	M	405
	21-Acetate	240	15,600	M	405
$C_{21}H_{29}O_4Cl$	6α-Chloro-17α,21-dihydroxy-4-pregnene-3,20-dione				
	21-Acetate	237	4.18	A	334
	6β-Chloro-17α,21-dihydroxy-4-pregnene-3,20-dione				
	21-Acetate	240	4.15	A	334
	12α-Chloro-11β,21-dihydroxy-4-pregnene-3,20-dione	240	16,400	M	405
	21-Acetate	240	15,600	M	405
		240	15,600	M	404
$C_{21}H_{29}O_4F$	6α-Fluoro-17α,21-dihydroxy-4-pregnene-3,20-dione	236	4.21	A	60
	Diacetate	236	4.17	A	60

TABLE V—*continued*

Formula	Compound	λ_{max}	Ext.	Sol.	Ref.
4-en-3-Ones (cont.)					
$C_{21}H_{29}O_4F$	6β-Fluoro-17α,21-dihydroxy-4-pregnene-3,20-dione	234	4.09	A	60
	Diacetate	233	4.05	A	60
	12α-Fluoro-11β,21-dihydroxy-4-pregnene-3,20-dione	241	15,500	M	405
	21-Acetate	241	16,600	M	405
		240.5	16,600	A	404
	21-Fluoro-11β,17α-dihydroxy-4-pregnene-3,20-dione	242	15,000	A	178
$C_{21}H_{29}O_5Br$	9α-Bromo-11β,17α,21-trihydroxy-4-pregnene-3,20-dione				
	21-Acetate	243	14,500	A	156
$C_{21}H_{29}O_5Cl$	4-Chloro-11β,17α,21-trihydroxy-4-pregnene-3,20-dione	254	4.12	A	331
	6α-Chloro-11β,17α,21-trihydroxy-4-pregnene-3,20-dione				
	21-Acetate	238	4.08	A	334
	9α-Chloro-11β,17α,21-trihydroxy-4-pregnene-3,20-dione	241	17,000	A	156
	21-Acetate	241	15,800	A	156
$C_{21}H_{29}O_5F$	6α-Fluoro-11β,17α,21-trihydroxy-4-pregnene-3,20-dione				
	21-Acetate	237	4.23	A	60
	9α-Fluoro-11β,17α,21-trihydroxy-4-pregnene-3,20-dione	239	17,600	A	156
	21-Acetate	238	16,800	A	156
		239	15,900	A	125
	21-Dihydrogenphosphate	244	16,600	W	327
		238	15,820	M	327
	21-Hemisuccinate	238	17,700	A	156
	21-Heptanoate	239	16,100	A	156
$C_{21}H_{29}O_5I$	11β,17α,21-Trihydroxy-9α-iodo-4-pregnene-3,20-dione				
	21-Acetate	243	11,000	A	156
$C_{21}H_{29}O_6Cl$	15β-Chloro-11β,14α,17α,21-tetrahydroxy-4-pregnene-3,20-dione				
	21-Acetate	240	4.22	A	7
$C_{21}H_{29}O_6F$	9α-Fluoro-1ξ,11β,17α,21-tetrahydroxy-4-pregnene-3,20-dione	237	16,850	M	268
	1,21-Diacetate	238	16,000	M	268
$C_{21}H_{30}O_2$	17α-Carboxy-17β-methyl-4-androsten-3-one				
	Methyl ester	241	4.21	A	131
	17β-Hydroxy-17α-allyl-19-nor-4-androsten-3-one	240	4.23		86

L

TABLE V—*continued*

Formula	Compound	λ_{max}	Ext.	Sol.	Ref.
4-en-3-Ones (cont.)					
$C_{21}H_{30}O_2$	17α,20-Epoxy-4-pregnen-3-one	240	4.23	A	36
	16α-Acetyl-4-androsten-3-one	241	15,510	A	146
		295	110	A	146
	4-Pregnene-3,20-dione	241	17,000	A	116
		234	17,300	E	116
	8α-4-Pregnene-3,20-dione	241	4.18	A	105
	1ξ-Methyl-19-nor-4-pregnene-3,20-dione	242.5	4.11	A	102
$C_{21}H_{30}O_2S$	21-Thio-4-pregnene-3,20-dione				
	Acetate	239	4.35		108
$C_{21}H_{30}O_3$	17β-Carboxy-17α-methyl-4-androsten-3-one	240	4.20	A	170
	Methyl ester	242	4.22	A	170
		241	4.16	A	131
	11β,17β-Dihydroxy-17α-vinyl-4-androsten-3-one				
	17-Acetate	241	15,200	M	261
	16α,17α-Epoxy-20β-hydroxy-4-pregnen-3-one	241	15,600		64
	11β,21-Dihydroxy-4,17(20)-*cis*-pregnadien-3-one	242.5	16,100	A	204
	21-Acetate	243	15,750		204
	16α,20ξ-Dihydroxy-17β-methyl-18-nor-17α-4,13-pregnadien-3-one	240	16,700	A	70
	Diacetate	240	17,400	A	70
	20β-Hydroxy-4-pregnene-3,11-dione	236	17,300	A	299
		238	16,570		87
	Acetate	236	17,800	A	299
	Benzoate	232	25,000		87
	17α-Ethyl-17β-hydroxy-4-androstene-3,11-dione	238	14,300	M	261
	11β,17β-Dihydroxy-17α-vinyl-4-androsten-3-one	242	15,000	M	261
	17α-Hydroxy-1ξ-methyl-19-nor-4-pregnene-3,20-dione	243	4.13	A	102
	1ξ-Hydroxy-4-pregnene-3,20-dione	241	15,800	M	304
		240.5	14,500	A	62
	2α-Hydroxy-4-pregnene-3,20-dione	242	4.22	A	381
	Acetate	240	4.24	A	381
	4-Hydroxy-4-pregnene-3,20-dione	277	4.06	M	50

TABLE V—*continued*

Formula	Compound	λ_{max}	Ext.	Sol.	Ref.
4-en-3-Ones (cont.)					
$C_{21}H_{30}O_3$	6α-Hydroxy-4-pregnene-3,20-dione	240	15,570	A	23
	Acetate	235.5	14,910	A	23
	6β-Hydroxy-4-pregnene-3,20-dione	235.5	12,390	A	23
		236–237	13,500	A	37
		235.5	12,390	A	282
	Acetate	235	13,970	A	23
	7β-Hydroxy-4-pregnene-3,20-dione	242	15,600	M	267
	11α-Hydroxy-4-pregnene-3,20-dione	242	4.19	A	324
	Tosylate	230	4.53	A	352
	11α-Hydroxy-17α-4-pregnene-3,20-dione	242	15,300	A	272
	11β-Hydroxy-4-pregnene-3,20-dione	242	4.26		355
	Formate	239	15,900	M	312
	Acetate	239	15,200	M	312
	12α-Hydroxy-4-pregnene-3,20-dione				
	Acetate	240	4.3	A	232
	Tosylate	228	4.4	A	232
		242(sh)	4.2	A	232
	15α-Hydroxy-4-pregnene-3,20-dione	240	15,560	A	68
	16α-Hydroxy-4-pregnene-3,20-dione	240	16,200	A	40
	Acetate	240.5	17,000	A	197
		239	16,900	A	40
	16β-Hydroxy-4-pregnene-3,20-dione	240	16,500	A	41
	Acetate	240	17,100	A	41
	17α-Hydroxy-4-pregnene-3,20-dione	242	16,500	A	116
	Caproate	240	4.23	A	34
	Cyclopentylpropionate	240	4.23	A	34
	Enanthianate	240	4.24	A	34
	19-Hydroxy-4-pregnene-3,20-dione	242	12,900	A	27
		242	12,900	A	26
	Acetate	239	17,300	A	27
		239	17,300	A	26

TABLE V—*continued*

Formula	Compound	λ_{max}	Ext.	Sol.	Ref.
4-en-3-Ones (cont.)					
$C_{21}H_{30}O_3$	19-Hydroxy-14β,17α-4-pregnene-3,20-dione	243	18,100	A	120
	21-Hydroxy-4-pregnene-3,20-dione	240	19,000	M	116
$C_{21}H_{30}O_3S$	17α-Hydroxy-21-thio-4-pregnene-3,20-dione				
	21-Acetate	239	4.35	A	108
$C_{21}H_{30}O_4$	17β-Carboxy-12α-hydroxy-17α-methyl-4-androsten-3-one				
	Tosylate, methyl ester	229	4.44	A	130
		242(sh)	4.2	A	130
	6α,11α-Dihydroxy-4-pregnene-3,20-dione	240	12,220	A	67
		241	13,200	A	152
	Diacetate	235	14,000	A	152
	6α,11α-Dihydroxy-17α-4-pregnene-3,20-dione				
	Diacetate	235	14,800	A	152
	6β,11α-Dihydroxy-4-pregnene-3,20-dione	238	13,590	A	67
	6β,15α-Dihydroxy-4-pregnene-3,20-dione	240	4.22	A	169
		285–300	1.98	A	169
	11α,15β-Dihydroxy-4-pregnene-3,20-dione	243	4.21	A	372
	12β,15β-Dihydroxy-4-pregnene-3,20-dione	241	4.23	A	372
	6α,17α-Dihydroxy-4-pregnene-3,20-dione	240	14,900	A	152
	6-Acetate	237	16,400	A	152
	6β,17α-Dihydroxy-4-pregnene-3,20-dione	236	14,000	A	152
		236	12,800	A	13
		238	12,600	A	273
	6-Acetate	236	12,500	A	273
		236	12,500	A	152
	11α,17α-Dihydroxy-4-pregnene-3,20-dione	242	4.19	A	346
	11-Acetate	240	16,300	A	311
	Diacetate	242	14,200	A	311

TABLE V—*continued*

Formula	Compound	λ_{max}	Ext.	Sol.	Ref.
4-en-3-Ones (cont.)					
$C_{21}H_{30}O_4$	11β,17α-Dihydroxy-4-pregnene-3,20-dione	242	14,200	M	310
	11-Acetate	240	15,100	M	310
	Diacetate	240	16,000	M	312
	11-Acetate,17-formate	238	17,200	M	312
	Diformate	238	12,900	M	312
	11-Acetate,17-caproate	239	16,100	M	312
	12α,17α-Dihydroxy-4-pregnene-3,20-dione	240	4.28	IP	3
	16α,17α-Dihydroxy-4-pregnene-3,20-dione	241–242	15,200	A	10
	16-Acetate	240	14,900	A	10
		240	4.20	A	351
	16β,17α-Dihydroxy-4-pregnene-3,20-dione				
	16-Acetate	240	4.21	A	351
		242	16,600	A	188
	2α,21-Dihydroxy-4-pregnene-3,20-dione				
	21-Trimethylacetate	241	13,300	M	24
	2-Acetate,21-trimethylacetate	241	16,900	M	24
	Diacetate	240	4.22	A	381
	6β,21-Dihydroxy-4-pregnene-3,20-dione				
	21-Acetate	236	4.12	A	347
		237	13,900	A	133
		236	12,900	A	13
	Diacetate	236	13,150	A	133
	7α,21-Dihydroxy-4-pregnene-3,20-dione	242	15,600	A	277
	21-Acetate	242	15,850	A	277
	9α,21-Dihydroxy-4-pregnene-3,20-dione	243	14,300	A	135
	21-Acetate	243	15,150	A	135
	11α,21-Dihydroxy-4-pregnene-3,20-dione				
	Diacetate	240	4.23	A	390
	11β,21-Dihydroxy-4-pregnene-3,20-dione	240	20,000	A	116
	14α,21-Dihydroxy-4-pregnene-3,20-dione	242	15,800	A	135
	15α,21-Dihydroxy-4-pregnene-3,20-dione	242	16,700	A	277

TABLE V—*continued*

Formula	Compound	λ_{max}	Ext.	Sol.	Ref.
4-en-3-Ones (cont.)					
$C_{21}H_{30}O_4$	15β,21-Dihydroxy-4-pregnene-3,20-dione	242	16,950	A	277
	16α,21-Dihydroxy-4-pregnene-3,20-dione	241	16,300	A	416
		241	16,600	M	82
	21-Acetate	241	16,300	M	82
	Diacetate	240	16,400		199
	17α,21-Dihydroxy-4-pregnene-3,20-dione	240	16,600	A	116
	20-Nitrimine	240	18,000	A	61
	18,21-Dihydroxy-4-pregnene-3,20-dione	240			233
	19,21-Dihydroxy-4-pregnene-3,20-dione	242	18,500	A	27
		242	18,500	A	26
	19-Acetate	239	16,000	A	26
		239	16,000	A	27
	21-Acetate	242	13,500	A	26
		242	13,500	A	27
	Diacetate	239	13,400	A	26
		239	13,400	A	27
	19,21-Dihydroxy-14β,17α-4-pregnene-3,20-dione	243	18,300	A	120
	21-Acetate	243	17,600	A	120
	11β,20β-Dihydroxy-4-pregnen-21-al-3-one				
	21,21-Dimethylacetal	242.5	4.18	M	406
	16β,17aβ-Dihydroxy-17aα-methyl-D-homo-4-androstene-3,17-dione	239	16,600		88
	17aβ-Hydroxymethyl-17aα-hydroxy-D-homo-4-androstene-3,17-dione	240	4.23	A	35
	17aβ-Acetate	240	4.22	A	35
$C_{21}H_{30}O_5$	1ξ,17α,21-Trihydroxy-4-pregnene-3,20-dione	241	16,500	M	168
	2α,17α,21-Trihydroxy-4-pregnene-3,20-dione	242	4.19	A	353
	2,21-Diacetate	242	4.19	A	353
	Triacetate	240	4.22	A	353
	2β,17α,21-Trihydroxy-4-pregnene-3,20-dione	243	14,500	M	183
		243	16,000	M	375
	2,21-Diacetate	244	16,200	M	183
		244	15,000	M	375

TABLE V—*continued*

Formula	Compound	λ_{max}	Ext.	Sol.	Ref.
4-en-3-Ones (cont.)					
$C_{21}H_{30}O_5$	6α,17α,21-Trihydroxy-4-pregnene-3,20-dione	240	14,500	A	152
	6,21-Diacetate	236	16,800	A	152
	6β,17α,21-Trihydroxy-4-pregnene-3,20-dione	238	12,900	A	275
		238	4.20		291
		236	4.14	A	383
	6,21-Diacetate	234.5	13,300	A	152
		236	4.12	A	383
	11α,17α,21-Trihydroxy-4-pregnene-3,20-dione	242	15,800	A	14
	11-Acetate	240	15,300	A	311
	21-Acetate	242	4.16	A	346
	11,21-Diacetate	240	16,800	A	311
		239–240	15,500	A	14
		240	4.24	A	346
	11β,17α,21-Trihydroxy-4-pregnene-3,20-dione	241	16,700		61
		242	15,400		61
	11-Acetate	240	16,250	A	310
	11-Formate	238	15,700		309
	21-Acetate,11-formate	239	15,000	A	308
		239	15,100		309
	11,21-Diacetate	240	17,200	A	310
		238	17,200	A	307
	21-Dimethylphosphate	241	15,800	M	327
	21-Nitrimine	240	17,200	A	61
	12α,17α,21-Trihydroxy-4-pregnene-3,20-dione				
	21-Acetate	240	4.21	IP	3
	12β,17α,21-Trihydroxy-4-pregnene-3,20-dione				
	12,21-Diacetate	239	4.19	IP	2
	15α,17α,21-Trihydroxy-4-pregnene-3,20-dione	241	16,400	M	38
	15β,17α,21-Trihydroxy-4-pregnene-3,20-dione	241	16,600	M	38

TABLE V—*continued*

Formula	Compound	λ_{max}	Ext.	Sol.	Ref.
4-en-3-Ones (cont.)					
$C_{21}H_{30}O_5$	16α,17α,21-Trihydroxy-4-pregnene-3,20-dione				
	21-Acetate	240	16,900		121
		240.5	17,500	A	10
	16,21-Diacetate	240	16,800	A	10
	16β,17α,21-Trihydroxy-4-pregnene-3,20-dione				
	16,21-Diacetate	241	16,800	A	351
		241	17,000		188
	17α,19,21-Trihydroxy-4-pregnene-3,20-dione	243	4.18		291
	6β,11β,21-Trihydroxy-4-pregnene-3,20-dione	237	4.13		291
	11β,12α,21-Trihydroxy-4-pregnene-3,20-dione	241	15,900	M	405
		241	15,900	M	404
	12,21-Diacetate	238	16,000	M	404
	11β,17aα-Dihydroxy-17aβ-hydroxymethyl-D-homo-4-androstene-3,17-dione				
	17aβ-Acetate	240	4.23	A	35
	11β,19,21-Trihydroxy-4-pregnene-3,20-dione	243	4.01		291
	19,21-Dibenzoate	231	4.59	A	291
	17α,20α,21-Trihydroxy-4-pregnene-3,11-dione	239	4.11	A	291
	17α,20β,21-Trihydroxy-4-pregnene-3,11-dione				
	20,21-Diacetate	237	16,500	A	14
		237.5	15,600	A	299
$C_{21}H_{30}O_6$	9α,11β,17α,21-Tetrahydroxy-4-pregnene-3,20-dione	242.5	16,200	A	252
		242	15,600	M	423
	21-Acetate	242–243	15,500	A	252
		242	15,570	M	423
		241	15,400	A	156
	11β,14α,17α,21-Tetrahydroxy-4-pregnene-3,20-dione	241	4.19	A	7
	11β,16α,17α,21-Tetrahydroxy-4-pregnene-3,20-dione	241–242	15,400	A	10
	21-Acetate	241	15,400	A	10
	16,21-Diacetate	240.5	15,000	A	10

TABLE V—*continued*

Formula	Compound	λ_{max}	Ext.	Sol.	Ref.
4-en-3-Ones (cont.)					
$C_{21}H_{31}O_2Br$	4-Bromo-17β-hydroxy-2,2-dimethyl-4-androsten-3-one				
	Acetate	262	4.07	A	335
$C_{21}H_{32}O_2$	20ξ-Hydroxy-1ξ-methyl-19-nor-4-pregnen-3-one	242.5	4.14	A	102
	17β-Hydroxy-17α-propyl-19-nor-4-androsten-3-one	241	4.21		86
	17β-Hydroxy-2,2-dimethyl-4-androsten-3-one				
	Acetate	240	4.19	A	335
	17β-Hydroxy-2α,17α-dimethyl-4-androsten-3-one	240	4.21	A	335
	17β-Hydroxy-6α,17α-dimethyl-4-androsten-3-one	242	15,600	A	72
		242	4.19	A	332
	17β-Hydroxy-6β,17α-dimethyl-4-androsten-3-one	242	15,500	A	72
	17β-Hydroxy-16β,17α-dimethyl-4-androsten-3-one	240	4.26	A	341
	17α-Hydroxy-4-pregnen-3-one	240	4.22	A	36
	17β-Hydroxy-17α-ethyl-4-androsten-3-one	243	14,300	Ch	116
	20β-Hydroxy-4-pregnen-3-one	240	4.23	A	378
		240.5	16,000	A	299
	Acetate	241	18,400	A	299
		240	4.22	A	378
	17aβ-Hydroxy-17aα-methyl-D-homo-4-androsten-3-one	241	4.225	A	409
$C_{21}H_{32}O_3$	11β,17β-Dihydroxy-17α-ethyl-4-androsten-3-one	242	14,400	M	261
	16α,20α-Dihydroxy-4-pregnen-3-one				
	Diacetate	240	16,100		65
	20β,21-Dihydroxy-4-pregnen-3-one	242	15,600	A	74
	Diacetate	242	21,000	A	74
		240.5	17,400	A	299
	17β,17aα-Dihydroxy-17aβ-methyl-D-homo-4-androsten-3-one	240	4.19	M	409
$C_{21}H_{32}O_4$	11β,17α,20α-Trihydroxy-4-pregnen-3-one	242	15,900	M	326
	11β,17α,20β-Trihydroxy-4-pregnen-3-one	242	15,650	M	326
$C_{21}H_{32}O_5$	11β,17α,20α,21-Tetrahydroxy-4-pregnen-3-one				
	20,21-Diacetate	242	12,600	A	325
	11β,17α,20β,21-Tetrahydroxy-4-pregnen-3-one				
	21-Acetate	242.5	$E^{1\%}_{1\,cm.}$ 399	A	207

TABLE V—*continued*

Formula	Compound	λ_{max}	Ext.	Sol.	Ref.
4-en-3-Ones (cont.)					
$C_{21}H_{32}O_5$	20,21-Diacetate	239.5	16,000	A	299
		241	15,300	A	14
$C_{22}H_{26}O_6$	17α,20,21-Trihydroxy-20-nor-4,20(22)-norcholadien-3-one-22-oic acid-22 → 17 lactone	242	22,400		247
	22-Imine	238	$E^{1\%}_{1cm.}$ 439		247
		286	$E^{1\%}_{1cm.}$ 383		247
$C_{22}H_{29}O_2N$	16α-Cyano-4-pregnene-3,20-dione	240	4.23	A	342
$C_{22}H_{29}O_5F$	9α-Fluoro-17α,21-dihydroxy-2α-methyl-4-pregnene-3,11,20-trione				
	21-Acetate	235.5	15,500	A	206
$C_{22}H_{30}O_2$	17α-Ethinyl-17β-hydroxy-2α-methyl-4-androsten-3-one	240	4.19	A	335
	17α-Ethinyl-17β-hydroxy-6α-methyl-4-androsten-3-one	241	4.19	IP	1
		242	15,475	A	72
	17α-Ethinyl-17β-hydroxy-6β-methyl-4-androsten-3-one	241.5	4.25	IP	1
		242	15,950	A	72
	Sulphate	241	4.2	IP	1
	17α-Methyl-4,11-pregnadiene-3,20-dione	239	4.23	A	130
$C_{22}H_{30}O_3$	17β-Hydroxy-17α-(3′-hydroxy-1′-propyn)-4-androsten-3-one	241	4.2	A	33
	20ξ,22ξ-Epoxy-17α,21-dihydroxy-4-bisnorcholen-3-one	242	16,800	M	303
$C_{22}H_{30}O_4$	17α,21-Dihydroxy-2α-methyl-4,9(11)-pregnadiene-3,20-dione				
	21-Acetate	240	16,750	A	206
	17α,21-Dihydroxy-6α-methyl-4,9(11)-pregnadiene-3,20-dione				
	21-Acetate	239.5	16,400	A	395
	17α,21-Dihydroxy-16α-methyl-4,9(11)-pregnadiene-3,20-dione				
	21-Acetate	239	17,300	M	18
	16α-Carboxy-4-pregnene-3,20-dione	240	4.23		124
		240	4.22	A	342
	Methyl ester	240	4.23	A	342
	17α-Hydroxy-6α-methyl-4-pregnene-3,11,20-trione	238–240	4.16	A	59
	21-Hydroxy-17α-methyl-4-pregnene-3,11,20-trione	238	4.2	A	127
	21-Acetate	237	4.44	A	126
		237	4.4	A	127

TABLE V—*continued*

Formula	Compound	λ_{max}	Ext.	Sol.	Ref.
4-en-3-Ones (cont.)					
$C_{22}H_{30}O_4$	17aβ-Hydroxy-D-homo-17aα-4-pregnene-3,11,20-trione	239	15,270	A	81
$C_{22}H_{30}O_4F_2$	9α,21-Difluoro-11β,17α-dihydroxy-6α-methyl-4-pregnene-3,20-dione	239	14,225	A	395
$C_{22}H_{30}O_5$	17α,21-Dihydroxy-4-methyl-4-pregnene-3,11,20-trione	249	4.15		398
	9β,11β-Epoxy-17α,21-dihydroxy-6α-methyl-4-pregnene-3,20-dione				
	21-Acetate	242	14,625	A	395
	17α,21-Dihydroxy-6α-methyl-4-pregnene-3,11,20-trione				
	21-Acetate	238	4.19	A	59
	9β,11β-Epoxy-17α,21-dihydroxy-16α-methyl-4-pregnene-3,20-dione				
	21-Acetate	244	14,600	M	18
	17α,21-Dihydroxy-16α-methyl-4-pregnene-3,11,20-trione				
	21-Acetate	238	15,400	M	19
	17α,21-Dihydroxy-16β-methyl-4-pregnene-3,11,20-trione	238	16,200	M	403
	21-Acetate	238	15,800	M	403
	17aα,21-Dihydroxy-D-homo-4-pregnene-3,11,20-trione				
	21-Acetate	238	14,900	A	81
	17aβ,21-Dihydroxy-D-homo-17aα-4-pregnene-3,11,20-trione				
	21-Acetate	238	15,200	A	81
	21-Hydroxy-12β-methoxy-4-pregnene-3,20-dione				
	Acetate	238	16,200	M	405
	17α-Hydroxy-21-methoxy-4-pregnene-3,11,20-trione	238	$E^{1\%}_{1cm.}$ 400		208
	20ξ,22-Epoxy-17α,21-dihydroxy-4-dinorcholene-3,11-dione	238	15,400		300
		238	15,400	M	303
$C_{22}H_{30}O_6$	17α,21-Dihydroxy-9α-methoxy-4-pregnene-3,11,20-trione				
	21-Acetate	238	16,500	A	156
$C_{22}H_{31}O_2Cl$	21-Chloro-17α-methyl-4-pregnene-3,20-dione	240	4.24	A	191
	21-Chloro-17β-methyl-17α-4-pregnene-3,20-dione	239	4.2		132
$C_{22}H_{31}O_2I$	21-Iodo-17α-methyl-4-pregnene-3,20-dione	240	4.27	A	191
$C_{22}H_{31}O_5Cl$	9α-Chloro-11β,17α,21-trihydroxy-16α-methyl-4-pregnene-3,20-dione				
	21-Acetate	241	16,750	M	18
$C_{22}H_{31}O_5Br$	9α-Bromo-11β,17α,21-trihydroxy-6α-methyl-4-pregnene-3,20-dione				
	21-Acetate	239.5	14,225	A	395

TABLE V—*continued*

Formula	Compound	λ_{max}	Ext.	Sol.	Ref.
4-en-3-Ones (cont.)					
$C_{22}H_{31}O_5Br$	9α-Bromo-11β,17α,21-trihydroxy-16α-methyl-4-pregnene-3,20-dione				
	21-Acetate	244	16,200	M	18
$C_{22}H_{31}O_5F$	9α-Fluoro-11β,17α,21-trihydroxy-2α-methyl-4-pregnene-3,20-dione	239	16,175	A	206
	21-Acetate	238.5	16,150	A	206
	9α-Fluoro-11β,17α,21-trihydroxy-6α-methyl-4-pregnene-3,20-dione	239	16,400	A	395
	21-Acetate	239	15,775	A	395
	9α-Fluoro-11β,17α,21-trihydroxy-16α-methyl-4-pregnene-3,20-dione				
	21-Acetate	239	16,700	M	18
$C_{22}H_{31}O_6F$	9α-Fluoro-11β,16α,17α,21-tetrahydroxy-2α-methyl-4-pregnene-3,20-dione	237–238	15,100	A	39
	16,21-Diacetate	237–238	16,300	A	39
$C_{22}H_{32}O_2$	4-Allyl-17β-hydroxy-4-androsten-3-one	250	15,000	M	21
	17β-Hydroxy-2α-methyl-17α-vinyl-4-androsten-3-one	240	4.20	A	335
	4-Methyl-4-pregnene-3,20-dione	251	4.18	A	386
	6α-Methyl-4-pregnene-3,20-dione	242	4.21	A	332
		241	15,700	A	63
	6α-Methyl-17α-4-pregnene-3,20-dione	241	16,040	A	63
	6β-Methyl-4-pregnene-3,20-dione	242	4.21	A	332
		242	19,040	A	63
	16α-Methyl-4-pregnene-3,20-dione	240	4.31	A	344
		241	17,300		234
	16β-Methyl-17α-4-pregnene-3,20-dione	242	4.35	A	344
	16β-Methyl-4-pregnene-3,20-dione	240	4.34	A	344
	17α-Methyl-4-pregnene-3,20-dione	240	4.22	A	170
	D-Homo-4-pregnene-3,20-dione	242	16,600		115
$C_{22}H_{32}O_3$	11α-Hydroxy-6α-methyl-4-pregnene-3,20-dione	241	4.17		89
	12α-Hydroxy-17α-methyl-4-pregnene-3,20-dione	241	4.2	A	130
	Tosylate	229	4.25	A	130
		242(sh)		A	130

TABLE V—*continued*

Formula	Compound	λ_{max}	Ext.	Sol.	Ref.
4-en-3-Ones (cont.)					
$C_{22}H_{32}O_3$	17α-Hydroxy-6α-methyl-4-pregnene-3,20-dione	241	16,150	A	22
	Acetate	240	15,950	A	22
	Caproate	240	15,300	A	22
	β-Cyclopentylpropionate	240.5	15,775	A	22
	Phenylacetate	240	16,125	A	22
	Propionate	240	16,075	A	22
	17α-Hydroxy-6β-methyl-4-pregnene-3,20-dione	242	16,500	A	22
	21-Hydroxy-17α-methyl-4-pregnene-3,20-dione				
	Acetate	240	4.26	A	131
		242	4.22	A	191
	21-Hydroxy-17β-methyl-17α-4-pregnene-3,20-dione	241	4.23		132
	Acetate	241	4.24		132
	16α-Hydroxymethyl-4-pregnene-3,20-dione	240–242	4.23	A	342
	21-Methoxy-4-pregnene-3,20-dione	240	4.22	A	448
	21-Hydroxy-D-homo-4-pregnene-3,20-dione				
	Acetate	241	16,200		115
	11β,21-Dihydroxy-2α-methyl-4,17(20)-pregnadien-3-one				
	21-Acetate	242	15,025	A	206
	11β,21-Dihydroxy-6α-methyl-4,17(20)-pregnadien-3-one	242	15,000	A	396
	21-Acetate	243	15,025	A	396
	20ξ,22-Epoxy-21-hydroxy-4-dinorcholen-3-one	242	17,000	M	303
$C_{22}H_{32}O_4$	11β,21-Dihydroxy-17α-methyl-4-pregnene-3,20-dione				
	21-Acetate	241	4.2	A	128
	21-Hydroxy-16α-methoxy-4-pregnene-3,20-dione				
	Acetate	240	16,800	IP	90
	20ξ,21-Dihydroxy-17α-methyl-4-pregnene-3,11,20-trione				
	Diacetate	238	4.5	A	128
	20ξ,22-Epoxy-17α,21-dihydroxy-4-dinorcholen-3-one				
	21-Acetate	242	15,800	M	303
$C_{22}H_{32}O_5$	11β,17α,21-Trihydroxy-2α-methyl-4-pregnene-3,20-dione	242	15,250	A	206
	21-Acetate	242	15,125	A	206

TABLE V—*continued*

Formula	Compound	λ_{max}	Ext.	Sol.	Ref.
4-en-3-Ones (cont.)					
$C_{22}H_{32}O_5$	11β,17α,21-Trihydroxy-4-methyl-4-pregnene-3,20-dione				
	21-Acetate	252	4.17		398
	11β,17α,21-Trihydroxy-6α-methyl-4-pregnene-3,20-dione	243	15,600	A	396
	21-Acetate	243	14,525	A	396
	11β,17α,21-Trihydroxy-9α-methyl-4-pregnene-3,20-dione	244	14,300	M	203
	21-Acetate	243	16,500	M	203
	11β,17α,21-Trihydroxy-11α-methyl-4-pregnene-3,20-dione				
	21-Acetate	243	16,350	A	153
	11β,17α,21-Trihydroxy-16α-methyl-4-pregnene-3,20-dione				
	21-Acetate	242	16,900	M	19
	11β,17α,21-Trihydroxy-16β-methyl-4-pregnene-3,20-dione				
	21-Acetate	242	15,800	M	403
$C_{22}H_{32}O_6$	11β,17α,21-Trihydroxy-9α-methoxy-4-pregnene-3,20-dione				
	21-Acetate	243	14,800	A	156
	11β,16α,17α,21-Tetrahydroxy-2α-methyl-4-pregnene-3,20-dione	240–241	16,600	A	39
	16,21-Diacetate	240–241	17,500	A	39
$C_{22}H_{34}O_2$	17α-Ethyl-17β-hydroxy-2α-methyl-4-androsten-3-one	240	4.21	A	335
	17α-*n*-Butyl-17β-hydroxy-19-nor-4-androsten-3-one	240.5	4.23		86
$C_{22}H_{34}O_3$	11α,21-Dihydroxy-20β-methyl-4-pregnen-3-one	242	12,700	A	274
	Diacetate	242	14,600	A	274
$C_{22}H_{34}O_4$	6β,11α,21-Dihydroxy-20β-methyl-4-pregnen-3-one	238	12,900	A	274
$C_{23}H_{29}O_6Br$	17α,20:20,21-Bismethylenedioxy-9α-bromo-4-pregnene-3,11-dione	238	15,800	M	203
$C_{23}H_{30}O_4$	16αβ-Carboxy-16,17-cyclopropano-4-pregnene-3,20-dione				
	Methyl ester	241	15,572	M	288
	20-Acetoxy-4,17(20)-pregnadiene-3,16-dione	242	26,400	A	41
		241	16,400	BA	41
		308	21,200	BA	41
$C_{23}H_{30}O_5$	20-Ethylenedioxy-17α,21-epoxy-4-pregnen-3,11-dione	238	16,600	A	12
$C_{23}H_{31}O_6Br$	17α,20:20,21-Bismethylenedioxy-9α-bromo-11β-hydroxy-4-pregnen-3-one	243	15,500	M	203
$C_{23}H_{32}O_3$	20-Ethylenedioxy-4,16-pregnadien-3-one	240	16,600	A	40

TABLE V—*continued*

Formula	Compound	λ_{max}	Ext.	Sol.	Ref.
4-en-3-Ones (cont.)					
$C_{23}H_{32}O_3$	20-Acetoxy-4,17(20)-pregnadien-3-one	240	4.18	A	98
$C_{23}H_{32}O_4$	16α,17α-Epoxy-20-ethylenedioxy-4-pregnen-3-one	240	14,600	A	40
$C_{23}H_{32}O_5$	20-Ethylenedioxy-17α,21-dihydroxy-4,7-pregnadien-3-one	239	14,300		15
	20-Ethylenedioxy-11β,21-dihydroxy-4,16-pregnadien-3-one	242	16,100	A	9
$C_{23}H_{32}O_6$	20-Ethylenedioxy-17α,21-dihydroxy-4-pregnene-3,11-dione	238	15,200	A	14
	21-Acetate	237	16,700	A	14
$C_{23}H_{34}O_3$	20-Ethylenedioxy-4-pregnen-3-one	242	16,800	A	171
	2α-Ethyl-11β,21-dihydroxy-4,17(20)-*cis*-pregnadien-3-one				
	21-Acetate	242	15,000	A	206
$C_{23}H_{34}O_4$	20-Ethylenedioxy-21-hydroxy-4-pregnen-3-one	242	4.24		138
	21-Acetate	242	4.24		138
	20-Ethylenedioxy-16α-hydroxy-4-pregnen-3-one	240	15,000	A	40
$C_{23}H_{34}O_6$	20-Ethylenedioxy-11α,17α,21-trihydroxy-4-pregnen-3-one	240	4.24	A	384
	20-Ethylenedioxy-11β,17α,21-trihydroxy-4-pregnen-3-one	241.5	15,400		139
$C_{23}H_{36}O_2$	4-*n*-Butyl-17β-hydroxy-4-androsten-3-one	251	15,000	M	21
$C_{24}H_{32}O_6$	16α-Malonoyl-4-pregnene-3,20-dione				
	Dimethyl ester	240	15,700	A	53
$C_{24}H_{36}O_3$	20β,21-iso-Propylidenedioxy-4-pregnen-3-one	240.5	18,200	A	299
$C_{24}H_{32}O_6ClF$	6α-Chloro-9α-fluoro-11β,21-dihydroxy-16α,17α-iso-propylidenedioxy-4-pregnene-3,20-dione				
	21-Acetate	234	4.17	A	334
	6β-Chloro-9α-fluoro-11β,21-dihydroxy-16α,17α-iso propylidenedioxy-4-pregnene-3,20-dione				
	21-Acetate	238	4.12	A	334
$C_{24}H_{34}O_6$	17α,20:20,21-Bismethylenedioxy-11β-hydroxy-9α-methyl-4-pregnen-3-one	244	14,800	M	203
$C_{25}H_{37}O_3N$	21-Morpholino-4-pregnene-3,20-dione	241	15,951		279
	Hydrochloride	240.5	14,150		279
$C_{25}H_{38}O_4$	11β-Hydroxy-20ξ,21-iso-propylidenedioxy-17α-methyl-4-pregnen-3-one	242	4.2	A	128
$C_{26}H_{42}O_2$	17β-Hydroxy-17α-octyl-19-nor-4-androsten-3-one	240	4.22		86

TABLE V—*continued*

Formula	Compound	λ_{max}	Ext.	Sol.	Ref.
4-en-3-Ones (cont.)					
$C_{27}H_{24}O_4$	17α-Hydroxy-21-phenoxy-4-pregnene-3,20-dione	240	4.25	A	338
		276	3.20	A	338
$C_{27}H_{34}O_8$	20,21,21-Trihydroxy-4,17(20)-pregnadiene-3,11-dione	237.5	17,000	M	48
$C_{30}H_{40}O_4$	16α-Benzyloxy-20-ethylenedioxy-4-pregnen-3-one	240	16,800	A	40
$C_{34}H_{46}O_{12}$	21-(Methyl-2,3,4-tri-O-acetyl-β-D-glucosiduronate)-4-pregnene-3,20-dione	240	4.2	A	447
$C_{40}H_{54}O_4$	Di-17α(17β-hydroxy-4-androsten-3-one)-acetylene	240	4.52	A	382
5-en-7-Ones					
$C_{19}H_{28}O_3$	3β,17β-Dihydroxy-5-androsten-7-one	240	4.18		189
	Diacetate	237	4.15		189
$C_{21}H_{30}O_3$	3β-Hydroxy-5-pregnene-7,20-dione	237.5	4.13	M	365
	Acetate	234	4.26	M	365
$C_{21}H_{30}O_4$	3-Ethylenedioxy-17β-hydroxy-5-androsten-7-one				
	Acetate	241	4.1	A	328
$C_{21}H_{32}O_2$	20β-Hydroxy-5-pregnen-7-one				
	Acetate	236	4.24	A	345
$C_{21}H_{32}O_3$	3β,20β-Dihydroxy-5-pregnen-7-one				
	Diacetate	236	4.24	A	345
$C_{25}H_{36}O_6$	3,20-Bisethylenedioxy-21-hydroxy-5-pregnen-7-one	240	12,400	A	251
	Acetate	240–241	12,700	A	251
$C_{28}H_{38}O_2S$	3β-Benzylthioxy-20β-hydroxy-5-pregnen-7-one				
	Acetate	236	4.29	A	345
7-en-6-Ones					
$C_{20}H_{22}O_3$	*d,l*-17a-Methoxy-D-homo-18-nor-7,13(17α),14,16-androstatetraene-3,6-dione	241	4.2	A	222
		301	4.4	A	222
$C_{22}H_{26}O_4$	*d,l*-17a-Methoxy-3-ethylenedioxy-D-homo-18-nor-7,13(17a),14,16-androstatetraen-6-one	241	4.1	A	222
		301	4.4	A	222

Table V—*continued*

Formula	Compound	λ_{max}	Ext.	Sol.	Ref.
8-en-7-Ones					
$C_{21}H_{26}O_4$	5α-8-Pregnene-3,7,11,20-tetraone	268	3.94	A	103
$C_{21}H_{28}O_3$	5α-8-Pregnene-3,7,20-trione	252	4.10	A	103
$C_{21}H_{28}O_4$	3β-Hydroxy-5α-8-pregnene-7,11,20-trione				
	Acetate	268	3.88	A	104
$C_{21}H_{28}O_5$	16α,17α-Epoxy-3β,11α-dihydroxy-5α-8-pregnene-7,20-dione	254	4.02	A	103
	Diacetate	252	4.07	A	103
$C_{21}H_{30}O_3$	3β-Hydroxy-5α-8-pregnene-7,20-dione	252	4.10	A	103
$C_{21}H_{30}O_4$	3β,11α-Dihydroxy-5α-8-pregnene-7,20-dione				
	3-Acetate	252	4.12	A	104
	Diacetate	252	4.09	A	104
		252	4.07	A	103
$C_{21}H_{32}O_4$	3β,11α,20β-Trihydroxy-5α-8-pregnen-7-one	254	4.11	A	103
	Triacetate	252	4.04	A	103
8-en-11-Ones					
$C_{19}H_{28}O_3$	3β,17β-Dihydroxy-8-androsten-11-one				
	Diacetate	252	3.96	A	192
$C_{20}H_{28}O_4$	17β-Carboxy-3α-hydroxy-8-etiocholen-11-one				
	Acetate, methyl ester	254	3.93	M	202
$C_{21}H_{28}O_5$	17α,21-Dihydroxy-8-pregnene-3,11,20-trione				
	21-Acetate	256	8175		167
		256	8175	M	423
	17α,21-Dihydroxy-14β-8-pregnene-3,11,20-trione				
	21-Acetate	248	8450	M	423
$C_{21}H_{30}O_3$	3β-Hydroxy-5α-8-pregnene-11,20-dione				
	Acetate	254	3.95	A	31
8(14)-en-15-ones					
$C_{20}H_{26}O_6$	17β-Carboxy-3β,11α-dihydroxy-8(14)-androstene-12,15-dione				
	Diacetate	252	3.88	A	366
	Diacetate, methyl ester	249	3.95	A	366

M

TABLE V—*continued*

Formula	Compound	λ_{max}	Ext.	Sol.	Ref.
9(11)-en-12-Ones					
$C_{21}H_{26}O_5$	17β-Carboxy-7α-hydroxy-9(11)-etiocholene-3,12-dione				
	Acetate, methyl ester	237	4.10	A	230
		290	2.29	A	230
$C_{20}H_{28}O_4$	17β-Carboxy-3α-hydroxy-9(11)-etiocholen-12-one				
	Methyl ester	242	4.10	A	73
	Acetate, methyl ester	240	4.22	A	230
		321	1.83	A	230
	3-Ethylcarbonate, methyl ester	239	4.07	A	73
	3-Methylsuccinate, methyl ester	239	4.14	A	73
$C_{20}H_{28}O_5$	17β-Carboxy-3α,7α-dihydroxy-9(11)-etiocholen-12-one				
	Methyl ester	240	4.09	A	230
	7-Acetate, methyl ester	238	4.07	A	230
		322	1.87	A	230
	Diacetate, methyl ester	237–238	4.11	A	230
		322	1.84	A	230
14-en-16-Ones					
$C_{21}H_{24}O_5$	*d,l*-3-Ethylenedioxy-11β-hydroxy-5,14-androstadien-16-one-18-oic acid-18 → 11-lactone	221	10,050	A	433
		241	11,800	A	433
$C_{21}H_{26}O_4$	*d,l*-3-Ethylenedioxy-D-homo-18-nor-18ξ-5,14-androstadiene-11,16-dione	238	12,600	A	432
$C_{21}H_{26}O_5$	*d,l*-3-Ethylenedioxy-11β-hydroxy-5,14-androstadien-18-al-16-one				
	Acetate	238	12,900	A	433
	d,l-11β,18-Epoxy-3-ethylenedioxy-18-hydroxy-5,14-androstadien-16-one				
	Acetate	232	16,600	A	433
$C_{21}H_{28}O_4$	*d,l*-3-Ethylenedioxy-11β-hydroxy-D-homo-18-nor-18ξ-5,14-androstadien-16-one	243	14,000	A	432
$C_{22}H_{26}O_5$	*d,l*-18-Carboxy-3-ethylenedioxy-11β-hydroxy-5,14-androstadien-16-one-18 → 11-lactone	229	17,100	A	187

TABLE V—*continued*

Formula	Compound	λ_{max}	Ext.	Sol.	Ref.
14-en-16-Ones (cont.)					
$C_{23}H_{30}O_6$	*d,l*-3,18-Bisethylenedioxy-11β-hydroxy-5,14-androstadien-16-one				
	Acetate	233	14,250	A	433
15-en-17-Ones					
$C_{19}H_{22}O_2$	3-Methoxy-1,3,5(10),15-estratetraen-17-one	223	4.15	A	218
	3-Methoxy-14β-1,3,5(10),15-estratetraen-17-one	221	4.23	A	218
$C_{19}H_{27}O_2Br$	16-Bromo-3β-hydroxy-15-androsten-17-one	254	6050	A	142
		324	76	A	142
$C_{19}H_{28}O_2$	3β-Hydroxy-15-androsten-17-one	233	3.84	A	141
	Acetate	233	3.84	A	141
16-en-20-Ones					
$C_{20}H_{24}O_2$	3-Methoxy-18,19-dinor-1,3,5(10),16-pregnatetraen-20-one	231	13,900	M	211
$C_{20}H_{24}O_3$	3,21-Dihydroxy-19-nor-1,3,5(10),16-pregnatetraen-20-one				
	Diacetate	238	4.03	A	101
$C_{21}H_{26}O_2$	4,6,16-Pregnatriene-3,20-dione	240	4.21	A	378a
	3-Methoxy-19-nor-1,3,5(10),16-pregnatetraen-20-one	230	4.19	A	389
$C_{21}H_{26}O_4Br_2$	4β,12α-Dibromo-21-hydroxy-16-pregnene-3,11,20-trione				
	Acetate	235	9600	A	269
	12α,15ξ-Dibromo-3α-hydroxy-16-pregnen-21-al-11,20-dione				
	Acetate, hydrate	241	10,500	E	84
$C_{21}H_{27}O_4Br_3$	12α,15ξ,21-Tribromo-3α,21-dihydroxy-16-pregnene-11,20-dione				
	Diacetate	251	8700	E	85
$C_{21}H_{28}O_4$	2ξ,3β-Dihydroxy-5,16-pregnadiene-12,20-dione				
	Diacetate	225	3.9		285
$C_{21}H_{28}O_4BrI$	12α-Bromo-3α,21-dihydroxy-15ξ-iodo-16-pregnene-11,20-dione				
	Diacetate	243	13,000	E	84
$C_{21}H_{28}O_4Br_2$	12α,15ξ-Dibromo-3α,21-dihydroxy-16-pregnene-11,20-dione				
	Diacetate	235	11,000	E	84

TABLE V—*continued*

Formula	Compound	λ_{max}	Ext.	Sol.	Ref.
16-en-20-Ones (cont.)					
$C_{21}H_{29}O_2I$	3β-Hydroxy-21-iodo-5,16-pregnadien-20-one				
	Formate	250	3.96	A	349
	Acetate	249.5	3.92	A	101
$C_{21}H_{29}O_4Br$	12α-Bromo-3α,21-dihydroxy-16-pregnene-11,20-dione	235	8600	M	85
	Diacetate	231	8700	E	85
$C_{21}H_{29}O_5Br$	12α-Bromo-3α,15ξ,21-trihydroxy-16-pregnene-11,20-dione				
	Triacetate	229	9800	E	84
$C_{21}H_{30}O_2$	3β-Hydroxy-5,16-pregnadien-20-one				
	Formate	238	4.05	A	349
	Acetate	240	9095	A	63
	3α-Hydroxy-7,16-pregnadien-20-one				
	Acetate	238	4.11	A	411
		318	1.83	A	411
	3β-Hydroxy-8(14),16-pregnadien-20-one				
	Acetate	230	4.07	A	258
	3α-Hydroxy-9(11),16-pregnadien-20-one				
	Acetate	238	7070	A	400
	16-Pregnene-3,20-dione	233	4.0		363
$C_{21}H_{30}O_3$	1ξ,3β-Dihydroxy-5,16-pregnadien-20-one	240	9100	M	304
	Diacetate	239.5	9250	A	62
	3β,21-Dihydroxy-5,16-pregnadien-20-one				
	21-Acetate	240	4.11	A	349
	3-Formate,21-acetate	240	4.10	A	349
	Diacetate	241	4.08	A	101
	3α-Hydroxy-16-pregnene-11,20-dione				
	Acetate	236	4.12		356
		312	1.79		356
		236	7400	A	400
	3β-Hydroxy-14β-16-pregnene-11,20-dione				
	Acetate	235	3.89	A	111

TABLE V—*continued*

Formula	Compound	λ_{max}	Ext.	Sol.	Ref.
16-en-20-Ones (cont.)					
$C_{21}H_{30}O_3$	3β-Hydroxy-5α-16-pregnene-11,20-dione				
	Acetate	237	4.13	A	96
		312	1.85	A	96
		235	9250	A	77
	n-Octanoate	235	9700	A	71
	3β-Hydroxy-5α-16-pregnene-12,20-dione				
	Acetate	227	3.82	A	286
$C_{21}H_{30}O_4$	3β,12β-Dihydroxy-5α-16-pregnene-11,20-dione				
	Diacetate	230	4.08	A	262
	3α,21-Dihydroxy-16-pregnene-11,20-dione				
	Diacetate	237	9900	M	377
	3β,13α-Dihydroxy-12,13-*seco*-5α-16-pregnen-20-one				
	12 → 13-lactone 3-Acetate,12-oic acid	227	4.0		357
$C_{21}H_{31}O_4I$	3β,6β-Dihydroxy-21-iodo-5α-16-pregnen-20-one				
	Diacetate	250	3.94	A	348
$C_{21}H_{32}O_2$	3β-Hydroxy-5α-16-pregnen-20-one				
	Acetate	242	4.2	A	66
	3β-Hydroxy-5α,14β-16-pregnen-20-one				
	Acetate	242	3.95	A	110
	3β-Hydroxy-5α,8α-16-pregnen-20-one				
	Acetate	240	4.0	A	105
	3β-Hydroxy-14β-16-pregnen-20-one				
	Acetate	242	3.95	A	111
$C_{21}H_{32}O_3$	2β,3β-Dihydroxy-16-pregnen-20-one				
	Diacetate	239	3.92	M	417
	3β,11α-Dihydroxy-5α-16-pregnen-20-one				
	Diacetate	237	4.12	A	96
	3α,11α-Dihydroxy-16-pregnen-20-one				
	Diacetate	236	9200	A	186
	3α,12α-Dihydroxy-16-pregnen-20-one				
	Diacetate	238	10,900	M	227

TABLE V—*continued*

Formula	Compound	λ_{max}	Ext.	Sol.	Ref.
16-en-20-Ones (cont.)					
$C_{21}H_{32}O_3$	3α,15β-Dihydroxy-5α-16-pregnen-20-one				
	Diacetate	231	4.00	A	99
		231	4.00	A	100
$C_{21}H_{32}O_4$	2α,3β,15β-Trihydroxy-5α-16-pregnen-20-one				
	Triacetate	231	3.97	A	99
	3β,6β,21-Trihydroxy-5α-16-pregnen-20-one				
	Triacetate	240	4.20	A	348
	3β,12β-Dihydroxy-5α-16-pregnene-11,20-dione				
	Diacetate	232	3.95	A	287
$C_{21}H_{34}O_3$	3β,6β-Dihydroxy-5α-16-pregnen-20-one				
	Diacetate	238	4.03	A	348
$C_{22}H_{32}O_2$	3β-Hydroxy-16-methyl-5,16-pregnadien-20-one	250	4.26	A	344
		252	4.25		288
	Acetate	250	4.28	A	344
$C_{22}H_{32}O_3$	3α-Hydroxy-16-methyl-16-pregnene-11,20-dione				
	Acetate	249	9300	M	403
		248	10,800	M	314
$C_{22}H_{34}O_2$	3β-Hydroxy-16-methyl-5α-16-pregnen-20-one	252	4.05	A	344
$C_{23}H_{28}O_5$	*d,l*-3-Ethylenedioxy-11β-hydroxy-5,16-pregnadien-20-one-18-oic acid-18 → 11-lactone	237	8000	A	370
	d,l-3-Ethylenedioxy-11β-hydroxy-14β-5,16-pregnadien-20-one-18-oic acid-18 → 11-lactone	236	7600	A	370
$C_{23}H_{30}O_2N$	21-Dimethylamino-3β-hydroxy-5,16-pregnadien-20-one				
	Acetate	240.5	6800	A	279
	Acetate, hydrochloride salt	246	8860	A	279
	Acetate, methiodide salt	243	8050	A	279
$C_{23}H_{31}O_3Cl$	4ξ-Chloro-3-ethylenedioxy-9(11),16-pregnadien-20-one	238	6820	A	400
$C_{23}H_{32}O_3$	3-Ethylenedioxy-5,16-pregnadien-20-one	238	4.03	A	391

TABLE V—*continued*

Formula	Compound	λ_{max}	Ext.	Sol.	Ref.
16-en-20-Ones (cont.)					
$C_{23}H_{32}O_4$	3-Ethylenedioxy-21-hydroxy-5,16-pregnadien-20-one				
	Acetate	239.5	8800	A	9
$C_{25}H_{37}O_3N$	3β-Hydroxy-21-morpholino-5,16-pregnadien-20-one				
	Acetate	240.5	6540		279
	Acetate, hydrochloride salt	245.5	8600		279
$C_{26}H_{36}O_5$	*d,l*-Ethylenedioxy-16-iso-propoxy-5,16-pregnadiene-11,20-dione	274	14,400	M	20
17(20)-Enones					
$C_{22}H_{32}O_2$	3β-Hydroxy-21-methyl-5,17(20)-*trans*-pregnadien-21-one	242	4.25	A	343
	Acetate	242	4.22	A	343
$C_{25}H_{32}O_6$	*d,l*-20-Acetoxy-3-ethylenedioxy-5,17(20)-pregnadiene-11,16-dione	246	14,000	M	20
$C_{26}H_{36}O_5$	*d,l*-3-Ethylenedioxy-20-iso-propoxy-5,17(20)-pregnadiene-11,16-dione	281	16,600	M	20
D-homo-enones					
$C_{19}H_{22}O_2$	*d,l*-3-Methoxy-D-homo-18-nor-1,3,5(10),13-estratetraen-17a-one	246	15,600	A	215
	3-Methoxy-D-homo-18-nor-1,3,5(10),13(17a)-estratetraen-17-one	238	13,000	A	399
$C_{19}H_{28}O_2$	*d,l*-3α-Hydroxy-D-homo-18-nor-13-etiocholen-17a-one	248	4.10	A	220
	d,l-3β-Hydroxy-D-homo-18-nor-13-androsten-17a-one	248.5	4.12	A	213
$C_{19}H_{28}O_3$	*d,l*-3α,11β-Dihydroxy-D-homo-18-nor-13-etiocholen-17a-one	248	4.11	A	220
	d,l-3β,11β-Dihydroxy-D-homo-18-nor-13-androsten-17a-one	248	4.14	A	220
	d,l-3β,11β-Dihydroxy-D-homo-18-nor-16-androsten-17a-one	224.7	3.94	A	220
$C_{20}H_{26}O_3$	3-Ethylenedioxy-D-homo-18,19-dinor-5,13-androstadien-17a-one	248.5	12,500	A	52
$C_{20}H_{28}O_3$	3β-Hydroxy-D-homo-16-androstene-11,17a-dione	225	8200	A	30
$C_{20}H_{28}O_4$	3α,17-Dihydroxy-D-homo-16-etiocholene-11,17a-dione	267	6200	M	426
	Diacetate	233	7500	M	426
$C_{21}H_{28}O_3$	*d,l*-3-Ethylenedioxy-D-homo-18-nor-5,16-androstadien-17a-one	225	3.94	A	214
	d,l-3-Ethylenedioxy-D-homo-18-nor-5,13-androstadien-17a-one	246.5	4.13	A	214
$C_{21}H_{30}O_3$	3α-Hydroxy-17-methyl-D-homo-16-etiocholene-11,17a-dione				
	Acetate	235	8300	M	429
		235	3.92	M	424

TABLE V—*continued*

Formula	Compound	λ_{max}	Ext.	Sol.	Ref.
D-homo-enones (cont.)					
$C_{21}H_{30}O_3$	3β,17-Dihydroxy-17a-methyl-D-homo-5,17-androstadien-16-one	277	9120		88
		276	3.97	A	351
	Diacetate	245	11,830		88
		244	4.08	A	351
$C_{21}H_{30}O_4$	3α,17-Dihydroxy-15-methyl-D-homo-16-etiocholene-11,17a-dione	273	8600	M	426
	Diacetate	239	10,850	M	426
	3α,17-Dihydroxy-17a-methyl-D-homo-17-etiocholene-11,16-dione	279	9450	M	428
	Diacetate	241	10,750	M	428
	16,17-Quinoxalone	238	32,600	M	428
		311(inf.)	8350	M	428
		329	10,700	M	428
$C_{22}H_{32}O_2$	3β-Hydroxy-D-homo-5,17(17a)-pregnadien-20-one	233	8930		115
$C_{22}H_{32}O_3$	3α-Hydroxy-D-homo-17,17a-pregnene-11,20-dione				
	Acetate	230	10,100	A	81
Enones (misc.)					
$C_{19}H_{27}O_2N$	16-Cyano-3β-hydroxy-13,17-*seco*-17-nor-14ξ-12-androsten-11-one				
	Acetate	234	7200	A	30
		311–315	27	A	30
$C_{19}H_{28}O_4$	3α-Hydroxy-13,17-*seco*-12-etiocholen-11-one-17-oic acid				
	Acetate	236	4.12		246
	3β-Hydroxy-13,17-*seco*-12-androsten-11-one-17-oic acid	239	13,600	A	30
$C_{20}H_{28}O_2$	3β-Hydroxy-16-methylene-5-androsten-17-one	228	3.91	A	297
$C_{20}H_{28}O_3$	3α-Hydroxy-16-methylene-etiocholane-11,17-dione				
	Acetate	228	8800	M	426
$C_{20}H_{30}O_2$	3α-Hydroxy-17,17-dimethyl-13-nor-12-etiocholen-11-one				
	Acetate	240	17,200	M	421
$C_{21}H_{28}O_6$	9aξ,17α,21-Trihydroxy-A-nor-B-homo-10-nor-9aξ-methyl-3(5)-pregnene-3,11,20-trione				
	21-Acetate	233	15,500	A	32
$C_{21}H_{30}O_2$	16-Acetyl-5,15-androstadien-3β-ol				
	Acetate	244	12,300	A	146

TABLE V—*continued*

Formula	Compound	λ_{max}	Ext.	Sol.	Ref.
Enones (misc.) (cont.)					
$C_{21}H_{30}O_2$	16-Acetyl-5,16-androstadien-3β-ol				
	Acetate	240	9780	A	146
		309	63	A	146
$C_{21}H_{30}O_3$	16-Acetyl-3α-hydroxy-16-etiocholen-11-one	237	12,300	M	425
	Acetate	237.5	10,500	M	425
$C_{22}H_{32}O_3$	16-Acetyl-3α-hydroxy-17-methyl-16-etiocholen-11-one	251	10,320	M	425
Enones-Cumulative					
$C_{18}H_{22}O_2$	18,19-Bisnor-D-homo-4,13-androstadien-17a-one	244.5	25,500	A	52
$C_{18}H_{22}O_3$	*d,l*-11β-Hydroxy-18-nor-13ξ-4,14-androstadiene-3,16-dione	238	31,700	A	433
$C_{20}H_{22}O_4$	18-Carboxy-11β-hydroxy-4,14-androstadiene-3,16-dione-18′→ 11-lactone	235	32,000	M	187
$C_{20}H_{24}O_5$	17β-Carboxy-17α-hydroxy-4,8(9)-androstadiene-3,11-dione	235	18,300	M	423
	17β-Carboxy-17α-hydroxy-14β-4,8(9)-androstadiene-3,11-dione	241	19,350	M	423
$C_{21}H_{24}O_2$	*d,l*-17a-Methoxy-4-methyl-D-homo-18-nor-4,8,13(17a),14,16-androstapentaen-3-one	221	4.41	A	223
		255	4.35	A	223
$C_{21}H_{24}O_3$	1,4,16-Pregnatriene-3,11,20-trione	236	4.38	A	238
$C_{21}H_{25}O_4Br$	12α-Bromo-21-hydroxy-4,16-pregnadiene-3,11,20-trione				
	Acetate	237–238	24,950	A	269
$C_{21}H_{26}O_2$	4,9(11),16-Pregnatriene-3,20-dione	239	22,200	A	400
$C_{21}H_{26}O_3$	21-Hydroxy-4,9,(11),16-pregnatriene-3,20-dione	238–239	24,500	A	9
	Acetate	239	24,000	A	9
	4,16-Pregnadiene-3,11,20-trione	231	27,225	E	257
		236	24,875	M	257
		238	24,552	M	228
$C_{21}H_{26}O_4$	17α,21-Dihydroxy-4,7,9(11)-pregnatriene-3,20-dione	243	18,000	A	156
		237(sh)	16,600	A	156
		250(sh)	14,700	A	156
	21-Acetate	243	21,900	A	156
		237	20,300	A	156

TABLE V—*continued*

Formula	Compound	λ_{max}	Ext.	Sol.	Ref.
Enones—Cumulative (cont.)					
$C_{21}H_{26}O_4$	21-Acetate	250	18,000	A	156
		242.5	26,200	M	423
		237.5(sh)	24,900	M	423
		250	22,100	M	423
	17α,21-Dihydroxy-4,8(14),9(11)-pregnatriene-3,20-dione				
	21-Acetate	241	21,600	M	423
		270	4700	M	423
		240	17,400	A	156
		275	4150	A	156
	17α,21-Dihydroxy-4,8,14-pregnatriene-3,20-dione				
	21-Acetate	242	37,400	M	423
	21-Hydroxy-4,16-pregnadiene-3,11,20-trione	238	23,900	M	9
	Acetate	238	24,600	M	9
		237–238	25,300	A	269
	21-Hydroxy-17β-methyl-18-nor-9ξ,14ξ,17α-4,12-pregnadiene-3,11,20-trione				
	Acetate	238	26,200	A	195
	4,17(20)-*cis*-Pregnadiene-3,11-dione-21-oic acid				
	Methyl ester	233	24,375	A	204
	4,17(20)-*trans*-Pregnadiene-3,11-dione-21-oic acid				
	Methyl ester	230	24,300	A	204
$C_{21}H_{26}O_5$	17α,21-Dihydroxy-4,8(9)-pregnadiene-3,11,20-trione	237	17,900	M	423
	21-Acetate	236.5	17,700	M	423
		235	17,200	A	156
		236.5	17,700	M	167
	17α,21-Dihydroxy-14β-4,8(9)-pregnadiene-3,11,20-trione				
	21-Acetate	237.5	19,700	M	423
		237.5	19,600	M	167
	Diacetate	237.5	19,900	M	423
		237.5	19,900	M	167

TABLE V—*continued*

Formula	Compound	λ_{max}	Ext.	Sol.	Re.
Enones—Cumulative (cont.)					
$C_{21}H_{27}O_3Br$	20-Bromo-4,17(20)-pregnadien-3-one-21-oic acid				
	Methyl ester	244	4.37	A	343
$C_{21}H_{28}O_2$	16-Acetyl-4,15-androstadien-3-one	244	17,380	A	146
		300	90	A	146
	16-Acetyl-4,16-androstadien-3-one	244	16,600	A	146
		300	90	A	146
$C_{21}H_{28}O_3$	11α-Hydroxy-4,16-pregnadiene-3,20-dione	235	25,725	A	257
	Acetate	239	25,775	A	257
	21-Hydroxy-4,16-pregnadiene-3,20-dione	240–241	23,600	A	9
	Acetate	238–241	24,200	A	9
		234	27,400	E	82
		241	25,200	M	82
		241	4.40	A	349
	4,17(20)-*cis*-Pregnadien-3-one-21-oic acid				
	Methyl ester	236–238	4.38	A	343
	4,17(20)-Pregnadien-3-one-21-oic acid				
	Ethyl ester	230	4.4	A	318
$C_{21}H_{28}O_4$	11β,21-Dihydroxy-4,16-pregnadiene-3,20-dione	241–242	22,600	A	9
	Acetate	240.5	24,400	A	9
	11α-Hydroxy-4,17(20)-*cis*-pregnadien-3-one-21-oic acid				
	Methyl ester	239	22,425	A	204
$C_{22}H_{26}O_5$	17-Acetoxy-D-homo-4,16-androstadiene-3,11,17a-trione	236	21,000	M	427
$C_{22}H_{28}O_4$	6α-Methyl-4,17(20)-pregnadiene-3,11-dione-21-oic acid				
	Methyl ester	234	23,100	A	396
$C_{22}H_{30}O_2$	6α-Methyl-4,16-pregnadiene-3,20-dione	240	28,400	A	63
$C_{23}H_{28}O_5$	20-Acetoxy-4,17(20)-pregnadien-21-al-3,11-dione	241	23,700	M	48
		238	26,600	E	48
$C_{23}H_{30}O_5$	20-Acetoxy-11β-hydroxy-4,17(20)-pregnadien-21-al-3-one	239	26,500	M	48

TABLE VI. CONJUGATED DIENONES

Formula	Compound	λ_{max}	Ext.	Sol.	Ref.
1,5(10)-dien-3-Ones					
$C_{22}H_{28}O_6$	4,4-Diacetoxy-1,5(10)-estradiene-3,17-dione (purity?)	335	3400	M	162
3,5-dien-7-Ones					
$C_{19}H_{24}O_3$	3-Hydroxy-3,5-androstadiene-7,17-dione	322	4.3	A	328
$C_{19}H_{26}O_2$	17β-Hydroxy-3,5-androstadien-7-one	392	4.7	BA	328
	Acetate	280	4.42	A	388
$C_{20}H_{26}O_3$	3-Methoxy-3,5-androstadiene-7,17-dione	311	4.35	A	328
$C_{20}H_{28}O_3$	17β-Hydroxy-3-methoxy-3,5-androstadien-7-one	311	4.35	A	328
$C_{21}H_{28}O_4$	3,21-Dihydroxy-3,5-pregnadiene-7,20-dione	320–321	23,600	A	251
		391–392	3800	A	251
		390–391	74,400	BA	251
$C_{21}H_{30}O_2$	20β-Hydroxy-3,5-pregnadien-7-one				
	Acetate	278	4.48	A	345
$C_{21}H_{30}O_4$	3-(β-Hydroxyethoxy)-17β-hydroxy-3,5-androstadien-7-one	311	4.39	A	328
$C_{25}H_{36}O_6$	20-Ethylenedioxy-3-(β-hydroxyethoxy)-21-hydroxy-3,5-pregnadien-7-one	309–310	32,800	A	251
	Diacetate	308	28,000	A	251
4,6-dien-3-Ones					
$C_{18}H_{24}O_2$	17β-Hydroxy-19-nor-4,6-androstadien-3-one				
	Acetate	282–284	4.29	A	445
		284	27,500	A	412
$C_{19}H_{24}O_2$	4,6-Androstadiene-3,17-dione	284	4.47	A	378a
$C_{19}H_{24}O_2Cl_2$	1α,2β-Dichloro-17β-hydroxy-4,6-androstadien-3-one				
	Propionate	296.5	4.36	A	239
$C_{19}H_{26}O_2$	17β-Hydroxy-4,6-androstadien-3-one	284	4.50	A	378a
$C_{21}H_{26}O_2$	4,6,16-Pregnatriene-3,20-dione	284	4.48	A	378a
$C_{21}H_{26}O_4$	17α-Hydroxy-4,6-pregnadiene-3,12,20-trione	281.5	19,940	A	358
$C_{21}H_{26}O_5$	17α,21-Dihydroxy-4,6-pregnadiene-3,11,20-trione	280.5	25,900	A	266
	21-Acetate	280	26,100	A	266

TABLE VI—*continued*

Formula	Compound	λ_{max}	Ext.	Sol.	Ref.
4,6-dien-3-Ones (cont.)					
$C_{21}H_{26}O_6$	14α,17α,21-Trihydroxy-4,6-pregnadiene-3,11,20-trione				
	21-Acetate	282	24,300	A	8
$C_{21}H_{27}O_4F$	9α-Fluoro-11β,17α-dihydroxy-4,6-pregnadiene-3,20-dione	281	26,000	A	154
$C_{21}H_{27}O_5F$	9α-Fluoro-11β,17α,21-trihydroxy-4,6-pregnadiene-3,20-dione	281	25,600	A	154
	21-Acetate	281	4.40	M	201
		281	23,000	A	154
	21-Mesylate	281	27,500	A	154
$C_{21}H_{28}O_2$	4,6-Pregnadiene-3,20-dione	284	4.30	M	364
		284	4.50	A	380
$C_{21}H_{28}O_3$	11α-Hydroxy-4,6-pregnadiene-3,20-dione	286	20,300	A	322
	11-Acetate	284	23,000	A	322
	21-Hydroxy-4,6-pregnadiene-3,20-dione	283	25,500	A	251
	21-Acetate	284	4.49	A	380
		284	27,300	A	277
		282	27,500		251
	17α-Hydroxy-4,6-pregnadiene-3,20-dione	284	4.48	A	380
	17β-Carboxy-4,6-androstadien-3-one				
	Methyl ester	283	26,900	A	277
$C_{21}H_{28}O_4$	17α,21-Dihydroxy-4,6-pregnadiene-3,20-dione				
	21-Acetate	284	4.47	A	380
$C_{21}H_{28}O_5$	17α,20β,21-Trihydroxy-4,6-pregnadiene-3,11-dione	282	22,800	M	164
	11β,17α,21-Trihydroxy-4,6-pregnadiene-3,20-dione	283	24,900	M	165
	21-Acetate	284	25,000	A	8
$C_{21}H_{28}O_6$	11β,14α,17α,21-Tetrahydroxy-4,6-pregnadiene-3,20-dione				
	21-Acetate	283	24,800	A	8
$C_{21}H_{30}O_2$	20β-Hydroxy-4,6-pregnadien-3-one	284	4.49	A	380
$C_{22}H_{28}O_5$	20ξ,22ξ-Epoxy-17α,21-dihydroxy-4,6-dinorcholadiene-3,11-dione	280.5	24,700	M	303
$C_{27}H_{36}O_7$	6-Methoxy-16α-dimethylmalonoyl-4,6-pregnadiene-3,20-dione	205	5100	A	53
		249	8540	A	53
		304	16,100	A	53

TABLE VI—*continued*

Formula	Compound	λ_{max}	Ext.	Sol.	Ref.
7,9(11)-dien-12-Ones					
$C_{20}H_{24}O_4$	17β-Carboxy-7,9(11)-etiocholadiene-3,12-dione				
	Methyl ester	289	4.16	A	230
$C_{20}H_{26}O_4$	17β-Carboxy-3α-hydroxy-7,9(11)-etiocholadien-12-one				
	Methyl ester	240	3.48	A	230
		292.5	4.12	A	230
8,11-dien-7-Ones					
$C_{21}H_{30}O_3$	3β,20β-Dihydroxy-5α-8,11-pregnadien-7-one	226	4.30	A	350
		298	3.81	A	350
	Diacetate	226	4.33	A	350
		297	3.88	A	350
8(14),15-dien-7-Ones					
$C_{21}H_{30}O_3$	3β,20β-Dihydroxy-5α-8(14),15-pregnadien-7-one				
	Diacetate	225	4.27	A	249
		298	3.80	A	249
14,16-dien-20-Ones					
$C_{21}H_{27}O_4Br$	12α-Bromo-3α,21-dihydroxy-14,16-pregnadiene-11,20-dione				
	Diacetate	305	9000	E	84
Dienones (Misc.)					
$C_{26}H_{32}O_4$	18-Benzylidene-3β-hydroxy-13,17-*seco*-12-androsten-11-one-17-oic acid	240	10,600	A	30
		325	34,200	A	30
$C_{27}H_{34}O_4$	18-Benzylidene-17β-carboxy-3β-hydroxy-13,17-*seco*-12-androsten-11-one	238	14,000	A	30
		325	35,200	A	30

TABLE VII. CROSS-CONJUGATED DIENONES

Formula	Compound	λ_{max}	Ext.	Sol.	Ref.
1,4-dien-3-Ones					
$C_{18}H_{22}O_3$	10ξ-Hydroxy-1,4-estradiene-3,17-dione	235	13,000	M	162
	Acetate	248	13,000	M	162
$C_{18}H_{24}O_3$	10ξ,17β-Dihydroxy-1,4-estradien-3-one	241	12,000	M	162
	10-Acetate	250	13,000	M	162
$C_{19}H_{20}O_4$	6α,7α-Epoxy-1,4-androstadiene-3,11,17-trione	240	14,300	M	302
$C_{19}H_{21}O_3Br$	6ξ-Bromo-1,4-androstadiene-3,11,17-trione	243	15,300	M	165
$C_{19}H_{22}O_3$	1,4-Androstadiene-3,11,17-trione	239	13,900	A	185
$C_{19}H_{24}O_3$	2-Hydroxy-1,4-androstadiene-3,17-dione	253	14,200	M	24
	11β-Hydroxy-1,4-androstadiene-3,17-dione	242	15,200	A	185
	1-Dehydrotestololactone	242	15,800	A	157
$C_{19}H_{24}O_2Cl_2$	1,2-Dichloro-17β-hydroxy-1,4-androstadien-3-one				
	Propionate	257.5	4.10	A	239
$C_{19}H_{25}O_2Cl$	2-Chloro-17β-hydroxy-1,4-androstadien-3-one				
	Propionate	251	4.21	A	239
	4-Chloro-17β-hydroxy-1,4-androstadien-3-one				
	Propionate	246	4.05	A	239
$C_{19}H_{26}O_2$	17β-Hydroxy-1,4-androstadien-3-one	244	4.18	A	337
		243	16,100	A	157
	Acetate	244.5	15,700	A	225
	Benzoate	235	25,450	A	225
$C_{19}H_{26}O_3$	2,17β-Dihydroxy-1,4-androstadien-3-one	254	15,400	M	24
	17-Acetate	253	17,100	M	24
	Diacetate	247.5	16,750	M	24
	2,3-Quinoxalone	224.5	27,800	M	24
		267	24,300	M	24
		347	16,000	M	24
		362	15,300	M	24
$C_{19}H_{26}O_4Se$	17β-Hydroxy-1,4-androstadien-3-one-2-seleninic acid	252	10,600	M	24
$C_{20}H_{25}O_2Br$	6ξ-Bromo-2-methyl-1,4-androstadiene-3,17-dione	246	4.2	A	209
$C_{20}H_{26}O_2$	2-Methyl-1,4-androstadiene-3,17-dione	247	4.20	A	209
$C_{20}H_{26}O_5$	17β-Carboxy-11β,17α-dihydroxy-1,4-androstadien-3-one	243	4.16	M	200

TABLE VII—*continued*

Formula	Compound	λ_{max}	Ext.	Sol.	Ref.
1,4-dien-3-Ones (cont.)					
$C_{20}H_{28}O_2$	17β-Hydroxy-2-methyl-1,4-androstadien-3-one	248	4.23	A	209
	17β-Hydroxy-4-methyl-1,4-androstadien-3-one	244	4.16	A	386
	Acetate	245	4.17	A	386
	17β-Hydroxy-17α-methyl-1,4-androstadien-3-one	245	15,600	A	415
$C_{20}H_{28}O_3$	17β-Hydroxy-2-methoxy-1,4-androstadien-3-one	254	16,000	M	24
	2,17β-Dihydroxy-17α-methyl-1,4-androstadien-3-one	254	14,300	M	24
$C_{21}H_{24}O_3$	17α-Ethinyl-17β-hydroxy-1,4-androstadiene-3,11-dione	238	13,600	A	413
$C_{21}H_{24}O_4$	1,4-Pregnadien-21-al-3,11,20-trione				
	21,21-Dimethylacetal	238	14,900	A	185
$C_{21}H_{24}O_5$	17α-Hydroxy-1,4-pregnadien-21-al-3,11,20-trione				
	Hydrate	238	15,800	A	182
$C_{21}H_{24}O_5ClF$	6α-Chloro-9α-fluoro-17α,21-dihydroxy-1,4-pregnadiene-3,11,20-trione				
	21-Acetate	235	4.18	A	334
$C_{21}H_{24}O_6$	6α,7α-Epoxy-17α,21-dihydroxy-1,4-pregnadiene-3,11,20-trione	240	14,800	M	302
	21-Acetate	240	15,600	M	302
$C_{21}H_{25}O_4F$	17α,21-Epoxy-9α-fluoro-11β-hydroxy-1,4-pregnadiene-3,20-dione	237	17,200	A	178
$C_{21}H_{25}O_5Br$	4-Bromo-17α,21-dihydroxy-1,4-pregnadiene-3,11,20-trione				
	21-Acetate	243	9700	M	316
	6ξ-Bromo-17α,21-dihydroxy-1,4-pregnadiene-3,11,20-trione				
	21-Acetate	245	16,300	A	165
$C_{21}H_{25}O_5Cl$	4-Chloro-17α,21-dihydroxy-1,4-pregnadiene-3,11,20-trione				
	21-Acetate	242	10,600	M	316
	6α-Chloro-17α,21-dihydroxy-1,4-pregnadiene-3,11,20-trione				
	21-Acetate	237	4.19	A	334
	6β-Chloro-17α,21-dihydroxy-1,4-pregnadiene-3,11,20-trione				
	21-Acetate	241	4.17	A	334
	9α-Chloro-17α,21-dihydroxy-1,4-pregnadiene-3,11,20-trione				
	21-Acetate	236	15,500	A	154
$C_{21}H_{25}O_5F$	6α-Fluoro-17α,21-dihydroxy-1,4-pregnadiene-3,11,20-trione				
	21-Acetate	237	4.23	A	60

N

TABLE VII—*continued*

Formula	Compound	λ_{max}	Ext.	Sol.	Ref.
1,4-dien-3-Ones (cont.)					
$C_{21}H_{25}O_5F$	9α-Fluoro-17α,21-dihydroxy-1,4-pregnadiene-3,11,20-trione				
	21-Acetate	235	15,600	A	154
$C_{21}H_{25}O_6Br$	6β-Bromo-7α,17α,21-trihydroxy-1,4-pregnadiene-3,11,20-trione				
	21-Acetate	244	16,770	M	302
	7,21-Diacetate	243	15,900	M	302
$C_{21}H_{25}O_6F$	6β-Fluoro-7α,17α,21-trihydroxy-1,4-pregnadiene-3,11,20-trione				
	21-Acetate	236	14,700	M	302
	7,21-Diacetate	236	15,100	M	302
	9α-Fluoro-16α,17α,21-trihydroxy-1,4-pregnadiene-3,11,20-trione				
	16,21-Diacetate	235	16,200	A	407
$C_{21}H_{26}O_2$	17α-Ethinyl-17β-hydroxy-1,4-androstadien-3-one	244	15,500	A	415
		244	4.20	A	392
	1,4,11-Pregnatriene-3,20-dione	245	17,750	A	415
$C_{21}H_{26}O_3$	17α-Ethinyl-11β,17β-dihydroxy-1,4-androstadien-3-one	242	14,650	A	413
$C_{21}H_{26}O_4$	17α,21-Dihydroxy-1,4,9(11)-pregnatriene-3,20-dione				
	21-Acetate	238	16,100	A	154
	17α-Hydroxy-1,4-pregnadiene-3,11,20-trione	239.5	14,650	A	225
	17α,21-Epoxy-11β-hydroxy-1,4-pregnadiene-3,20-dione	243	15,400	A	178
	13α,21-Epoxy-11β-hydroxy-17β-methyl-18-nor-17α-1,4-pregnadiene-3,20-dione	243	15,900	A	178
	11α-Hydroxy-1,4,17(20)-pregnatrien-3-one-21-oic acid				
	Acetate, methyl ester	239	23,925	A	255
$C_{21}H_{26}O_4F_2$	9α,21-Difluoro-11β,17α-dihydroxy-1,4-pregnadiene-3,20-dione	237	15,500	A	178
$C_{21}H_{26}O_5$	11β,17α-Dihydroxy-1,4-pregnadien-21-al-3,20-dione	242	15,300	M	78
	9β,11β-Epoxy-17α,21-dihydroxy-1,4-pregnadiene-3,20-dione				
	21-Acetate	249	15,800	A	154
	17α,21-Dihydroxy-1,4-pregnadiene-3,11,20-trione	238	15,500	M	185
	21-Acetate	238	16,100	A	185
	21-Dihydrogenphosphate	244	15,300	W	327
	21-Trimethylacetate	240	15,600	A	415

TABLE VII—*continued*

Formula	Compound	λ_{max}	Ext.	Sol.	Ref.
1,4-dien-3-Ones (cont.)					
$C_{21}H_{26}O_5ClF$	6α-Chloro-9α-fluoro-11β,17α,21-trihydroxy-1,4-pregnadiene-3,20-dione				
	21-Acetate	238	4.19	A	334
$C_{21}H_{26}O_6$	2,17α,21-Trihydroxy-1,4-pregnadiene-3,11,20-trione				
	21-Trimethylacetate	252.5	12,100	M	24
	7α,17α,21-Trihydroxy-1,4-pregnadiene-3,11,20-trione				
	21-Acetate	237	14,500	M	302
	7,21-Diacetate	237	15,200	M	302
$C_{21}H_{27}O_3F$	6α-Fluoro-17α-hydroxy-1,4-pregnadiene-3,20-dione				
	Acetate	241	4.18	A	60
$C_{21}H_{27}O_4Cl$	6α-Chloro-17α,21-dihydroxy-1,4-pregnadiene-3,20-dione				
	21-Acetate	243	4.21	A	334
$C_{21}H_{27}O_4F$	6α-Fluoro-17α,21-dihydroxy-1,4-pregnadiene-3,20-dione	241	4.22	A	60
	Diacetate	242	4.23	A	60
	9α-Fluoro-11β,17α-dihydroxy-1,4-pregnadiene-3,20-dione	238	15,500	A	154
	12α-Fluoro-11β,21-dihydroxy-1,4-pregnadiene-3,20-dione				
	21-Acetate	242	15,700	M	404
		242	15,700	M	405
	21-Fluoro-11β,17α-dihydroxy-1,4-pregnadiene-3,20-dione	243	15,100	A	178
$C_{21}H_{27}O_5Br$	9α-Bromo-11β,17α,21-trihydroxy-1,4-pregnadiene-3,20-dione				
	21-Acetate	241	13,400	A	154
$C_{21}H_{27}O_5Cl$	6α-Chloro-11β,17α,21-trihydroxy-1,4-pregnadiene-3,20-dione	242	4.19	A	334
	21-Acetate	242	4.17	A	334
	9α-Chloro-11β,17α,21-trihydroxy-1,4-pregnadiene-3,20-dione				
	21-Acetate	238	15,000	A	154
$C_{21}H_{27}O_5F$	6α-Fluoro-11β,17α,21-trihydroxy-1,4-pregnadiene-3,20-dione				
	21-Acetate	242	4.25	A	60
	9α-Fluoro-11β,17α,21-trihydroxy-1,4-pregnadiene-3,20-dione	238	15,500	A	154
		239	14,800	M	298
		240	15,800	A	415
	21-Acetate	238	15,400	M	125
		240	16,250	A	415

TABLE VII—*continued*

Formula	Compound	λ_{max}	Ext.	Sol.	Ref.
1,4-dien-3-Ones (cont.)					
$C_{21}H_{27}O_5F$	21-Acetate	239	4.19	M	201
		238	14,500	A	154
	21-Mesylate	238	15,000	A	154
$C_{21}H_{28}O_2$	1,4-Pregnadiene-3,20-dione	244	4.25	A	392
		245	16,150	A	414
$C_{21}H_{28}O_3$	2-Hydroxy-1,4-pregnadiene-3,20-dione	253.5	14,500	M	24
	21-Hydroxy-1,4-pregnadiene-3,20-dione	244	14,100	A	414
	Acetate	243	15,800	M	298
		243	16,550	A	414
		243	4.19	A	146
	Trimethylacetate	244	16,000	A	278
$C_{21}H_{28}O_4$	2,21-Dihydroxy-1,4-pregnadiene-3,20-dione				
	21-Trimethylacetate	253.5	15,600	M	24
	11β,21-Dihydroxy-1,4-pregnadiene-3,20-dione	244	15,300	A	414
	21-Acetate	243	14,800	A	414
	17α,21-Dihydroxy-1,4-pregnadiene-3,20-dione	244	4.16	A	338
		244	15,900	M	298
	Diacetate	244	4.16	A	338
$C_{21}H_{28}O_5$	11β,17α,21-Trihydroxy-1,4-pregnadiene-3,20-dione	243	15,000	M	185
		243	14,300	M	298
	21-Acetate	242	15,255	A	205
		243	15,000	M	185
	21-Dimethylphosphate	242.5	15,100	M	327
	21-Trimethylacetate	244	14,700	A	415
	17α,20β,21-Trihydroxy-1,4-pregnadiene-3,11-dione	238	4.15	A	401
	21-Acetate	239	4.2	A	401
	20,21-Diacetate	238	4.16	A	401
	11β,20ξ-Dihydroxy-1,4-pregnadien-3-one-21-oic acid	242	4.15	Ch	200
$C_{21}H_{30}O_2$	20β-Hydroxy-1,4-pregnadien-3-one	244	4.24	A	392
	Acetate	244	4.24	A	392

TABLE VII—*continued*

Formula	Compound	λ_{max}	Ext.	Sol.	Ref.
1,4-dien-3-Ones (cont.)					
$C_{21}H_{30}O_4$	17α,20β,21-Trihydroxy-1,4-pregnadien-3-one	244.5	14,200	A	289
	20,21-Diacetate	243.5	15,900	A	289
$C_{22}H_{28}O_4$	17α,21-Dihydroxy-6α-methyl-1,4,9(11)-pregnatriene-3,20-dione				
	21-Acetate	239	15,450	A	395
	17α,21-Dihydroxy-16α-methyl-1,4,9(11)-pregnatriene-3,20-dione				
	21-Acetate	238	15,500	M	315
	17α,21-Dihydroxy-16β-methyl-1,4,9(11)-pregnatriene-3,20-dione				
	21-Acetate	239	19,300	M	313
	21-Hydroxy-17α-methyl-1,4-pregnadiene-3,11,20-trione	240	14,600	A	415
	21-Acetate	240	14,800	A	415
$C_{22}H_{28}O_4F_2$	9α,21-Difluoro-11β,17α-dihydroxy-6α-methyl-1,4-pregnadiene-3,20-dione	239	15,000	A	395
$C_{22}H_{28}O_5$	9β,11β-Epoxy-17α,21-dihydroxy-6α-methyl-1,4-pregnadiene-3,20-dione				
	21-Acetate	249	16,150	A	395
	9β,11β-Epoxy-17α,21-dihydroxy-16α-methyl-1,4-pregnadiene-3,20-dione				
	21-Acetate	249	15,600	M	315
	9β,11β-Epoxy-17α,21-dihydroxy-16β-methyl-1,4-pregnadiene-3,20-dione				
	21-Acetate	249	15,600	M	313
	17α,21-Dihydroxy-16α-methyl-1,4-pregnadiene-3,11,20-trione				
	21-Acetate	238	15,500	M	314
		238	15,400	M	19
	17α,21-Dihydroxy-16β-methyl-1,4-pregnadiene-3,11,20-trione	238	14,900	M	403
		238	14,700	M	314
	21-Acetate	238	15,100	M	403
		238	14,200	M	314
	20ξ,21-Epoxy-17α,21-dihydroxy-1,4-dinorcholadiene-3,11-dione	239	16,200		300
		239	15,600	M	303
$C_{22}H_{29}O_5F$	9α-Fluoro-11β,17α,21-trihydroxy-6α-methyl-1,4-pregnadiene-3,20-dione	238	15,150	A	395
	21-Acetate	239	15,250	A	395

TABLE VII—*continued*

Formula	Compound	λ_{max}	Ext.	Sol.	Ref.
1,4-dien-3-Ones (cont.)					
$C_{22}H_{29}O_5F$	9α-Fluoro,11β,17α,21-trihydroxy-16α-methyl-1,4-pregnadiene-3,20-dione				
	21-Acetate	239	14,500	M	315
		239	14,900	M	18
	9α-Fluoro-11β,17α,21-trihydroxy-16β-methyl-1,4-pregnadiene-3,20-dione				
	21-Acetate	239	25,200	M	313
$C_{22}H_{30}O_3$	11β,21-Dihydroxy-6α-methyl-1,4,17(20)-pregnatrien-3-one				
	21-Acetate	243	15,000	A	396
$C_{22}H_{30}O_4$	17α,21-Dihydroxy-16α-methyl-1,4-pregnadiene-3,20 dione	244	14,900	M	315
$C_{22}H_{30}O_5$	11β,17α,21-Trihydroxy-6α-methyl-1,4-pregnadiene-3,20-dione	243	14,875	A	396
	21-Acetate	243	14,825	A	396
	11β,17α,21-Trihydroxy-9α-methyl-1,4-pregnadiene-3,20-dione				
	21-Acetate	245	14,000	M	203
	11α,17α,21-Trihydroxy-16α-methyl-1,4-pregnadiene-3,20-dione	247	18,200	M	315
	21-Acetate	247	19,000	M	315
	11-Tosylate,21-acetate	229.5	22,200	M	315
	11α,17α,21-Trihydroxy-16β-methyl-1,4-pregnadiene-3,20-dione				
	21-Acetate	247	16,700	M	313
	11β,17α,21-Trihydroxy-16α-methyl-1,4-pregnadiene-3,20-dione				
	21-Acetate	242	15,200	M	19
	11β,17α,21-Trihydroxy-16β-methyl-1,4-pregnadiene-3,20-dione	243	14,600	M	403
	21-Acetate	243	15,000	M	403
	20ξ,22-Epoxy-11β,17α,21-trihydroxy-1,4-dinorcholadien-3-one	244	15,000	A	300
		244	15,000	M	303
	21-Acetate	243	15,000	M	303
$C_{24}H_{30}O_6ClF$	6α-Chloro-9α-fluoro-11β,21-dihydroxy-16α,17α-iso-propylidenedioxy-1,4-pregnadiene-3,20-dione	238	4.17	A	334
$C_{26}H_{30}O_4ClN$	17α-Hydroxy-21-pyridinium-1,4-pregnadiene-3,11,20-trione Chloride	241	18,600	M	182

TABLE VII—*continued*

Formula	Compound	λ_{max}	Ext.	Sol.	Ref.
Cross-conjugated dienones (Misc.)					
$C_{18}H_{20}O_3$	2,5(10)-Estradiene-1,4,17-trione	250	16,000	M	162
		340	1200	M	162
$C_{18}H_{20}O_4$	3-Hydroxy-2,5(10)-estradiene-1,4,17-trione	277	14,000	M	162
		275	16,000	AcM	162
		284	11,000	BM	162
$C_{20}H_{28}O_3$	17β-Hydroxy-2-hydroxymethylene-4-androsten-3-one	252	4.06	A	418
		307	3.76	A	418
$C_{23}H_{30}O_4$	17-Acetoxy-3β-hydroxy-17a-methyl-D-homo-5,14,17-androstatrien-16-one				
	3-Acetate	246.5	17,600		121

TABLE VIII. CONJUGATED TRIENONES

Formula	Compound	λ_{max}	Ext.	Sol.	Ref.
4,6,8(14)-trien-3-Ones					
$C_{21}H_{24}O_5$	17α,21-Dihydroxy-4,6,8(14)-pregnatriene-3,11,20-trione	337	25,800	M	423
	21-Acetate	334	27,500	M	423
4,6,8-trien-3-Ones					
$C_{21}H_{26}O_4$	17α,21-Dihydroxy-4,6,8-pregnatriene-3,20-dione				
	21-Acetate	244	14,300	A	156
		285–300	3100	A	156
		385	6700	A	156

TABLE IX. CROSS-CONJUGATED TRIENONES

Formula	Compound	λ_{max}	Ext.	Sol.	Ref.
1,4,6-trien-3-Ones					
$C_{19}H_{20}O_3$	1,4,6-Androstatriene-3,11,17-trione	222	11,300	M	165
		255	9900	M	165
		296	11,900	M	165
$C_{19}H_{23}O_2Cl$	2-Chloro-17β-hydroxy-1,4,6-androstatrien-3-one				
	Propionate	267.5	4.04	A	239
		305	4.01	A	239
	4-Chloro-17β-hydroxy-1,4,6-androstatrien-3-one				
	Propionate	229	4.12	A	239
		255(inf.)	3.85	A	239
		310.5	4.11	A	239
$C_{20}H_{24}O_2$	2-Methyl-1,4,6-androstatriene-3,17-dione	266	4.04	A	209
		301	3.98	A	209
$C_{20}H_{24}O_3$	17β-Carboxy-1,4,6-androstatrien-3-one				
	Methyl ester	222	4.15	A	394
		254	4.08	A	394
		296	4.20	A	394
$C_{21}H_{24}O_5$	17α,21-Dihydroxy-1,4,6-pregnatriene-3,11,20-trione	222	11,100	M	165
		255	9900	M	165
		296	11,700	M	165
	21-Acetate	222	11,400	A	165
		255	10,300	A	165
		297	12,100	A	165
		223	10,700	A	8
		255	9800	A	8
		297	12,100	A	8
$C_{21}H_{26}O_3$	21-Hydroxy-1,4,6-pregnatriene-3,20-dione				
	Acetate	223	11,600	A	415
		256	9900	A	415
		300	12,800	A	415

TABLE IX—*continued*

Formula	Compound	λ_{max}	Ext.	Sol.	Ref.
1,4,6-trien-3-Ones (cont.)					
$C_{21}H_{26}O_5$	11β,17α,21-Trihydroxy-1,4,6-pregnatriene-3,20-dione	221	11,500	A	8
		255	9300	A	8
		298	12,400	A	8
		222	11,600	M	165
		256	9600	M	165
		298	12,200	M	165
	21-Acetate	223	13,400	A	8
		253	10,500	A	8
		301	13,300	A	8

TABLE X. α,β-UNSATURATED ALDEHYDES

Formula	Compound	λ_{max}	Ext.	Sol.	Ref.
$C_{20}H_{28}O_2$	16-Formyl-5,16-androstadien-3β-ol	chart			145
		232(chart)			143
$C_{21}H_{30}O_2$	3β-Hydroxy-5,17(20)-pregnadien-21-al				
	Acetate	244	4.25	A	343
		244	4.36	A	378
$C_{21}H_{30}O_4$	3α,20-Dihydroxy-17(20)-pregnen-21-al-11-one				
	3-Acetate	284	12,800	A	265

TABLE XI. α,β-UNSATURATED ACIDS AND ESTERS

Formula	Compound	λ_{max}	Ext.	Sol.	Ref.
$C_{19}H_{28}O_5$	2,3-Dicarboxy-2,3-*seco*-4-androsten-17β-ol	222	4.06	A	418
$C_{20}H_{24}O_4$	3,11α-Dihydroxy-19-nor-1,3,5(10),17(20)-pregnatetraen-21-oic acid				
	Methyl ester	224	17,375	A	255
$C_{20}H_{28}O_3$	16-Carboxy-5,16-androstadien-3β-ol	chart			145
		chart			143
	Methyl ester	chart			145
		chart			143
$C_{20}H_{30}O_3$	17-Carboxy-14β-16-androsten-3β-ol				
	Acetate, methyl ester	226	3.89	A	319
$C_{21}H_{29}O_3Br$	20-Bromo-3β-hydroxy-5,17(20)-pregnadien-21-oic acid	248	3.8	A	343
	Methyl ester	222–224	3.72	A	343
		250	3.85	A	343
	Acetate, methyl ester	222–224	3.78	A	343
		248	3.84	A	343
$C_{21}H_{30}O_3$	3β-Hydroxy-5,17(20)-*cis*-pregnadien-21-oic acid	224	4.04	A	343
	Methyl ester	224	4.09	A	343
	Acetate, methyl ester	224–226	4.10	A	343
	3β-Hydroxy-5,17(20)-*trans*-pregnadien-21-oic acid	222	4.22	A	343
	Methyl ester	222	4.24	A	343
	Acetate, methyl ester	222	4.22	A	343
$C_{21}H_{30}O_4$	3α-Hydroxy-17(20)-pregnen-11-one-21-oic acid	220	4.2	A	127
	Methyl ester	221	3.9	A	127
	Acetate, methyl ester	222	4.1	A	127
$C_{21}H_{31}O_3Br_2$	16ξ-Bromo-3β-hydroxy-5α-17(20)-pregnen-20-oic acid				
	Hexahydrobenzoate, ethyl ester	235(chart)	3.9	A	76
	Benzoate, ethyl ester	229(chart)	4.4	D	76
$C_{21}H_{32}O_3$	3β-Hydroxy-5α-17(20)-pregnen-21-oic acid				
	Ethyl ester	227(chart)	4.3	D	76
	Hexahydrobenzoate, ethyl ester	225(chart)	4.2	A	76
$C_{21}H_{32}O_4$	3α,12α-Dihydroxy-17(20)-pregnen-21-oic acid				
	Diacetate, methyl ester	222	4.23	A	130
$C_{23}H_{30}O_5$	3-Ethylenedioxy-5,17(20)-*cis*-pregnadien-11-one-21-oic acid				
	Methyl ester	225	13,525	A	204

TABLE XI—*continued*

Formula	Compound	λ_{max}	Ext.	Sol.	Ref.
α,β-Unsaturated Acid and Esters (cont.)					
$C_{23}H_{32}O_3$	3-Ethoxy-3,5,17(20)-pregnatrien-21-oic acid				
	Ethyl ester	232	4.5	A	318
$C_{24}H_{36}O_5$	3β,20ξ,21-Trihydroxy-5,22-choladienic acid				
	t-Butyl ester	208	9800	IP	380

TABLE XII. α,β-UNSATURATED NITRILES

Formula	Compound	λ_{max}	Ext.	Sol.	Ref.
$C_{20}H_{27}ON$	16-Cyano-5,15-androstadien-3β-ol				
	Acetate	chart			144
		224	7400	A	146
	16-Cyano-5,16-androstadien-3β-ol				
	Acetate	chart			144
		220	7600	A	146
	17-Cyano-5,16-androstadien-3β-ol				
	Acetate	218	7180	A	146
$C_{21}H_{29}O_2N$	17a-Cyano-3α-hydroxy-D-homo-17(17a)-etiocholen-11-one				
	Acetate	213	9800	A	81
$C_{22}H_{29}O_2N$	20-Cyano-21-hydroxy-9(11),17(20)-pregnadien-3-one				
	Acetate	222	$E^{1\%}_{1\,cm.}$ 413	M	166
$C_{22}H_{29}O_3N$	20-Cyano-3β-hydroxy-5,17(20)-pregnadien-21-oic acid				
	Acetate, ethyl ester	238	4.1	A	318
	20-Cyano-21-hydroxy-17(20)-pregnene-3,11-dione	223	13,680	M	226
	iso-compound	222	11,050	M	226
	Acetate	222	14,650	M	226
	Acetate iso-compound	222	13,300	M	226
$C_{22}H_{31}O_2N$	20-Cyano-3β-hydroxy-5α-17(20)-pregnen-11-one				
	Acetate	221	12,300	A	54
$C_{22}H_{31}O_3N$	20-Cyano-11β,21-dihydroxy-17(20)-pregnen-3-one	222.5	$E^{1\%}_{1\,cm.}$ 396	M	422
	21-Acetate	222.5	$E^{1\%}_{1\,cm.}$ 370	M	422
$C_{24}H_{35}O_4N$	20-Cyano-3,3-dimethoxy-21-hydroxy-17(20)-pregnen-11-one	222.5	$E^{1\%}_{1\,cm.}$ 357	M	422
	21-Acetate	222.5	$E^{1\%}_{1\,cm.}$ 328	M	422
$C_{26}H_{39}O_4N$	20-Cyano-3,3-diethoxy-21-hydroxy-17(20)-pregnen-11-one				
	Acetate	222.5	$E^{1\%}_{1\,cm.}$ 307	M	422

TABLE XIII. β-DIKETONES AND β-KETOESTERS

Formula	Compound	λ_{max}	Ext.	Sol.	Ref.
$C_{19}H_{24}O_3$	4-Androstene-3,15,17-trione	242	15,600	BM	420
		277	19,700	BM	420
$C_{21}H_{30}O_4$	16β-Acetyl-3α-hydroxy-etiocholane-11,17-dione	282	8300	M	419
$C_{20}H_{30}O_4$	17β-Carboxy-3β-hydroxy-etiocholan-16-one				
	Acetate, methyl ester	259	78	A	196
		293(sh)	34	A	196
$C_{21}H_{28}O_3$	4-Pregnene-3,16,20-trione	285	5430	A	41
		308	20,100	BA	41
$C_{23}H_{30}O_5$	*d,l*-3-Ethylenedioxy-13α-5-pregnene-11,16,20-trione	285	9100	M	20
	d,l-3-Ethylenedioxy-14β-5-pregnene-11,16,20-trione	286	7900	M	20

TABLE XIV. AROMATIC RING A

Formula	Compound	λ_{max}	Ext.	Sol.	Ref.
$C_{18}H_{20}O_2$	3-Hydroxy-1,3,5(10),7-estratetraen-17-one	282	3.36	A	445
$C_{18}H_{20}O_3$	3-Hydroxy-1,3,5(10)-estratriene-7,17-dione	282	3.32	A	210
	Benzoate	232	4.27	A	210
$C_{18}H_{20}O_6N_2$	3-Hydroxy-2,4-dinitro-1,3,5(10)-estratrien-17-one	276	6890	A	431
		353	3405	A	431
		430	1050	A	431
$C_{18}H_{21}O_4N$	3-Hydroxy-2-nitro-1,3,5(10)-estratrien-17-one	293–294	8220	A	431
		364–366	3710	A	431
	3-Hydroxy-4-nitro-1,3,5(10)-estratrien-17-one	278	1720	A	431
$C_{18}H_{22}O_2$	3-Hydroxy-1,3,5(10)-estratrien-17-one	280	3.37	A	209
		280	2300	A	116
$C_{18}H_{22}O_3$	1,3-Dihydroxy-1,3,5(10)-estratrien-17-one	280–287	2060	M	162
	1-Acetate	282	1700	M	162
	Diacetate	267	440	M	162
	1,4-Dihydroxy-1,3,5(10)-estratrien-17-one	295	3600	M	162
	Diacetate	265	340	M	162
	3,4-Dihydroxy-1,3,5(10)-estratrien-17-one				
	Diacetate	263	310	M	162
	3,7α-Dihydroxy-1,3,5(10)-estratrien-17-one	281	3.35	A	210
	Diacetate	268	2.82	A	210
		274	2.80	A	210
	3-Benzoate	232	4.29	A	210
	3-Benzoate, 7-mesylate	232	4.28	A	210
	3,7β-Dihydroxy-1,3,5(10)-estratrien-17-one	280	3.37	A	210
	Diacetate	268	2.96	A	210
		276	2.94	A	210
	3,13α-Dihydroxy-13,17-*seco*-1,3,5(10)-estratrien-17-oic acid-17,13-lactone	267	1080	A	157
	3-Acetate	275	950	A	157
	6α,7α-Epoxy-1,3,5(10)-estratriene-3,17β-diol	269	2.84	A	210
	Diacetate	276	2.84	A	210

TABLE XIV—*continued*

Formula	Compound	λ_{max}	Ext.	Sol.	Ref.
Aromatic Ring A (cont.)					
$C_{18}H_{22}O_4$	3,6α,7α-Trihydroxy-1,3,5(10)-estratrien-17-one	282	3.29	A	210
	Triacetate	267	2.86	A	210
		275	2.81	A	210
	3,6β,7α-Trihydroxy-1,3,5(10)-estratrien-17-one				
	Triacetate	268	2.81	A	210
		276	2.81	A	210
$C_{18}H_{22}O_5N_2$	2,4-Dinitro-1,3,5(10)-estratrien-3-ol	278–279	6760	A	431
		353–354	3575	A	431
$C_{18}H_{22}O_6N_2$	2,4-Dinitro-1,3,5(10)-estratriene-3,17β-diol	277	6655	A	430
		352–354	3340	A	430
		424–426(inf)	910	A	430
$C_{18}H_{24}O_2$	1,3,5(10)-Estratriene-3,17β-diol	280	3.33	A	209
		280	2000	A	116
	d,l-8α-1,3,5(10)-Estratriene-3,17β-diol	280	3.31	A	215
$C_{18}H_{24}O_3$	1,3,5(10)-Estratriene-3,7α,17β-triol	282	3.23	A	210
	7,17-Diacetate	282	3.29	A	210
	Triacetate	268	2.86	A	210
	3-Benzoate	231	4.28	A	210
	1,3,5(10)-Estratriene-3,16α,17β-triol	280	2300	A	116
		280	2090	A	248
$C_{18}H_{24}O_4$	1,3,5(10)-Estratriene-3,6α,7α,17β-tetraol	282	3.28	A	210
	Tetraacetate	268	2.81	A	210
		274	2.76	A	210
	1,3,5(10)-Estratriene-3,6β,7α,17β-tetraol				
	3,17-Diacetate	268	2.75	A	210
		276	2.71	A	210
$C_{19}H_{22}O_2$	*d,l*-3-Methoxy-D-homo-18-nor-1,3,5(10),13-estratetraen-17a-one	229	13,400	A	215
		246	15,600	A	215
		286	2360	A	215
	3-Methoxy-1,3,5(10),14-estratetraen-17-one	276	3.35	A	218
		286	3.32	A	218

TABLE XIV—*continued*

Formula	Compound	λ_{max}	Ext.	Sol.	Ref.
Aromatic Ring A (cont.)					
$C_{19}H_{22}O_2$	3-Methoxy-1,3,5(10),15-estratetraen-17-one	223	4.15	A	218
		277	3.3	A	218
		286	3.24	A	218
	3-Methoxy-14β-1,3,5(10),15-estratetraen-17-one	221	4.23	A	218
		277	3.43	A	218
		286	3.37	A	218
$C_{19}H_{22}O_5$	17β-Carboxy-3,14β-dihydroxy-1,3,5(10)-estratrien-11-one	215–222(sh)	3.91–3.88	A	402
		280	3.21	A	402
	Methyl ester	215–220(sh)	3.9	A	402
		280	3.25	A	402
$C_{19}H_{23}O_2Br$	16ξ-Bromo-3-methoxy-1,3,5(10)-estratrien-17-one	278	3.29	A	218
		286	3.26	A	218
		313	2.10	A	218
$C_{19}H_{24}O$	17-Methyl-1,3,5(10),16-estratetraen-3-ol	280	3.3	A	296
$C_{19}H_{24}O_2$	3-Hydroxy-1-methyl-1,3,5(10)-estratrien-17-one	287	3.23	A	209
	3-Hydroxy-2-methyl-1,3,5(10)-estratrien-17-one	283	3.41	A	209
	Benzoate	226	4.36	A	209
		270	3.54	A	209
	3-Methoxy-14β-1,3,5(10)-estratrien-17-one	277	3.33	A	218
		286	3.29	A	218
	d,l-3-Methoxy-D-homo-18-nor-18α-1,3,5(10)-estratrien-17a-one	278	2270	A	215
		287	2140	A	215
$C_{19}H_{24}O_3$	17β-Carboxy-1,3,5(10)-estratrien-3-ol				
	Methyl ester	280	3.38	A	394
	3-Hydroxy-2-methoxy-1,3,5(10)-estratrien-17-one	284.5–288.5	4000	A	242
					243
	Acetate	278	2360	A	242
		281(inf.)	2300	A	242
		287(inf.)	2050	A	242
	1-Hydroxy-4-methyl-1,3,5(10)-estratrien-17-one				
	Acetate	268	320		117

TABLE XIV—*continued*

Formula	Compound	λ_{max}	Ext.	Sol.	Ref.
Aromatic Ring A (cont.)					
$C_{19}H_{24}O_3$	3-Hydroxy-9,10-*seco*-1-3,5(10)-androstatriene-9,17-dione	280	2320	M	113
	Acetate	266	650	M	113
		273	650	M	113
	3-Hydroxy-9,10-*seco*-1,3,5(10)-androstatriene-11,17-dione	281	2250	A	254
		286(inf.)		A	254
$C_{19}H_{26}O$	1- *or* 4-Methyl-1,3,5(10)-estratrien-17β-ol	262.5	2.49	A	94
	Acetate	263	2.50	A	94
	17α-Methyl-1,3,5(10)-estratrien-3-ol	280	3.3	A	296
	17β-Methyl-1,3,5(10)-estratrien-3-ol	280	3.3	A	296
$C_{19}H_{26}O_2$	3-Methoxy-1,3,5(10)-estratrien-17-ol	278	1930	A	437
		286.5	1780	A	437
	1-Methyl-1,3,5(10)-estratriene-3,17β-diol	284	3.28	A	209
	2-Methyl-1,3,5(10)-estratriene-3,17β-diol	284	3.38	A	209
	3-Benzoate	226	4.37	A	209
		270	3.58	A	209
$C_{19}H_{26}O_3$	2-Methoxy-1,3,5(10)-estratriene-3,17β-diol	286	3640	A	149
$C_{19}H_{26}O_4$	2-Methoxy-1,3,5(10)-estratriene-3,16α,17β-triol	286	3700	A	151
$C_{20}H_{22}O_4$	17β-Carboxy-3-methoxy-1,3,5(10),14-estratetraen-11-one				
	Methyl ester	220–230(sh)	4.1–4.0	A	402
		280	3.31	A	402
		285(sh)	3.29	A	402
$C_{20}H_{23}O_2I$	3-Hydroxy-21-iodo-19-nor-1,3,5(10),16-pregnatetraen-20-one				
	Acetate	249	3.91	A	101
$C_{20}H_{24}O_2$	17α-Ethinyl-1,3,5(10)-estratriene-3,17β-diol	280	2140	A	116
	3-Methoxy-18,19-dinor-1,3,5(10),16-pregnatetraen-20-one	231	13,900	M	211
		278	2010	M	211
		287	1990	M	211
$C_{20}H_{24}O_3$	16α,17α-Epoxy-3-hydroxy-19-nor-1,3,5(10)-pregnatrien-20-one	280	3.49		264
		280	3.49	A	444
	Acetate	268	2.68		264
		276	2.98		264

TABLE XIV—*continued*

Formula	Compound	λ_{max}	Ext.	Sol.	Ref.
Aromatic Ring A (cont.)					
$C_{20}H_{24}O_3$	3-Methoxy-1,3,5(10)-estratrien-17β-carboxylic acid				
	Methyl ester	220–225(sh)	3.9	A	402
		278	3.31	A	402
		286.5	3.30	A	402
		307.5	1.85	A	402
		323	1.72	A	402
$C_{20}H_{24}O_4$	3-Carboxymethoxy-1,3,5(10)-estratrien-17-one	277	3.34	A	235
		286	3.33	A	235
	17-Ethylenedioxy-6α,7α-epoxy-1,3,5(10)-estratrien-3-ol	229	3.80	A	210
		284	3.24	A	210
	Acetate	269	2.69	A	210
		276	2.64	A	210
	3,11α-Dihydroxy-19-nor-1,3,5(10),17(20)-pregnatetraen-21-oic acid				
	Methyl ester	224	17,375	A	225
		279	2275	A	255
		287	1175	A	255
$C_{20}H_{24}O_5$	17β-Carboxy-14β-hydroxy-3-methoxy-1,3,5(10)-estratrien-11-one				
	Methyl ester	215–225(sh)	3.92–3.86	A	402
		278	3.14	A	402
		285	3.10	A	402
$C_{20}H_{26}O_2$	3-Hydroxy-1,2-dimethyl-1,3,5(10)-estratrien-17-one	288	3.36	A	209
	3-Hydroxy-19-nor-1,3,5(10)-pregnatrien-20-one	280	3.36	A	392
		280–282	3.30	A	57
$C_{20}H_{26}O_3$	3-(2′-hydroxyethoxy)-1,3,5(10)-estratrien-17-one				
	2′-Acetate	277	3.28	A	235
		286	3.25	A	235
	3-Hydroxy-1-methyl-1,3,5(10)-estratrien-17β-carboxylic acid				
	Acetate, methyl ester	270	2.54	A	394
	3-Methoxy-1,3,5(10)-estratrien-17β-carboxylic acid	215–225(sh)	3.92	A	402
	Methyl ester	278	3.34	A	402

TABLE XIV—*continued*

Formula	Compound	λ_{max}	Ext.	Sol.	Ref.
Aromatic Ring A (cont.)					
		286.5	3.32	A	402
		305–310(sh)	1.5	A	402
$C_{20}H_{26}O_3$	19-Nor-1,3,5(10),17(20)-pregnatetraene-3,11β,21-triol	281	2000	A	253
	3,17α-Dihydroxy-19-nor-1,3,5(10)-pregnatrien-20-one	282	3.37		264
	3-Acetate	276	2.88		264
	3,21-Dihydroxy-19-nor-1,3,5(10)-pregnatrien-20-one				
	Diacetate	267	2.93	A	101
		274	2.91	A	101
$C_{20}H_{28}O_2$	1,2-Dimethyl-1,3,5(10)-estratriene-3,17β-diol	288	3.25	A	209
	1,4-Dimethyl-1,3,5(10)-estratriene-3,17β-diol	288	3.23	A	386
$C_{21}H_{25}O_2N$	17β-Acetyl-16α-cyano-1,3,5(10)-estratrien-3-ol	280–282	3.36	A	342
	Acetate	268	3.30	A	342
		276	3.22	A	342
$C_{21}H_{26}O_2$	17α-Ethinyl-4-methyl-1,3,5(10)-estratriene-1,17β-diol				
	Diacetate	266	2.55	A	392
	3-Methoxy-17α-ethyl-1,3,5(10)-estratrien-17β-ol	278	3.35		86
	3-Methoxy-19-nor-1,3,5(10),16-pregnatetraen-20-one	278	3.45	A	389
$C_{21}H_{26}O_3$	16α,17α-Epoxy-3-methoxy-19-nor-1,3,5(10)-pregnatrien-20-one	278	3.29		264
		286	3.25		264
$C_{21}H_{28}O_2$	3-Methoxy-19-nor-1,3,5(10)-pregnatrien-20-one	278	3.42	A	389
$C_{21}H_{28}O_3$	17α-Hydroxy-3-methoxy-19-nor-1,3,5(10)-pregnatrien-20-one	278	3.27		264
	1,21-Dihydroxy-4-methyl-19-nor-1,3,5(10)-pregnatrien-20-one				
	Diacetate	267	2.54	A	79
	3-Hydroxy-9,10-*seco*-1,3,5(10)-pregnatriene-11,20-dione	281	2225	A	254
		287	1975	A	254
	Acetate	268	558	A	254
		274.5	548	A	254
	3-Hydroxy-9,10-*seco*-17α-1,3,5(10)-pregnatriene-11,20-dione	281	2225	A	254
		287	1975	A	254
	Acetate	268	555	A	254
		274.5	540	A	254

TABLE XIV—*continued*

Formula	Compound	λ_{max}	Ext.	Sol.	Ref.
Aromatic Ring A (cont.)					
$C_{21}H_{30}O_2$	4-Methyl-19-nor-1,3,5(10)-pregnatriene-1,20β-diol				
	Diacetate	266	2.50	A	292
$C_{22}H_{26}O_2$	3-Hydroxy-1,2-dimethyl-1,3,5(10)-estratrien-17-one				
	Acetate	272	2.73	A	209
		280	2.73	A	209
$C_{22}H_{30}O_2$	3-Methoxy-17α-allyl-1,3,5(10)-estratrien-17β-ol	278	3.32		86
	3-Methoxy-1-methyl-19-nor-1,3,5(10)-pregnatrien-20-one	280–286	3.20	A	102
$C_{22}H_{30}O_3$	17α-Hydroxy-3-methoxy-1-methyl-19-nor-1,3,5(10)-pregnatrien-20-one	283	3.15	A	102
$C_{22}H_{32}O_2$	3-Methoxy-17α-n-propyl-1,3,5(10)-estratrien-17β-ol	278	3.32		86
$C_{23}H_{30}O_3$	20-Acetoxy-4-methyl-19-nor-1,3,5(10),17(20)-pregnatetraen-1-ol				
	Acetate	266	2.53	A	392
$C_{31}H_{29}O_5N$	3-(2′-Benzoyl-4′-nitro)-phenoxy-1,3,5(10)-estratrien-17-one	254	18,000	A	149
		296	12,000	A	149
$C_{31}H_{31}O_5N$	3-(2′-Benzoyl-4′-nitro)-phenoxy-1,3,5(10)-estratrien-17β-ol	254.5	17,000	A	149
		296	11,300	A	149
$C_{31}H_{31}O_6N$	3-(2′-Benzoyl-4′-nitro)-phenoxy-1,3,5(10)-estratriene-2,17β-diol				
	17β-Acetate	255	17,250	A	149
		289	14,620	A	149
$C_{32}H_{33}O_6N$	3-(2′-Benzoyl-4′-nitro)-phenoxy-2-methoxy-1,3,5(10)-estratrien-17β-ol	254	15,960	A	149
	Acetate	287	13,350	A	149

TABLE XV. AROMATIC RING B

Formula	Compound	λ_{max}	Ext.	Sol.	Ref.
$C_{18}H_{22}O_2$	3β-Hydroxy-5,7,9-estratrien-17-one				
	Acetate	269	395		161

TABLE XIV. AROMATIC RING D-HOMO

Formula	Compound	λ_{max}	Ext.	Sol.	Ref.
$C_{19}H_{24}O_2$	*d,l*-17a-Hydroxy-D-homo-18-nor-8α-13,15,17(17a)-androstatrien-3-one				
	Acetate	262	2.85	A	221
$C_{19}H_{26}O_2$	*d,l*-D-homo-18-nor-13,15,17(17a)-androstatriene-3β,17a-diol				
	Diacetate	261	2.45	A	221
	d,l-D-homo-18-nor-8α-13,15,17(17a)-androstatriene-3β,17a-diol	273	3.16	A	221
		279	3.15	A	221
$C_{20}H_{24}O_2$	*d,l*-17a-Methoxy-D-homo-18-nor-4,13,15,17(17a)-androstatetraen-3-one	232	4.32	A	222
		278(sh)	3.35	A	222
	d,l-17a-Methoxy-D-homo-18-nor-8α-4,13,15,17(17a)-androstatetraen-3-one	231	4.21	A	222
		241	4.20	A	222
		278(sh)	3.28	A	222
	d,l-17a-Methoxy-D-homo-18-nor-9β-4,13,15,17(17a)-androstatetraen-3-one	232	4.27	A	212
		240	4.26	A	212
		278	3.30	A	212
	d,l-17a-Methoxy-D-homo-18-nor-8α,9β-4,13,15,17(17a)-androstatetraen-3-one	231	4.21	A	222
		243	4.21	A	222
		278(sh)	3.31	A	222
$C_{20}H_{24}O_3$	*d,l*-17a-Methoxy-D-homo-18-nor-9β-13,15,17(17a)-androstatriene-3,6-dione	272	3.23	A	212
		279	3.24	A	212
$C_{20}H_{26}O_2$	*d,l*-17a-Methoxy-D-homo-18-nor-13,15,17(17a)-androstatrien-3-one	271	3.13	A	222
		278.5	3.14	A	222
	d,l-17a-Methoxy-D-homo-18-nor-8α-13,15,17(17a)-androstatrien-3-one	271.5	3.09	A	222
		278.5	3.13	A	222
	d,l-17a-Methoxy-D-homo-18-nor-9β-13,15,17(17a)-androstatrien-3-one	271	3.14	A	212
		278	3.16	A	212
	d,l-17a-Methoxy-D-homo-18-nor-13,15,17(17a)-etiocholatrien-3-one	271	3.14	A	222
		278	3.15	A	222

TABLE XVI—*continued*

Formula	Compound	λ_{max}	Ext.	Sol.	Ref.
Aromatic Ring D-homo (cont.)					
$C_{20}H_{26}O_2$	*d,l*-17a-Methoxy-D-homo-18-nor-9β-13,15,17(17a)-etiocholatrien-3-one	271	3.16	A	222
		278	3.19	A	222
	d,l-17a-Methoxy-D-homo-18-nor-8α,9β-13,15,17(17a)-etiocholatrien-3-one	271	3.2	A	222
		278.5	3.2	A	222
	d,l-3β-Hydroxy-17a-methoxy-D-homo-18-nor-13,15,17(17a)-etiocholatrien-11-one	273	3.24	A	219
		279	3.26	A	219
	Acetate	272	3.23	A	219
		279	3.24	A	219
	d,l-5α-Hydroxy-17a-methoxy-D-homo-18-nor-9β-13,15,17(17a)-androstatrien-3-one	272	3.27	A	212
		278	3.30	A	212
	Acetate	272	3.26	A	212
		279	3.28	A	212
	d,l-5β-Hydroxy-17a-methoxy-D-homo-18-nor-9β-13,15,17(17a)-androstatrien-3-one				
	Acetate	272	3.22	A	212
		279	3.28	A	212
$C_{20}H_{28}O_2$	*d,l*-17a-Methoxy-D-homo-18-nor-8α-13,15,17(17a)-androstatrien-3β-ol	271	3.14	A	222
		278	3.15	A	222
	d,l-17a-Methoxy-D-homo-18-nor-13,15,17(17a)-etiocholatrien-3α-ol	272	3.13	A	222
		278	3.13	A	222
$C_{20}H_{28}O_3$	*d,l*-17a-Methoxy-D-homo-18-nor-9β-13,15,17(17a)-androstatriene-3β,5α-diol	272	3.23	A	212
		278	3.30	A	212
	d,l-17a-Methoxy-D-homo-18-nor-13,15,17(17a)-androstatriene-3β,12ξ-diol				
	Diacetate	275	3.38	A	219
		281	3.38	A	219

TABLE XVI—*continued*

Formula	Compound	λ_{max}	Ext.	Sol.	Ref.
Aromatic Ring D-homo (cont.)					
$C_{20}H_{28}O_3$	*d,l*-17a-Methoxy-D-homo-18-nor-9β-13,15,17(17a)-androstatriene-3β,12ξ-diol				
	Diacetate	275	3.44	A	219
		282	3.45	A	219
$C_{20}H_{28}O_3$	*d,l*-17a-Methoxy-D-homo-18-nor-13,15,17(17a)-etiocholatriene-3α,12ξ-diol				
	Diacetate	274	3.39	A	219
		282	3.38	A	219
$C_{20}H_{28}O_4$	*d,l*-17a-Methoxy-D-homo-18-nor-9β-13,15,17(17a)-androstatriene-3β,11ξ,12ξ-triol				
	3-Acetate	272	3.24	A	219
		279	3.29	A	219
	3-Acetate,12ξ-benzoate	226	4.31	A	219
		274	3.58	A	219
		281	3.56	A	219
$C_{22}H_{28}O_2$	*d,l*-Ethoxy-17a-methoxy-D-homo-18-nor-9β-3,5,13,15,17(17a)-androstapentaene	241	4.37	A	212
		278	3.23	A	212
$C_{22}H_{28}O_3$	*d,l*-3-Ethylenedioxy-17a-methoxy-D-homo-18-nor-5,13,15,17(17a)-androstatetraene	271	3.15	A	222
		277.5	3.18	A	222
	d,l-3-Ethylenedioxy-17a-methoxy-D-homo-18-nor-8α-5,13,15,17(17a)-androstatetraene	270	3.12	A	222
		277.5	3.15	A	222
	d,l-3-Ethylenedioxy-17a-methoxy-D-homo-18-nor-8α,9β-5,13,15,17(17a)-androstatetraene	271	3.25	A	222
		278	3.28	A	222
$C_{22}H_{30}O_3$	*d,l*-3-Ethylenedioxy-17a-methoxy-D-homo-18-nor-8α-13,15,17(17a)-androstatriene	270.5	3.12	A	222
		278.5	3.14	A	222

TABLE XVII. CONJUGATED AROMATIC RING A

Formula	Compound	λ_{max}	Ext.	Sol.	Ref.
6-Enes					
$C_{18}H_{20}O_2$	3-Hydroxy-1,3,5(10),6-estratetraen-17-one	221	4.49	A	209
		262	3.95	A	209
		306	3.40	A	209
$C_{18}H_{20}O_3$	3,7-Dihydroxy-1,3,5(10),6-estratetraen-17-one				
	Diacetate	266	4.02	A	210
$C_{18}H_{22}O_2$	1,3,5(10),6-Estratetraene-3,17β-diol	222	4.50	A	209
		263	3.98	A	209
		306	3.52	A	209
$C_{19}H_{22}O_2$	3-Hydroxy-1-methyl-1,3,5(10),6-estratetraen-17-one	228	4.49	A	209
		267	3.92	A	209
		276	3.82	A	209
		304	3.29	A	209
$C_{19}H_{22}O_3$	17β-Carboxy-1,3,5(10),6-estratetraen-3-ol	222	4.48	A	394
	Methyl ester	264	3.95	A	394
		302	3.42	A	394
$C_{19}H_{24}O_2$	1-Methyl-1,3,5(10),6-estratetraene-3,17β-diol	227	4.57	A	209
		266	3.95	A	209
		276	3.74	A	209
		305	3.20	A	209
$C_{20}H_{24}O_2$	3-Hydroxy-1,2-dimethyl-1,3,5(10),6-estratetraen-17-one	231	4.45	A	209
		272	3.94	A	209
		306	3.38	A	209
	Acetate	225	4.45	A	209
		266	3.11	A	209
$C_{20}H_{24}O_3$	17β-Carboxy-1-methyl-1,3,5(10),6-estratetraen-3-ol				
	Acetate, methyl ester	224	4.43	A	394
		264	3.90	A	394

TABLE XVII—*continued*

Formula	Compound	λ_{max}	Ext.	Sol.	Ref.
6-Enes (cont.)					
$C_{20}H_{24}O_3$	17-Ethylenedioxy-1,3,5(10),6-estratetraen-3-ol	222	4.40	A	210
		263	3.87	A	210
		272	3.80	A	210
		305	3.40	A	210
	Acetate	220	4.40	A	210
		262	3.94	A	210
$C_{20}H_{26}O_2$	1,2-Dimethyl-1,3,5(10),6-estratetraene-3,17β-diol	230	4.49	A	209
		270–272	3.99	A	209
		306–308	3.41	A	209
9(11)-Enes					
$C_{18}H_{20}O_2$	3-Hydroxy-1,3,5(10),9(11)-estratetraen-17-one	263	18,050	A	255
		298	3125	A	255
$C_{19}H_{22}O_2$	1-Hydroxy-4-methyl-1,3,5(10),9(11)-estratetraen-17-one	255.5	13,200	M	113
		300	3830	M	113

TABLE XVIII. CONJUGATED AROMATIC RING D-HOMO

Formula	Compound	λ_{max}	Ext.	Sol.	Ref.
8-Enes					
$C_{20}H_{24}O_2$	*d,l*-17a-Methoxy-D-homo-18-nor-5,8,13,15,17(17a)-androstapentaen-3-ol				
	Acetate	267	3.96	A	222
		272.5	3.98	A	222
	d,l-17a-Methoxy-D-homo-18-nor-8,13,15,17(17a)-androstatraen-3-one	222	4.49	A	222
		265.5	4.14	A	222
	d,l-17a-Methoxy-D-homo-18-nor-8,13,15,17(17a)-etiocholatetraen-3-one	221.5	4.39	A	222
		267.5	4.07	A	222
$C_{20}H_{24}O_3$	*d,l*-5α-Hydroxy-17a-methoxy-D-homo-18-nor-8,13,15,17(17a)-androstatetraen-3-one	221	4.42	A	212
		269	4.06	A	212
	d,l-5β-Hydroxy-17a-methoxy-D-homo-18-nor-8,13,15,17(17a)-androstatetraen-3-one	222	4.44	A	212
		270	4.10	A	212
$C_{20}H_{26}O_2$	*d,l*-17a-Methoxy-D-homo-18-nor-8,13,15,17(17a)-etiocholatetraen-3α-ol	222.5	4.37	A	222
		269	4.06	A	222
$C_{22}H_{26}O_3$	*d,l*-17a-Methoxy-3-ethylenedioxy-D-homo-18-nor-5,8,13,15,17(17a)-androstapentaene	220	4.44	A	222
		266	4.03	A	222
		272	4.04	A	222
$C_{22}H_{28}O_2$	*d,l*-3-Ethoxy-17a-methoxy-D-homo-18-nor-2,8,13,15,17(17a)-androstapentaene	217	4.46	A	222
		269	4.09	A	222
11-Enes					
$C_{20}H_{24}O_2$	*d,l*-17a-Methoxy-D-homo-18-nor-9β-5,11,13,15,17(17a)-androstapentaen-3β-ol				
	Acetate	268	3.79	A	219
		298	3.54	A	219
		308	3.50	A	219

TABLE XVIII—*continued*

Formula	Compound	λ_{max}	Ext.	Sol.	Ref.
11-Enes (cont.)					
$C_{20}H_{26}O_2$	*d,l*-17a-Methoxy-D-homo-18-nor-11,13,15,17(17a)-androstatetraen-3β-ol				
	Acetate	268	3.95	A	219
		298	3.68	A	219
		309	3.65	A	219
	d,l-17a-Methoxy-D-homo-18-nor-9β-11,13,15,17(17a)-androstatetraen-3β-ol				
	Acetate	269	4.01	A	219
		298	3.75	A	219
		309	3.71	A	219
	d,l-17a-Methoxy-D-homo-18-nor-11,13,15,17(17a)-etiocholatetraen-3α-ol				
	Acetate	214	4.22	A	219
		225	4.19	A	219
		268	3.97	A	219
		298	3.71	A	219
		308	3.67	A	219
	d,l-17a-Methoxy-D-homo-18-nor-9β-11,13,15,17(17a)-etiocholatetraen-3α-ol				
	Acetate	221	4.25	A	219
		227	4.25	A	219
		271	3.91	A	219
		300	3.65	A	219
		312	3.62	A	219
$C_{20}H_{26}O_3$	*d,l*-17a-Methoxy-D-homo-18-nor-9β-11,13,15,17(17a)-androstatetraene-3β,5α-diol				
	Diacetate	268	3.99	A	219
		298	3.75	A	219
		308	3.70	A	219

TABLE XIX. AROMATIC RINGS AB

Formula	Compound	λ_{max}	Ext.	Sol.	Ref.
$C_{18}H_{18}O_2$	3-Hydroxy-1,3,5(10),6,8-estrapentaen-17-one	230			116
		270	7080	A	116
		282	7420	A	116
		292	5500	A	116
		328	3800	A	116
		340	4790	A	116
$C_{18}H_{20}O$	1,3,5(10),6,8-Estrapentaen-17β-ol Acetate	230	4.99		438
		286	3.75		438
		322	2.94		438
$C_{19}H_{20}O$	4-Methyl-14β-1,3,5(10),6,8-estrapentaen-17-one	249	3800	A	117
		255	3480	A	117
		277	6610	A	117
		287	7400	A	117
		294	5900	A	117
		309	1520	A	117
		315(inf).	1000	A	117
		325	1260	A	117
$C_{20}H_{22}O_2$	1-Methoxy-4-methyl-14β-1,3,5(10),6,8-estrapentaen-17-one	223	50,880	A	117
		238(inf.)	38,470	A	117
		302	6990	A	117
		320	5080	A	117
		334	4470	A	117
$C_{20}H_{22}O_3$	3-Methoxy-14ξ-1,3,5(10),6,8-estrapentaen-17β-carboxylic acid Methyl ester	230	4.76	A	402
		267	3.70	A	402
		278	3.72	A	402
		288	3.56	A	402
		310	3.05	A	402
		312	3.36	A	402
		321	3.31	A	402
		328	3.43	A	402

TABLE XX. CONJUGATED AROMATIC RINGS AB

Formula	Compound	λ_{max}	Ext.	Sol.	Ref.
11-Ones					
$C_{18}H_{20}O_3$	3-Hydroxy-13α,14β-1,3,5(10),6,8,estrapentaene-11,17-dione				
	Acetate	246	4.40	M	270
		314	3.86	M	270
$C_{19}H_{20}O_2$	3-Methoxy-1,3,5(10),6,8-estrapentaen-11-one	220	4.7	A	118
		250	4.5	A	118
		315	3.82	A	118
	3-Methoxy-14β-1,3,5(10),6,8-estrapentaen-11-one	246	4.6	A	118
		313	3.93	A	118
		345	3.64	A	118
14-en-11-Ones					
$C_{19}H_{18}O_2$	3-Methoxy-1,3,5(10),6,8,14-estrahexaen-11-one	235	4.4	A	118
		275	4.5	A	118
		315	3.74	A	118

TABLE XXI. CONJUGATED AROMATIC RINGS CD-HOMO

Formula	Compound	λ_{max}	Ext.	Sol.	Ref.
$C_{20}H_{22}O_3$	*d,l*-5α-Hydroxy-17a-methoxy-D-homo-8,11,13,15,17(17a)-androstapentaen-3-one				
	Acetate	224	4.71	A	212
		287	3.83	A	212
		298	3.87	A	212
		312	3.74	A	212
		325	3.60	A	212
$C_{20}H_{24}O_2$	*d,l*-17a-Methoxy-D-homo-18-nor-8,11,13,15,17(17a)-etiocholapentaen-3α-ol				
	Acetate	227.5	4.70	A	212
		285	3.74	A	212
		295.5	3.84	A	212
		310	3.67	A	212
		323	3.46	A	212
	ANTHRA STEROIDS				
$C_{19}H_{24}O$	5,7,9,14-Anthrastatetraen-17β-ol	221	24,400	A	295
		227	25,600	A	295
		266	17,200	A	295
		297	2500	A	295
		308	2100	A	295
	Benzoate	227	39,300	A	295
		266	19,000	A	295
		296	2500	A	295
		308	2100	A	295
$C_{21}H_{26}O$	5,7,9,14-Anthrapregnatetraen-20-one	221	24,600	I	294
		226	25,300	I	294
		266	16,300	I	294
		296	2400	I	294
		308	1900	I	294

TABLE XXII. STEROIDS CONTAINING AROMATIC CHROMOPHORES

Formula	Compound	λ_{max}	Ext.	Sol.	Ref.
Phenyl Ring					
$C_{27}H_{38}O_4$	16α-Benzyloxy-17β-carboxy-pregnan-3β-ol	252	2.27	A	284
		258	2.30	A	284
		264	2.21	A	284
$C_{28}H_{38}O_3$	16α-Benzyloxy-3β-hydroxy-5-pregnen-20-one	252.5	198	A	198
		258	227	A	198
		264	184	A	198
		287	67	A	198
$C_{30}H_{42}O_4$	16α-Benzyloxy-20-ethylenedioxy-5-pregnen-3β-ol	247(sh)	112	A	40
		252	156	A	40
		258	196	A	40
		264	149	A	40
		267(sh)	86	A	40
	Acetate	247(sh)	122	A	40
		252	163	A	40
		258	201	A	40
		264	155	A	40
		267(sh)	86	A	40
$C_{32}H_{44}O_5$	16α-Benzyloxy-3,20-bisethylenedioxy-5-pregnene	248(sh)	120	A	40
		252	163	A	40
		258	198	A	40
		264	152	A	40
		268(sh)	92	A	40

TABLE XXIII. STEROIDS CONTAINING CONJUGATED AROMATIC CHROMOPHORES

Formula	Compound	λ_{max}	Ext.	Sol.	Ref.
Conjugated phenyl ring					
$C_{28}H_{36}O_3$	18-Benzylidene-3β-hydroxy-5α,14β,17α-pregnane-11,20-dione	255(inf.)	20,900	A	30
		284	2600	A	30
		293	1800	A	30
$C_{28}H_{38}O_3$	21-Benzylidene-3α,20β-dihydroxy-pregnan-11-one	254	20,700	A	306
$C_{28}H_{40}O_3$	18-Benzylidene-5α,14β,17α-pregnane-3β,11β,20ξ-triol	255	20,800	A	30
	21-Benzylidene-pregnane-3α,11β,20β-triol	254	18,900	A	306
	Triacetate	254	18,900	A	306
Pyridine Ring					
$C_{25}H_{33}ON$	20-(2′-Pyridyl)-21-nor-5,17-pregnadien-3β-ol				
	Acetate	250	19,100		175
$C_{26}H_{35}ON$	20-(2′-Pyridyl)-5,20-pregnadien-3β-ol				
	Acetate	230	7350		175

TABLE XXIV. BENZYLIDENE DERIVATIVES

Formula	Compound	λ_{max}	Ext.	Sol.	Ref.
$C_{26}H_{28}O_2$	16-Benzylidene-3-methoxy-1,3,5(10)-estratrien-17-one	295	21,000		408
$C_{26}H_{34}O_2$	*d,l*-17-Benzylidene-3β-hydroxy-D-homo-18-nor-androstan-17a-one (transoid)	222	3.77	A	221
		286.5	4.20	A	221
	d,l-17-Benzylidene-3β-hydroxy-D-homo-18-nor-androstan-17a-one (cisoid)	220	4.06	A	221
		269	3.93	A	221
	d,l-17-Benzylidene-3β-hydroxy-D-homo-18-nor-14β-androstan-17a-one (transoid)	222	3.86	A	221
		292	4.24	A	221
	d,l-17-Benzylidene-3β-hydroxy-D-homo-18-nor-14β-androstan-17a-one (cisoid)	221	4.12	A	221
		278	3.91	A	221
$C_{27}H_{36}O_2$	17-Benzylidene-3β-hydroxy-D-homo-androstan-17a-one	218	4.06	A	319
		283	4.24	A	319
	d,l-17-Benzylidene-3β-hydroxy-D-homo-14β-androstan-17a-one (transoid)	222	3.9	A	221
		290	4.19	A	221
	d,l-17-Benzylidene-3β-hydroxy-D-homo-14β-androstan-17a-one (cisoid)	219	4.08	A	221
		274	3.95	A	221
	Acetate (transoid)	222	3.82	A	221
		292	4.22	A	221
	Acetate (cisoid)	220	4.08	A	221
		275	3.89	A	221
$C_{28}H_{36}O_4$	16-Benzylidene-3α,17aβ-dihydroxy-17aα-methyl-D-homo-androstane-11,17-dione				
	3-Acetate	220	3.9	M	424
		285	4.36	M	424

TABLE XXIV—*continued*

Formula	Compound	λ_{max}	Ext.	Sol.	Ref.
Benzylidene Derivatives (cont.)					
$C_{30}H_{38}O_4$	21-Benzylidene-3α-hydroxy-pregnane-3,20-dione	294	21,800	A	306
$C_{30}H_{42}O_3$	21-Benzylidene-16α-ethoxy-3β-hydroxy-pregnan-20-one				
	Acetate	223	4.23	A	284
		294	4.43	A	284
$C_{35}H_{44}O_3$	21-Benzylidene-16α-benzyloxy-3β-hydroxy-pregnan-20-one				
	3-Acetate	225(sh)	4.2	A	284
		295.5	4.39	A	284

TABLE XXV. FURFURYLIDENES

Formula	Compound	λ_{max}	Ext.	Sol.	Ref.
$C_{24}H_{26}O_3$	*d,l*-17-Furfurylidene-3-methoxy-D-homo-18-nor-8α-1,3,5(10)-estratrien-17a-one	326.7	26,300	A	215
	d,l-17-Furfurylidene-3β-hydroxy-D-homo-18-nor-androstan-17a-one	324.5	4.41	A	213
$C_{24}H_{32}O_4$	*d,l*-17-Furfurylidene-3β,11β-dihydroxy-D-homo-18-nor-androstan-17a-one	324	4.34	A	220
$C_{25}H_{28}O_3$	*d,l*-17-Furfurylidene-3-methoxy-D-homo-8α-1,3,5(10)-estratrien-17a-one	321.9	22,400	A	215
	d,l-17-Furfurylidene-3-methoxy-D-homo-8α,13α-1,3,5(10)-estratrien-17a-one	326.2	24,600	A	215
$C_{25}H_{34}O_3$	*d,l*-17-Furfurylidene-3β-hydroxy-D-homo-androstan-17a-one	323	4.34	A	213
	Acetate	322.5	4.34	A	213
	17-Furfurylidene-3β-hydroxy-D-homo-androstan-17a-one				
	Acetate	322.5	4.33	A	319
	d,l-17-Furyfurylidene-3β-hydroxy-D-homo-13α-androstan-17a-one	326.5	4.33	A	213
$C_{25}H_{34}O_4$	*d,l*-17-Furfurylidene-3β,11β-hihydroxy-D-homo-androstan-17a-one				
	3-Acetate	320.7	4.33	A	220
	Diacetate	322	4.33	A	220
	d,l-17-Furfurylidene-3β,11β-dihydroxy-D-homo-13α-androstan-17a-one				
	Diacetate	329.5	4.40	A	220
$C_{26}H_{32}O_4$	*d,l*-3-Ethylenedioxy-17-furfurylidene-D-homo-18-nor-5-androsten-17a-one	325	4.32	A	214
$C_{27}H_{34}O_4$	*d,l*-3-Ethylenedioxy-17-furfurylidene-D-homo-5-androsten-17a-one	323	4.35	A	214
	d,l-3-Ethylenedioxy-17-furfurylidene-D-homo-13α-5-androsten-17a-one	327	4.36	A	214

TABLE XXVI. CHROMOPHORIC ESTERS

Formula	Compound	λ_{max}	Ext.	Sol.	Ref.
Benzoate Esters					
$C_{17}H_{24}O_3$	5,17β-Dihydroxy-4-nor-5(x)-estren-3-oic acid-3,5-lactone				
	17-Benzoate	230	15,790	A	173
		270(inf.)	1050	A	173
		278(inf.)	790	A	173
$C_{19}H_{30}O_2$	5-Androstene-3β,17β-diol				
	17-Benzoate	229	14,000	A	295
		273	890	A	295
		280	710	A	295
$C_{20}H_{28}O$	3β-Hydroxy-17β-methyl-5-androstene				
	Benzoate	229	14,200	A	176
		273	950	A	176
		280	750	A	176
$C_{21}H_{28}O_6$	*d,l*-11β,18-Epoxy-3-ethylenedioxy-11β,14ξ,18-trihydroxy-5-androsten-16-one				
	18-Benzoate	231	12,100	A	433
$C_{21}H_{32}O_3$	3-Ethylenedioxy-5-androsten-17β-ol				
	Benzoate	229	14,500	A	17
		271–172	690	A	17
		280–281	670	A	17
$C_{21}H_{32}O_4$	3β-Hydroxy-5α-pregnan-16-one-21-oic acid				
	Benzoate, ethyl ester	(chart)	4.2	A	76
	11α,21-Dihydroxy-5α-pregnane-3,20-dione				
	11-Acetate, 21-benzoate	230	4.25	A	390
Tosylate Esters					
$C_{21}H_{30}O_4$	17β-Carboxy-12α-hydroxy-17α-methyl-androstan-3-one				
	Tosylate, methyl ester	226	4.1	A	130
$C_{22}H_{34}O_3$	12α-Hydroxy-17α-methyl-pregnane-3,20-dione				
	Tosylate	226	3.93	A	130

TABLE XXVI—*continued*

Formula	Compound	λ_{max}	Ext.	Sol.	Ref.
Tosylate Esters (cont.)					
$C_{25}H_{36}O_7$	3,20-Bisethylenedioxy-17α,21-dihydroxy-5-pregnen-11-one 21-Tosylate	225	11,500	A	12
		262	660	A	12
$C_{25}H_{38}O_5$	3,20-Bisethylenedioxy-5-pregnen-21-ol Tosylate	225.5	11,600	A	12
		262	570	A	12
$C_{25}H_{38}O_7$	3,20-Bisethylenedioxy-5-pregnene-11α,17α,21-triol 11,21-Ditosylate	261	1100	E	12
	3,20-Bisethylenedioxy-5-pregnene-11β,17α,21-triol 21-Tosylate	225	10,700	A	12
		262	415	A	12

TABLE XXVII. STEROIDS CONTAINING CARBONYL "C=N" DERIVATIVES

Formula	Compound	λ_{max}	Ext.	Sol.	Ref.
Hydrazone					
$C_{21}H_{28}O_4N_2$	11β,17α-Dihydroxy-3,20-dioxo-1,4-pregnadien-21-al-21-hydrazone	244	16,100	M	78
2,4-Dinitrophenylhydrazones					
$C_{25}H_{32}O_5N_4$	3β-Hydroxy-5-androsten-17-one-17-(2,4-dinitrophenylhydrazone)	367		Ch	330a
$C_{25}H_{32}O_6N_4$	3β,17β-Dihydroxy-5-androsten-16-one-16-(2,4-dinitrophenylhydrazone)	368		Ch	330a
	Diacetate	362–363		Ch	330a
$C_{25}H_{34}O_5N_4$	3α-Hydroxy-androstan-17-one-17-(2,4-dinitrophenylhydrazone)	368		Ch	330a
	Acetate	367		Ch	330a
	3β-Hydroxy-androstan-17-one-17-(2,4-dinitrophenylhydrazone)	368		Ch	330a
$C_{27}H_{34}O_5N_4$	4-Pregnene-3,20-dione-20-(2-4,dinitrophenylhydrazone)	367		Ch	330a
$C_{27}H_{36}O_5N_4$	3β-Hydroxy-5-pregnen-20-one-20-(2,4-dinitrophenylhydrazone)	368		Ch	330a
	Acetate	368		Ch	330a
$C_{27}H_{36}O_6N_4$	3α-Hydroxy-pregnane-11,20-dione-20-(2,4-dinitrophenylhydrazone)	365		Ch	330b
	3β,21-Dihydroxy-5-pregnen-20-one-20-(2,4-dinitrophenylhydrazone)	372	24,855	Ch	330b
	21-Acetate	365		Ch	330b
	Diacetate	364		Ch	330b
$C_{27}H_{36}O_7N_4$	3β,17α,21-Trihydroxy-5-pregnen-20-one-20-(2,4-dinitrophenylhydrazone)				
	3,21-Diacetate	357		Ch	330b
$C_{27}H_{38}O_5N_4$	3α-Hydroxy-pregnan-20-one-20-(2,4-dinitrophenylhydrazone)	367–368		Ch	330a

TABLE XXVII—*continued*

Formula	Compound	λ_{max}	Ext.	Sol.	Ref.
2,4-Dinitrophenylhydrazones (cont.)					
	3β-Hydroxy-5α-pregnan-20-one-20-(2,4-dinitrophenylhydrazone)	368		Ch	330a
$C_{27}H_{38}O_6N_4$	3α,12α-Dihydroxy-pregnan-20-one-20-(2,4-dinitrophenylhydrazone)				
	Diacetate	366		Ch	330a
	3β,16α-Dihydroxy-5α-pregnan-20-one-20-(2,4-dinitrophenylhydrazone)	262	11,400	Ch	290
		363	24,300	Ch	290
		432	21,900	BA	290
		542	12,500	BA	290
	3β,17α-Dihydroxy-5α-pregnan-20-one-20-(2,4-dinitrophenylhydrazone)	362		Ch	330a
	3-Acetate	362		Ch	330a
$C_{33}H_{40}O_8N_8$	Pregnane-3,20-dione-3,20-bis(2,4-dinitrophenylhydrazone)	368–369		Ch	330a
Conjugated 2,4-dinitrophenylhydrazones					
$C_{25}H_{32}O_5N_4$	17β-Hydroxy-4-androsten-3-one-3-(2,4-dinitrophenylhydrazone)	390		Ch	330a
	Acetate	390		Ch	330a
$C_{27}H_{32}O_8N_4$	17α,21-Dihydroxy-4-pregnene-3,11,20-trione-3-(2,4-dinitrophenylhydrazone)				
	21-Acetate	387		Ch	330a
$C_{27}H_{34}O_5N_4$	4-Pregnene-3,20-dione-3-(2,4-dinitrophenylhydrazone)	390		Ch	330a
	3β-Hydroxy-5,16-pregnadien-20-one-20-(2,4-dinitrophenylhydrazone)	385		Ch	330a
	Acetate	385		Ch	330a
$C_{27}H_{34}O_6N_4$	21-Hydroxy-4-pregnene-3,20-dione-(2,4-dinitrophenylhydrazone)				
	Acetate	389		Ch	330a

TABLE XXVII—*continued*

Formula	Compound	λ_{max}	Ext.	Sol.	Ref.
Conjugated 2,4-dinitrophenylhydrazones (cont.),					
	3β,21-Dihydroxy-5,16-pregnadien-20-one-20-(2,4-dinitrophenylhydrazone)	381		Ch	330b
$C_{27}H_{34}O_7N_4$	17α,21-Dihydroxy-4-pregnene-3,20-dione-3-(2,4-dinitrophenylhydrazone)			Ch	330c
	21-Acetate	389			
$C_{27}H_{34}O_8N_4$	11β,17α,21-Trihydroxy-4-pregnene-3,20-dione-3-(2,4-dinitrophenylhydrazone)				
	21-Acetate	389		Ch	330c
$C_{27}H_{36}O_5N_4$	3β-Hydroxy-5α-16-pregnen-20-one-20-(2,4-dinitrophenylhydrazone)	260	17,700	Ch	290
		384	25,300	Ch	290
		260	9700	BA	290
		455	14,800	BA	290
	Acetate	386		Ch	330b
$C_{27}H_{36}O_8N_4$	11β,17α,20β,21-Tetrahydroxy-4-pregnen-3-one-3-(2,4-dinitrophenylhydrazone)	390		Ch	330a
$C_{31}H_{32}O_9N_8$	4-Androstene-3,11,17-trione-3,17-bis(2,4-dinitrophenylhydrazone)	375		Ch	330a
$C_{31}H_{34}O_8N_8$	4-Androstene-3,17-dione-3,17-bis(2,4-dinitrophenylhydrazone)	380		Ch	330a
$C_{31}H_{34}O_9N_8$	11β-Hydroxy-4-androstene-3,17-dione-3,17-bis(2,4-dinitrophenylhydrazone)	377		Ch	330a
$C_{33}H_{32}O_9N_8$	1,4,16-Pregnatriene-3,20-dione-3,20-bis(2,4-dinitrophenylhydrazone)	385–386	4.7	A	238
$C_{33}H_{36}O_8N_8$	4,16-Pregnadiene-3,20-dione-3,20-bis(2,4-dinitrophenylhydrazone)	386–387		Ch	330a
$C_{33}H_{36}O_9N_8$	4-Pregnene-3,11,20-trione-3,20-bis(2,4-dinitrophenylhydrazone)	375		Ch	330a

TABLE XXVII—*continued*

Formula	Compound	λ_{max}	Ext.	Sol.	Ref.
Conjugated 2,4-Dinitrophenylhydrazones (cont.)					
$C_{33}H_{36}O_{11}N_8$	17α,21-Dihydroxy-4-pregnene-3,11,20-trione-3,20-bis(2,4-dinitrophenylhydrazone)	380		Ch	330c
	21-Acetate	258	27,801	Ch	330c
		376	43,227	Ch	330c
$C_{33}H_{38}O_8N_8$	4-Pregnene-3,20-dione-3,20-bis(2,4-dinitrophenylhydrazone)	380		Ch	330a
$C_{33}H_{38}O_9N_8$	3β-Hydroxy-20-keto-5-pregnen-21-al-20,21-bis(2,4-dinitrophenylhydrazone)	350		Ch	330b
		398		Ch	330b
		445		Ch	330b
	11β-Hydroxy-4-pregnene-3,20-dione-3,20-bis(2,4-dinitrophenylhydrazone)	380		Ch	330a
	17α-Hydroxy-4-pregnene-3,20-dione-3,20-bis(2,4-dinitrophenylhydrazone)	376–377		Ch	330a
	21-Hydroxy-4-pregnene-3,20-dione-3,20-bis(2,4-dinitrophenylhydrazone)	257	29,838	Ch	330c
		383	53,322	Ch	330c
	Acetate	256	32,312	Ch	330c
		378	49,740	Ch	330c
$C_{33}H_{38}O_{10}N_8$	17α,21-Dihydroxy-4-pregnene-3,20-dione-3,20-bis(2,4-dinitrophenylhydrazone)				
	21-Acetate	257	29,616	Ch	330c
		376	46,275	Ch	330c
$C_{33}H_{38}O_{11}N_8$	11β,17α,21-Trihydroxy-4-pregnene-3,20-dione-3,20-bis(2,4-dinitrophenylhydrazone)	382		Ch	330c
	21-Acetate	259	27,175	Ch	330c
		376	42,715	Ch	330c
$C_{39}H_{40}O_{12}N_{12}$	3,20-Diketo-4-pregnen-21-al-3,20,21-tri(2,4-dinitrophenylhydrazone)	394		Ch	330c
Oximes					
$C_{20}H_{29}O_3N$	3β-Hydroxy-D-homo-16-androsten-17a-one-17a-oxime				
	Acetate	236	8400	A	30

TABLE XXVII—*continued*

Formula	Compound	λ_{max}	Ext.	Sol.	Ref.
Oximes (cont.)					
$C_{21}H_{29}O_5N$	17α,21-Dihydroxy-4-pregnene-3,11,20-trione-3-oxime	240	18,400	A	61
	21-Acetate	240	20,400	A	61
$C_{21}H_{30}O_5N_2$	17α,21-Dihydroxy-4-pregnene-3,11,20-trione-3,20-dioxime	240	20,700	A	61
	21-Acetate	240	22,600	A	61
$C_{21}H_{31}O_3N$	1ξ,3β-Dihydroxy-5,16-pregnadien-20-one-20-oxime				
	Diacetate	236	14,930	A	62
$C_{21}H_{31}O_5N_2$	11β,17α,21-Trihydroxy-4-pregnene-3,20-dione-3,20-dioxime	240	18,500	A	61
$C_{21}H_{32}O_4N$	17α,21-Dihydroxy-4-pregnene-3,20-dione-3-dioxime	241	19,200	A	61
	21-Acetate	240	21,400	A	61
$C_{21}H_{32}O_5N_2$	11β,17α,21-Trihydroxy-4-pregnene-3,20-dione-3,20-dioxime	240	22,700	A	61
$C_{23}H_{34}O_5N_2$	17α,21-Dihydroxy-4-pregnene-3,11,20-trione-3,20-dioxime dimethyl ether				
	21-Acetate	249	20,200	A	61
$C_{23}H_{36}O_4N_2$	17α,21-Dihydroxy-4-pregnene-3,20-dione-3,20-dioxime-dimethyl ether	249	23,000	A	61
$C_{23}H_{36}O_5N_2$	11β,17α,21-Trihydroxy-4-pregnene-3,20-dione-3,20-dioxime-dimethyl ether	249	30,000	A	61
Semicarbazones					
$C_{22}H_{35}O_3N_3$	3β,21-Dihydroxy-4-pregnen-20-one-20-semicarbazone				
	21-Acetate	236		A	330b
$C_{22}H_{35}O_5N_3$	3β,17α,21-Trihydroxy-5α-pregnane-11,20-dione-20-semicarbazone	239.5	9960	A	61
$C_{23}H_{36}O_5N_6$	17α,21-Dihydroxy-5α-pregnane-3,11,20-trione-3,20-bis-semicarbazone	229	22,860	A	61
	21-Acetate	231	24,250	A	61
Conjugated Semicarbazones					
$C_{21}H_{25}O_2N_3$	*d,l*-17a-Methoxy-D-homo-18-nor-4,8,13,15,17(17a)-androstapentaen-3-one-3-semicarbazone	223.5	4.47	A	223
		271	4.62	A	223
$C_{22}H_{31}O_5N_3$	17α,21-Dihydroxy-4-pregnene-3,11,20-trione-3-semicarbazone				
	21-Acetate	270	30,800	A	61

TABLE XXVII—*continued*

Formula	Compound	λ_{max}	Ext.	Sol.	Ref.
Conjugated Semicarbazones (cont.)					
$C_{22}H_{33}O_4N_3$	17α,21-Dihydroxy-4-pregnene-3,20-dione-3-semicarbazone				
	21-Acetate	269	30,500	A	61
$C_{23}H_{31}O_4N_6$	17α,21-Dihydroxy-4,6-pregnadiene-3,11,20-trione-3,20-bis-semicarbazone				
	21-Acetate	242	14,500	M	165
		301	40,200	M	165
$C_{23}H_{33}O_4N_6$	11β,17α,21-Trihydroxy-4,6-pregnadiene-3,20-dione-3,20-bis-semicarbazone	236	11,100		165
		298	37,400		165
$C_{23}H_{33}O_4BrN_6$	12α-Bromo-21-hydroxy-4-pregnene-3,11,20-trione-3,20-bis-semicarbazone	245–250(sh)	25,200	M	405
	21-Acetate	269	30,300	M	405
$C_{23}H_{33}O_5N_3$	17α,21-Dihydroxy-16α-methyl-4-pregnene-3,11,20-trione-3-semicarbazone				
	21-Acetate	269	28,400	M	19
$C_{23}H_{34}O_5N_6$	17α,21-Dihydroxy-4-pregnene-3,11,20-trione-3,20-bis-semicarbazone	240(sh)	19,500	A	61
		270	31,200	A	61
	21-Acetate	242.5	22,400	A	61
		269	28,950	A	61
$C_{23}H_{36}O_4N_6$	17α,21-Dihydroxy-4-pregnene-3,20-dione-3,20-bis-semicarbazone	269	34,100	A	61
	21-Acetate	269	34,100	A	61

TABLE XXVIII. MISCELLANEOUS COMPOUNDS

Formula	Compound	λ_{max}	Ext.	Sol.	Ref.
$C_{16}H_{14}O_5$	6-Thia-B-nor-1,3,5(10),8,14-estrapentaen-17-one	235.5	4.18		83
		255	4.09		83
		261.5	4.1		83
		292	4.35,4.37		83
$C_{16}H_{15}ON$	6-Aza-D-homo-B-nor-18-nor-1,3,5(10),8,13-estrapentaen-17a-one	255	4.041		49
		393	4.2492		49
$C_{16}H_{16}OS$	6-Thia-B-nor-1,3,5(10),8-estratetraen-17-one	233	4.47		83
		264	3.95		83
		290	3.56		83
		300	3.47		83
$C_{16}H_{17}ON$	6-Aza-D-homo-B-nor-18-nor-1,3,5(10),8-estratetraen-17a-one	225	4.528	A	49
$C_{17}H_{14}O_3S$	15-Carboxy-6-thia-B-nor-1,3,5(10),8,15-estrapentaen-17-one	234	4.64		83
		261	4.09		83
		299.5	3.45		83
	15-Carboxy-6-thia-B-nor-1,3,5(10),8,14-estrapentaen-17-one				
	Ethyl ester	222	4.45		83
		263	4.07		83
		328.5	4.45		83
$C_{17}H_{26}O_2N_2$	17β-Hydroxy-3,4-diaza-4-androsten-2-one	244	3.90	A	418
$C_{19}H_{29}ON$	17-Amino-5,16-androstadien-3β-ol				
	Diacetate	240	3.82	A	354
$C_{23}H_{32}O_4N_2$	16,17-[3,1-(3-carboxy-2-pyrazolino)]-3β-hydroxy-5-pregnen-20-one	285	6809	M	288
		316	5207	M	288
	3-Acetate	286	7300	M	288
		316	5710	M	288
	3-Acetate, ethyl ester	290	7577	M	288
		317	6777	M	288

TABLE XXIX. ISOLATED DOUBLE BONDS

Formula	Compound	λ_{max}	Ext.	Sol.	Ref.
$C_{19}H_{28}O$	3-Androsten-17-one	205	1450	A	526
$C_{19}H_{28}O_2$	11β-Hydroxy-5ξ-3-androsten-17-one	205	1500	A	526
$C_{19}H_{28}O_3$	3-Methoxy-19-nor-2,5(10)-androstadiene-16α,17β-diol	197	3.93	A	551
		277	1.91	A	551
		285.5	1.86	A	551
		198	4.02	C	551
		277	2.50	C	551
		286	2.86	C	551
$C_{19}H_{30}O$	3-Androsten-17β-ol				
	Acetate	205	1200	A	526
$C_{20}H_{28}O_4$	17β-Carboxy-3β-hydroxy-14-etiocholen-11-one				
	Acetate, methyl ester	191.5	3.91	C	562
		196	3.80	A	562
	17β-Carboxy-3β-hydroxy-14-etiocholen-12-one				
	Acetate, methyl ester	192	3.75	C	562
		195.5	3.80	A	562
$C_{20}H_{30}O_2$	17β-Carboxy-8(14)-androstene				
	Methyl ester	215	3.84		573
$C_{20}H_{30}O_3$	17β-Carboxy-7-etiocholen-3α-ol				
	Acetate, methyl ester	191.5(190.5)	3.90(3.92)	C	562
		196(195.5)	3.79(3.80)	A	562
	17β-Carboxy-8(14)-etiocholen-3α-ol				
	Acetate, methyl ester	202(202)	3.79(3.79)	C	562
		201(201)	3.78(3.78)	A	562
	17β-Carboxy-8(14)-etiocholen-3β-ol				
	Acetate, methyl ester	203(203)	4.10(4.10)	C	562
		201.5(201.5)	4.08(4.08)	A	562
	17β-Carboxy-9(11)-etiocholen-3α-ol				
	Acetate, methyl ester	196(195)	3.84(3.84)	C	562
		197.5(196.5)	3.81(3.81)	A	562

TABLE XXIX—*continued*

Formula	Compound	λ_{max}	Ext.	Sol.	Ref.
$C_{20}H_{30}O_3$ (cont.)					
	17β-Carboxy-11-etiocholen-3α-ol				
	Acetate, methyl ester	192.5(191.5)	4.01(4.02)	C	562
		196(196)	3.92(3.92)	A	562
	17β-Carboxy-14-etiocholen-3β-ol				
	Acetate, methyl ester	194(194)	3.92(3.93)	C	562
		196.5(196)	3.86(3.87)	A	562
$C_{20}H_{30}O_4$	17β-Carboxy-8(14)-etiocholene-3β,11α-diol				
	Diacetate, methyl ester	202(202)	4.07(4.07)	C	562
		201(201)	4.08(4.08)	A	562
	17β-Carboxy-14-etiocholene-3β,11α-diol				
	Diacetate, methyl ester	193.5(192.5)	3.91(3.92)	C	562
		197.5(197)	3.82(3.83)	A	562
$C_{21}H_{30}O_4$	17α,21-Dihydroxy-3-pregnene-11,20-dione				
	21-Acetate	206.5	3100	A	526
	17α,21-Dihydroxy-5α-3-pregnene-11,20-dione				
	21-Acetate	206.5	2900	A	526

TABLE XXX. DIENES

Formula	Compound	λ_{max}	Ext.	Sol.	Ref.
3,5-Dienes					
$C_{19}H_{26}O_2$	17β-Hydroxy-3,5-androstadien-11-one				
	Acetate	188.5	3.64	C	562
		227	4.28	C	562
		234	4.31	C	562
		243	4.07	C	562
		197	3.62	A	562
		226	4.27	A	562
		233	4.29	A	562
		241	4.08	A	562
$C_{21}H_{30}O$	3,5-Pregnadien-20-one	228	19,100	A	560
		235	20,400	A	560
	3,5-Pregnadiene-18,20β-epoxide	228	4.32	A	483
		235	4.34	A	483
		243	4.16	A	483
$C_{21}H_{32}O_3$	3,5-Pregnadiene-20β,21-diol				
	Diacetate	228	17,000		560
$C_{22}H_{29}ON$	6-Cyano-3,5-pregnadien-20-one	260	20,890	A	467
3,5-Dienol Acetates					
$C_{20}H_{28}O_3$	3-Acetoxy-19-nor-3,5-androstadien-17β-ol				
	Acetate	235	4.32	A	570
$C_{21}H_{30}O_3$	3-Acetoxy-16β-methyl-19-nor-3,5-androstadien-17β-ol				
	Acetate	234–236	4.24	A	515
$C_{22}H_{28}O_3$	3-Acetoxy-17α-ethinyl-19-nor-3,5-androstadien-17β-ol				
	Acetate	235	4.27	A	511
$C_{22}H_{29}O_3N$	3-Acetoxy-6-cyano-3,5-androstadien-17β-ol				
	Acetate	262–264	17,400	A	467
$C_{23}H_{29}O_4Br$	3-Acetoxy-16β-bromo-17α-hydroxy-3,5,9(11)-pregnatrien-20-one				
	Acetate	236	19,700	M	449
$C_{23}H_{30}O_5$	3-Acetoxy-17α,21-dihydroxy-3,5,9(11)-pregnatrien-20-one				
	Diacetate	236	17,400	A	464

TABLE XXX—*continued*

Formula	Compound	λ_{max}	Ext.	Sol.	Ref.
Dienol Acetates (cont.)					
$C_{23}H_{30}O_6$	3-Acetoxy-17α,21-dihydroxy-3,5-pregnadien-20-one Diacetate	234	20,890	A	469
$C_{23}H_{32}O_4$	3-Acetoxy-17α-hydroxy-3,5-pregnadien-20-one Acetate	234	20,000	A	469
$C_{24}H_{31}O_3N$	3-Acetoxy-6-cyano-3,5-pregnadien-20-one	264	18,200	A	467
$C_{24}H_{31}O_4N$	3-Acetoxy-6-cyano-17α-hydroxy-3,5-pregnadien-20-one Acetate	262–264	18,620	A	467
$C_{24}H_{34}O_4$	3-Acetoxy-17α-hydroxy-6-methyl-3,5-pregnadien-20-one Acetate	244	19,950	A	542
3,5-Dienol Ethers					
$C_{21}H_{32}O_2$	3-Ethoxy-6-methyl-19-nor-3,5-androstadien-17β-ol	247	4.25	A	570
$C_{22}H_{31}O_3N$	6-Cyano-3-(2′-hydroxyethoxy)-3,5-androstadien-17β-ol	284	18,620	A	467
$C_{23}H_{33}O_3Cl$	6-Chloro-3-ethoxy-17α-hydroxy-3,5-pregnadien-20-one Acetate	251	4.35		540
$C_{23}H_{34}O_3$	3-Ethoxy-17α-hydroxy-3,5-pregnadien-20-one Acetate	241	4.32	A	540
$C_{24}H_{33}O_7N$	6-Cyano-17α-hydroxy-3-(2′-hydroxyethoxy)-3,5-pregnadien-20-one	282–284	19,500	A	467
$C_{26}H_{33}O_7N$	17,20:20,21-Bismethylenedioxy-6-cyano-3-(2′-hydroxyethoxy)-3,5-pregnadien-11-one	284–286	18,200	A	467
$C_{26}H_{35}O_7N$	6-Cyano-20-ethylenedioxy-17α,21-dihydroxy-3-(2′-hydroxyethoxy)-3,5-pregnadien-11-one	284–286	17,800	A	467
$C_{26}H_{37}O_4N$	6-Cyano-20-ethylenedioxy-3-(2′-hydroxyethoxy)-3,5-pregnadien	282–284	23,990	A	467
$C_{26}H_{37}O_5N$	6-Cyano-20-ethylenedioxy-3-(2′-hydroxyethoxy)-3,5-pregnadien-17α-ol	282–284	19,500	A	467
8,14-Dienes					
$C_{20}H_{28}O_2$	8,14-Androstadien-17β-oic acid Methyl ester	247	4.22		573
Dienes-Cumulative					
$C_{22}H_{28}O_4$	11-Keto-3-methoxy-3,5,17(20)-pregnatrien-21-oic acid Methyl ester	235	27,075	A	480

TABLE XXX—*continued*

Formula	Compound	λ_{max}	Ext.	Sol.	Ref.
Dienes-Cumulative (Cont.)					
$C_{23}H_{28}O_5$	3-Acetoxy-11-keto-3,5,17(20)-pregnatrien-21-oic acid	238	28,850	A	480
Dienes (one double bond exocyclic)					
$C_{21}H_{26}O$	20-Methylene-19-nor-1,3,5(10),16-pregnatetraen-3-ol				
	Acetate	239	4.22	H	561
	Maleic Anhydride Addition Product	268	2.98	A	561
$C_{22}H_{32}O_3$	3-Ethylenedioxy-7-methylene-5-androsten-17β-ol				
	Acetate	238	4.25	A	579
$C_{22}H_{34}O_2$	7-Methylene-5-pregnene-3β,20β-diol	237	20,000	M	545
	TRIENES				
3,5,7-Trienes					
$C_{25}H_{35}O_2N$	3-(1-Pyrrolidinyl)-3,5,7,17(20)-pregnatetraene-11β,21-diol				
	21-Acetate	324		A	480
		284		E	480

TABLE XXXI. SIMPLE KETONES

Formula	Compound	λ_{max}	Ext.	Sol.	Ref.
3-Ones					
$C_{20}H_{30}O_6$	17β-Carboxy-11α,14β,19-trihydroxy-etiocholan-3-one				
	11,19-Diacetate, methyl ester	283	2.19	A	571
$C_{20}H_{30}O_7$	17β-Carboxy-5β,11α,14β,19-tetrahydroxy-etiocholan-3-one				
	11,19-Diacetate, methyl ester	285	1.56	A	524
		280	1.30	A	571
11-Ones					
$C_{20}H_{30}O_4$	17β-Carboxy-3β-hydroxy-etiocholan-11-one				
	Acetate, methyl ester	189.5(189)	3.43(3.44)	C	562
		195(193)	3.20(3.22)	A	562
$C_{20}H_{30}O_5$	17β-Carboxy-3β,19-dihydroxy-etiocholan-11-one				
	Diacetate, methyl ester	295	1.54	A	571
$C_{20}H_{30}O_6$	17β-Carboxy-3β,14β,19-trihydroxy-etiocholan-11-one				
	19-Acetate, methyl ester	300(ca.)	1.49	A	571
	3,19-Diacetate, methyl ester	298	1.54	A	571
	17β-Carboxy-3α,14β,19-trihydroxy-etiocholan-11-one				
	3,19-Diacetate, methyl ester	295	1.67	A	571
$C_{20}H_{30}O_7$	17β-Carboxy-3α,5β,14β,19-tetrahydroxy-etiocholan-11-one				
	19-Acetate, methyl ester	290	1.55	A	572
$C_{26}H_{38}O_7$	3,20-Bisethylenedioxy-17α,21-dihydroxy-7β-methyl-5-pregnen-11-one	290–298	1.65	A	579
12-Ones					
$C_{20}H_{30}O_4$	17β-Carboxy-3β-hydroxy-etiocholan-12-one				
	Acetate, methyl ester	189(189)	3.46(3.48)	C	562
15-Ones					
$C_{20}H_{30}O_5$	17β-Carboxy-3β,5β-dihydroxy-etiocholan-15-one				
	Methyl ester	292	1.43	A	553
	3-Acetate, methyl ester	295	1.42		521

TABLE XXXI—*continued*

Formula	Compound	λ_{max}	Ext.	Sol.	Ref.
20-Ones					
$C_{22}H_{33}O_3N$	6β-Cyano-3β,5α-dihydroxy-5α-pregnan-20-one	240–246	21	A	467
		280–288	34	A	467
α-Haloketones					
$C_{19}H_{29}O_2F$	2α-Fluoro-17β-hydroxy-androstan-3-one				
	Acetate	283	1.44	A	491
$C_{20}H_{31}O_2F$	2α-Fluoro-17β-hydroxy-17α-methyl-androstan-3-one	283	1.52	A	491
$C_{21}H_{33}O_2Br$	17α-Bromo-3β-hydroxy-5α-pregnan-20-one				
	Acetate	296–298	2.04	M	490
	21-Bromo-3β-hydroxy-5α-pregnan-20-one				
	Acetate	292–294	1.95	M	490
		306–308	2.01	H	490
$C_{21}H_{33}O_2Cl$	21-Chloro-3β-hydroxy-5α-pregnan-20-one				
	Acetate	282	1.84	M	490
		294–298	1.81	H	490
$C_{21}H_{33}O_2F$	21-Fluoro-3β-hydroxy-5α-pregnan-20-one	284	1.88	M	490
$C_{21}H_{33}O_2I$	21-Iodo-3β-hydroxy-5α-pregnan-20-one	268–270	2.62	M	490
		274–276	2.61	H	490
$C_{21}H_{33}O_3Br$	9α-Bromo-3α,20β-dihydroxy-pregnan-11-one				
	Diacetate	320	100	A	512
	12α-Bromo-3α,20β-dihydroxy-pregnan-11-one				
	Diacetate	319	150	A	512
3,11-Diones					
$C_{20}H_{28}O_6$	17β-Carboxy-14β,19-dihydroxy-etiocholane-3,11-dione				
	19-Acetate, methyl ester	290	1.71	A	571
$C_{20}H_{28}O_7$	17β-Carboxy-5β,14β,19-trihydroxy-etiocholane-3,11-dione				
	19-Acetate, methyl ester	297–298	1.44	A	572
$C_{23}H_{32}O_8$	17β-Carboxy-5β,14β-dihydroxy-1β,19-iso-Propylidenedioxy-etiocholane-3,11-dione				
	Methyl ester	300	1.67	A	572

TABLE XXXI—*continued*

Formula	Compound	λ_{max}	Ext.	Sol.	Ref.
3,15-Diones					
$C_{20}H_{28}O_5$	17β-Carboxy-5β-hydroxy-etiocholane-3,15-dione				
	Methyl ester	282–286	1.61	A	553
3,17-Diones					
$C_{20}H_{27}O_3N$	6α-Cyano-5α-hydroxy-androstane-3,17-dione	286–292	54	A	467
3,20-Diones					
$C_{21}H_{31}O_4F$	6β-Fluoro-5α,17α-dihydroxy-pregnane-3,20-dione				
	17-Acetate	280–286	72	M	470
$C_{22}H_{31}O_3N$	6β-Cyano-5α-hydroxy-5α-pregnane-3,20-dione	278–288	53	A	467
8,14-Diones					
$C_{20}H_{28}O_6$	17β-Carboxy-3β,6β-dihydroxy-8,14-*seco*-4-androstene-8,14-dione				
	Diacetate, methyl ester	280	2.66	M	573
11,20-Diones					
$C_{21}H_{30}O_4$	17α,21-Dihydroxy-5α-3-pregnene-11,20-dione				
	21-Acetate	294	110	A	526
	17α,21-Dihydroxy-3-pregnene-11,20-dione				
	21-Acetate	294	110	A	526
$C_{21}H_{32}O_4$	3α,17α-Dihydroxy-5α-pregnane-11,20-dione	Chart			530
	3-Acetate				

TABLE XXXII. ENONES

Formula	Compound	λ_{max}	Ext.	Sol.	Ref.
1-en-3-Ones					
$C_{19}H_{24}O_2$	1,5-Androstadiene-3,17-dione	224	11,800	A	534
$C_{20}H_{28}O_7$	17β-Carboxy-5β,11α,14β,19-tetrahydroxy-1-etiocholen-3-one				
	11-Acetate, methyl ester	233	4.06	A	571
$C_{21}H_{26}O_5$	17α,21-Dihydroxy-1,5-pregnadiene-3,11,20-trione				
	21-Acetate	224	13,000	A	534
$C_{21}H_{26}O_6$	7α,17α,21-Trihydroxy-1,5-pregnadiene-3,11,20-trione				
	21-Acetate	224	12,000	A	534
$C_{21}H_{28}O_5$	11β,17α,21-Trihydroxy-1,5-pregnadiene-3,20-dione				
	21-Acetate	224	11,800	A	534
$C_{22}H_{29}O_5F$	9α,Fluoro-11β,17α,21-trihydroxy-16α-methyl-1,5-pregnadiene-3,20-dione				
	21-Acetate	220	14,800	A	534
3(5)-en-2-Ones					
$C_{18}H_{24}O_2$	A-Nor-3(5)-androstene-2,17-dione	232	15,600	A	574
$C_{18}H_{26}O_2$	17β-Hydroxy-A-nor-3(5)-androsten-2-one	234	15,200	A	574
$C_{20}H_{26}O_5$	17α,21-Dihydroxy-A-nor-3(5)-pregnene-2,11,20-trione	229	4.12		509
$C_{20}H_{28}O_2$	A-nor-3(5)-pregnene-2,20-dione	233	15,800	A	574
$C_{20}H_{30}O_2$	20β-Hydroxy-A-nor-3(5)-pregnen-2-one	234	15,000	A	574
$C_{22}H_{28}O_6$	17,20 : 20,21-Bismethylenedioxy-A-nor-3(5)-pregnene-2,11-dione	229	4.16		509
$C_{22}H_{30}O_6$	17,20 : 20,21-Bismethylenedioxy-11α-hydroxy-A-nor-3(5)-pregnen-3-one	233	4.20	M	509
	17,20 : 20,21-Bismethylenedioxy-11β-hydroxy-A-nor-3(5)-pregnen-3-one	234	4.18	M	509
4-en-3-Ones					
$C_{18}H_{26}O_3$	2α,17β-Dihydroxy-19-nor-4-androsten-3-one				
	17-Acetate	239.5	15,920	M	451
	Diacetate	240	14,230	M	451
	2β,17β-Dihydroxy-19-nor-4-androsten-3-one				
	Diacetate	242	16,530	M	451

TABLE XXXII—*continued*

Formula	Compound	λ_{max}	Ext.	Sol.	Ref.
4-en-3-Ones (cont.)					
$C_{18}H_{26}O_3$	16α,17β-Dihydroxy-19-nor-4-androsten-3-one	240	4.21	A	551
$C_{19}H_{22}O_5$	*d,l*-11β,18 : 14ξ,15ξ-Diepoxy-18-hydroxy-4-androstene-3,16-dione	238	15,200	A	507
$C_{19}H_{24}O_3$	4-Androstene-3,15,17-trione	241	17,300	M	505
$C_{19}H_{25}O_2Br$	16α-Bromo-4-androstene-3,17-dione	239	4.179	A	496
	16β-Bromo-4-androstene-3,17-dione	239	4.214	A	496
$C_{19}H_{25}O_4N$	6α-Nitro-4-androstene-3,17-dione	232	14,790	A	474
	6β-Nitro-4-androstene-3,17-dione	232–234	11,750	A	474
$C_{19}H_{26}O_2$	6α-Methyl-19-nor-4-androstene-3,17-dione	240	4.17	A	570
	6β-Methyl-19-nor-4-androstene-3,17-dione	240	4.16	A	570
	16β-Methyl-19-nor-4-androstene-3,17-dione	240	4.21	A	515
	4-Androstene-3,16-dione	240	4.22	A	547
$C_{19}H_{26}O_3$	7α-Hydroxy-4-androstene-3,17-dione	241–242	16,800	A	455
	15β-Hydroxy-4-androstene-3,17-dione	240	16,900	M	505
	13,17-Seco-4,13(18)-androstadien-3-one-17-oic acid	242	4.26	A	508
$C_{19}H_{26}O_3S$	1α-Thiol-13α-hydroxy-13,17-*seco*-4-androsten-3-one-17-oic acid-lactone				
	S-Acetyl	239.5	17,900	M	488
$C_{19}H_{26}O_4$	13ξ,18-Epoxy-13,17-*seco*-4-androsten-3-one-17-oic acid	240	4.24	A	508
	13α,18-Dihydroxy-13,17-*seco*-4-androsten-3-one-17-oic acid-17 → 13-lactone	238	4.24	A	508
$C_{19}H_{27}O_2Br$	16α-Bromo-17β-hydroxy-4-androsten-3-one	239	4.303	A	496
	Acetate	239	4.208	A	496
	16β-Bromo-17β-hydroxy-4-androsten-3-one	239	4.186	A	496
	Acetate	239	4.190	A	496
$C_{19}H_{27}O_2Cl$	4-Chloro-17β-hydroxy-17α-methyl-19-nor-4-androsten-3-one	255	4.12	A	523
$C_{19}H_{27}O_2F$	2α-Fluoro-17β-hydroxy-4-androsten-3-one	242	4.15	A	491
	6α-Fluoro-17β-hydroxy-4-androsten-3-one				
	Acetate	236	15,500	A	471
$C_{19}H_{27}O_4N$	17β-Hydroxy-6α-nitro-4-androsten-3-one	234	13,180	A	474
	17β-Hydroxy-6β-nitro-4-androsten-3-one	234–236	10,720	A	474
		234–236	10,800	A	469
	Acetate	234–236	10,000	A	469

TABLE XXXII—*continued*

Formula	Compound	λ_{max}	Ext.	Sol.	Ref.
4-en-3-Ones (cont.)					
$C_{19}H_{28}O_2$	17β-Hydroxy-6α-methyl-19-nor-4-androsten-3-one	241	4.13	A	570
	Acetate	241	4.27	A	570
	17β-Hydroxy-6β-methyl-19-nor-4-androsten-3-one	240	4.22	A	570
	Acetate	240	4.26	A	570
	17β-Hydroxy-16β-methyl-19-nor-4-androsten-3-one	240	4.21	A	515
$C_{19}H_{28}O_2S$	17β-Hydroxy-1α-thiol-4-androsten-3-one				
	S-Acetyl, 3-acetate	240.5	16,800	M	488
$C_{19}H_{28}O_2S_2$	17β-Hydroxy-1α,17α-dithiol-4-androsten-3-one				
	S,S-Diacetyl, 17-acetate	237.5	20,100	M	565
$C_{19}H_{28}O_3$	15β,17β-Dihydroxy-4-androsten-3-one	242	15,000	M	505
	17β,19-Dihydroxy-4-androsten-3-one	243	14,900	A	494
	Diacetate	239	18,800	A	494
$C_{19}H_{28}O_5$	13α,18-Dihydroxy-13,17-*seco*-4-androsten-3-one-17-oic acid	244	4.21	A	508
$C_{20}H_{23}O_3NS$	9α-Thiocyano-4-androstene-3,11,17-trione	236	14,270	A	514
$C_{20}H_{25}O_2Cl$	4-Chloro-17α-ethinyl-17β-hydroxy-19-nor-4-androsten-3-one	255	4.11	A	523
$C_{20}H_{25}O_2N$	6α-Cyano-4-androstene-3,17-dione	228–230	5120	A	467
		288–290	11,750	A	467
		338–340	19,950	BA	467
$C_{20}H_{25}O_2F$	17α-Ethinyl-6β-fluoro-17β-hydroxy-19-nor-4-androsten-3-one	234	4.10	A	581
$C_{20}H_{25}O_3NS$	11β-Hydroxy-9α-thiocyano-4-androstene-3,17-dione	242	14,200	A	514
$C_{20}H_{26}O_2$	17α-Ethinyl-17β-hydroxy-19-nor-4-androsten-3-one	240	4.20	A	511
$C_{20}H_{26}O_4$	17β-Carboxy-4-androstene-3,15-dione				
	Methyl ester	238	4.21	A	553
$C_{20}H_{26}O_6$	17β-Carboxy-14β,19-dihydroxy-4-androstene-3,11-dione				
	19-Acetate, methyl ester	235–236	4.22–4.23	A	571
$C_{20}H_{27}O_2Cl$	4-Chloro-17β-hydroxy-17α-vinyl-19-nor-4-androsten-3-one	255	4.13	A	523
	4-Chloro-19-nor-4-pregnene-3,20-dione	256	4.11	A	523

TABLE XXXII—*continued*

Formula	Compound	λ_{max}	Ext.	Sol.	Ref.
4-en-3-Ones (cont.)					
$C_{20}H_{27}O_2N$	6α-Cyano-17β-hydroxy-4-androsten-3-one				
	Acetate	230	4900	A	467
		288–290	11,500	A	467
		340–342	18,200	BA	467
$C_{20}H_{28}O_2$	18-Nor-4-pregnene-3,20-dione	242	4.2	A	450
$C_{20}H_{28}O_2Br_2$	2α,6β-Dibromo-17β-hydroxy-4-methyl-4-androsten-3-one				
	Acetate	263.5	4.14	A	489
	2β,6β-Dibromo-17β-hydroxy-2α-methyl-4-androsten-3-one	253	12,100	A	516
		352	16.1	C	516
$C_{20}H_{28}O_3$	17β-Carboxy-4-androsten-3-one				
	Methyl ester	231	4.31	C	562
		240	4.25	A	562
$C_{20}H_{28}O_5$	17β-Carboxy-15β,17α-dihydroxy-4-androsten-3-one	241	16,400	M	505
	Methyl ester	242	15,500	M	505
$C_{20}H_{28}O_6$	17β-Carboxy-11α,14β,19-trihydroxy-4-androsten-3-one				
	11,19-Diacetate, methyl ester	240	4.10	A	524
		238	4.22	A	571
$C_{20}H_{29}O_2Cl$	4-Chloro-17α-ethyl-17β-hydroxy-19-nor-4-androsten-3-one	256	4.14	A	523
$C_{20}H_{29}O_2F$	2α-Fluoro-17β-hydroxy-17α-methyl-4-androsten-3-one	242	4.22	A	491
$C_{20}H_{30}O_2$	2α-Methyl-17β-hydroxy-4-androsten-3-one	242	4.19	A	541
	4-Methyl-17β-hydroxy-4-androsten-3-one	251	14,100	A	478
	7α-Methyl-17β-hydroxy-4-androsten-3-one	242	16,050	A	480
	7β-Methyl-17β-hydroxy-4-androsten-3-one	244	4.21	A	579
$C_{21}H_{25}O_3F$	16α,17α-Epoxy-6β-fluoro-4,9(11)-pregnadiene-3,20-dione	232	11,200	A	466
$C_{21}H_{26}O_3$	16α,17α-Epoxy-4,9(11)-pregnadiene-3,20-dione	239	17,150	M	449
		240	16,950	A	479
		239	16,900	M	454
$C_{21}H_{26}O_3ClF$	4-Chloro-9α-fluoro-4-pregnene-3,11,20-trione	252	13,300	A	479
$C_{21}H_{26}O_4$	9β,11β : 16α,17α-Diepoxy-4-pregnene-3,20-dione	244	13,000	M	456
$C_{21}H_{26}O_4ClF$	4-Chloro-9α-fluoro-17α-hydroxy-4-pregnene-3,11,20-trione	252	14,000	A	479

TABLE XXXII—*continued*

Formula	Compound	λ_{max}	Ext.	Sol.	Ref.
4-en-3-Ones (cont.)					
$C_{21}H_{26}O_5$	16α,17α-Epoxy-21-hydroxy-4-pregnene-3,11,20-trione	238	4.19	A	495
	Acetate	238	4.20	A	495
	Hemisuccinate	238	4.19	A	495
$C_{21}H_{26}O_6$	*d,l*-11β,18-Epoxy-18-hydroxy-4-androstene-3,20-dione-21-oic acid				
	Methyl ester	240	10,750	A	507
$C_{21}H_{27}O_2Cl$	4-Chloro-4,9(11)-pregnadiene-3,20-dione	256	14,800	A	479
$C_{21}H_{27}O_2F$	17α-Ethinyl-2α-fluoro-17β-hydroxy-4-androsten-3-one	242	4.28		491
$C_{21}H_{27}O_3Br$	16β-Bromo-17α-hydroxy-4,9(11)-pregnadiene-3,20-dione	238	17,900	M	449
$C_{21}H_{27}O_3Cl$	4-Chloro-17α-hydroxy-4,9(11)-pregnadiene-3,20-dione	255	13,600	A	479
	4-Chloro-9β,11β-epoxy-4-pregnene-3,20-dione	256	9600	A	479
$C_{21}H_{27}O_3I$	16β-Iodo-17α-hydroxy-4,9(11)-pregnadiene-3,20-dione	238	17,300	M	449
		238.5	17,800	M	454
$C_{21}H_{27}O_4Br$	9α-Bromo-16α,17α-epoxy-11β-hydroxy-4-pregnene-3,20-dione	242	16,700	M	456
$C_{21}H_{27}O_4Cl$	4-Chloro-9β,11β-epoxy-17α-hydroxy-4-pregnene-3,20-dione	256	12,150	A	479
$C_{21}H_{27}O_4F$	6α-Fluoro-17α,21-dihydroxy-4,9(11)-pregnadiene-3,20-dione				
	21-Acetate	234–236	15,850	A	468
	Diacetate	234	16,800	A	464
	9α-Fluoro-16α,17α-epoxy-11β-hydroxy-4-pregnene-3,20-dione	238	18,600	M	456
	9α-Fluoro-17α-hydroxy-4-pregnene-3,11,20-trione				
	Acetate	235	16,990	M	454
$C_{21}H_{27}O_4N$	10β-Cyano-14β,21-dihydroxy-4-pregnene-3,20-dione	230	17,300	M	536
	21-Acetate	229	17,600	M	536
$C_{21}H_{27}O_5F$	2ξ-Fluoro-17α,21-dihydroxy-4-pregnene-3,11,20-trione	237	14,175		531
	9β,11β-Epoxy-6α-fluoro-17α,21-dihydroxy-4-pregnene-3,20-dione				
	21-Acetate	236–238	12,600	A	468
	6α-Fluoro-17α,21-dihydroxy-4-pregnene-3,11,20-trione				
	21-Acetate	233	16,220	A	468
	Diacetate	232–234	16,000	A	468
	6β-Fluoro-17α,21-dihydroxy-4-pregnene-3,11,20-trione				
	Diacetate	232–234	11,480	A	468

TABLE XXXII—*continued*

Formula	Compound	λ_{max}	Ext.	Sol.	Ref.
4-en-3-Ones (cont.)					
$C_{21}H_{27}O_6Br$	12α-Bromo-16α,17α,21-trihydroxy-4-pregnene-3,11,20-trione				
	21-Acetate	237	16,400	M	462
	16,21-Diacetate	237	13,700	A	462
$C_{21}H_{27}O_6Cl$	9α-Chloro-16α,17α,21-trihydroxy-4-pregnene-3,11,20-trione				
	16,21-Diacetate	235.5	15,400	A	459
$C_{21}H_{27}O_6F$	9α-Fluoro-16α,17α,21-trihydroxy-4-pregnene-3,11,20-trione				
	16,21-Diacetate	234.5	16,100	A	459
$C_{21}H_{27}O_7N$	17α,21-Dihydroxy-6α-nitro-4-pregnene-3,11,20-trione	228–230	14,130	A	469
	17α,21-Dihydroxy-6β-nitro-4-pregnene-3,11,20-trione				
	Diacetate	226–228	11,480	A	469
$C_{21}H_{28}O_2F_2$	21,21-Difluoro-4-pregnene-3,20-dione	241	4.22	A	491
$C_{21}H_{28}O_3$	16α-Hydroxy-17β-methyl-18-nor-17α-4,13-pregnadiene-3,20-dione	238	18,500		555
	16β-Hydroxy-17β-methyl-18-nor-17α-4,13-pregnadiene-3,20-dione	238	17,300	A	555
	Acetate	238	17,200	A	555
	Tosylate	228	25,400	A	555
	4-Pregnene-3,11,20-trione	239	15,500	A	522
	17α-Hydroxy-4,9(11)-pregnadiene-3,20-dione				
	Acetate	239	18,150	M	454
	16β,17β-Epoxy-17α-4-pregnene-3,20-dione	241	16,200	A	555
$C_{21}H_{28}O_3ClF$	4-Chloro-9α-fluoro-11β-hydroxy-4-pregnene-3,20-dione	255	12,700	A	479
$C_{21}H_{28}O_3S$	7α-Thiol-4-pregnene-3,11,20-trione				
	S-Acetyl	236	18,000	M	488
	21-Carboxy-17β-hydroxy-7α-thiol-19-nor-17α-4-pregnen-3-one-21′ → 17-lactone				
	S-Acetyl	237	21,000	M	482
$C_{21}H_{28}O_4$	17α-Hydroxy-4-pregnene-3,11,20-trione	239	15,300	M	456
		238–240	4.20	A	501
	9β,11β-Epoxy-17α-hydroxy-4-pregnene-3,20-dione				
	Acetate	243.5	15,100	M	454
	16α,17α-Epoxy-11α-hydroxy-4-pregnene-3,20-dione				
	Mesylate	238.5	15,300	M	449

TABLE XXXII—*continued*

Formula	Compound	λ_{max}	Ext.	Sol.	Ref.
4-en-3-Ones (cont.)					
	16α,17α-Dihydroxy-4,9(11)-pregnadiene-3,20-dione	240	17,100	M	456
		239	17,200	M	449
	16-Acetate	238	17,200	M	456
		240	16,300	M	449
	16α,17α-Dihydroxy-17β-methyl-D-homo-4,9(11)-androstadien-3,17a-one	239	17,700	M	456
	16-Acetate	237	18,300	M	456
$C_{21}H_{28}O_4BrF$	7α-Bromo-6β-fluoro-17α,21-dihydroxy-4-pregnene-3,20-dione				
	Diacetate	234–236	10,500	A	466
	9α-Bromo-11β-fluoro-17α,21-dihydroxy-4-pregnene-3,20-dione				
	21-Acetate	241	15,500	A	466
$C_{21}H_{28}O_4ClF$	4-Chloro-9α-fluoro-11β,17α-dihydroxy-4-pregnene-3,20-dione	255	11,150	A	479
$C_{21}H_{28}O_5$	17α,21-Dihydroxy-4-pregnene-3,11,20-trione				
	Diacetate	238	16,600	A	468
		238	15,000	M	548
	17α,21-Dihydroxy-4-pregnene-3,15,20-trione				
	21-Acetate	240	17,300	A	505
	16α,17α-Epoxy-11α,21-dihydroxy-4-pregnene-3,20-dione	242	4.19	A	495
	21-Hemisuccinate	241.5	4.22	A	495
	11,21-Diacetate	239	4.22	A	495
	16α,17α,21-Trihydroxy-4,9(11)-pregnadiene-3,20-dione				
	21-Acetate	238.5	16,700	A	459
	16,21-Diacetate	238–239	17,400	A	459
		239	14,200	A	460
	16β,17α,21-Trihydroxy-4,9(11)-pregnadiene-3,20-dione				
	16,21-Diacetate	239	15,700	A	458
	20β-Hydroxy-4-pregnene-3,11-dione-21-oic acid				
	Acetate	237.5	15,300	M	563
$C_{21}H_{28}O_5F_2$	6α,9α-Difluoro-11β,17α,21-trihydroxy-4-pregnene-3,20-dione				
	21-Acetate	234	19,900	M	468

TABLE XXXII—*continued*

Formula	Compound	λ_{max}	Ext.	Sol.	Ref.
4-en-3-Ones (cont.)					
$C_{21}H_{28}O_5S$	17α,21-Dihydroxy-7α-thiol-4-pregnene-3,11,20-trione				
	S-Acetyl, 21-acetate	235.5	17,400	M	488
$C_{21}H_{28}O_5S_2$	17α,21-Dihydroxy-1α,7α-dithiol-4-pregnene-3,11,20-trione				
	S,S-Diacetyl, 21-acetate	235.5	18,500	M	565
$C_{21}H_{28}O_6$	9β,11β-Epoxy-16α,17α,21-trihydroxy-4-pregnene-3,20-dione	243.5	15,000	A	459
	16,21-Diacetate	243–243.5	15,000	A	459
	9β,11β-Epoxy-16β,17α,21-trihydroxy-4-pregnene-3,20-dione				
	16,21-Diacetate	243–244	15,200	A	458
$C_{21}H_{28}O_6F_2$	6α,9α-Difluoro-11β,16α,17α,21-tetrahydroxy-4-pregnene-3,20-dione	234	4.18	A	528
$C_{21}H_{28}O_7$	6α,7α,17α,21-Tetrahydroxy-4-pregnene-3,11,20-trione				
	21-Acetate	238–240	4.00	A	578
	9α,16α,17α,21-Tetrahydroxy-4-pregnene-3,11,20-trione				
	16,21-Diacetate	237	14,200	A	459
$C_{21}H_{29}ON$	18,20-Imino-4,20(N)-pregnadien-3-one	240	4.21	A	477
$C_{21}H_{29}O_2Cl$	6α-Chloro-4-pregnene-3,20-dione	237	4.19	A	540
$C_{21}H_{29}O_3Br$	6α-Bromo-17α-hydroxy-4-pregnene-3,20-dione				
	Acetate	236	4.12	A	540
	6β-Bromo-17α-hydroxy-4-pregnene-3,20-dione				
	Acetate	246	4.14	A	540
	17α-Bromo-16β-hydroxy-4-pregnene-3,20-dione	241	16,600	A	555
$C_{21}H_{29}O_3Cl$	6α-Chloro-17α-hydroxy-4-pregnene-3,20-dione				
	Acetate	236	4.20	A	540
	Caproate	238	4.15	A	540
	6β-Chloro-17α-hydroxy-4-pregnene-3,20-dione				
	Acetate	239	4.19	A	540
$C_{21}H_{29}O_3F$	6α-Fluoro-17α-hydroxy-4-pregnene-3,20-dione				
	Acetate	236	15,900	A	470
	6β-Fluoro-17α-hydroxy-4-pregnene-3,20-dione				
	Acetate	232–234	13,000	A	466
	6α-Fluoro-21-hydroxy-4-pregnene-3,20-dione				
	Acetate	236	15,500	M	471

TABLE XXXII—*continued*

Formula	Compound	λ_{max}	Ext.	Sol.	Ref.
4-en-3-Ones (cont.)					
$C_{21}H_{29}O_3F$	6β-Fluoro-21-hydroxy-4-pregnene-3,20-dione				
	Acetate	234	10,000	A	471
$C_{21}H_{29}O_4Br$	9α-Bromo-11β,17α-dihydroxy-4-pregnene-3,20-dione				
	17-Acetate	242.5	15,900	M	454
	16β-Bromo-11α,17α-dihydroxy-4-pregnene-3,20-dione				
	11-Mesylate	238	17,600	M	449
$C_{21}H_{29}O_4Cl$	6α-Chloro-17α,21-dihydroxy-4-pregnene-3,20-dione				
	Diacetate	237	4.19	A	540
$C_{21}H_{29}O_4F$	6α-Fluoro-17α,21-dihydroxy-4-pregnene-3,20-dione	236	16,220	A	471
	21-Acetate	236	16,100	A	471
	Diacetate	236	15,490	A	471
	6β-Fluoro-17α,21-dihydroxy-4-pregnene-3,20-dione				
	Diacetate	234	11,220	A	471
	9α-Fluoro-11β,17α-dihydroxy-4-pregnene-3,20-dione				
	17-Acetate	238	17,500	M	454
	Diacetate	236.5	17,400	M	454
$C_{21}H_{29}O_4N$	6α-Nitro-4-pregnene-3,20-dione	232–234	15,850	A	474
	6β-Nitro-4-pregnene-3,20-dione	234–236	12,020	A	474
	21-Nitro-4-pregnene-3,20-dione	240	19,000	A	473
		312–316	813	A	473
		240	20,400	BA	473
		332–334	18,600	BA	473
$C_{21}H_{29}O_5Br$	9α-Bromo-11β,16α,17α-trihydroxy-4-pregnene-3,20-dione				
	16-Acetate	242	16,100	M	456
$C_{21}H_{29}O_5Cl$	9α-Chloro-11β,16α,17α-trihydroxy-4-pregnene-3,20-dione				
	16-Acetate	240	18,000	M	456
$C_{21}H_{29}O_5D$	11α-Deutero-11β,17α,21-trihydroxy-4-pregnene-3,20-dione	242	18,000	M	465
	21-Acetate	242	16,200	M	465
$C_{21}H_{29}O_5F$	2α-Fluoro-11β,17α,21-trihydroxy-4-pregnene-3,20-dione	241	14,800	M	517
	2ξ-Fluoro-11β,17α,21-trihydroxy-4-pregnene-3,20-dione				
	21-Acetate	243	14,100		531

TABLE XXXII—*continued*

Formula	Compound	λ_{max}	Ext.	Sol.	Ref.
4-en-3-Ones (cont.)					
$C_{21}H_{29}O_5F$	6α-Fluoro-11β,17α,21-trihydroxy-4-pregnene-3,20-dione				
	21-Acetate	236–238	16,600	A	468
	9α-Fluoro-11β,16α,17α-trihydroxy-4-pregnene-3,20-dione	238	17,800	M	456
	16-Acetate	238	19,600	M	456
$C_{21}H_{29}O_5N$	6α-Nitro-17α-hydroxy-4-pregnene-3,20-dione				
	17-Acetate	232–234	14,130	A	469
$C_{21}H_{29}O_6Br$	9α-Bromo-11β,16α,17α,21-tetrahydroxy-4-pregnene-3,20-dione				
	16,21-Diacetate	243	14,100	A	459
$C_{21}H_{29}O_6Cl$	9α-Chloro-11β,16α,17α,21-tetrahydroxy-4-pregnene-3,20-dione	240–240.5	15,900	A	459
	16,21-Diacetate	240.5	15,800	A	459
$C_{21}H_{29}O_6F$	6α-Fluoro-11β,16α,17α,21-tetrahydroxy-4-pregnene-3,20-dione	237	4.18	A	528
	9α-Fluoro-11β,16α,17α,21-tetrahydroxy-4-pregnene-3,20-dione	238.5	16,300	A	459
	21-Trimethylacetate	238.5	16,100	A	459
	16,21-Diacetate	237.5–238.5	17,600	A	459
	9α-Fluoro-11β,16β,17α,21-tetrahydroxy-4-pregnene-3,20-dione				
	16,21-Diacetate	239	16,500	A	458
$C_{21}H_{29}O_7F$	9α-Fluoro-6α,7α,11β,17α,21-pentahydroxy-4-pregnene-3,20-dione				
	21-Acetate	238	3.95	A	578
$C_{21}H_{30}O_2$	20ξ-Hydroxy-18,21-cyclo-4-pregnen-3-one	243	4.16		475
	16α-Hydroxy-17β-methyl-18-nor-17α-4,13-pregnadien-3-one	238–240	4.17	A	547
	13,17-Seco-4,13(18)-pregnadiene-3,20-dione	240	4.22	A	508
$C_{21}H_{30}O_3$	1β-Hydroxy-4-pregnene-3,20-dione	241	14,000	M	532
		244.5	17,700	BM	532
	18-Hydroxy-4-pregnene-3,20-dione	242	4.16	A	477
	13,18-Epoxy-13,17-*seco*-4-pregnene-3,20-dione	240	4.21	A	508
	18,20-Epoxy-20ξ-hydroxy-4-pregnen-3-one	242	4.175	A	519
	13α,20 : 18,20-Diepoxy-13,17-*seco*-4-pregnene-3-one	240	4.2	A	508
$C_{21}H_{30}O_3S$	17α-Hydroxy-7α-thiol-4-pregnene-3,20-dione				
	S-Acetyl	238.5	19,200	M	488
$C_{21}H_{30}O_5$	7α,17α,21-Trihydroxy-4-pregnene-3,20-dione	242–243	14,800	A	455
	21-Acetate	242	15,300	A	455

TABLE XXXII—*continued*

Formula	Compound	λ_{max}	Ext.	Sol.	Ref.
4-en-3-Ones (cont.)					
$C_{21}H_{30}O_5$	7,21-Diacetate	238	16,100	A	455
	11α,16α,17α-Trihydroxy-4-pregnene-3,20-dione	241	14,600	M	449
	14β,19,21-Trihydroxy-4-pregnene-3,20-dione				
	19,21-Diacetate	239	16,600	M	535
	15β,17α,21-Trihydroxy-4-pregnene-3,20-dione	242	16,600	M	505
	21-Acetate	242	17,700	A	505
	15,21-Diacetate	239	16,800	A	505
	17α,20α,21-Trihydroxy-4-pregnene-3,11-dione				
	20,21-Diacetate	238	15,500	M	481
	17α,20β,21-Trihydroxy-4-pregnene-3,11-dione				
	21-Acetate	238	15,300	M	563
$C_{21}H_{30}O_5S_2$	11β,17α,21-Trihydroxy-1α,7α-dithiol-4-pregnene-3,20-dione				
	S,S-Dipropionyl, 21-acetate	239	21,200	M	565
$C_{21}H_{30}O_7$	9α,11β,16α,17α,21-Pentahydroxy-4-pregnene-3,20-dione	241–242	14,300	A	459
	16,21-Diacetate	242	16,100	A	459
$C_{21}H_{31}O_2Br$	4-Bromo-17β-hydroxy-2,2-dimethyl-4-androsten-3-one				
	Acetate	262	4.07	A	541
$C_{21}H_{31}O_2N$	16α-Acetyl-17β-amino-4-androsten-3-one				
	N-Acetyl	239–240	4.09	A	547
$C_{21}H_{32}O_2$	17β-Hydroxy-2,2-dimethyl-4-androsten-3-one				
	Acetate	240	4.19	A	541
	17β-Hydroxy-2α,17α-dimethyl-4-androsten-3-one	240	4.21	A	541
	17β-Hydroxy-7α,17α-dimethyl-4-androsten-3-one	243	16,250	A	480
	17β-Hydroxy-7β,17α-dimethyl-4-androsten-3-one	243	16,650	A	480
	4-Ethyl-17β-hydroxy-4-androsten-3-one	251	13,150	A	478
$C_{21}H_{32}O_3$	11β,17β-Dihydroxy-7α,17α-dimethyl-4-androsten-3-one	243	15,825	A	480
	11β,17β-Dihydroxy-7β,17α-dimethyl-4-androsten-3-one	244	15,175	A	480
	20β,21-Dihydroxy-4-pregnen-3-one				
	Diacetate	241	16,000	A	560
$C_{21}H_{32}O_4$	17α,20α,21-Trihydroxy-4-pregnen-3-one				
	20,21-Diacetate	242	16,100	M	481

TABLE XXXII—*continued*

Formula	Compound	λ_{max}	Ext.	Sol.	Ref.
4-en-3-Ones (cont.)					
$C_{21}H_{32}O_4$	17α,20β,21-Trihydroxy-4-pregnen-3-one	242	16,300	A	481
	20,21-Diacetate	241	16,600	A	481
	11β,20β,21-Trihydroxy-4-pregnen-3-one	242	15,600	M	563
	20-Acetate	243	14,800	C : M	563
	21-Acetate	242.5	15,700	M	563
	20,21-Diacetate	242	15,800	M	563
	20-Acetate, 21-mesylate	242	15,500	M	563
$C_{22}H_{27}O_5N$	6α-Cyano-17α,21-dihydroxy-4-pregnene-3,11,20-trione	220–222	4300	A	467
		286–288	10,800	A	467
$C_{22}H_{27}O_5NS$	17α,21-Dihydroxy-9α-thiocyano-4-pregnene-3,11,20-trione	238	16,310	A	514
$C_{22}H_{29}O_2N$	6α-Cyano-4-pregnene-3,20-dione	230	5130	A	467
		288–290	10,250	A	467
		338–340	18,200	BA	467
	16α-Cyano-4-pregnene-3,20-dione	240	17,300	M	525
$C_{22}H_{29}O_3N$	6α-Cyano-17α-hydroxy-4-pregnene-3,20-dione				
	Acetate	220–230	2700	A	467
		288–290	14,790	A	467
$C_{22}H_{29}O_4F$	6α-Fluoro-17α,21-dihydroxy-16α-methyl-4,9(11)-pregnadiene-3,20-dione				
	21-Acetate	235	4.17	A	492
$C_{22}H_{29}O_5F$	2ξ-Fluoro-17α,21-dihydroxy-6α-methyl-4-pregnene-3,11,20-trione				
	21-Acetate	237	14,250		531
$C_{22}H_{29}O_5NS$	11β,17α,21-Trihydroxy-9α-thiocyano-4-pregnene-3,20-dione	243	13,430	A	514
	21-Acetate	243	14,000	A	514
$C_{22}H_{29}O_6F$	9α-Fluoro-16α,17α,21-trihydroxy-2α-methyl-4-pregnene-3,11,20-trione				
	16,21-Diacetate	235	15,000	A	457
$C_{22}H_{30}O_2$	17α-Ethinyl-17β-hydroxy-2α-methyl-4-androsten-3-one	240	4.19	A	541
	17β-Hydroxy-2α-propargyl-4-androsten-3-one	241	4.19	A	476
	Acetate	241	4.18	A	476
	17β-Hydroxy-6α-propargyl-4-androsten-3-one	239.5	4.19	A	476
	17β-Hydroxy-17α-prop-1′-ynyl-4-androsten-3-one	240	4.2	A	452

TABLE XXXII—*continued*

Formula	Compound	λ_{max}	Ext.	Sol.	Ref.
4-en-3-Ones (cont.)					
$C_{22}H_{30}O_3$	16α-Methyl-4-pregnene-3,11,20-trione	238	15,850		552
	16β-Carboxy-20β-hydroxy-4-pregnen-3-one-lactone	241	17,000	M	525
$C_{22}H_{30}O_3S$	21-Carboxy-17β-hydroxy-1α-thiol-17α-4-pregnen-3-one-21′ → 17-lactone				
	S-Acetyl	240.5	16,200	M	482
	21-Carboxy-17β-hydroxy-7α-thiol-17α-4-pregnen-3-one-21′ → 17-lactone				
	S-Acetyl	238	20,200	M	482
$C_{22}H_{30}O_5$	16α,17α,21-Trihydroxy-2α-methyl-4,9(11)-pregnadiene-3,20-dione				
	21-Acetate	237–238	17,400	A	457
	16,21-Diacetate	238–239	16,900	A	457
	17α,21-Dihydroxy-6α-methyl-4-pregnene-3,11,20-trione	242	14,600		554
	17α,21-Dihydroxy-7β-methyl-4-pregnene-3,11,20-trione	240	4.23	A	579
	21-Acetate	240	4.23	A	579
		239	13,800	A	546
$C_{22}H_{30}O_5F_2$	6α,9α-Difluoro-16α-methyl-11β,17α,21-trihydroxy-4-pregnene-3,20-dione				
	21-Acetate	234	4.22	A	492
$C_{22}H_{30}O_6$	9β,11β-Epoxy-16α,17α,21-trihydroxy-2α-methyl-4-pregnene-3,20-dione				
	16,21-Diacetate	242–243	14,100	A	457
	16α,17α,21-Trihydroxy-2α-methyl-4-pregnene-3,11,20-trione				
	16,21-Diacetate	237	15,200	A	457
$C_{22}H_{31}O_2Cl$	4-Chloro-16α-methyl-4-pregnene-3,20-dione	254–256	13,900	A	539
	21-Chloro-16α-methyl-4-pregnene-3,20-dione	243	14,350	A	539
$C_{22}H_{31}O_2F$	21-Fluoro-16α-methyl-4-pregnene-3,20-dione	240	16,350	A	539
$C_{22}H_{31}O_2N$	16α-Cyano-20β-hydroxy-4-pregnen-3-one	240.5	16,500	M	525
	Acetate	240	17,200	M	525
$C_{22}H_{31}O_3F$	2ξ-Fluoro-11β,21-dihydroxy-6α-methyl-4,17(20)-*cis*-pregnadien-3-one	243			531
$C_{22}H_{31}O_5F$	2ξ-Fluoro-11β,17α,21-trihydroxy-6α-methyl-4-pregnene-3,20-dione				
	21-Acetate	242	13,280		531

TABLE XXXII—*continued*

Formula	Compound	λ_{max}	Ext.	Sol.	Ref.
4-en-3-Ones (cont.)					
$C_{22}H_{31}O_5F$	6α-Fluoro-11β,17α,21-trihydroxy-16α-methyl-4-pregnene-3,20-dione	237	14,800	A	513
	21-Acetate	236	14,700	A	513
		237	14,950		552
$C_{22}H_{31}O_6D$	17,20 : 20,21-Bismethylenedioxy-11α-deutero-11β-hydroxy-4-pregnen-3-one	242	12,000		465
$C_{22}H_{31}O_6F$	9α-Fluoro-11β,16α,17α,21-tetrahydroxy-2α-methyl-4-pregnene-3,20-dione	237–238	15,300	A	457
	16,21-Diacetate	237–238	16,300	A	457
$C_{22}H_{32}O_2$	17β-Hydroxy-2α-methyl-17α-vinyl-4-androsten-3-one	240	4.20	A	541
	4-Methyl-4-pregnene-3,20-dione	251	15,500	A	478
	7α-Methyl-4-pregnene-3,20-dione	242	16,900	A	480
	7β-Methyl-4-pregnene-3,20-dione	242	16,500	M	545
	16α-Methyl-4-pregnene-3,20-dione	241	14,400	A	506
	17a,17a-Dimethyl-D-homo-4-androsten-17-one	242		M	568
$C_{22}H_{32}O_3$	7β-Hydroxy-7α-methyl-4-pregnene-3,20-dione	244	15,700	M	545
	11β-Hydroxy-11α-methyl-4-pregnene-3,20-dione	245	13,400	A	497
	17α-Hydroxy-6α-methyl-4-pregnene-3,20-dione	242	15,200	A	469
		241	16,150	A	542
	Acetate	241	15,500	A	542
		239	4.19	A	453
	17α-Hydroxy-16α-methyl-4-pregnene-3,20-dione	242	16,600	A	506
	21-Hydroxy-16α-methyl-4-pregnene-3,20-dione				
	21-Acetate	240	16,155	A	539
	11β,21-Dihydroxy-7β-methyl-4,17(20)-*cis*-pregnadien-3-one				
	21-Acetate	244	15,825	A	480
	11β,21-Dihydroxy-11α-methyl-4,17(20)-*cis*-pregnadien-3-one				
	21-Acetate	244	16,075	A	497
$C_{22}H_{32}O_4$	17α,21-Dihydroxy-6α-methyl-4-pregnene-3,20-dione				
	21-Acetate	241	15,500	A	542
	Diacetate	241	16,600	A	542

R

TABLE XXXII—*continued*

Formula	Compound	λ_{max}	Ext.	Sol.	Ref.
4-en-3-Ones (cont.)					
$C_{22}H_{32}O_4$	16α-Carboxy-20β-hydroxy-4-pregnene-3-one				
	Acetate	241	16,400	M	525
	Methyl ester	241	15,700	M	525
$C_{22}H_{32}O_5$	11α,17α,21-Trihydroxy-6α-methyl-4-pregnene-3,20-dione	242	14,500		554
	11β,17α,21-Trihydroxy-6α-methyl-4-pregnene-3,20-dione				
	21-Acetate	242	14,800		498
	11β,17α,21-Trihydroxy-7β-methyl-4-pregnene-3,20-dione	244	4.22	A	579
		292–294	2.66	A	579
	21-Acetate	243	15,000	M	546
		245	16,425	A	480
		244	4.18	A	579
	11β,17α,21-Trihydroxy-11α-methyl-4-pregnene-3,20-dione				
	21-Acetate	243	16,350	A	497
$C_{22}H_{32}O_6$	11β,16α,17α,21-Tetrahydroxy-2α-methyl-4-pregnene-3,20-dione	240–241	16,600	A	457
	16,21-Diacetate	240–241	17,500	A	457
$C_{22}H_{32}O_7$	11β,16α,17α,21-Tetrahydroxy-9α-methoxy-4-pregnene-3,20-dione				
	16,21-Diacetate	243-244	15,800	A	459
$C_{22}H_{34}O_2$	17α-Ethyl-17β-hydroxy-2α-methyl-4-androsten-3-one	240	4.21	A	541
$C_{22}H_{23}O_3S$	21-Carboxy-17β-hydroxy-7α-thiol-17α-4-pregnen-3-one-21′ → 17-lactone				
	S-Propionyl	238	19,800	M	482
$C_{23}H_{30}O_8$	17,20 : 20,21-Bismethylenedioxy-1ξ,2ξ-dihydroxy-4-pregnene-3,11-dione	236	4.15	M	509
$C_{23}H_{31}O_2N$	16α-Cyanomethyl-4-pregnene-3,20-dione	240	16,300	M	525
$C_{23}H_{32}O_2$	17β-Hydroxy-6α-methyl-17α-prop-1′-ynyl-4-androsten-3-one	241	4.16	A	452
	17α-But-1′-ynyl-17β-hydroxy-4-androsten-3-one	240.5	4.2	A	452
$C_{23}H_{32}O_6$	20-Ethylenedioxy-16α,17α,21-trihydroxy-4,9(11)-pregnadien-3-one				
	16,21-Diacetate	239–240	16,700	A	457
$C_{23}H_{33}O_6F$	20-Ethylendioxy-2α-fluoro-11β,17α,21-trihydroxy-4-pregnen-3-one	242	14,000	M	517
$C_{23}H_{34}O_7$	9α-Ethoxy-11β,16α,17α,21-tetrahydroxy-4-pregnene-3,20-dione				
	16,21-Diacetate	243–244	15,300	A	459

TABLE XXXII—*continued*

Formula	Compound	λ_{max}	Ext.	Sol.	Ref.
4-en-3-Ones (cont.)					
$C_{23}H_{24}O_7$	20-Ethylenedioxy-11β,16α,17α,21-tetrahydroxy-4-pregnen-3-one				
	21-Acetate	241–242	14,400	A	457
$C_{24}H_{30}O_2N_2$	16α-Dicyanomethyl-4-pregnene-3,20-dione	240	16,300	M	525
$C_{24}H_{30}O_4Br_2$	2α,21-Dibromo-16α,17α-iso-propylidenedioxy-4,9(11)-pregnadiene-3,20-dione	240	15,500	M	449
$C_{24}H_{31}O_4Br$	2α-Bromo-16α,17α-iso-propylidenedioxy-4,9(11)-pregnadiene-3,20-dione	241	16,300	M	449
$C_{24}H_{32}O_2$	6α-Propargyl-4-pregnene-3,20-dione	240	4.17	A	476
		323	43	C	476
		338	41	C	476
		351	30	C	476
		369	10	C	476
$C_{24}H_{32}O_3$	17α-Hydroxy-6α-propargyl-4-pregnene-3,20-dione	240	4.17	A	476
	Acetate	239	4.18	A	476
$C_{24}H_{32}O_4$	16α,17α-iso-Propylidenedioxy-4,9(11)-pregnadiene-3,20-dione	238	18,300	M	449
		239	17,700	M	456
	16α,17α-iso-Propylidenedioxy-17β-methyl-D-homo-4,9(11)-androstadiene-3,17a-dione	238	17,100	M	456
$C_{24}H_{32}O_5$	9β,11β-Epoxy-16α,17α-iso-propylidenedioxy-4-pregnene-3,20-dione	242	15,600	M	456
$C_{24}H_{32}O_6$	17,20 : 20,21-Bismethylenedioxy-16α-methyl-4-pregnene-3,11-dione	238	15,200	M	513
$C_{24}H_{32}O_7$	17α,21-Dihydroxy-6α,7α-iso-propylidenedioxy-4-pregnene-3,11,20-trione				
	21-Acetate	240	4.11	A	578
$C_{24}H_{33}O_5Br$	9α-Bromo-11β-hydroxy-16α,17α-iso-propylidenedioxy-4-pregnene-3,20-dione	242	16,850	M	456
$C_{24}H_{33}O_5F$	6α-Fluoro-21-hydroxy-16α,17α-iso-propylidenedioxy-4-pregnene-3,20-dione				
	Acetate	236	4.19	A	528
	9α-Fluoro-11β-hydroxy-16α,17α-iso-propylidenedioxy-4-pregnene-3,20-dione	238	17,100	M	456

TABLE XXXII—*continued*

Formula	Compound	λ_{max}	Ext.	Sol.	Ref.
4-en-3-Ones (cont.)					
$C_{24}H_{33}O_6F$	17,20 : 20,21-Bismethylenedioxy-6α-fluoro-11β-hydroxy-16α-methyl-4-pregnen-3-one	237	14,850	A	513
	6α-Fluoro-11β,21-dihydroxy-16α,17α-iso-propylidenedioxy-4-pregnene-3,20-dione				
	21-Acetate	237	4.18	A	528
	9α-Fluoro-11β,21-dihydroxy-16α,17α-iso-propylidenedioxy-4-pregnene-3,20-dione	238–239	16,100	A	459
$C_{24}H_{34}O_2$	17α-But-1′-ynyl-17β-hydroxy-6α-methyl-4-androsten-3-one	241	4.16	A	452
	17β-Hydroxy-17α-pent-1′-ynyl-4-androsten-3-one	241	4.2	A	452
	20-Acetoxy-16α-methyl-4,17(20)-pregnadien-3-one	239	15,500	A	506
$C_{24}H_{34}O_5$	11α-Hydroxy-16α,17α-iso-propylidenedioxy-4-pregnene-3,20-dione	241	16,200	M	449
	Mesylate	238	17,100	M	449
$C_{24}H_{34}O_6$	11β,21-Dihydroxy-16α,17α-iso-propylidenedioxy-4-pregnene-3,20-dione	240	16,100	M	461
	17,20 : 20,21-Bismethylenedioxy-11β-hydroxy-6α-methyl-4-pregnen-3-one	242	13,700		498
$C_{25}H_{32}O_2$	17β-Hydroxy-4-phenyl-4-androsten-3-one	241	11,840	A	478
	Acetate	240	11,200	A	478
$C_{25}H_{36}O_2$	17β-Hydroxy-6α-methyl-17α-pent-1′-ynyl-4-androsten-3-one	240.5	4.13	A	452
	17α-Hex-1′-ynyl-17β-hydroxy-4-androsten-3-one	241	4.2	A	452
$C_{25}H_{36}O_6$	11β,21-Dihydroxy-16α,17α-iso-propylidenedioxy-6α-methyl-4-pregnene-3,20-dione	241	15,400	M	461
$C_{26}H_{35}O_4N$	16α-Carboethoxycyanomethyl-4-pregnene-3,20-dione	240	16,500	M	525
$C_{27}H_{34}O_2$	6α-Phenyl-4-pregnene-3,20-dione	244–246	4.11	A	580
	6β-Phenyl-4-pregnene-3,20-dione	242	4.14	A	580
$C_{27}H_{34}O_3$	17α-Hydroxy-6α-phenyl-4-pregnene-3,20-dione	244–246	4.18	A	580
$C_{29}H_{36}O_6$	20-Ethylenedioxy-17α,21-dihydroxy-6α-phenyl-4-pregnene-3,11-dione	236–238	4.19	A	580
$C_{29}H_{44}O_2$	17β-Hydroxy-17α-non-1′-ynyl-4-androsten-3-one	241	4.17	A	452
5-en-7-Ones					
$C_{19}H_{26}O_3$	3β-Hydroxy-5-androstene-7,17-dione	238	13,500	M	487

TABLE XXXII—*continued*

Formula	Compound	λ_{max}	Ext.	Sol.	Ref.
5-en-7-Ones (cont.)					
$C_{20}H_{30}O_3$	3β,17β-Dihydroxy-17α-methyl-5-androsten-7-one				
	3-Acetate, 17-trifluoroacetate	235	13,150	A	480
$C_{21}H_{30}O_3$	3β-Hydroxy-5-pregnene-7,20-dione				
	Acetate	235	13,450	M	486
$C_{25}H_{34}O_8$	3,20-Bisethylenedioxy-17α,21-dihydroxy-5-pregnene-7,11-dione				
	21-Acetate	238–240	4.03	A	579
		237	11,000	M	546
$C_{25}H_{36}O_7$	3,20-Bisethylenedioxy-17α,21-dihydroxy-5-pregnen-7-one				
	21-Acetate	240	13,000	A	455
8-en-11-Ones					
$C_{20}H_{28}O_4$	17α-Carboxy-3α-hydroxy-8-etiocholen-11-one				
	Acetate, methyl ester	187.5	3.64	C	562
		241	3.94	C	562
		327	1.32	C	562
		194	3.48	A	562
		248	3.93	A	562
		318	1.59	A	562
$C_{21}H_{28}O_3$	8-Pregnene-3,11,20-trione	253	8000	A	512
$C_{21}H_{32}O_3$	3α,20β-Dihydroxy-8-pregnen-11-one	254	8000	A	512
	Diacetate	254	8000	A	512
13(17)-en-20-Ones					
$C_{23}H_{30}O_3$	3-Ethylenedioxy-5,13(17)-pregnadien-20-one	256	4.05	A	450
14-en-16-Ones					
$C_{21}H_{26}O_5$	*d,l*-11β,18-Epoxy-3-ethylenedioxy-18-hydroxy-5,14-androstadien-16-one				
	Tetrahydropyranylate	234	16,300	A	507

TABLE XXXII—*continued*

Formula	Compound	λ_{max}	Ext.	Sol.	Ref.
14-en-16-Ones (cont.)					
$C_{21}H_{26}O_5$	*d,l*-11β,18-Epoxy-3-ethylenedioxy-18-hydroxy-5,14-pregnadiene-16,20-dione-21-oic acid	236	9800	A	507
		294	4600	A	507
	Tetrahydropyranylate, methyl ester	237	14,300	BA	507
		339	11,100	BA	507
	Tetrahydropyranylate, morpholine amide	249	12,500	A	507
		290(sh)	6100	A	507
		325	3400	A	507
15-en-17-Ones					
$C_{19}H_{28}O_2$	3β-Hydroxy-14β-15-androsten-17-one	230	7200		559
$C_{19}H_{28}O_3$	3β,14β-Dihydroxy-15-androsten-17-one				
	3-Acetate	213	13,500	A	559
16-en-20-Ones					
$C_{21}H_{28}O_3$	3β-Hydroxy-5,16-pregnadiene-11,20-dione				
	Acetate	234	3.93	M	548
	21-Hydroxy-9(11),16-pregnadiene-3,20-dione				
	Acetate	238–239	8050	A	460
$C_{21}H_{30}O_3$	1β,3β-Dihydroxy-5,16-pregnadien-20-one	240	9100	A	532
	3β,11α-Dihydroxy-5,16-pregnadien-20-one	238	8230	M	548
	11-Acetate	235	8180	M	548
	Diacetate	236–238	4.01	A	501
		234	8875	M	548
$C_{22}H_{32}O_3$	3α-Hydroxy-16-methyl-16-pregnene-11,20-dione	248	9300	M	556
	Acetate	248	9300	M	556
$C_{23}H_{28}O_7$	*d,l*-11β,18-Epoxy-3-ethylenedioxy-18-hydroxy-5,16-pregnadien-20-one-21-oic acid				
	Tetrahydropyranylate, methyl ester	252	6200	A	507
	Tetrahydropyranylate, morpholine amide	248	7300	A	507

TABLE XXXII—*continued*

Formula	Compound	λ_{max}	Ext.	Sol.	Ref.
D-Homo-Enones					
$C_{19}H_{26}O_2$	3β-Hydroxy-D-homo-5,13(17a)-androstadien-17-one				
	Acetate	244	4.23	A	508
$C_{20}H_{28}O_4$	3α,17-Dihydroxy-D-homo-16-etiocholene-11,17a-dione	267	16,200	M	575
	Diacetate	233	7500	A	575
$C_{21}H_{34}O_4$	3α,17-Dihydroxy-16-methyl-D-homo-16-etiocholene-11,17a-dione	273	8600	A	575
	Diacetate	239	10,850	A	575
$C_{22}H_{32}O_3$	3β,16-Dihydroxy-17a,17a-dimethyl-D-homo-5,15-androstadien-17-one				
	3-Acetate	272		M	568
	Diacetate	234		M	568
$C_{22}H_{34}O_2$	3β-Hydroxy-17a,17a-dimethyl-D-homo-15-androsten-17-one	233	6134	M	568
$C_{22}H_{34}O_3$	3β,16-Dihydroxy-17a,17a-dimethyl-D-homo-15-androsten-17-one				
	16-Acetate	271		M	568
$C_{44}H_{66}O_4Se_2$	16-Bis(3β-hydroxy-17a,17a-dimethyl-D-homo-15-androsten-17-one)				
	Diselenide	302	2040	M	568
	Diacetate	302	5183	M	568
Enones (misc.)					
$C_{20}H_{28}O_3$	3α-Hydroxy-16-methylene-etiocholane-11,17-dione				
	Acetate	228	8800	A	575
$C_{21}H_{30}O_2$	16-Acetyl-5,16-androstadien-3β-ol	240–242	4.16	A	547
	Acetate	240–242	4.07	A	547
$C_{21}H_{31}O_2N$	16-Acetyl-17-amino-5,16-androstadien-3β-ol	314	4.22	A	547
$C_{25}H_{30}O_9$	*d,l*-20-Acetoxy-11β,18-epoxy-3-ethylenedioxy-5,17(20)-pregnadien-16-one-21-oic acid				
	Tetrahydropyranylate, methyl ester	260	7200	A	507

TABLE XXXII—*continued*

Formula	Compound	λ_{max}	Ext.	Sol.	Ref.
Enones-Cumulative					
$C_{20}H_{24}O_4$	17β-Carboxy-4,9(11)-androstadiene-3,12-dione				
	Methyl ester	188	4.00	C	562
		232	4.42	C	562
		332(*ca.*)	1.98	C	562
		239.5	4.41	A	562
		318	2.07	A	562
$C_{20}H_{28}O$	17β-Hydroxy-2-hydroxymethylene-17α-methyl-19-nor-4-androsten-3-one	281	3.96	A	541
$C_{21}H_{24}O_2Br_2$	2α,21-Dibromo-4,9(11),16-pregnatriene-3,20-dione	242	24,200	M	550
$C_{21}H_{25}O_3Br$	2α-Bromo-21-hydroxy-4,9(11),16-pregnatriene-3,20-dione				
	Acetate	250	24,500	M	550
$C_{21}H_{25}O_4Br$	6ξ-Bromo-4,17(20)-*cis*-pregnadiene-3,11-dione-21-oic acid				
	Methyl ester	232	20,300	A	480
$C_{21}H_{26}O_2Br_2$	4,9(11),16-Pregnatriene-3,20-dione	238	26,100	M	456
$C_{21}H_{26}O_3F_3$	2α,21-Dibromo-11α-hydroxy-4,16-pregnadiene-3,20-dione	244	14,400	M	550
$C_{21}H_{27}O_3$	9α-Fluoro-11β-hydroxy-4,16-pregnadiene-3,20-dione	238	26,800	M	456
$C_{21}H_{28}O_3$	11α-Hydroxy-4,16-pregnadiene-3,20-dione	240	24,800	M	449
$C_{21}H_{28}O_4$	11α,21-Dihydroxy-4,16-pregnadiene-3,20-dione				
	11-Tosylate, 21-acetate	229	30,800	M	550
$C_{22}H_{28}O_4$	16α-Methyl-4,17(20)-*cis*-pregnadiene-3,11-dione-21-oic acid				
	Methyl ester	232.5	23,750		552
	16αMethyl-4,17(20)-*trans*-pregnadiene-3,11-dione-21-oic acid				
	Methyl ester	232.5	24,100		552
$C_{21}H_{29}O_2N$	16-Acetyl-17-amino-4,16-androstadien-3-one	238–240	4.22	A	547
	N-Benzoate	310	4.10	A	547
$C_{21}H_{30}O_3$	17β-Hydroxy-2-hydroxymethylene-17α-methyl-4-androsten-3-one	252	12,000	A	485
		307	6030	A	485
		251	4.07	A	541
		309	3.73	A	541
$C_{21}H_{30}O_4$	11β-Hydroxy-11α-methyl-4,17(20)-*cis*-pregnadien-3-one-21-oic acid				
	Methyl ester	238	23,100	A	497

TABLE XXXII—*continued*

Formula	Compound	λ_{max}	Ext.	Sol.	Ref.
Enones-Cumulative (cont.)					
$C_{22}H_{32}O_3$	20β-Hydroxy-2-hydroxymethylene-4-pregnen-3-one	251	10,000	A	574
$C_{25}H_{28}O_9$	*d,l*-Acetoxy-11β,18-epoxy-3-ethylenedioxy-18-hydroxy-5,15,17(20)-pregnatrien-16-one-21-oic acid				
	Tetrahydropyranylate, methyl ester	265	15,900	A	507
	Tetrahydropyranylate, morpholine amide	270	13,600	A	507
$C_{25}H_{29}O_5I$	21-Iodo-2ξ-ethoxyoxalyl-4,9(11),16-pregnatriene-3,20-dione	242	17,700	M	550
		228	21,600	BM	550
		340	7800	BM	550
		248	17,700	AcM	550
$C_{29}H_{34}O_8$	2ξ,21-Diethoxyoxalyl-4,9(11),16-pregnatriene-3,20-dione	242	16,900	M	550
		315	13,300	M	550
		249	20,000	BM	550
		315	10,400	BM	550
$C_{29}H_{36}O_9$	2ξ,21-Diethoxyoxalyl-11α-hydroxy-4,16-pregnadiene-3,20-dione	244	15,600	M	550
		313	12,900	M	550
		250	18,100	BM	550
		335	20,100	BM	550

TABLE XXXIII. CONJUGATED DIENONES

Formula	Compound	λ_{max}	Ext.	Sol.	Ref.
4,6-dien-3-Ones					
$C_{19}H_{24}O_2S$	1α-Thiol-4,6-androstadiene-3,17-dione				
	S-Acetyl	287	23,400	M	565
$C_{19}H_{26}O_2$	17β-Hydroxy-4,6-androstadien-3-one				
	Acetate	284	27,600	A	470
$C_{20}H_{27}O_2Br$	2α-Bromo-17β-hydroxy-4-methyl-4,6-androstadien-3-one				
	Acetate	294	4.26	A	489
$C_{20}H_{28}O_2$	17β-Hydroxy-7-methyl-4,6-androstadien-3-one	296–298	4.43	A	579
	Acetate	294–296	4.34	A	579
	17β-Hydroxy-17α-methyl-4,6-androstadien-3-one	283	25,990	A	485
		285	26,850	A	480
$C_{20}H_{28}O_3$	11β,17β-Dihydroxy-17α-methyl-4,6-androstadien-3-one	284	25,800	A	480
$C_{21}H_{24}O_4$	4,6,17(20)-*cis*-Pregnatriene-3,11-dione-21-oic acid				
	Methyl ester	282	26,500	A	480
$C_{21}H_{26}O_3$	4,6-Pregnadiene-3,11,20-trione	281	24,300	M	488
	21-Hydroxy-4,6,17(20)-*cis*-pregnatriene-3,11-dione				
	Acetate	286	26,350	A	480
	21-Carboxy-17β-hydroxy-19-nor-4,6-pregnadien-3-one-21′ → 17-lactone	283	27,000	M	482
$C_{21}H_{26}O_7$	1α,2α,17α,21-Tetrahydroxy-4,6-pregnadiene-3,11,20-trione				
	21-Acetate	280	4.32	A	578
$C_{21}H_{27}O_3Cl$	6-Chloro-17α-hydroxy-4,6-pregnadiene-3,20-dione				
	Acetate	285	4.36	A	540
$C_{21}H_{27}O_3F$	6-Fluoro-17α-hydroxy-4,6-pregnadiene-3,20-dione				
	Acetate	282–284	24,500	A	470
$C_{21}H_{27}O_4Cl$	6-Chloro-17α,21-dihydroxy-4,6-pregnadiene-3,20-dione				
	Diacetate	285	4.31	A	540
$C_{21}H_{28}O_3$	17α-Hydroxy-4,6-pregnadiene-3,20-dione				
	Propionate	284	27,000	M	488
	11β,21-Dihydroxy-4,6,17(20)-*cis*-pregnatrien-3-one	286	23,400	A	480

TABLE XXXIII—*continued*

Formula	Compound	λ_{max}	Ext.	Sol.	Ref.
4,6-dien-3-Ones (cont.)					
$C_{21}H_{28}O_4$	17α,21-Dihydroxy-4,6-pregnadiene-3,20-dione	283	26,400	A	455
	21-Acetate	283	29,000	A	455
	Diacetate	284	27,500	A	466
$C_{21}H_{30}O_2$	17β-Hydroxy-7,17α-dimethyl-4,6-androstadien-3-one	296.5	27,700	A	480
$C_{21}H_{30}O_3$	11β,17β-Dihydroxy-7,17α-dimethyl-4,6-androstadien-3-one	296	23,250	A	480
$C_{22}H_{28}O_3$	21-Carboxy-17β-hydroxy-4,6-pregnadien-3-one-21′ → 17-lactone	283	26,700	M	482
$C_{22}H_{28}O_5$	17α,21-Dihydroxy-7-methyl-4,6-pregnadiene-3,11,20-trione	294	4.45	A	579
	21-Acetate	292–294	4.41	A	579
		293	25,000	M	546
$C_{22}H_{29}O_3F$	21-Fluoro-17α-hydroxy-6-methyl-4,6-pregnadiene-3,20-dione				
	Acetate	288	23,300	M	558
$C_{22}H_{30}O_2$	7-Methyl-4,6-pregnadiene-3,20-dione	297	28,000	M	545
$C_{22}H_{30}O_3$	17α-Hydroxy-6-methyl-4,6-pregnadiene-3,20-dione				
	Acetate	289	24,000	A	542
$C_{22}H_{30}O_5$	11β,17α,21-Trihydroxy-7-methyl-4,6-pregnadiene-3,20-dione	296–298	4.48	A	579
$C_{22}H_{32}O_2$	20β-Hydroxy-7-methyl-4,6-pregnadien-3-one	297	28,000	M	545
$C_{23}H_{32}O_5$	20-Ethylenedioxy-17α,21-dihydroxy-4,6-pregnadien-3-one				
	21-Acetate	283–284	25,100	M	455
$C_{24}H_{31}O_5F$	9α-Fluoro-11β-hydroxy-16α,17α-iso-propylidenedioxy-4,6-pregnadiene-3,20-dione	281	23,800	M	456
4,6-dien-8-Ones					
$C_{20}H_{26}O_5$	17β-Carboxy-3β-hydroxy-8,14-*seco*-4,6-androstadiene-8,14-dione				
	Acetate, methyl ester	279	4.2	M	573

Dear Librarian:

This book has been supplied without Library of Congress Catalog Cards because they are presently unavailable and we did not want to delay shipment.

Bro-Dart Books, Inc.
P.O. Box 923
Williamsport, Pa.

TABLE XXXIV. CROSS-CONJUGATED DIENONES

Formula	Compound	λ_{max}	Ext.	Sol.	Ref.
1,4-dien-3-Ones					
$C_{18}H_{21}O_2Cl$	2,4,10β-Trichloro-17β-hydroxy-1,4-androstadien-3-one				
	Acetate	258	15,400	A	529
		300		BA	529
$C_{18}H_{22}O_3$	10ξ-Hydroxy-19-nor-1,4-androstadiene-3,17-dione	238	11,900	A	504
	Acetate	248	13,000	A	504
$C_{18}H_{23}O_2Cl$	10β-Chloro-17β-hydroxy-19-nor-1,4-androstadien-3-one				
	Acetate	248	16,000	A	529
$C_{18}H_{23}O_2F$	10β-Fluoro-17β-hydroxy-19-nor-1,4-androstadien-3-one	240	4.06	A	527
$C_{18}H_{24}O_3$	10ξ,17β-Dihydroxy-19-nor-1,4-androstadien-3-one	242	10,680	A	502
	10-Acetate	250	12,800	A	502
	17-Acetate	242	11,480	A	502
	Diacetate	249	13,400	A	502
$C_{19}H_{22}O_2$	1,4,9(11)-Androstatriene-3,17-dione	238	15,200	M	544
$C_{19}H_{22}O_2BrF$	9α-Bromo-11β-fluoro-1,4-androstadiene-3,17-dione	239	14,000	M	544
$C_{19}H_{22}O_2Cl_2$	9α,11β-Dichloro-1,4-androstadiene-3,17-dione	235	15,600	M	544
$C_{19}H_{26}O_3$	2,17β-Dihydroxy-1,4-androstadien-3-one	253		M	500
		284(sh)		M	500
	2,17-Diacetate	246		M	500
	17β,19-Dihydroxy-1,4-androstadien-3-one				
	Diacetate	243	13,700	A	494
$C_{20}H_{24}O_6$	17β-Carboxy-14β,19-dihydroxy-1,4-androstadiene-3,11-dione				
	Methyl ester	240	3.97	A	572
$C_{20}H_{25}O_2F$	10β-Fluoro-19-nor-1,4-pregnadiene-3,20-dione	241	4.04	A	527
$C_{21}H_{25}O_4BrCl_2$	6ξ-Bromo-9α,11β-dichloro-17α,21-dihydroxy-1,4-pregnadiene-3,20-dione				
	21-Acetate	243	14,000	M	544
$C_{21}H_{25}O_5F$	6β-Fluoro-17α,21-dihydroxy-1,4-pregnadiene-3,11,20-trione				
	21-Acetate	238	15,500	A	468
	Diacetate	236–238	15,100	A	468
$C_{21}H_{25}O_6Cl$	9β-Chloro-16α,17α,21-trihydroxy-1,4-pregnadiene-3,11,20-trione				
	16,21-Diacetate	237	15,800	M	459

TABLE XXXIV—*continued*

Formula	Compound	λ_{max}	Ext.	Sol.	Ref.
1,4-dien-3-Ones (cont.)					
$C_{21}H_{25}O_6F$	9α-Fluoro-16α,17α,21-trihydroxy-1,4,-pregnadiene-3,11,20-trione				
	16,21-Diacetate	235	17,000	A	459
$C_{21}H_{26}O_4$	17α.21-Dihydroxy-1,4,9(11)-pregnatriene-3,20-dione				
	21-Acetate	238	15,000	M	544
$C_{21}H_{26}O_4BrCl$	9α-Bromo-11β-chloro-17α,21-dihydroxy-1,4-pregnadiene-3,20-dione	240	13,500	M	544
	21-Acetate	239	14,500	M	544
$C_{21}H_{26}O_4BrF$	9α-Bromo-11β-fluoro-17α,21-dihydroxy-1,4-pregnadiene-3,20-dione	239	14,300	M	544
	21-Acetate	240	13,800	M	544
$C_{21}H_{26}O_4Br_2$	9α,11β-Dibromo-17α,21-dihydroxy-1,4-pregnadiene-3,20-dione				
	21-Acetate	240	14,100	M	544
$C_{21}H_{26}O_4Cl_2$	9α,11β-Dichloro-17α,21-dihydroxy-1,4-pregnadiene-3,20-dione	237	15,400	M	544
	21-Acetate	237	15,000	M	544
	21-Ethylcarbonate	237	14,800	M	544
	21-Hemisuccinate	237	14,600	M	544
$C_{21}H_{26}O_5$	16α,17α,21-Trihydroxy-1,4,9(11)-pregnatriene-3,20-dione				
	21-Acetate	238	16,400	M	550
	16,21-Diacetate	238	16,400	M	550
		238	15,800	M	459
$C_{21}H_{26}O_5F_2$	6α,9α-Difluoro-17α,21-dihydroxy-1,4-pregnadiene-3,20-dione				
	21-Acetate	238	15,100	A	468
$C_{21}H_{26}O_6$	16α,17α,21-Trihydroxy-1,4-pregnadiene-3,11,20-trione				
	16,21-Diacetate	238	14,700	M	459
	9β,11β-Epoxy-16α,17α,21-trihydroxy-1,4-pregnadiene-3,20-dione				
	16,21-Diacetate	247	16,200	M	459
$C_{21}H_{26}O_7$	6α,7α,17α,21-Tetrahydroxy-1,4-pregnadiene-3,11,20-trione				
	21-Acetate	238	4.11	A	578
$C_{21}H_{27}O_3Br$	6α-Bromo-17α-hydroxy-1,4-pregnadiene-3,20-dione				
	Acetate	244	4.15	A	540
	6β-Bromo-17α-hydroxy-1,4-pregnadiene-3,20-dione				
	Acetate	250	4.24		540

TABLE XXXIV—*continued*

Formula	Compound	λ_{max}	Ext.	Sol.	Ref.
1,4-dien-3-Ones (cont.)					
$C_{21}H_{27}O_3Cl$	6α-Chloro-17α-hydroxy-1,4-pregnadiene-3,20-dione				
	Acetate	242	4.21	A	540
$C_{21}H_{27}O_3F$	6α-Fluoro-17α-hydroxy-1,4-pregnadiene-3,20-dione				
	Acetate	240–242	15,900	A	470
$C_{21}H_{27}O_4F$	6α-Fluoro-17α,21-dihydroxy-1,4-pregnadiene-3,20-dione	240–242	16,600	M	471
	21-Acetate	240	16,000	A	471
	Diacetate	242	16,950	A	471
$C_{21}H_{27}O_5Br$	9α-Bromo-11β,17α,21-trihydroxy-1,4-pregnadiene-3,20-dione				
	11,21-Diacetate	240	14,000	M	543
	11-Formate, 21-acetate	239	13,800	M	543
	11-Trifluoroacetate, 21-acetate	240	13,900	M	543
	11-Diethylacetate	240	14,600	M	543
	11-Diethylacetate, 21-acetate	240	14,600	M	543
	Triacetate	241	14,300	M	543
$C_{21}H_{27}O_5Cl$	9α-Chloro-11β,16α,17α-trihydroxy-1,4-pregnadiene-3,20-dione	238	15,300	M	449
	9α-Chloro-11β,17α,21-trihydroxy-1,4-pregnadiene-3,20-dione				
	11,21-Diacetate	236	15,600	M	543
	11-Formate, 21-acetate	237	14,500	A	543
$C_{21}H_{27}O_5F$	6α-Fluoro-11β,17α,21-trihydroxy-1,4-pregnadiene-3,20-dione				
	21-Acetate	242	17,750	A	468
	9α-Fluoro-11β,16α,17α-trihydroxy-1,4-pregnadiene-3,20-dione	238	15,700	M	449
		238	15,100	M	456
	16-Acetate	239	16,200	M	456
	9α-Fluoro-11β,16α,17α-trihydroxy-17β-methyl-D-homo-1,4-androstadiene-3,17a-dione	238	14,800	M	449
$C_{21}H_{27}O_6Cl$	9α-Chloro-11β,16α,17α,21-tetrahydroxy-1,4-pregnadiene-3,20-dione	239	15,800	A	459
	16,21-Diacetate	239	14,600	M	459

TABLE XXXIV—*continued*

Formula	Compound	λ_{max}	Ext.	Sol.	Ref.
1,4-dien-3-Ones (cont.)					
$C_{21}H_{27}O_6F$	9α-Fluoro-11β,16α,17α,21-tetrahydroxy-1,4-pregnadiene-3,20-dione	239	15,224 ± 122	A	557
		238	15,800	A	459
		240	14,500	BA	557
		264(inf.)	7800	BA	557
		310	2270	BA	557
	16,21-Diacetate	239	15,270	A	557
		239	15,200	A	459
		240	13,800	BA	557
		265(inf.)	7150	BA	557
		310	2000	BA	557
	9α-Fluoro-11β,16β,17α,21-tetrahydroxy-1,4-pregnadiene-3,20-dione				
	16,21-Diacetate	238	13,000	A	458
$C_{21}H_{28}O_3$	17α-Hydroxy-1,4-pregnadiene-3,20-dione				
	Acetate	243	4.20		540
$C_{21}H_{28}O_5$	17α,20α,21-Trihydroxy-1,4-pregnadiene-3,11-dione	239	14,900	M	463
		239	15,400	M	481
	20,21-Diacetate	239	15,100	M	481
	17α,20β,21-Trihydroxy-1,4-pregnadiene-3,11-dione	238	15,300	M	481
$C_{21}H_{28}O_6$	11β,16α,17α,21-Tetrahydroxy-1,4-pregnadiene-3,20-dione	241–242	14,800	A	459
	16,21-Diacetate	242	14,200	A	459
$C_{22}H_{28}O_3$	21-Carboxy-17β-hydroxy-17α-1,4-pregnadien-3-one-21′ → 17-lactone	245	14,900	M	482
$C_{22}H_{28}O_4$	17α,21-Dihydroxy-16α-methyl-1,4,9(11)-pregnatriene-3,20-dione				
	21-Acetate	240	15,700	A	493
$C_{22}H_{28}O_5F_2$	6α,9α-Difluoro-17α,21-dihydroxy-16α-methyl-1,4-pregnadiene-3,20-dione				
	21-Acetate	237	4.16	A	492
		238	16,500		552
$C_{22}H_{28}O_6$	16α,17α,21-Trihydroxy-2-methyl-1,4-pregnadiene-3,11,20-trione				
	16,21-Diacetate	243	13,800	A	457
$C_{22}H_{29}O_6F$	9α-Fluoro-11β,16α,17α,21-tetrahydroxy-2-methyl-1,4-pregnadiene-3,20-dione	245	15,500	A	457

TABLE XXXIV—*continued*

Formula	Compound	λ_{max}	Ext.	Sol.	Ref.
1,4-dien-3-Ones (cont.)					
$C_{22}H_{30}O_3$	17α-Hydroxy-6α-methyl-1,4-pregnadiene-3,20-dione				
	Acetate	244	14,100	A	542
$C_{22}H_{30}O_5$	11β,17α,21-Trihydroxy-6α-methyl-1,4-pregnadiene-3,20-dione	244	14,500		498
	21-Acetate	243	14,685		498
$C_{22}H_{30}O_6$	11β,16α,17α,21-Tetrahydroxy-2-methyl-1,4-pregnadiene-3,20-dione				
	16,21-Diacetate	247	15,900	M	457
$C_{23}H_{28}O_7$	17,20 : 20,21-Bismethylenedioxy-2-hydroxy-1,4-pregnadiene-3,11-dione	252	4.05	M	509
	Sodium salt	315	3.69	M	509
$C_{23}H_{30}O_5$	17α,21-Dihydroxy-16,16-dimethyl-1,4-pregnadiene-3,11,20-trione				
	21-Acetate	238	14,200	M	510
$C_{24}H_{30}O_4$	16α,17α-iso-Propylidenedioxy-1,4,9(11)-pregnadiene-3,20-dione	238	15,600	M	449
$C_{24}H_{30}O_5$	9β,11β-Epoxy-16α,17α-iso-propylidenedioxy-1,4-pregnadiene-3,20-dione	247	15,700	M	449
$C_{24}H_{31}O_5Br$	9α-Bromo-11β-hydroxy-16α,17α-iso-propylidenedioxy-1,4-pregnadiene-3,20-dione	242	14,700	M	449
$C_{24}H_{31}O_5Cl$	9α-Chloro-11β-hydroxy-16α,17α-iso-propylidenedioxy-1,4-pregnadiene-3,20-dione	238	15,200	M	449
$C_{24}H_{31}O_5F$	9α-Fluoro-11β-hydroxy-16α,17α-iso-propylidenedioxy-1,4-pregnadiene-3,20-dione	238	15,500	M	449
		238	15,500	M	456
	9α-Fluoro-11β-hydroxy-16α,17α-iso-propylidenedioxy-17β-methyl-D-homo-1,4-androstadiene-3,17a-dione	237	16,100	M	449
$C_{24}H_{31}O_6F$	6α-Fluoro-11β,21-dihydroxy-16α,17α-iso-propylidenedioxy-1,4-pregnadiene-3,20-dione				
	21-Acetate	241	4.16	A	528
	9α-Fluoro-11β,21-dihydroxy-16α,17α-iso-propylidenedioxy-1,4-pregnadiene-3,20-dione	238–239	14,600	A	459
$C_{24}H_{32}O_6$	11β,21-Dihydroxy-16α,17α-iso-propylidenedioxy-1,4-pregnadiene-3,20-dione	242	15,800	M	461
	17,20 : 20,21-Bismethylenedioxy-11β-hydroxy-6α-methyl-1,4-pregnadien-3-one	244	13,550		498

TABLE XXXIV—*continued*

Formula	Compound	λ_{max}	Ext.	Sol.	Ref.
1,4-dien-3-Ones (cont.)					
$C_{25}H_{34}O_6$	11β,21-Dihydroxy-6α-methyl-16α,17α-iso-propylidenedioxy-1,4-pregnadiene-3,20-dione	241	15,500	M	461
	CUMULATIVE EFFECT				
$C_{21}H_{24}O_3$	21-Hydroxy-1,4,9(11),16-pregnatetraene-3,20-dione Acetate	238	24,000	M	550

TABLE XXXV. CROSS-CONJUGATED TRIENONES

Formula	Compound	λ_{max}	Ext.	Sol.	Ref.
1,4,6-trien-3-Ones					
$C_{20}H_{26}O_2$	17β-Hydroxy-2-methyl-1,4,6-androstatrien-3-one				
	Acetate	265.5	11,900	A	516
		300	10,320	A	516
	17β-Hydroxy-4-methyl-1,4,6-androstatrien-3-one				
	Acetate	226	4.10	A	489
		255(sh)	3.84	A	489
		306	4.04	A	489
$C_{21}H_{25}O_3Cl$	6-Chloro-17α-hydroxy-1,4,6-pregnatriene-3,20-dione				
	Acetate	229	4.00	A	540
		258	4.00	A	540
		297	4.03	A	540
$C_{21}H_{25}O_3F$	6-Fluoro-17α-hydroxy-1,4,6-pregnatriene-3,20-dione				
	Acetate	225	10,580	A	470
		254	10,000	A	470
		298	10,230	A	470
$C_{21}H_{25}O_4Cl$	6-Chloro-17α,21-dihydroxy-1,4,6-pregnatriene-3,20-dione				
	Diacetate	228	4.00	A	540
		260	4.03	A	540
		295	4.07	A	540
$C_{22}H_{26}O_3$	21-Carboxy-17β-hydroxy-17α-1,4,6-pregnatrien-3-one-lactone	222	11,100	M	482
		266	10,700	M	482
		296	13,700	M	482
$C_{22}H_{28}O_3$	17α-Hydroxy-6-methyl-1,4,6-pregnatriene-3,20-dione				
	Acetate	228	13,500	A	542
		253	9102	A	542
		304	11,700	A	542

TABLE XXXVI. AROMATIC RING A

Formula	Compound	λ_{max}	Ext.	Sol.	Ref.
$C_{18}H_{22}O_6N_2$	2,4-Dinitro-1,3,5(10)-estratriene-3,17β-diol	277	6490	A	538
		352	3430	A	538
		430	1040	A	538
$C_{18}H_{23}ON$	3-Amino-1,3,5(10)-estratrien-17-one	238	9100	M	499
	N-Acetyl	247	15,500	M	499
		289	1100	M	499
$C_{18}H_{23}O_2N$	2-Amino-3-hydroxy-1,3,5(10)-estratrien-17-one	297	4190	A	518
	4-Amino-3-hydroxy-1,3,5(10)-estratrien-17-one	289	2710	A	518
$C_{18}H_{23}O_4N$	2-Nitro-1,3,5(10)-estratriene-3,17β-diol	293	8100	A	538
		364–366	3690	A	538
	4-Nitro-1,3,5(10)-estratriene-3,17β-diol	278	1810	A	538
$C_{18}H_{24}O_2$	1,3,5(10)-Estratriene-3,17β-diol				
	17-Heptanoate	281	2000	A	577
$C_{18}H_{24}O_3$	1,3,5(10)-Estratriene-2,3,17β-triol	288	4042	M	451
	17-Acetate	288	4213	M	451
	1,3,5(10)-Estratriene-3,6α,17β-triol	282	2350	A	576
		287	2130	A	576
	17-Acetate	282	2150	A	576
		287	1980	A	576
	Triacetate	268	730	A	576
		275	670	A	576
	1,3,5(10)-Estratriene-3,6β,17β-triol				
	Triacetate	268		A	576
$C_{18}H_{25}ON$	3-Amino-1,3,5(10)-estratrien-17β-ol	275		A	576
		237	7900	M	499
		238	8600	A	503
		291–292	1712	A	503
		266	621	AcA	503
		274	638	AcA	503
	Acetate	239	9200	A	503
		292	1810	A	503

TABLE XXXVI—*continued*

Formula	Compound	λ_{max}	Ext.	Sol.	Ref.
Aromatic Ring A (cont.)					
		266	688	AcA	503
		274	688	AcA	503
	Acetate, N-acetyl	249	15,000	M	499
		209	28,800	A	503
		248	16,200	A	503
$C_{19}H_{22}O_2$	3-Hydroxy-16-methylene-1,3,5(10)-estratrien-17-one	224	4.15	A	515
		284–286	3.28	A	515
$C_{19}H_{23}O_4N$	2-Nitro-3-methoxy-1,3,5(10)-estratrien-17-one	272.5	4510	A	518
		336	3130	A	518
	4-Nitro-3-methoxy-1,3,5(10)-estratrien-17-one	275.5	1570	A	518
		250–257	1220	A	518
$C_{19}H_{24}O_2$	1-Hydroxy-4-methyl-1,3,5(10)-estratrien-17-one	281–286	2250	M	484
	3-Hydroxy-2-methyl-1,3,5(10)-estratrien-17-one	283	2660	A	537
	3-Hydroxy-6β-methyl-1,3,5(10)-estratrien-17-one	281	3.32	A	569
	3-Hydroxy-16β-methyl-1,3,5(10)-estratrien-17-one	284–286	3.19	A	515
$C_{19}H_{24}O_3$	3-Hydroxy-2-hydroxymethyl-1,3,5(10)-estratrien-17-one				
	2′,3-Diacetate	269	872	A	537
		278	872	A	537
	2-Hydroxy-3-methoxy-1,3,5(10)-estratrien-17-one	287.5	4200	A	518
	3-Hydroxy-4-methoxy-1,3,5(10)-estratrien-17-one	278	1820	A	518
	4-Hydroxy-3-methoxy-1,3,5(10)-estratrien-17-one	277–283	2110	A	518
	3,7α-Dihydroxy-6β-methyl-estratrien-17-one	280	3.41	A	569
$C_{19}H_{25}O_2Cl$	2-Chloro-1-methyl-1,3,5(10)-estratriene-1,17β-diol	274	554	A	516
	Dipropionate	282	550	A	516
	2-Chloro-4-methyl-1,3,5(10)-estratriene-1,17β-diol				
	Dipropionate	274	485	A	516
	4-Chloro-1-methyl-1,3,5(10)-estratriene-3,17β-diol				
	Dipropionate	285(inf.)	1875	A	516
		290	1940	A	516
$C_{19}H_{25}O_2N$	2-Amino-3-methoxy-1,3,5(10)-estratrien-17-one	239	6980	A	518
		295.5	4480	A	518

TABLE XXXVI—*continued*

Formula	Compound	λ_{max}	Ext.	Sol.	Ref.
Aromatic Ring A (cont.)					
$C_{19}H_{26}O_2$	2-Methyl-1,3,5(10)-estratriene-3,17β-diol	283	2680	A	537
	6β-Methyl-1,3,5(10)-estratriene-3,17β-diol	281	3.29	A	569
	16β-Methyl-1,3,5(10)-estratriene-3,17β-diol	286	3.13	A	515
$C_{19}H_{29}O_2N$	4-Amino-3-methoxy-1,3,5(10)-estratrien-17-one	287.5	2820	A	518
$C_{20}H_{24}O_2$	3-Methoxy-16-methylene-1,3,5(10)-estratrien-17-one	224–226	4.15	A	515
		278	3.32	A	515
		286	3.27	A	515
$C_{20}H_{26}O_2$	3-Methoxy-16β-methyl-1,3,5(10)-estratrien-17-one	278	3.31	A	515
		286	3.27	A	515
$C_{20}H_{28}O_2$	3-Methoxy-16β-methyl-1,3,5(10)-estratrien-17β-ol	278	3.27	A	515
		286	3.23	A	515
	1,2-Dimethyl-1,3,5(10)-estratriene-3,17β-diol				
	Diacetate	272	540	A	516
		280	530	A	516
$C_{21}H_{28}O_4$	17-Ethylenedioxy-6β-methyl-1,3,5(10)-estratriene-3,7α-diol	280	3.32	A	569
$C_{21}H_{29}O_2N$	3-Hydroxy-2-dimethylaminomethyl-1,3,5(10)-estratrien-17-one	286	2530	A	537
	3-Hydroxy-16ξ-dimethylaminomethyl-1,3,5(10)-estratrien-17-one	284–286	3.36	A	515
$C_{23}H_{33}O_2N$	2-Diethylaminomethyl-3-hydroxy-1,3,5(10)-estratrien-17-one	286	2800	A	537
$C_{24}H_{33}O_2N$	3-Hydroxy-2-piperidinomethyl-1,3,5(10)-estratrien-17-one	286	2850	A	537
$C_{24}H_{35}O_2N$	2-Piperidinomethyl-1,3,5(10)-estratriene-3,17β-diol	286	2620	A	537

TABLE XXXVII. CONJUGATED AROMATIC RING A

Formula	Compound	λ_{max}	Ext.	Sol.	Ref.
$C_{19}H_{22}O_2$	3-Hydroxy-6-methyl-1,3,5(10),6-estratetraen-17-one	222	4.37	A	569
		262	3.83	A	569
		305	3.42	A	569
$C_{19}H_{25}O_2Cl$	2-Chloro-1-methyl-1,3,5(10),6-estratetraene-3,17β-diol Dipropionate	226	29,450	A	516
		232	25,450	A	516
		271	12,700	A	516
	4-Chloro-1-methyl-1,3,5(10),6-estratetraene-3,17β-diol Dipropionate	227	30,800	A	516
		269.5	9900	A	516
$C_{19}H_{26}O_2$	6-Methyl-1,3,5(10),6-estratetraene-3,17β-diol	221	4.35	A	569
		262	3.86	A	569
		304	3.45	A	569
$C_{20}H_{28}O_2$	1,2-Dimethyl-1,3,5(10),6-estratetraene-3,17β-diol Diacetate	225	27,950	A	516
		232(inf.)	22,000	A	516
		268	11,500	A	516

TABLE XXXVIII. STEROIDS CONTAINING AROMATIC CHROMOPHORES

Formula	Compound	λ_{max}	Ext.	Sol.	Ref.
$C_{27}H_{36}O_3$	5α-Hydroxy-6β-phenyl-pregnane-3,20-dione	254	2.34	A	580
		260	2.38	A	580
$C_{27}H_{36}O_4$	5α,17α-Dihydroxy-6β-phenyl-pregnane-3,20-dione	254	2.31	A	580
		260	2.38	A	580
		266	2.29	A	580
$C_{29}H_{38}O_7$	20-Ethylenedioxy-5α,17α,21-trihydroxy-6β-phenyl-pregnane-3,11-dione	254	2.28	A	580
		260	2.33	A	580
$C_{31}H_{42}O_8$	3,20-Bisethylenedioxy-5α,17α,21-trihydroxy-6β-phenyl-pregnan-11-one	254	2.28	A	580
		260	2.34	A	580
		266	2.22	A	580
$C_{31}H_{44}O_5$	3,20-Bisethylenedioxy-6β-phenyl-pregnan-5α-ol	254	2.24	A	580
		260	2.31	A	580
$C_{31}H_{44}O_6$	3,20-Bisethylenedioxy-6β-phenyl-pregnane-5α,17α-diol	254	2.26	A	580
		260	2.32	A	580
		266	2.17	A	580
	CHROMOPHORIC ESTERS				
$C_{20}H_{32}O_2$	17β-Hydroxy-2α-methyl-androstan-3-one β-Phenylpropionate	254	2.33	A	541
		258	2.38	A	541
$C_{22}H_{38}O_3$	6α-Hydroxymethyl-pregnane-3β,20β-diol 3,20-Diacetate,6′-tosylate	225	12,000	M	533

TABLE XXXIX. STEROIDS CONTAINING C=N DERIVATIVES

Formula	Compound	λ_{max}	Ext.	Sol.	Ref.
2,4-Dinitrophenylhydrazones					
$C_{27}H_{31}O_9FN_4$	9α-Fluoro-11β,16α,17α,21-tetrahydroxy-1,4-pregnadiene-3,20-dione-3-(2,4-dinitrophenylhydrazone)				
	16,21-Diacetate	259	16,100	Ch	459
		305	6600	Ch	459
		398–400	32,400	Ch	459
$C_{27}H_{32}O_9N_4$	11β,16α,17α,21-Tetrahydroxy-1,4-pregnadiene-3,20-dione-3-(2,4-dinitrophenylhydrazone)				
	16,21-Diacetate	258	18,000	A	459
		291	8920	A	459
		393	32,400	A	459
$C_{27}H_{33}O_9FN_4$	9α-Fluoro-11β,16α,17α,21-tetrahydroxy-4-pregnene-3,20-dione-3-(2,4-dinitrophenylhydrazone)				
	16,21-Diacetate	261	16,200	Ch	459
		292	11,100	Ch	459
		391	29,800	Ch	459
$C_{27}H_{34}O_9F_4$	11β,16α,17α,21-Tetrahydroxy-4-pregnene-3,20-dione-3-(2,4-dinitrophenylhydrazone)				
	16,21-Diacetate	258	17,600	Ch	459
		292	10,300	Ch	459
		386	28,600	Ch	459
Semicarbazones					
$C_{25}H_{33}O_4N_3$	16α,17α-iso-Propylidenedioxy-1,4,9(11)-pregnatriene-3,20-dione-3-semicarbazone	241	10,300	M	449
		298	25,800	M	449
$C_{25}H_{35}O_4N_3$	16α,17α-iso-Propylidenedioxy-4,9(11)-pregnadiene-3,20-dione-3-semicarbazone	269	33,700	M	449

TABLE XL. α,β-UNSATURATED ACIDS AND ESTERS

Formula	Compound	λ_{max}	Ext.	Sol.	Ref.
$C_{19}H_{28}O_5$	2,3-Dicarboxy-2,3-*seco*-4-androsten-17β-ol				
	Dimethyl ester	222	14,200	A	574
$C_{20}H_{28}O_4$	17β-Carboxy-3β-hydroxy-14β-methyl-18-nor-13(17)-etiocholen-15-one				
	Methyl ester	231	3.98	A	520
	Methyl ester, oxime	236	4.00	A	520
$C_{21}H_{24}O_4$	21-Carboxy-4,6,17(20)-pregnatriene-3,11-dione				
	Methyl ester	224	12,650	A	480
$C_{22}H_{31}O_4F$	21-Carboxy-6β-fluoro-5α-hydroxy-6α-methyl-17(20)-*trans*-pregnen-3-one				
	Methyl ester	224	13,850		552
$C_{23}H_{32}O_5$	21-Carboxy-3-ethylenedioxy-16α-methyl-5,17(20)-*trans*-pregnen-11-one				
	Methyl ester	225	13,850		552
$C_{30}H_{40}O_9$	*d,l*-20-Acetoxy-11β,18-epoxy-3-ethylenedioxy-18-tetrahydropyranyloxy-5,17(20)-pregnadien-21-oic acid				
	Methyl ester	228	12,500	A	507
$C_{30}H_{40}O_{12}$	*d,l*-20-Acetoxy-11β,18-epoxy-3-ethylenedioxy-15ξ-hydroxy-18-tetrahydropyranyloxy-5,17(20)-pregnadien-21-oic acid				
	Morpholine amide	221	11,900	A	507

TABLE XLI. UNSATURATED NITRILES

Formula	Compound	λ_{max}	Ext.	Sol.	Ref.
Mono-enes					
$C_{21}H_{27}O_2N$	17-Cyano-3-ethylenedioxy-18-nor-5,13(17)-androstadiene	227	4.16	A	450
$C_{22}H_{31}O_2N$	6-Cyano-3β-hydroxy-5-pregnen-20-one	220–222	10,000	A	467
$C_{22}H_{31}O_3N$	6-Cyano-3-ethylenedioxy-5-androsten-17β-ol	224	13,180	A	467
$C_{26}H_{33}O_7N$	17,20:20,21-Bismethylenedioxy-6-cyano-3-ethylenedioxy-5-pregnen-11-one	224	10,075	A	467
$C_{26}H_{35}O_7N$	6-Cyano-3,20-bisethylenedioxy-17α,21-dihydroxy-5-pregnen-11-one	224	11,000	A	467
$C_{26}H_{37}O_4N$	6-Cyano-3,20-bisethylenedioxy-5-pregnene	224	9590	A	467
$C_{26}H_{37}O_5N$	6-Cyano-3,20-bisethylenedioxy-5-pregnen-17α-ol	224	10,200	A	467
Dienes					
$C_{22}H_{29}ON$	6-Cyano-3,5-pregnadien-20-one	260	20,890	A	467
$C_{22}H_{29}O_3N$	3-Acetoxy-6-cyano-3,5-androstadien-17β-ol Acetate	262–264	17,400	A	467
$C_{22}H_{31}O_3N$	6-Cyano-3-(2′-hydroxyethoxy)-3,5-androstadien-17β-ol	284	18,620	A	467
$C_{24}H_{31}O_3N$	3-Acetoxy-6-cyano-3,5-pregnadien-20-one	264	18,200	A	467
$C_{24}H_{31}O_4N$	3-Acetoxy-6-cyano-17α-hydroxy-3,5-pregnadien-20-one Acetate	262–264	18,620	A	467
$C_{24}H_{33}O_3N$	6-Cyano-17α-hydroxy-3-(2′-hydroxyethoxy)-3,5-pregnadien-20-one	282–284	19,500	A	467
$C_{26}H_{33}O_7N$	17,20 : 20,21-Bismethylenedioxy-6-cyano-3-(2′-hydroxyethoxy)-3,5-pregnadien-11-one	284-288	18,200	A	467
$C_{26}H_{35}O_7N$	6-Cyano-20-ethylenedioxy-17α,21-dihydroxy-3-(2′-hydroxyethoxy)-3,5-pregnadien-11-one	284–286	17,800	A	467
$C_{26}H_{37}O_4N$	6-Cyano-20-ethylenedioxy-3-(2′-hydroxyethoxy)-3,5-pregnadiene	282–284	23,990	A	467
$C_{26}H_{37}O_5N$	6-Cyano-20-ethylenedioxy-3-(2′-hydroxyethoxy)-3,5-pregnadien-17α-ol	282–284	19,500	A	467

TABLE XLII. β-DIKETONES AND β-KETOESTERS

Formula	Compound	λ_{max}	Ext.	Sol.	Ref.
$C_{20}H_{30}O_3$	17β-Hydroxy-2-hydroxymethylene-androstan-3-one	282	10,300	A	485
		282	3.94	A	491
		275	11,200	A	574
$C_{21}H_{30}O_3$	17β-Hydroxy-2-hydroxymethylene-4,4-dimethyl-19-nor-5-androsten-3-one	288–292	3.82	A	472
$C_{21}H_{32}O_3$	17β-Hydroxy-2-hydroxymethylene-17α-methyl-androstan-3-one	285	3.99	A	541
	2′-Acetate	255	4.09	A	541
	2′-Propionate	257	4.11	A	541
	2′-Benzoate	252	4.06	A	541
		305	3.75	A	541
$C_{23}H_{36}O_5$	17β-Hydroxy-4-hydroxymethylene-2,2,17α-trimethyl-androstan-3-one	294–296	3.78	A	472
$C_{25}H_{36}O_5$	3β-Hydroxy-21-methoxyoxalyl-16α-methyl-5-pregnen-20-one	293	10,250	A	506
	Acetate	291	9700	A	506
$C_{25}H_{38}O_5$	3β,11α-Dihydroxy-21-methoxyoxalyl-16α-methyl-5α-pregnan-20-one Diacetate	294	10,800	A	506
$C_{26}H_{36}O_8$	11β-Hydroxy-2ξ,21-dimethoxyoxalyl-11α-methyl-4-pregnene-3,20-dione	289	14,400	A	497
$C_{28}H_{36}O_7$	16α,17α-iso-Propylidenedioxy-2ξ-methoxyoxalyl-4,9(11)-pregnadiene-3,20-dione	242	14,200	M	449
		244	14,500	AcM	449
		320	2230	AcM	449
		244	14,500	BM	449
		352	11,000	BM	449
$C_{32}H_{40}O_{10}$	16α,17α-iso-Propylidenedioxy-2ξ,21-dimethoxyoxalyl-4,9(11)-pregnadiene-3,20-dione	244	13,000	M	449
		330	4390	M	449
		244	13,000	AcM	449
		320	2400	AcM	449
		244	14,500	BM	449
		350	11,100	BM	449

TABLE XLIII. MISCELLANEOUS COMPOUNDS

Formula	Compound	λ_{max}	Ext.	Sol.	Ref.
$C_{17}H_{23}O_2N$	4-Aza-1,3,5(10)-estratriene-3,17β-diol				
	17-Acetate	226	6460	M	567
		289	6220	M	567
$C_{18}H_{27}O_2N$	17β-Hydroxy-4-aza-5-androsten-3-one	233	13,790	M	567
	Acetate	233	13,630	M	567
$C_{19}H_{26}O_2S_2$	1α,5α-Epidithio-androstane-3,17-dione	268	240	M	566
$C_{19}H_{28}O_2S$	1α-Thiol-androstane-3,17-diol				
	S-Acetyl	232	4350	M	488
$C_{19}H_{29}O_4N$	6β-Nitro-4-androstene-3β,17β-diol	280–286	115	A	474
	6-Nitro-5-androstene-3β,17β-diol	264–266	2,140	A	474
	Diacetate	260	1,820	A	474
$C_{19}H_{30}OS$	3β-Thiol-androstan-17-one				
	S-Acetyl	233	4020	A	564
	3α-Thiol-androstan-17-one				
	S-Acetyl	233	3800	A	564
$C_{19}H_{32}O_2S_2$	1α,5α-Dithiol-androstane-3α,17β-diol				
	S,S-Diacetyl, diacetate	238	9750	M	566
$C_{20}H_{29}O_2N$	4-Aza-5-pregnene-3,20-dione	233	13,430	M	567
$C_{21}H_{28}ON_2$	17β-Hydroxy-17α-methyl-androsta-4,6-dieno[3,2-c]pyrazole	226	9190	A	485
		232	8240	A	485
		297	24,330	A	485
		308	18,350	A	485
	N-Acetyl	237	7100	A	485
		255	4900	A	485
		289	24,200	A	485
$C_{21}H_{31}O_4N$	3β-Hydroxy-6-nitro-5-pregnen-20-one	262–264	1905	A	474
	Acetate	258–260	1950	A	474
$C_{21}H_{32}ON_2$	17β-Hydroxy-17α-methyl-androstano[3,2-c]pyrazole	223	4740	A	485
	N-Acetyl	258	19,000	A	485
$C_{22}H_{30}O_3$	3α,20ξ-Dihydroxy-16′,20ξ-epoxy-16-methyl-16-pregnen-11-one				
	3-Acetate	222	6000	M	556

V. REFERENCES

[1] ACKROYD, M., ADAMS, W. J., ELLIS, B., PETROW, V. and STUART-WEBB, I. A., *J. Chem. Soc.* 4099 (1957).
[2] ADAMS, W. J., KIRK, D. N., PATEL, D. K., PETROW, V. and STUART-WEBB, I. A., *J. Chem. Soc.* 870 (1955).
[3] ADAMS, W. J., PATEL, D. K., PETROW, V. and STUART-WEBB, I. A., *J. Chem. Soc.* 1825 (1954).
[4] ADAMS, W. J., PATEL, D. K. and PETROW, V., *J. Chem. Soc.* 4688 (1954).
[5] ADAMS, W. J., PATEL, D. K., PETROW, V. and STUART-WEBB, I. A., *J. Chem. Soc.* 297 (1956).
[6] ADAMS, W. J., PATEL, D. K., PETROW, V., STUART-WEBB, I. A. and STURGEON, B., *J. Chem. Soc.* 4490 (1956).
[7] AGNELLO, E. J., BLOOM, B. L. and LAUBACH, G. D., *J. Amer. Chem. Soc.* **77**, 4684 (1955).
[8] AGNELLO, E. J. and LAUBACH, G. D., *J. Amer. Chem. Soc.* **79**, 1257 (1957).
[9] ALLEN, W. S. and BERNSTEIN, S., *J. Amer. Chem. Soc.* **77**, 1028 (1955).
[10] ALLEN, W. S. and BERNSTEIN, S., *J. Amer. Chem. Soc.* **78**, 1909 (1956).
[11] ALLEN, W. S. and BERNSTEIN, S., *J. Amer. Chem. Soc.* **78**, 3223 (1956).
[12] ALLEN, W. S., BERNSTEIN, S., HELLER, M. and LITTELL, R., *J. Amer. Chem. Soc.* **77**, 4784 (1955).
[13] AMENDOLLA, C., ROSENKRANZ, G. and SONDHEIMER, F., *J. Chem. Soc.* 1226 (1954).
[14] ANTONUCCI, R., BERNSTEIN, S., HELLER, M., LENHARD, R. H., LITTELL, R. and WILLIAMS, J. H., *J. Org. Chem.* **18**, 70 (1953).
[15] ANTONUCCI, R., BERNSTEIN, S. and LENHARD, R. H., *J. Amer. Chem. Soc.* **76**, 2956 (1954).
[16] ANTONUCCI, R., BERNSTEIN, S., LENHARD, R. H., SAX, K. J. and WILLIAMS, J. H., *J. Org. Chem.* **17**, 1369 (1952).
[17] ANTONUCCI, R., BERNSTEIN, S., LITTELL, R., SAX, K. J. and WILLIAMS, J. H., *J. Org. Chem.* **17**, 1341 (1952).
[18] ARTH, G. E., FRIED, J., JOHNSTON, D. B. R., HOFF, D. R., SARETT, L. H., SILBER, R. H., STOERK, H. C. and WINTER, C. A., *J. Amer. Chem. Soc.* **80**, 3161 (1958).
[19] ARTH, G. E., JOHNSTON, D. B. R., FRIED, J., SPOONCER, W. W., HOFF, D. R. and SARETT, L. H., *J. Amer. Chem. Soc.* **80**, 3160 (1958).
[20] ARTH, G. E., POOS, G. I. and SARETT, L. H., *J. Amer. Chem. Soc.* **77**, 3834 (1955).
[21] ATWATER, N. W., *J. Amer. Chem. Soc.* **79**, 5315 (1957).
[22] BABCOCK, J. C., GUTSELL, E. S., HERR, M. E., HOGG, J. A., STUCKI, J. C., BARNES, L. E. and DULIN, W. E., *J. Amer. Chem. Soc.* **80**, 2904 (1958).
[23] BALANT, C. P. and EHRENSTEIN, M., *J. Org. Chem.* **17**, 1587 (1952).
[24] BARAN, J. S., *J. Amer. Chem. Soc.* **80**, 1687 (1958).
[25] BARBER, G. W. and EHRENSTEIN, M., *J. Org. Chem.* **19**, 365 (1954).
[26] BARBER, G. W. and EHRENSTEIN, M., *J. Org. Chem.* **19**, 1758 (1954).
[27] BARBER, G. W. and EHRENSTEIN, M., *J. Amer. Chem. Soc.* **76**, 2026 (1954).
[28] BARBER, G. W. and EHRENSTEIN, M., *J. Org. Chem.* **20**, 1253 (1955).
[29] BARBER, G. W. and EHRENSTEIN, M., *Liebigs Ann.* **603**, 89 (1957).
[30] BARTON, D. H. R., CAMPOS-NEVES, A. DA S. and SCOTT, A. I., *J. Chem. Soc.* 2698 (1957).
[31] BARTON, D. H. R., EVANS, R. M., HAMLET, J. C., JONES, P. G. and WALKER, T., *J. Chem. Soc.* 747 (1954).
[32] BARTON, D. H. R. and TAYLOR, W. C., *Proc. Chem. Soc.* 147 (1957).
[33] BARTON, S. P., COOLEY, G., ELLIS, B. and PETROW, V., *J. Chem. Soc.* 5094 (1957).
[34] BATRES, E., GOMEZ, R., ROSENKRANZ, G. and SONDHEIMER, F., *J. Org. Chem.* **21**, 240 (1956).
[35] BATRES, E., ROSENKRANZ, G. and SONDHEIMER, F., *J. Amer. Chem. Soc.* **76**, 5171 (1954).
[36] BATRES, E., ROSENKRANZ, G. and SONDHEIMER, F., *J. Amer. Chem. Soc.* **77**, 4155 (1955).
[37] BERNSTEIN, S., ALLEN, W. S., LINDEN, C. E. and CLEMENTE, J., *J. Amer. Chem. Soc.* **77**, 6612 (1955).
[38] BERNSTEIN, S., FELDMAN, L. I., ALLEN, W. S., BLANK, R. H. and LINDEN, C. E., *Chem. & Ind.* 111 (1956).
[39] BERNSTEIN, S., HELLER, M., LITTELL, R., STOLAR, S. M., LENHARD, R. H. and ALLEN, W. S., *J. Amer. Chem. Soc.* **79**, 4555 (1957).
[40] BERNSTEIN, S., HELLER, M. and STOLAR, S. M., *J. Amer. Chem. Soc.* **76**, 5674 (1954).
[41] BERNSTEIN, S., HELLER, M. and STOLAR, S. M., *J. Amer. Chem. Soc.* **77**, 5327 (1955).
[42] BERNSTEIN, S., HELLER, M. and WILLIAMS, J. H., *J. Amer. Chem. Soc.* **75**, 1480 (1953).
[43] BERNSTEIN, S., LENHARD, R. H. and WILLIAMS, J. H., *J. Org. Chem.* **18**, 1166 (1953).
[44] BERNSTEIN, S., LENHARD, R. H. and WILLIAMS, J. H., *J. Org. Chem.* **19**, 41 (1954).
[45] BERNSTEIN, S., LITTELL, R. and WILLIAMS, J. H., *J. Amer. Chem. Soc.* **75**, 1481 (1953).
[46] BERNSTEIN, S., LITTELL, R. and WILLIAMS, J. H., *J. Amer. Chem. Soc.* **75**, 4830 (1953).
[47] BEYLER, R. E. and HOFFMAN, F., *J. Org. Chem.* **21**, 572 (1956).
[48] BEYLER, R. E. and HOFFMAN, F., *J. Amer. Chem. Soc.* **79**, 5297 (1957).
[49] BHIDE, G. V., PAI, N. R., TIKOTVAR, N. L. and TILAK, B. D., *Tetrahedron* **4**, 420 (1958).

[50] BIBLE, R. H., Jr., PLACEK, C. and MUIR, R. D., *J. Org. Chem.* **22**, 607 (1957).
[51] BIRCH, A. J. and HARRISON, R. J., *Aust. J. Chem.* **8**, 519 (1955).
[52] BIRCH, A. J. and SMITH, H., *J. Chem. Soc.* 4909 (1956).
[53] BLADON, P., *J. Chem. Soc.* 3723 (1958).
[54] BLADON, P., HENBEST, H. B., JONES, E. R. H., LOVELL, B. J. and WOODS, G. F., *J. Chem. Soc.* 125 (1954).
[55] BLOOM, B. M. and SHULL, G. M., *J. Amer. Chem. Soc.* **77**, 5767 (1955).
[56] BOTS, J. P. L., *Rec. Trav. Chim. Pays-Bas* **77**, 1010 (1958).
[57] BOWERS, A., CASAS-CAMPILLO, C. and DJERASSI, C., *Tetrahedron* **2**, 165 (1958).
[58] BOWERS, A. and RINGOLD, H. J., *Tetrahedron* **3**, 14 (1958).
[59] BOWERS, A. and RINGOLD, H. J., *J. Amer. Chem. Soc.* **80**, 3091 (1958).
[60] BOWERS, A. and RINGOLD, H. J., *J. Amer. Chem. Soc.* **80**, 4423 (1958).
[61] BROOKS, S. G., EVANS, R. M., GREEN, G. F. H., HUNT, J. S., LONG, A. G., MOONEY, B. and WYMAN, L. J., *J. Chem. Soc.* 4614 (1958).
[62] BURN, D., ELLIS, B. and PETROW, V., *J. Chem. Soc.* 795 (1958).
[63] BURN, D., ELLIS, B., PETROW, V., STUART-WEBB, I. A. and WILLIAMSON, D. M., *J. Chem. Soc.* 4092 (1957).
[64] CAMERINO, B. and ALBERTI, C. G., *Gazz. Chim. Ital.* **85**, 51 (1955).
[65] CAMERINO, B. and ALBERTI, C. G., *Gazz. Chim. Ital.* **85**, 56 (1955).
[66] CAMERINO, B., ALBERTI, C. G. and VERCELLONE, A., *Gazz. Chim. Ital.* **83**, 795 (1953).
[67] CAMERINO, B., ALBERTI. C. G., VERCELLONE, A. and AMMANNATI, F., *Gazz. Chim. Ital.* **84**, 301 (1954).
[68] CAMERINO, B., MODELLI, R. and SPALLA, C., *Gazz. Chim. Ital.* **86**, 1226 (1956).
[69] CAMERINO, B., PATELLI, B. and VERCELLONE, A., *J. Amer. Chem. Soc.* **78**, 3540 (1956).
[70] CAMERINO, B. and VERCELLONE, A., *Gazz. Chim. Ital.* **86**, 260 (1956).
[71] CAMERON, A. F. B., EVANS, R. M., HAMLET, J. C., HUNT, J. S., JONES, P. G. and LONG, A. G., *J. Chem. Soc.* 2807 (1955).
[72] CAMPBELL, J. A., BABCOCK, J. C. and HOGG, J. A., *J. Amer. Chem. Soc.* **80**, 4717 (1958).
[73] CASANOVA, R., SHOPPEE, C. W. and SUMMERS, G. H. R., *J. Chem. Soc.* 2983 (1953).
[74] CASPI, E., *J. Org. Chem.* **21**, 729 (1956).
[75] CASPI, E. and PECHET, M. M., *J. Biol. Chem.* **230**, 843 (1958).
[76] CERNEY, V. and SORM, F., *Chem. Listy* **50**, 1134 (1956).
[77] CHAMBERLIN, E. M., RUYLE, W. V., ERICKSON, A. E., CHEMERDA, J. M., ALIMINOSA, L. M., ERICKSON, R. L., SITA, G. E. and TISHLER, M., *J. Amer. Chem. Soc.* **75**, 3477 (1953).
[78] CHRISTENSEN, B. G., STEINBERG, N. G. and HIRSCHMANN, R., *Chem. & Ind.* 1259 (1958).
[79] CLARKE, R. L., DOBRINER, K., MOORADIAN, A. and MARTINI, C. M., *J. Amer. Chem. Soc.* **77**, 661 (1955).
[80] CLINTON, R. O., CHRISTIANSEN, R. G., NEUMANN, H. C. and LASKOWSKI, S. C., *J. Amer. Chem. Soc.* **79**, 6475 (1957).
[81] CLINTON, R. O., NEUMANN, H. C., MANSON, A. J., LASKOWSKI, S. C. and CHRISTIANSEN, R. G., *J. Amer. Chem. Soc.* **80**, 3395 (1958).
[82] COLE, W. and JULIAN, P. L., *J. Org. Chem.* **19**, 131 (1954).
[83] COLLINS, R. J. and BROWN, E. V., *J. Amer. Chem. Soc.* **79**, 1103 (1957).
[84] COLTON, F. B. and KENDALL, E. C., *J. Biol. Chem.* **194**, 247 (1952).
[85] COLTON, F. B., NES, W. R., VAN DORP, D. A., MASON, H. L. and KENDALL, E. C., *J. Biol. Chem.* **194**, 235 (1952).
[86] COLTON, F. B., NYSTED, L. N., RIEGEL, B. and RAYMOND, A. L., *J. Amer. Chem. Soc.* **79**, 1123 (1957).
[87] CONSTANTIN, J. M., HAVEN, A. C., Jr. and SARETT, L. H., *J. Amer. Chem. Soc.* **75**, 1716 (1953).
[88] COOLEY, G., ELLIS, B., HARTLEY, F. and PETROW, V., *J. Chem. Soc.* 4377 (1955).
[89] COOLEY, G., ELLIS, B., KIRK, D. N. and PETROW, V., *J. Chem. Soc.* 4112 (1957).
[90] COOLEY, G., ELLIS, B. and PETROW, V., *J. Chem. Soc.* 1813 (1954).
[91] CRABBÉ, P., OURISSON, G. and TAKAHASHI, T., *Tetrahedron* **3**, 279 (1958).
[92] CUTLER, F. A., Jr., CONBERE, J. P., LUKES, R. M., FISHER, J. F., MERTEL, H. E., HIRSCHMANN, R., CHEMERDA, J. M., SARETT, L. H. and PFISTER, K., III, *J. Amer. Chem. Soc.* **80**, 6300 (1958).
[93] DANNENBERG, H., *Abh. Preuss. Akad. Wiss. Math. Naturw. Kl.* **21**, 3 (1939).
[94] DANNENBERG, H. and DOERING, C. H., *Hoppe-Seyl. Z.* **311**, 84 (1958).
[95] DERUGGIERI, P., *Gazz. Chim. Ital.* **87**, 795 (1957).
[96] DJERASSI, C., BATRES, E., ROMO, J. and ROSENKRANZ, G., *J. Amer. Chem. Soc.* **74**, 3634 (1952).
[97] DJERASSI, C., BENDAS, H. and SEGALOFF, A., *J. Org. Chem.* **21**, 1056 (1956).
[98] DJERASSI, C., GROSSMAN, J. and THOMAS, G. H., *J. Amer. Chem. Soc.* **77**, 3826 (1955).

99 DJERASSI, C., GROSSNICKLE, T. T. and HIGH, L. B., *J. Amer. Chem. Soc.* **78**, 3166 (1956).
100 DJERASSI, C., HIGH, L. B., FRIED, J. and SABO, E., *J. Amer. Chem. Soc.* **77**, 3673 (1955).
101 DJERASSI, C. and LENK, C. T., *J. Amer. Chem. Soc.* **76**, 1722 (1954).
102 DJERASSI, C., LIPPMAN, A. E. and GROSSMAN, J., *J. Amer. Chem. Soc.* **78**, 2479 (1956).
103 DJERASSI, C., MANCERA, O., ROMO, J. and ROSENKRANZ, G., *J. Amer. Chem. Soc.* **75**, 3505 (1953).
104 DJERASSI, C., MANCERA, O., VELASCO, M., STORK, G. and ROSENKRANZ, G., *J. Amer. Chem. Soc.* **74**, 3321 (1952).
105 DJERASSI, C., MANSON, A. J. and BENDAS, H., *Tetrahedron* **1**, 22 (1957).
106 DJERASSI, C., MIRAMONTES, L., ROSENKRANZ, G. and SONDHEIMER, F., *J. Amer. Chem. Soc.* **76**, 4092 (1954).
107 DJERASSI, C., MIRAMONTES, L. and ROSENKRANZ, G., *J. Amer. Chem. Soc.* **75**, 4440 (1953).
108 DJERASSI, C. and NUSSBAUM, A. L., *J. Amer. Chem. Soc.* **75**, 3700 (1953).
109 DJERASSI, C., ROMO, J. and ROSENKRANZ, G., *J. Org. Chem.* **17**, 641 (1952).
110 DJERASSI, C. and THOMAS, G. H., *Chem. & Ind.* 1228 (1954).
111 DJERASSI, C. and THOMAS, G. H., *J. Amer. Chem. Soc.* **79**, 3835 (1957).
112 DODSON, R. M., GOLDKAMP, A. H. and MUIR, R. D., *J. Amer. Chem. Soc.* **79**, 3921 (1957).
113 DODSON, R. M. and MUIR, R. D., *J. Amer. Chem. Soc.* **80**, 5004 (1958).
114 DODSON, R. M. and MUIR, R. D., *J. Amer. Chem. Soc.* **80**, 6148 (1958).
115 DODSON, R. M., SOLLMAN, P. B. and RIEGEL, B., *J. Amer. Chem. Soc.* **75**, 5132 (1953).
116 DORFMAN, L., *Chem. Rev.* **53**, 47 (1953).
117 DREIDING, A. S. and VOLTMAN, A., *J. Amer. Chem. Soc.* **76**, 537 (1954).
118 EGLINTON, G., NEVENZEL, J. C., NEWMAN, M. S. and SCOTT, A. I., *Chem. & Ind.* 686 (1953).
119 EHRENSTEIN, M. and DÜNNENBERGER, M., *J. Org. Chem.* **21**, 774 (1956).
120 EHRENSTEIN, M. and DÜNNENBERGER, M., *J. Org. Chem.* **21**, 783 (1956).
121 ELLIS, B., HARTLEY, F., PETROW, V. and WEDLAKE, D., *J. Chem. Soc.* 4383 (1955).
122 ELLIS, B., PATEL, D. and PETROW, V., *J. Chem. Soc.* 800 (1958).
123 ELLIS, B. and PETROW, V., *J. Chem. Soc.* 1179 (1956).
124 ELLIS, B., PETROW, V. and WEDLAKE, D., *J. Chem. Soc.* 3748 (1958).
125 ELKS, J., PHILLIPS, G. H. and WALL, W. F., *J. Chem. Soc.* 4001 (1958).
126 ENGEL, CH. R., *J. Amer. Chem. Soc.* **77**, 1064 (1955).
127 ENGEL, CH. R., *J. Amer. Chem. Soc.* **78**, 4727 (1956).
128 ENGEL, CH. R., *Canad. J. Chem.* **53**, 131 (1957).
129 ENGEL, CH. R. and JAHNKE, H., *Canad. J. Biochem. and Physiol.* **35**, 1047 (1957).
130 ENGEL, CH. R., JENNINGS, K. F. and JUST, G., *J. Amer. Chem. Soc.* **78**, 6153 (1956).
131 ENGEL, CH. R. and JUST, G., *J. Amer. Chem. Soc.* **76**, 4909 (1954).
132 ENGEL, CH. R. and JUST, G., *Canad. J. Chem.* **33**, 1515 (1955).
133 EPPSTEIN, S. H., MEISTER, P. D., PETERSON, D. H., MURRAY, H. C., LEIGH, H. M., LYTTLE, D. A., REINEKE, L. M. and WEINTRAUB, A., *J. Amer. Chem. Soc.* **75**, 408 (1953).
134 EPPSTEIN, S. H., MEISTER, P. D., LEIGH, H. M., PETERSON, D. H., MURRAY, H. C., REINEKE, L. M. and WEINTRAUB, A., *J. Amer. Chem. Soc.* **76**, 3174 (1954).
135 EPPSTEIN, S. H., MEISTER, P. D., PETERSON, D. H., MURRAY, H. C., OSBORN, H. M. L., WEINTRAUB, A., REINEKE, L. M. and MEEKS, R. C., *J. Amer. Chem. Soc.* **80**, 3382 (1958).
136 ERCOLI, A. and DERUGGIERI, P., *J. Amer. Chem. Soc.* **75**, 650 (1953).
137 ERCOLI, A., DERUGGIERI, P. and DELLA MORTE, D., *Gazz. Chim. Ital.* **85**, 628 (1955).
138 VON EUW, J., NEHER, R. and REICHSTEIN, T., *Helv. Chim Acta* **38**, 1423 (1955).
139 EVANS, R. M., GREEN, G. F. H., HUNT, J. S., LONG, A. G., MOONEY, B. and PHILLIPPS, G. H., *J. Chem. Soc.* 1529 (1958).
140 EVANS, R. M., HAMLET, J. C., HUNT, J. S., JONES, P. G., LONG, A. G., OUGHTON, J. F., STEPHENSON, L., WALKER, T. and WILSON, B. M., *J. Chem. Soc.* 4356 (1956).
141 FAJKOŠ, J., *Coll. Trav. Chim. Tchécosl.* **23**, 1559 (1958).
142 FAJKOŠ, J., *Coll. Trav. Chim. Tchécosl.* **23**, 2155 (1958).
143 FAJKOŠ, J. and ŠORM, F., *Chem. Listy* **47**, 712 (1953).
144 FAJKOŠ, J. and ŠORM, F., *Chem. Listy* **47**, 1836 (1953).
145 FAJKOŠ, J. and ŠORM, F., *Coll. Trav. Chim. Tchécosl.* **19**, 91 (1954).
146 FAJKOŠ, J. and ŠORM, F., *Coll. Trav. Chim. Tchécosl.* **22**, 1873 (1957).
147 FAJKOŠ, J. and ŠORM, F., *Chem. Listy* **52**, 505 (1958).
148 FIESER, L. F. and FIESER, M., *Steroids* p. 15. Reinhold, New York (1959).
149 FISHMAN, J., *J. Amer. Chem. Soc.* **80**, 1213 (1958).
150 FISHMAN, J., *Chem. & Ind.* 1556 (1958).
151 FISHMAN, J. and GALLAGHER, T. F., *Arch. Biochem. Biophys.* **77**, 511 (1958).
152 FLOREY, K. and EHRENSTEIN, M., *J. Org. Chem.* **19**, 1331 (1954).
153 FONKEN, G. S. and HOGG, J. A., *Tetrahedron* **2**, 365 (1958).

[154] FRIED, J., FLOREY, K., SABO, E. F., HERZ, J. E., RESTIVO, A. R., BORMAN, A. and SINGER, F. M., *J. Amer. Chem. Soc.* **77**, 4181 (1955).
[155] FRIED, J., HERZ, J. E., SABO, E. F. and MORRISSON, M. H., *Chem. & Ind.* 1232 (1956).
[156] FRIED, J. and SABO, E. F., *J. Amer. Chem. Soc.* **79**, 1130 (1957).
[157] FRIED, J., THOMA, R. W. and KLINGSBERG, R., *J. Amer. Chem. Soc.* **75**, 5764 (1953).
[158] GALINOVSKY, F., KERSCHBAUM, E. and JANISCH, H., *Mh. Chem.* **84**, 193 (1953).
[159] GENSLER, W. J. and MAHADEVAN, A. P., *J. Amer. Chem. Soc.* **76**, 6192 (1954).
[160] GILLAM, A. E. and STERN, E. S., *An Introduction to Electronic Absorption Spectroscopy in Organic Chemistry*. Arnold, London (1954).
[161] GLEN, W. L., BARBER, R. and PAPINEAU-COUTURE, G., *Nature, Lond.* **182**, 1308 (1958).
[162] GOLD, A. M. and SCHWENK, E., *J. Amer. Chem. Soc.* **80**, 5683 (1958).
[163] GOULD, D. and HERSHBERG, E. B., *J. Amer. Chem. Soc.* **75**, 3593 (1953).
[164] GOULD, D., ILAVSKY, J., GUTEKUNST, R. and HERSHBERG, E. B., *J. Org. Chem.* **22**, 829 (1957).
[165] GOULD, D., SHAPIRO, E. L., HERZOG, H. L., GENTLES, M. J., HERSHBERG, E. B., CHARNEY, W., GILMORE, M., TOLKSDORF, S., EISLER, M., PERLMAN, P. L. and PECHET, M. M., *J. Amer. Chem. Soc.* **79**, 502 (1957).
[166] GRABER, R. P., HAVEN, A. C., Jr. and WENDLER, N. L., *J. Amer. Chem. Soc.* **75**, 4722 (1953).
[167] GRABER, R. P., SNODDY, C. S., Jr. and WENDLER, N. L., *Chem. & Ind.* 57 (1956).
[168] GREENSPAN, G., SCHAFFNER, C. P., CHARNEY, W., HERZOG, H. L. and HERSHBERG, E. B., *J. Amer. Chem. Soc.* **79**, 3922 (1957).
[169] GUBLER, A. and TAMM, CH., *Helv. Chim. Acta* **41**, 301 (1958)
[170] GÜNTHARD, H. H., BERIGER, E., ENGEL, CH. R. and HEUSSER, H., *Helv. Chim. Acta* **35**, 2437, (1952).
[171] GUT, M., *J. Org. Chem.* **21**, 1327 (1956).
[172] HAM, E. A., HARMAN, R. E., BRINK, N. G. and SARETT, L. H., *J. Amer. Chem. Soc.* **77**, 1637 (1955).
[173] HARTMAN, J. A., TOMASEWSKI, A. J. and DREIDING, A. S., *J. Amer. Chem. Soc.* **78**, 5662 (1956).
[174] HEER, J. and HOFFMANN, K., *Helv. Chim. Acta* **39**, 1804 (1956).
[175] HEER, J. and HOFFMANN, K., *Helv. Chim. Acta* **39**, 1814 (1956).
[176] HELLER, M. and BERNSTEIN, S., *J. Amer. Chem. Soc.* **78**, 1161 (1956).
[177] HERR, M. E., HOGG, J. A. and LEVIN, R. H., *J. Amer. Chem. Soc.* **78**, 500 (1956).
[178] HERZ, J. E., FRIED, J., GRABOWICH, P. and SABO, E. F., *J. Amer. Chem. Soc.* **78**, 4812 (1956).
[179] HERZ, J. E., FRIED, J. and SABO, E. F., *J. Amer. Chem. Soc.* **78**, 2017 (1956).
[180] HERZIG, P. Th. and EHRENSTEIN, M., *J. Org. Chem.* **17**, 713 (1952).
[181] HERZIG, P. Th. and EHRENSTEIN, M., *J. Org. Chem.* **17**, 724 (1952).
[182] HERZOG, H. L., GENTLES, M. J. and HERSHBERG, E. B., *J. Org. Chem.* **21**, 688 (1956).
[183] HERZOG, H. L. GENTLES, M. J., HERSHBERG, E. B., CARVAJAL, F., SUTTER, D., CHARNEY, W. and SCHAFFNER, C. P., *J. Amer. Chem. Soc.* **79**, 3921 (1957).
[184] HERZOG, H. L., JEVNIK, M. A., PERLMAN, P. L., NOBILE, A. and HERSHBERG, E. B., *J. Amer. Chem. Soc.* **75**, 266 (1953).
[185] HERZOG, H. L., PAYNE, C. C., JEVNIK, M. A., GOULD, D., SHAPIRO, E. L., OLIVETO, E. P. and HERSHBERG, E. B., *J. Amer. Chem. Soc.* **77**, 4781 (1955).
[186] HERZOG, H. L., PAYNE, C. C., TULLY, M. E. and HERSHBERG, E. B., *J. Amer. Chem. Soc.* **75**, 5751 (1953).
[187] HEUSLER, K., UEBERWASSER, H., WIELAND, P. and WETTSTEIN, A., *Helv. Chim. Acta* **40**, 787 (1957).
[188] HEUSLER, K. and WETTSTEIN, A., *Chem. Ber.* **87**, 1301 (1954).
[189] HEUSLER, K. and WETTSTEIN, A., *Helv. Chim. Acta* **35**, 284 (1952).
[190] HEUSLER, K. and WETTSTEIN, A., *Helv. Chim. Acta* **36**, 398 (1953).
[191] HEUSSER, H., BERIGER, E. and ENGEL, CH. R., *Helv. Chim. Acta* **37**, 2166 (1954).
[192] HEUSSER, H., HEUSLER, K., EICHENBERGER, K., HONEGGER, C. G., and JEGER, O., *Helv. Chim. Acta* **35**, 295 (1952).
[193] HEYL, F. W. and HERR, M. E., *J. Amer. Chem. Soc.* **75**, 1918 (1953).
[194] HEYL, F. W. and HERR, M. E., *J. Amer. Chem. Soc.* **77**, 488 (1955).
[195] HIRSCHMANN, R., BAILEY, G. A., POOS, G. I., WALKER, R. and CHEMERDA, J. M., *J. Amer. Chem. Soc.* **78**, 4814 (1956).
[196] HIRSCHMANN, H. and HIRSCHMANN, F. B., *J. Amer. Chem. Soc.* **78**, 3755 (1956).
[197] HIRSCHMANN, H., HIRSCHMANN, F. B. and CORCORAN, J. W., *J. Org. Chem.* **20**, 572 (1955).
[198] HIRSCHMANN, H., HIRSCHMANN, F. B. and DAUS, M. A., *J. Amer. Chem. Soc.* **74**. 539 (1952).
[199] HIRSCHMANN, H., HIRSCHMANN, F. B. and FARREL, G. L., *J. Amer. Chem. Soc.* **75**, 4862 (1953).
[200] HIRSCHMANN, R., BAILEY, G. and CHEMERDA, J. M., *Chem. & Ind.* 682 (1958).

[201] HIRSCHMANN, R. F., MILLER, R., BEYLER, R. E., SARETT, L. H. and TISHLER, M., *J. Amer. Chem. Soc.* **77**, 3166 (1955).
[202] HIRSCHMANN, R. and WENDLER, N. L., *J. Amer. Chem. Soc.* **75**, 2361 (1953).
[203] HOFFMAN, F., BEYLER, R. E. and TISHLER, M., *J. Amer. Chem. Soc.* **80**, 5322 (1958).
[204] HOGG, J. A., BEAL, P. F., NATHAN, A. H., LINCOLN, F. H., SCHNEIDER, W. P., MAGERLEIN, B. J., HANZE, A. R. and JACKSON, R. W., *J. Amer. Chem. Soc.* **77**, 4436 (1955).
[205] HOGG, J. A., LINCOLN, F. H., NATHAN, A. H., HANZE, A. R., SCHNEIDER, W. P., BEAL, P. F. and KORMAN, J., *J. Amer. Chem. Soc.* **77**, 4438 (1955).
[206] HOGG, J. A., LINCOLN, F. H., JACKSON, R. W. and SCHNEIDER, W. P., *J. Amer. Chem. Soc.* **77**, 6401 (1955).
[207] HUANG-MINLON and PETTEBONE, R. H., *J. Amer. Chem. Soc.* **74**, 1562 (1952).
[208] HUANG-MINLON, TULL, R. and BABCOCK, J., *J. Amer. Chem. Soc.* **76**, 2396 (1954).
[209] IRIARTE, J. and RINGOLD, H. J., *Tetrahedron* **3**, 28 (1958).
[210] IRIARTE, J., RINGOLD, H. J. and DJERASSI, C., *J. Amer. Chem. Soc.* **80**, 6105 (1958).
[211] JOHNS, W. F., *J. Amer. Chem. Soc.* **80**, 6456 (1958).
[212] JOHNSON, W. S., ACKERMAN, J., EASTHAM, J. F. and DEWALT, H. A., Jr., *J. Amer. Chem. Soc.* **78**, 6302 (1956).
[213] JOHNSON, W. S., BANNISTER, B. and PAPPO, R., *J. Amer. Chem. Soc.* **78**, 6331 (1956).
[214] JOHNSON, W. S., BANNISTER, B., PAPPO, R. and PIKE, J. E., *J. Amer. Chem. Soc.* **78**, 6354 (1956).
[215] JOHNSON, W. S., DAVID, I. A., DEHM, H. C., HIGHET, R. J., WARNHOFF, E. W., WOOD, W. D. and JONES, E. T., *J. Amer. Chem. Soc.* **80**, 661 (1958).
[216] JOHNSON, W. S., DEHM, H. C. and CHINN, L. J., *J. Org. Chem.* **19**, 670 (1954).
[217] JOHNSON, W. S., GASTAMBIDE, B. and PAPPO, R., *J. Amer. Chem. Soc.* **79**, 1991 (1957).
[218] JOHNSON, W. S. and JOHNS, W. F., *J. Amer. Chem. Soc.* **79**, 2005 (1957).
[219] JOHNSON, W. S., KEMP, A. D., PAPPO, R., ACKERMAN, J. and JOHNS, W. F., *J. Amer. Chem. Soc.* **78**, 6312 (1956).
[220] JOHNSON, W. S., PAPPO, R. and JOHNS, W. F., *J. Amer. Chem. Soc.* **78**, 6339 (1956).
[221] JOHNSON, W. S., ROGIER, E. R. and ACKERMAN, J., *J. Amer. Chem. Soc.* **78**, 6322 (1956).
[222] JOHNSON, W. S., ROGIER, E. R., SZMUSZKOVICZ, J., HADLER, H. I., ACKERMAN, J., BHATTACHARYYA, B. K., BLOOM, B. M., STALMANN, L., CLEMENT, R. A., BANNISTER, B. and WYNBERG, H., *J. Amer. Chem. Soc.* **78**, 6289 (1956).
[223] JOHNSON, W. S., SZMUSZKOVICZ, J., ROGIER, E. R., HADLER, H. I. and WYNBERG, H., *J. Amer. Chem. Soc.* **78**, 6285 (1956).
[224] JOLY, R. and WARNANT, J., *Bull. Soc. Chim. Fr.* 367 (1958).
[225] JOLY, R., WARNANT, J., NOMINÉ, G. and BERTIN, D., *Bull. Soc. Chim. Fr.* 366 (1958).
[226] JONES, R. E. and KOCHER, F. W., *J. Amer. Chem. Soc.* **76**, 3682 (1954).
[227] JULIAN, P. L., COCHRANE, C. C., MAGNANI, A. and KARPEL, W. J., *J. Amer. Chem. Soc.* **78**, 3153 (1956).
[228] JULIAN, P. L., COLE, W., MEYER, E. W. and REGAN, B. M., *J. Amer. Chem. Soc.* **77**, 4601 (1955).
[229] JUNGMANN, R., SCHINDLER, O. and REICHSTEIN, T., *Helv. Chim. Acta* **41**, 1234 (1958).
[230] JUNGMANN, R., SCHINDLER, O. and REICHSTEIN, T., *Helv. Chim. Acta* **41**, 1247 (1958).
[231] JUNGMANN, R., SIGG, H. P., SCHINDLER, O. and REICHSTEIN, T., *Helv. Chim. Acta* **41**, 1206 (1958).
[232] JUST, G., and ENGEL, CH. R., *J. Org. Chem.* **23**, 12 (1958).
[233] KAHNT, F. W., NEHER, R. and WETTSTEIN, A., *Helv. Chim. Acta* **38**, 1237 (1955).
[234] KASPAR, E. and WIECHART, R., *Chem. Ber.* **91**, 2664 (1958).
[235] KINCL, F. A., RINGOLD, H. J. and ROSENKRANZ, G., *J. Org. Chem.* **22**, 1127 (1957).
[236] KIRK, D. N., PATEL, D. K. and PETROW, V., *J. Chem. Soc.* 627 (1956).
[237] KIRK, D. N., PATEL, D. K. and PETROW, V., *J. Chem. Soc.* 1184 (1956).
[238] KIRK, D. N., PATEL, D. K. and PETROW, V., *J. Chem. Soc.* 1046 (1957).
[239] KIRK, D. N. and PETROW, V., *J. Chem. Soc.* 1334 (1958).
[240] KLYNE, W. and PALMER, S., *J. Chem. Soc.* 4545 (1958).
[241] KOCH, H. P., *Chem. & Ind.* **61**, 273 (1942).
[242] KRAYCHY, S. and GALLAGHER, T. F., *J. Biol. Chem.* **229**, 519 (1957).
[243] KRAYCHY, S. and GALLAGHER, T. F., *J. Amer. Chem. Soc.* **79**, 754 (1957).
[244] KÜNDIG-HEGEDÜS, H. and SCHINDLER, O., *Helv. Chim. Acta* **39**, 904 (1956).
[245] LARDON, A. and REICHSTEIN, T., *Helv. Chim. Acta* **41**, 904 (1958).
[246] LARDON, A., SCHMIDLIN, J., WETTSTEIN, A. and REICHSTEIN, T., *Helv. Chim. Acta* **40**, 662 (1957).
[247] LEANZA, W. J., CONBERE, J. P., ROGERS, E. F. and PFISTER, K., III, *J. Amer. Chem. Soc.* **76**, 1691 (1954).

[248] LEEDS, N. S., FUKUSHIMA, D. K. and GALLAGHER, T. F., *J. Amer. Chem. Soc.* **76**, 2943 (1954).
[249] LEMIN, A. J., ROSENKRANZ, G. and DJERASSI, C., *J. Amer. Chem. Soc.* **75**, 1745 (1953).
[250] LENHARD, R. H. and BERNSTEIN, S., *J. Amer. Chem. Soc.* **77**, 6665 (1955).
[251] LENHARD, R. H. and BERNSTEIN, S., *J. Amer. Chem. Soc.* **78**, 989 (1956).
[252] LITTELL, R. and BERNSTEIN, S., *J. Amer. Chem. Soc.* **78**, 984 (1956).
[253] MAGERLEIN, B. J. and HOGG, J. A., *J. Amer. Chem. Soc.* **79**, 1508 (1957).
[254] MAGERLEIN, B. J. and HOGG, J. A., *Tetrahedron* **2**, 80 (1958).
[255] MAGERLEIN, B. J. and HOGG, J. A., *J. Amer. Chem. Soc.* **80**, 2220 (1958).
[256] MAGERLEIN, B. J. and HOGG, J. A., *J. Amer. Chem. Soc.* **80**, 2226 (1958).
[257] MAGERLEIN, B. J., LYTTLE, D. A. and LEVIN, R. H., *J. Org. Chem.* **20**, 1709 (1955).
[258] MANCERA, O., BARTON, D. H. R., ROSENKRANZ, G. and DJERASSI, C., *J. Chem. Soc.* 1021 (1952).
[259] MANCERA, O., ROSENKRANZ, G. and SONDHEIMER, F., *J. Chem. Soc.* 2189 (1953).
[260] MANCERA, O., ROSENKRANZ, G. and SONDHEIMER, F., *J. Amer. Chem. Soc.* **77**, 5669 (1955).
[261] MARSHALL, C. W., RALLS, J. W., SAUNDERS, F. J. and RIEGEL, B., *J. Biol. Chem.* **228**, 339 (1957).
[262] MARTINEZ, H., RINGOLD, H. J., ROSENKRANZ, G. and DJERASSI, C., *J. Amer. Chem. Soc.* **75**, 239 (1953).
[263] MARTIN-SMITH, M., *J. Chem. Soc.* 523 (1958).
[264] MATEOS FERNANDEZ, J. L. and MIRAMONTES, L., *Bol. Inst. Quím. Univ. Nac. Autón, Méx.* **5**, 3 (1953).
[265] MATTOX, V. R., *J. Amer. Chem. Soc.* **74**, 4340 (1952).
[266] MATTOX, V. R., WOROCH, E. L., FLEISHER, G. A. and KENDALL, E. C., *J. Biol. Chem.* **197**, 261 (1952).
[267] MCALEER, W. J., KOZLOWSKI, M. A., STOUDT, T. H. and CHEMERDA, J. M., *J. Org. Chem.* **23**, 958 (1958).
[268] MCALEER, W. J., KOZLOWSKI, M. A., STOUDT, T. H. and CHEMERDA, J. M., *J. Org. Chem.* **23**, 508 (1958).
[269] MCGUCKIN, W. F. and MASON, H. L., *J. Amer. Chem. Soc.* **77**, 1822 (1955).
[270] MCNIVEN, N. L., *J. Amer. Chem. Soc.* **76**, 1725 (1954).
[271] MEEKS, R. C., MEISTER, P. D., EPPSTEIN, S. H., ROSSELET, J. P., WEINTRAUB, A., MURRAY, H. C., SEBEK, O. K., REINEKE, L. M. and PETERSON, D. H., *Chem. & Ind.* 391 (1958).
[272] MEISTER, P. D., PETERSON, D. H., MURRAY, H. C., EPPSTEIN, S. H., REINEKE, L. M., WEINTRAUB, A. and LEIGH, H. M., *J. Amer. Chem. Soc.* **75**, 55 (1953).
[273] MEISTER, P. D., PETERSON, D. H., MURRAY, H. C., SPERO, G. B., EPPSTEIN, S. H., WEINTRAUB, A., REINEKE, L. M. and LEIGH, H. M., *J. Amer. Chem. Soc.* **75**, 416 (1953).
[274] MEISTER, P. D., PETERSON, D. H., EPPSTEIN, S. H., MURRAY, H. C., REINEKE, L. M., WEINTRAUB, A. and OSBORN, H. M. L., *J. Amer. Chem. Soc.* **76**, 5679 (1954).
[275] MEISTER, P. D., REINEKE, L. M., MEEKS, R. C., MURRAY, H. C., EPPSTEIN, S. H., OSBORN, H. M. L., WEINTRAUB, A. and PETERSON, D. H., *J. Amer. Chem. Soc.* **76**, 4050 (1954).
[276] MEYER, A. S. and LINDBERG, M. C., *J. Amer. Chem. Soc.* **76**, 3033 (1954).
[277] MEYSTRE, CH., VISCHER, E. and WETTSTEIN, A., *Helv. Chim. Acta* **38**, 381 (1955).
[278] MEYSTRE, CH., FREY, H., VOSER, W. and WETTSTEIN, A., *Helv. Chim. Acta* **39**, 734 (1956).
[279] MICHELI, R. A. and BRADSHER, C. K., *J. Amer. Chem. Soc.* **77**, 4788 (1955).
[280] MILLS, J. S., RINGOLD, H. J. and DJERASSI, C., *J. Amer. Chem. Soc.* **80**, 6118 (1958).
[281] MOFFETT, R. B. and ANDERSON, H. V., *J. Amer. Chem. Soc.* **76**, 747 (1954).
[282] MOFFETT, R. B. and SLOMP, G., Jr., *J. Amer. Chem. Soc.* **76**, 3678 (1954).
[283] MOFFETT, R. B. and WEISBLAT, D. I., *J. Amer. Chem. Soc.* **74**, 2183 (1952).
[284] MOORE, J. A., *Helv. Chim. Acta* **37**, 659 (1954).
[285] MOORE, J. A. and WITTLE, E. L., *J. Amer. Chem. Soc.* **74**, 6287 (1952).
[286] MUELLER, G. P. and NORTON, L. L., *J. Amer. Chem. Soc.* **77**, 143 (1955).
[287] MUELLER, G. P., NORTON, L. L., STOBAUGH, R. E., TSAI, L. and WINNIFORD, R. S., *J. Amer. Chem. Soc.* **75**, 4892 (1953).
[288] MUELLER, G. P. and RIEGEL, B., *J. Amer. Chem. Soc.* **76**, 3686 (1954).
[289] NAWA, H., UCHIBAYASHI, M., TAKEDA, R., NAKANISHI, I., KUSAKA, T., TERUMICHI, J., UCHIDA, M., KATSUMATA, M., YOSHINO, K. and FUJITANI, H., *Tetrahedron* **4**, 201 (1958).
[290] NEHER, R., DESAULLES, P., VISCHER, E., WIELAND, P. and WETTSTEIN, A., *Helv. Chim. Acta* **41**, 1667 (1958).
[291] NEHER, R. and WETTSTEIN, A., *Helv. Chim. Acta* **39**, 2062 (1956).
[292] NELSON, N. A. and GARLAND, R. B., *J. Amer. Chem. Soc.* **79**, 6313 (1957).
[293] NES, W. R., KOSTIC, R. B. and MOSETTIG, E., *J. Amer. Chem. Soc.* **78**, 436 (1956).
[294] NES, W. R., STEELE, J. A. and MOSETTIG, E., *J. Amer. Chem. Soc.* **80**, 5230 (1958).
[295] NES, W. R., STEELE, J. A. and MOSETTIG, E., *J. Amer. Chem. Soc.* **80**, 5233 (1958).

[296] NICHOLAS, H. J., *J. Org. Chem.* **23**, 1747 (1958).
[297] NEUMANN, F., MANCERA, O., ROSENKRANZ, G. and SONDHEIMER, F., *J. Amer. Chem. Soc.* **77**, 5676 (1955).
[298] NOBILE, A., CHARNEY, W., PERLMAN, P. L., HERZOG, H. L., PAYNE, C. C., TULLY, M. E., JEVNIK, M. A. and HERSHBERG E. B., *J. Amer. Chem Soc.* **77**, 4184 (1955).
[299] NORYMBERSKI, J. K. and WOODS, G. F., *J. Chem. Soc.* 3426 (1955).
[300] NUSSBAUM, A. L., *Chem. & Ind.* 1313 (1956).
[301] NUSSBAUM, A. L., BRABAZON, G., OLIVETO, E. P. and HERSHBERG, E. B., *J. Org. Chem.* **22**, 977 (1957).
[302] NUSSBAUM, A. L., BRABAZON, G., POPPER, T. L. and OLIVETO, E. P., *J. Amer. Chem. Soc.* **80**, 2722 (1958).
[303] NUSSBAUM, A. L. and CARLON, F. E., *J. Amer. Chem. Soc.* **79**, 3831 (1957).
[304] NUSSBAUM, A. L., CARLON, F. E., GOULD, D., OLIVETO, E. P., HERSHBERG, E. B., GILMORE, M. L. and CHARNEY, W., *J. Amer. Chem. Soc.* **79**, 4814 (1957).
[305] OLIVETO, E. P., GEROLD, C. and HERSHBERG, E. B., *J. Amer. Chem. Soc.* **74**, 2248 (1952).
[306] OLIVETO, E. P., GEROLD, C. and HERSHBERG, E. B., *J. Amer. Chem. Soc.* **76**, 6111 (1954).
[307] OLIVETO, E. P., GEROLD, C. and HERSHBERG, E. B., *Arch. Biochem. Biophys.* **43**, 234 (1953).
[308] OLIVETO, E. P., GEROLD, C. and HERSHBERG, E. B., *Arch. Biochem. Biophys.* **49**, 244 (1954).
[309] OLIVETO, E. P., GEROLD, C., RAUSSER, R. and HERSHBERG, E. B., *J. Amer. Chem. Soc.* **77**, 3564 (1955).
[310] OLIVETO, E. P., GEROLD, C., WEBER, L., JORGENSEN, H. E., RAUSSER, R. and HERSHBERG, E. B., *J. Amer. Chem. Soc.* **75**, 5486 (1953).
[311] OLIVETO, E. P., HERZOG, H. L., JEVNIK, M. A., JORGENSEN, H. E. and HERSHBERG, E. B., *J. Amer. Chem. Soc.* **75**, 3651 (1953).
[312] OLIVETO, E. P., RAUSSER, R., GEROLD, C., HERSHBERG, E. B., EISLER, M., NERI, R. and PERLMAN, P. L., *J. Org. Chem.* **23**, 121 (1958).
[313] OLIVETO, E. P., RAUSSER, R., HERZOG, H. L., HERSHBERG, E. B., TOLKSDORF, S., EISLER, M., PERLMAN, P. L. and PECHET, M. M., *J. Amer. Chem. Soc.* **80**, 6687 (1958).
[314] OLIVETO, E. P., RAUSSER, R., NUSSBAUM, A. L., GEBERT, W., HERSHBERG, E. B., TOLKSDORF, S., EISLER, M., PERLMAN, P. L. and PECHET, M. M., *J. Amer. Chem. Soc.* **80**, 4428 (1958).
[315] OLIVETO, E. P., RAUSSER, R., WEBER, L., NUSSBAUM, A. L., GEBERT, W., CONIGLIO, C. T., HERSHBERG, E. B., TOLKSDORF, S., EISLER, M., PERLMAN, P. L. and PECHET, M. M., *J. Amer. Chem. Soc.* **80**, 4431 (1958).
[316] OLIVETO, E. P., WEBER, L., GEROLD, C., PECHET, M. M. and HERSHBERG, E. B., *J. Org. Chem.* **22**, 1720 (1957).
[317] PATAKI, J., ROSENKRANZ, G. and DJERASSI, C., *J. Amer. Chem. Soc.* **74**, 3436 (1952).
[318] PATEL, D. K., PETROW, V., ROYER, R. and STUART-WEBB, I. A., *J. Chem. Soc.* 161 (1952).
[319] PAPPO, R., BLOOM, B. M. and JOHNSON, W. S., *J. Amer. Chem. Soc.* **78**, 6347 (1956).
[320] PEDERSON, R. L., CAMPBELL, J. A., BABCOCK, J. C., EPPSTEIN, S. H., MURRAY, H. C., WEINTRAUB, A., MEEKS, R. C., MEISTER, P. D., REINEKE, L. M. and PETERSON, D. H., *J. Amer. Chem. Soc.* **78**, 1512 (1956).
[321] PÉRON, F. G. and DORFMAN, R. I., *Arch. Biochem. Biophys.* **67**, 490 (1957).
[322] PETERSON, D. H., NATHAN, A. H., MEISTER, P. D., EPPSTEIN, S. H., MURRAY, H. C., WEINTRAUB, A., REINEKE, L. M. and LEIGH, H. M., *J. Amer. Chem. Soc.* **75**, 419 (1953).
[323] PETERSON, D. H., MEISTER, P. D., WEINTRAUB, A., REINEKE, L. M., EPPSTEIN, S. H., MURRAY, H. C. and OSBORN, H. M. L., *J. Amer. Chem. Soc.* **77**, 4428 (1955).
[324] PETERSON, D. H. and MURRAY, H. C., *J. Amer. Chem. Soc.* **74**, 1871 (1952).
[325] PETERSON, R. E., PIERCE, C. E. and KLIMAN, B., *Arch. Biochem. Biophys.* **70**, 614 (1957).
[326] POOS, G. I., *J. Amer. Chem. Soc.* **77**, 4932 (1955).
[327] POOS, G. I., HIRSCHMANN, R., BAILEY, G. A., CUTLER, F. A., Jr., SARETT, L. H. and CHEMERDA, J. M., *Chem. & Ind.* 1260 (1958).
[328] RAO, P. N. and KURATH, P., *J. Amer. Chem. Soc.* **78**, 5660 (1956).
[329] RAPALA, R. T. and FARKAS, E., *J. Amer. Chem. Soc.* **80**, 1008 (1958).
[330] REBER, F., LARDON, A. and REICHSTEIN, T., *Helv. Chim. Acta* **37**, 45 (1954).
[330a] REICH, H., CRANE, K. F., and SANFILIPPO, S. J., *J. Org. Chem.* **18**, 822 (1953).
[330b] REICH, H. and SAMUELS, B. K., *J. Org. Chem.* **19**, 1041 (1954).
[330c] REICH, H. and SAMUELS, B. K., *J. Org. Chem.* **21**, 65 (1956).
[331] RINGOLD, H. J., BATRES, E., MANCERA, O. and ROSENKRANZ, G., *J. Org. Chem.* **21**, 1432 (1956).
[332] RINGOLD, H. J., BATRES, E. and ROSENKRANZ, G., *J. Org. Chem.* **22**, 99 (1957).
[333] RINGOLD, H. J., BATRES, E. and ZDERIC, J. A., *Tetrahedron* **2**, 164 (1958).
[334] RINGOLD, H. J., MANCERA, O., DJERASSI, C., BOWERS, A., BATRES, E., MARTÍNEZ, H., NECOECHEA, E., EDWARDS, J., VELASCO, M., CAMPILLO, C. C. and DORFMAN, R. I., *J. Amer. Chem. Soc.* **80**, 6464 (1958).
[335] RINGOLD, H. J. and ROSENKRANZ, G., *J. Org. Chem.* **21**, 1333 (1956).

[336] RINGOLD, H. J. and ROSENKRANZ, G., *J. Org. Chem.* **22**, 602 (1957).
[337] RINGOLD, H. J., ROSENKRANZ, G. and SONDHEIMER, F., *J. Org. Chem.* **21**, 239 (1956).
[338] RINGOLD, H. J., ROSENKRANZ, G. and SONDHEIMER, F., *J. Amer. Chem. Soc.* **78**, 820 (1956).
[339] RINGOLD, H. J., ROSENKRANZ, G. and SONDHEIMER, F., *J. Amer. Chem. Soc.* **78**, 2477 (1956).
[340] ROGERS, E. F., LEANZA, W. J., CONBERE, J. P. and PFISTER, K., III, *J. Amer. Chem. Soc.* **74**, 2947 (1952).
[341] ROMERO, M., ROMO, J. and LEPE, J., *Bol. Inst. Quím. Univ. Nac. Autón. Méx.* **4**, 115 (1952).
[342] ROMO, J., *Tetrahedron* **3**, 37 (1958).
[343] ROMO, J. and DEVIVAR, A. R., *J. Amer. Chem. Soc.* **79**, 1118 (1957).
[344] ROMO, J., LEPE, J. and ROMERO, M., *Bol. Inst. Quím. Univ. Nac. Autón. Méx.* **4**, 125 (1952).
[345] ROMO, J., ROSENKRANZ, G. and DJERASSI, C., *J. Org. Chem.* **17**, 1413 (1952).
[346] ROMO, J., ROSENKRANZ, G., DJERASSI, C. and SONDHEIMER, F., *J. Amer. Chem. Soc.* **75**, 1277 (1953).
[347] ROMO, J., ROSENKRANZ, G., DJERASSI, C. and SONDHEIMER, F., *J. Org. Chem.* **19**, 1509 (1954).
[348] ROMO, J., ROSENKRANZ, G. and SONDHEIMER, F., *J. Amer. Chem. Soc.* **76**, 5169 (1954).
[349] ROMO, J., ROSENKRANZ, G. and SONDHEIMER, F., *J. Amer. Chem. Soc.* **79**, 5034 (1957).
[350] ROMO, J., STORK, G., ROSENKRANZ, G. and DJERASSI, C., *J. Amer. Chem. Soc.* **74**, 2918 (1952).
[351] ROMO, J. and DEVIVAR, A. R., *J. Org. Chem.* **21**, 902 (1956).
[352] ROSENKRANZ, G., MANCERA, O. and SONDHEIMER, F., *J. Amer. Chem. Soc.* **76**, 2227 (1954).
[353] ROSENKRANZ, G., MANCERA, O. and SONDHEIMER, F., *J. Amer. Chem. Soc.* **77**, 145 (1955).
[354] ROSENKRANZ, G., MANCERA, O., SONDHEIMER, F. and DJERASSI, C., *J. Org. Chem.* **21**, 520 (1956).
[355] ROSENKRANZ, G., PATAKI, J. and DJERASSI, C., *J. Org. Chem.* **17**, 290 (1952).
[356] ROSENKRANZ, G., VELASCO, M., DJERASSI, C. and SONDHEIMER, F., *J. Amer. Chem. Soc.* **75**, 4430 (1953).
[357] ROTHMAN, E. S. and WALL, M. E., *J. Amer. Chem. Soc.* **77**, 2228 (1955).
[358] ROTHMAN, E. S. and WALL, M. E., *J. Amer. Chem. Soc.* **78**, 1744 (1956).
[359] RUELAS, J. P., IRIARTE, J., KINCL, F. and DJERASSI, C., *J. Org. Chem.* **23**, 1744 (1958).
[360] RUFF, A., SHOPPEE, C. W. and SUMMERS, G. H. R., *J. Chem. Soc.* 3683 (1953).
[361] RUYLE, W. V., JACOB, T. A., CHEMERDA, J. M., CHAMBERLIN, E. M., ROSENBURG, D. W., SITA, G. E., ERICKSON, R. L., ALIMINOSA, L. M. and TISHLER, M., *J. Amer. Chem. Soc.* **75**, 2604 (1953).
[362] SALLMANN, F. and TAMM, CH., *Helv. Chim. Acta* **39**, 1340 (1956).
[363] SCHEER, I., KOSTIC, R. B. and MOSETTIG, E., *J. Amer. Chem. Soc.* **77**, 641 (1955).
[364] SCHENCK, G. O. and NEUMÜLLER, O. A., *Liebigs Ann.* **618**, 194 (1958).
[365] SCHENCK, G. O., NEUMÜLLER, O. A. and EISFELD, W., *Liebigs Ann.* **618**, 202 (1958).
[366] SCHINDLER, O., *Helv. Chim. Acta* **39**, 375 (1956).
[367] SCHINDLER, O., *Helv. Chim. Acta* **39**, 1698 (1956).
[368] SCHLEGEL, W. and TAMM, CH., *Helv. Chim. Acta* **40**, 160 (1957).
[369] SCHLEGEL, W., TAMM, CH. and REICHSTEIN, T., *Helv. Chim. Acta* **38**, 1013 (1955).
[370] SCHMIDLIN, J., ANNER, G., BILLETER, J. R., HEUSLER, K., UEBERWASSER, H., WIELAND, P. and WETTSTEIN, A., *Helv. Chim. Acta* **40**, 1438 (1957).
[371] SCHMIDLIN, J., ANNER, G., BILLETER, J. R., HEUSLER, K., UEBERWASSER, H., WIELAND, P. and WETTSTEIN, A., *Helv. Chim. Acta* **40**, 2291 (1957).
[372] SCHUBERT, A., LANGBEIN, G. and SIEBERT, R., *Chem. Ber.* **90**, 2576 (1957).
[373] SCHÜTT, W. and TAMM, CH., *Chem. & Ind.* 42 (1958).
[374] SCHÜTT, W. and TAMM, CH., *Helv. Chim. Acta* **41**, 1730 (1958).
[375] SHIRASAKA, M., TSURUTA, M. and NAKAMURA, M., *Bull. Agric. Chem. Soc. Japan* **22**, 273 (1958).
[376] SHOPPEE, C. W., JENKINS, R. H. and SUMMERS, G. H. R., *J. Chem. Soc.* 3048 (1958).
[377] SLATES, H. L. and WENDLER, N. L., *J. Org. Chem.* **22**, 498 (1957).
[378] SONDHEIMER, F., AMENDOLLA, C. and ROSENKRANZ, G., *J. Amer. Chem. Soc.* **75**, 5930 (1953).
[378a] SONDHEIMER, F., AMENDOLLA, C. and ROSENKRANZ, G., *J. Amer. Chem. Soc.* **75**, 5932 (1953).
[379] SONDHEIMER, F., DANIELI, N. and MAZUR, Y., *J. Org. Chem.* **24**, 1278 (1959).
[380] SONDHEIMER, F., STJERNSTRÖM, N. and ROSENTHAL, D., *J. Org. Chem.* **24**, 1280 (1959).
[381] SONDHEIMER, F., KAUFMANN, ST., ROMO, J., MARTINEZ, H. and ROSENKRANZ, G., *J. Amer. Chem. Soc.* **75**, 4712 (1953).
[382] SONDHEIMER, F., MANCERA, O., FLORES, H. and ROSENKRANZ, G., *J. Amer. Chem. Soc.* **78**, 1742 (1956).
[383] SONDHEIMER, F., MANCERA, O. and ROSENKRANZ, G., *J. Amer. Chem. Soc.* **76**, 5020 (1954).
[384] SONDHEIMER, F., MANCERA, O., ROSENKRANZ, G. and DJERASSI, C., *J. Amer. Chem. Soc.* **75**, 1282 (1953).
[385] SONDHEIMER, F., MANCERA, O., URQUIZA, M. and ROSENKRANZ, G., *J. Amer. Chem. Soc.* **77**, 4145 (1955).

[386] SONDHEIMER, F. and MAZUR, Y., *J. Amer. Chem. Soc.* **79**, 2906 (1957).
[387] SONDHEIMER, F. and MECHOULAM, R., *J. Amer. Chem. Soc.* **79**, 5029 (1957).
[388] SONDHEIMER, F. and MECHOULAM, R., *J. Amer. Chem. Soc.* **80**, 3087 (1958).
[389] SONDHEIMER, F., NEUMANN, F., RINGOLD, H. J. and ROSENKRANZ, G., *J. Amer. Chem. Soc.* **76**, 2230 (1954).
[390] SONDHEIMER, F., ROSENKRANZ, G., MANCERA, O. and DJERASSI, C., *J. Amer. Chem. Soc.* **75**, 2601 (1953).
[391] SONDHEIMER, F., VELASCO, M. and ROSENKRANZ, G., *J. Amer. Chem. Soc.* **77**, 192 (1955).
[392] SONDHEIMER, F., VELASCO, M. and ROSENKRANZ, G., *J. Amer. Chem. Soc.* **77**, 5673 (1955).
[393] SANDOVAL, A., MIRAMONTES, L., ROSENKRANZ, G., DJERASSI, C. and SONDHEIMER, F., *J. Amer. Chem. Soc.* **75**, 4117 (1953).
[394] SANDOVAL, A., THOMAS, G. H., DJERASSI, C., ROSENKRANZ, G. and SONDHEIMER, F., *J. Amer. Chem. Soc.* **77**, 148 (1955).
[395] SPERO, G. B., THOMPSON, J. L., LINCOLN, F. H., SCHNEIDER, W. P. and HOGG, J. A., *J. Amer. Chem. Soc.* **79**, 1515 (1957).
[396] SPERO, G. B., THOMPSON, J. L., MAGERLEIN, B. J., HANZE, A. R., MURRAY, H. C., SEBEK, O. K. and HOGG, J. A., *J. Amer. Chem. Soc.* **78**, 6213 (1956).
[397] ST. ANDRÉ, A. F., MACPHILLAMY, H. B., NELSON, J. A., SHABICA, A. C. and SCHOLZ, C. R., *J. Amer. Chem. Soc.* **74**, 5506 (1952).
[398] STEINBERG, N. G., HIRSCHMANN, R. and CHEMERDA, J. M. *Chem. & Ind.* 975 (1958).
[399] STORK, G., KHASTGIR, H. N. and SOLO, A. J., *J. Amer. Chem. Soc.* **80**, 6457 (1958).
[400] SZPILFOGEL, S. A. and GERRIS, V., *Rec. Trav. Chim. Pays-Bas* **74**, 1462 (1955).
[401] SZPILFOGEL, S. A., VAN HEMERT, P. A. and DEWINTER, M. S., *Rec. Trav. Chim. Pays-Bas* **75**, 1227 (1956).
[402] TAMM, CH., VOLPP, G. and BAUMGARTNER, G., *Helv. Chim. Acta* **40**, 1469 (1957).
[403] TAUB, D., HOFFSOMMER, R. D., SLATES, H. L. and WENDLER, N. L., *J. Amer. Chem. Soc.* **80**, 4435 (1958).
[404] TAUB, D., HOFFSOMMER, R. D. and WENDLER, N. L., *J. Amer. Chem. Soc.* **78**, 2912 (1956).
[405] TAUB, D., HOFFSOMMER, R. D. and WENDLER, N. L., *J. Amer. Chem. Soc.* **79**, 452 (1957).
[406] TAUB, D., PETTEBONE, R. H., WENDLER, N. L. and TISHLER, M., *J. Amer. Chem. Soc.* **76**, 4094 (1954).
[407] THOMA, R. W., FRIED, J., BONANNO, S. and GRABOWICH, P., *J. Amer. Chem. Soc.* **79**, 4818 (1957).
[408] TOUCHSTONE, J. C., ELLIOTT, W. H., THAYER, S. A. and DOISY, E. A., *J. Amer. Chem. Soc.* **77**, 3562 (1955).
[409] TURNER, R. B., ANLIKER, R., HELBLING, R., MEIER, J. and HEUSSER, H., *Helv. Chim. Acta* **38**, 411 (1955).
[410] TURNER, R. B. and VOITLE, D. M., *J. Amer. Chem. Soc.* **73**, 1403 (1951).
[411] VELASCO, M., RIVERA, J., ROSENKRANZ, G., SONDHEIMER, F. and DJERASSI, C., *J. Org. Chem.* **18**, 92 (1953).
[412] VELLUZ, L., GOFFINET, B. and AMIARD, G., *Tetrahedron* **4**, 241 (1958).
[413] VELLUZ, L., MULLER, G., JEQUIER, R. and PLOTKA, C., *J. Amer. Chem. Soc.* **80**, 2026 (1958).
[414] VISCHER, E., MEYSTRE, CH. and WETTSTEIN, A., *Helv. Chim. Acta* **38**, 835 (1955).
[415] VISCHER, E., MEYSTRE, CH. and WETTSTEIN, A., *Helv. Chim. Acta* **38**, 1502 (1955).
[416] VISCHER, E., SCHMIDLIN, J. and WETTSTEIN, A., *Helv. Chim. Acta* **37**, 321 (1954).
[417] WALL, M. E., KENNEY, H. E. and ROTHMAN, E. S., *J. Amer. Chem. Soc.* **77**, 5665 (1955).
[418] WEISENBORN, F. L., REMY, D. C. and JACOBS, T. L., *J. Amer. Chem. Soc.* **76**, 552 (1954).
[419] WENDLER, N. L., *Chem. & Ind.* 1662 (1958).
[420] WENDLER, N. L., GRABER, R. P. and BOLLINGER, F. W., *Chem. & Ind.* 1312 (1956).
[421] WENDLER, N. L., GRABER, R. P. and HAZEN, G. G., *Tetrahedron* **3**, 144 (1958).
[422] WENDLER, N. L., GRABER, R. P., JONES, R. E. and TISHLER, M., *J. Amer. Chem. Soc.* **74**, 3630 (1952).
[423] WENDLER, N. L., GRABER, R. P., SNODDY, C. S., Jr. and BOLLINGER, F. W., *J. Amer. Chem. Soc.* **79**, 4476 (1957).
[424] WENDLER, N. L. and TAUB, D., *Chem. & Ind.* 505 (1955).
[425] WENDLER, N. L. and TAUB, D., *J. Org. Chem.* **23**, 953 (1958).
[426] WENDLER, N. L. and TAUB, D., *Chem. & Ind.* 415 (1958).
[427] WENDLER, N. L. and TAUB, D., *J. Amer. Chem. Soc.* **80**, 3402 (1958).
[428] WENDLER, N. L. and TAUB, D., *Chem. & Ind.* 1237 (1957).
[429] WENDLER, N. L., TAUB, D., DOBRINER, S. and FUKUSHIMA, D. K., *J. Amer. Chem. Soc.* **78**, 5027 (1956).
[430] WERBIN, H., *J. Org. Chem.* **21**, 1532 (1956).
[431] WERBIN, H. and HOLOWAY, C., *J. Biol. Chem.* **223**, 651 (1957).

[432] WETTSTEIN, A., HEUSLER, K., UEBERWASSER, H. and WIELAND, P., *Helv. Chim. Acta* **40**, 323 (1957).
[433] WIELAND, P., HEUSLER, K., UEBERWASSER, H. and WETTSTEIN, A., *Helv. Chim. Acta* **41**, 74 (1958).
[434] WIELAND, P., HEUSLER, K., UEBERWASSER, H. and WETTSTEIN, A., *Helv. Chim. Acta* **41**, 416 (1958).
[435] WIELAND, P., HEUSLER, K. and WETTSTEIN, A., *Helv. Chim. Acta* **41**, 1561 (1958).
[436] WIELAND, P., HEUSLER, K. and WETTSTEIN, A., *Helv. Chim. Acta* **41**, 1657 (1958).
[437] WILDS, A. L. and NELSON, N. A., *J. Amer. Chem. Soc.* **75**, 5366 (1953).
[438] WILDS, A. L., ZEITSCHEL, R. H., SUTTON, R. E. and JOHNSON, J. A., Jr., *J. Org. Chem.* **19**, 255 (1954).
[439] WILSON, E. and TISHLER, M., *J. Amer. Chem. Soc.* **74**, 1609 (1952).
[440] WOODWARD, R. B., *J. Amer. Chem. Soc.*, **63**, 1123 (1941).
[441] WOODWARD, R. B., *J. Amer. Chem. Soc.* **64**, 72 (1942).
[442] WOODWARD, R. B., *J. Amer. Chem. Soc.* **64**, 76 (1942).
[443] ZAFFARONI, A., RINGOLD, H. J., ROSENKRANZ, G., SONDHEIMER, F., THOMAS, G. H. and DJERASSI, C., *J. Amer. Chem. Soc.* **76**, 6210 (1954).
[444] ZAFFARONI, A., RINGOLD, H. J., ROSENKRANZ, G., SONDHEIMER, F., THOMAS, G. H. and DJERASSI, C., *J. Amer. Chem. Soc.* **80**, 6110 (1958).
[445] ZDERIC, J. A., BOWERS, A., CARPIO, H. and DJERASSI, C., *J. Amer. Chem. Soc.* **80**, 2596 (1958).
[446] ZORBACH, W. W., *J. Amer. Chem. Soc.* **75**, 6344 (1953).
[447] ZORBACH, W. W., *J. Org. Chem.* **23**, 1797 (1958).
[448] ZORBACH, W. W. and TAMORRIA, C. R., *J. Org. Chem.* **22**, 1127 (1957).

References for 1959 Literature

[449] ALLEN, G. R., Jr. and WEISS, M. J., *J. Amer. Chem. Soc.* **81**, 4968 (1959).
[450] ANLIKER, R., MÜLLER, M., PERELMAN, M., WOHLFAHRT, J. and HEUSSER, H., *Helv. Chim. Acta* **42**, 1071 (1959).
[451] AXELROD, L. R. and RAO, P. N., *Chem. & Ind.* 1454 (1959).
[452] BARTON, S. P., BURN, D., COOLEY, G., ELLIS, B. and PETROW, V., *J. Chem. Soc.* 1957 (1959).
[453] BARTON, S. P., ELLIS, B. and PETROW, V., *J. Chem. Soc.* 478 (1959).
[454] BERGSTROM, C. G., NICHOLSON, R. T., ELTON, R. L. and DODSON, R. M., *J. Amer. Chem. Soc.* **81**, 4432 (1959).
[455] BERNSTEIN, S., ALLEN, W. S., HELLER, M., LENHARD, R. H., FELDMAN, L. I. and BLANK, R. H., *J. Org. Chem.* **24**, 286 (1959).
[456] BERNSTEIN, S., BROWN, J. J., FELDMAN, L. I. and RIGLER, N. E., *J. Amer. Chem. Soc.* **81**, 4956 (1959).
[457] BERNSTEIN, S., HELLER, M., LITTELL, R., STOLAR, S. M., LENHARD, R. H., ALLEN, W. S. and RINGLER, I., *J. Amer. Chem. Soc.* **81**, 1696 (1959).
[458] BERNSTEIN, S., HELLER, M. and STOLAR, S. M., *J. Amer. Chem. Soc.* **81**, 1256 (1959).
[459] BERNSTEIN, S., LENHARD, R. H., ALLEN, W. S., HELLER, M., LITTELL, R., STOLAR, S. M., FELDMAN, L. I. and BLANK, R. H., *J. Amer. Chem. Soc.* **81**, 1689 (1959).
[460] BERNSTEIN, S. and LITTELL, R., *J. Org. Chem.* **24**, 429 (1959).
[461] BERNSTEIN, S., LITTELL, R., BROWN, J. J. and RINGLER, I., *J. Amer. Chem. Soc.* **81**, 4573 (1959).
[462] BERNSTEIN, S. and LITTELL, R., *J. Org. Chem.* **24**, 871 (1959).
[463] BEYLER, R. E., HOFFMAN, F. and SARETT, L. H., *J. Org. Chem.* **24**, 1386 (1959).
[464] BLOOM, B. M., BOGERT, V. V. and PINSON, R., Jr., *Chem. & Ind.* 1317 (1959).
[465] BOLLINGER, F. W. and WENDLER, N. L., *J. Org. Chem.* **24**, 1139 (1959).
[466] BOWERS, A., *J. Amer. Chem. Soc.* **81**, 4107 (1959).
[467] BOWERS, A., DENOT, E., SÁNCHEZ, M. B., SÁNCHEZ-HIDALGO, L. M. and RINGOLD, H. J., *J. Amer. Chem. Soc.* **81**, 5233 (1959).
[468] BOWERS, A., DENOT, E., SÁNCHEZ, M. B. and RINGOLD, H. J., *Tetrahedron* **7**, 153 (1959).
[469] BOWERS, A., IBÁNEZ, L. C. and RINGOLD, H. J., *J. Amer. Chem. Soc.* **81**, 3707 (1959).
[470] BOWERS, A., IBÁNEZ, L. C. and RINGOLD, H. J., *J. Amer. Chem. Soc.* **81**, 5991 (1959).
[471] BOWERS, A., IBÁNEZ, L. C. and RINGOLD, H. J., *Tetrahedron* **7**, 138 (1959).
[472] BOWERS, A. and RINGOLD, H. J., *J. Amer. Chem. Soc.* **81**, 424 (1959).
[473] BOWERS, A. and RINGOLD, H. J., *J. Amer. Chem. Soc.* **81**, 3710 (1959).
[474] BOWERS, A., SÁNCHEZ, M. B. and RINGOLD, H. J., *J. Amer. Chem. Soc.* **81**, 3702 (1959).
[475] BUCHSCHACHER, P., CEREGHETT, M., WEHRLI, H., SCHAFFNER, K. and JEGER, O., *Helv. Chim. Acta* **42**, 2122 (1959).
[476] BURN, D., COOLEY, G., PETROW, V. and WESTON, G. O., *J. Chem. Soc.* 3808 (1959).
[477] BUZZETTI, F., WICKI, W., KALVODA, J. and JEGER, O., *Helv. Chim. Acta* **42**, 388 (1959).

[478] CAMERINO, B., CATTAPAN, D., VALCAVI, U. and PATELLI, B., *Gazz. Chim. Ital.* **89**, 674 (1959).
[479] CAMERINO, B. and SCIAKY, R., *Gazz. Chim. Ital.* **89**, 663 (1959).
[480] CAMPBELL, J. A. and BABCOCK, J. C., *J. Amer. Chem. Soc.* **81**, 4069 (1959).
[481] CARVAJAL, F., VITALE, O. F., GENTLES, M. J., HERZOG, H. L. and HERSHBERG, E. B., *J. Org. Chem.* **24**, 695 (1959).
[482] CELLA, J. A. and TWEIT, R. C., *J. Org. Chem.* **24**, 1109 (1959).
[483] ČERNÝ, V., LÁBLER, L. and ŠORM, F., *Coll. Trav. Chim. Tchécosl.* **24**, 378 (1959).
[484] CHINN, L. J. and DODSON, R. M., *J. Org. Chem.* **24**, 879 (1959).
[485] CLINTON, R. O., MANSON, A. J., STONNER, F. W., BEYLER, A. L., POTTS, G. O. and ARNOLD, A., *J. Amer. Chem. Soc.* **81**, 1513 (1959).
[486] CUTLER, F. A., Jr., MANDELL, L., SHEW, D., FISHER, J. F. and CHEMERDA, J. M., *J. Org. Chem.* **24**, 1621 (1959).
[487] DODSON, R. M., NICHOLSON, R. T. and MUIR, R. D., *J. Amer. Chem. Soc.* **81**, 6295 (1959).
[488] DODSON, R. M. and TWEIT, R. C., *J. Amer. Chem. Soc.* **81**, 1224 (1959).
[489] DJERASSI, C. and BURSTEIN, S., *Tetrahedron* **7**, 37 (1959).
[490] DJERASSI, C., FORNAGUERA, I. and MANCERA, O., *J. Amer. Chem. Soc.* **81**, 2383 (1959).
[491] EDWARDS, J. and RINGOLD, H. J., *J. Amer. Chem. Soc.* **81**, 5262 (1959).
[492] EDWARDS, J. A., RINGOLD, H. J. and DJERASSI, C., *J. Amer. Chem. Soc.* **81**, 3156 (1959).
[493] EHMANN, L., HEUSLER, K., MEYSTRE, CH., WIELAND, P., ANNER, G. and WETTSTEIN, A., *Helv. Chim. Acta* **42**, 2548 (1959).
[494] EHRENSTEIN, M. and OTTO, K., *J. Org. Chem.* **24**, 2006 (1959).
[495] ERCOLI, A., GARDI, R. and DELLAMORTE, D., *Gazz. Chim. Ital.* **89**, 1382 (1959).
[496] FAJKOŠ, J. and ŠORM, F., *Coll. Trav. Chim. Tchécosl.* **24**, 766 (1959).
[497] FONKEN, G. S., HOGG, J. A. and MCINTOSH, A. V., Jr., *J. Org. Chem.* **24**, 1600 (1959).
[498] FRIED, J. H., ARTH, G. E. and SARETT, L. H., *J. Amer. Chem. Soc.* **81**, 1235 (1959).
[499] GOLD, A. M. and SCHWENK, E., *J. Amer. Chem. Soc.* **81**, 2198 (1959).
[500] GUAL, C., STITCH, S. R., GUT, M. and DORFMAN, R. I., *J. Org. Chem.* **24**, 418 (1959).
[501] HALPERN, O. and DJERASSI, C., *J. Amer. Chem. Soc.* **81**, 439 (1959).
[502] HECKER, E., *Chem. Ber.* **92**, 1386 (1959).
[503] HECKER, E., *Chem. Ber.* **92**, 3198 (1959).
[504] HECKER, E., *Naturwissenschaften* **46**, 514 (1959).
[505] HERZOG, H. L., GENTLES, M. J., CHARNEY, W., SUTTER, D., TOWNLEY, E., YUDIS, M., KABASAKALIAN, P. and HERSHBERG, E. B., *J. Org. Chem.* **24**, 691 (1959).
[506] HEUSLER, K., KEBRLE, J., MEYSTRE, CH., UEBERWASSER, H., WIELAND, P., ANNER, G. and WETTSTEIN, A., *Helv. Chim. Acta* **42**, 2043 (1959).
[507] HEUSLER, K., WIELAND, P. and WETTSTEIN, A., *Helv. Chim. Acta* **42**, 1586 (1959).
[508] HEUSSER, H., WOHLFAHRT, J., MÜLLER, M. and ANLIKER, R., *Helv. Chim. Acta* **42**, 2140 (1959).
[509] HIRSCHMANN, R., BAILEY, G. A., WALKER, R. and CHEMERDA, J. M., *J. Amer. Chem. Soc.* **81**, 2822 (1959).
[510] HOFFSOMMER, R. D., SLATES, H. L., TAUB, D. and WENDLER, N. L., *J. Org. Chem.* **24**, 1617 (1959).
[511] IRIARTE, J., DJERASSI, C. and RINGOLD, H. J., *J. Amer. Chem. Soc.* **81**, 436 (1959).
[512] JONES, E. R. H. and WLUKA, D. J., *J. Chem. Soc.* 907 (1959).
[513] KARADY, S. and SLETZINGER, M., *Chem. & Ind.* 1159 (1959).
[514] KAWASAKI, T. and MOSETTIG, E., *J. Org. Chem.* **24**, 2071 (1959).
[515] KINCL, F. A. and GARCÍA, M., *Chem. Ber.* **92**, 595 (1959).
[516] KIRK, D. N. and PETROW, V., *J. Chem. Soc.* 788 (1959).
[517] KISSMANN, H. M., SMALL, A. M. and WEISS, M. J., *J. Amer. Chem. Soc.* **81**, 1262 (1959).
[518] KRAYCHY, S., *J. Amer. Chem. Soc.* **81**, 1702 (1959).
[519] LÁBLER, L. and ŠORM, F., *Chem. & Ind.* 598 (1959).
[520] LARDON, A., SIGG, H. P. and REICHSTEIN, T., *Helv. Chim. Acta* **42**, 1457 (1959).
[521] LINDE, H. and MEYER, K., *Helv. Chim. Acta* **42**, 807 (1959).
[522] MAGERLEIN, B. J., *J. Org. Chem.* **24**, 1564 (1959).
[523] MANCERA, O. and RINGOLD, H. J., *Canad. J. Chem.* **37**, 1785 (1959).
[524] MARTIN, R. P. and TAMM, CH., *Helv. Chim. Acta* **42**, 696 (1959).
[525] MAZUR, R. H. and CELLA, J. A., *Tetrahedron* **7**, 130 (1959).
[526] MCKENNA, J., NORYMBERSKI, J. K. and STUBBS, R. D., *J. Chem. Soc.* 2502 (1959).
[527] MILLS, J. S., *J. Amer. Chem. Soc.* **81**, 5515 (1959).
[528] MILLS, J. S., BOWERS, A., CASAS CAMPILLO, C., DJERASSI, C. and RINGOLD, H. J., *J. Amer. Chem. Soc.* **81**, 1264 (1959).
[529] MUKAWA, F., *Tetrahedron Letters* No. 14, 17 (1959).
[530] NAGATA, W., TAMM, CH. and REICHSTEIN, T., *Helv. Chim. Acta* **42**, 1399 (1959).
[531] NATHAN, A. H., MAGERLEIN, B. J. and HOGG, J. A., *J. Org. Chem.* **24**, 1517 (1959).

[532] NUSSBAUM, A. L., CARLON, F. E., GOULD, D., OLIVETO, E. P., HERSHBERG, E. B., GILMORE, M. L. and CHARNEY, W., *J. Amer. Chem. Soc.* **81**, 5230 (1959).
[533] NUSSBAUM, A. L., POPPER, T. L., OLIVETO, E. P., FRIEDMAN, S. and WENDER, I., *J. Amer. Chem. Soc.* **81**, 1228 (1959).
[534] NUSSBAUM, A. L., TOPLISS, G. B., POPPER, T. L. and OLIVETO, E. P., *J. Amer. Chem. Soc.* **81**, 4574 (1959).
[535] OLIVETO, E. P., WEBER, L., FINCKENOR, C. G., PECHET, M. M. and HERSHBERG, E. B., *J. Amer. Chem. Soc.* **81**, 2831 (1959).
[536] OLIVETO, E. P., WEBER, L., PECHET, M. M. and HERSHBERG, E. B., *J. Amer. Chem. Soc.* **81**, 2833 (1959).
[537] PATTON, T. L., *Chem. & Ind.* 923 (1959).
[538] PATTON, T. L., *J. Org. Chem.* **24**, 1795 (1959).
[539] PETROW, V. and WILLIAMSON, D. M., *J. Chem. Soc.* 3595 (1959).
[540] RINGOLD, H. J., BATRES, E., BOWERS, A., EDWARDS, J. and ZDERIC, J., *J. Amer. Chem. Soc.* **81**, 3485 (1959).
[541] RINGOLD, H. J., BATRES, E., HALPERN, O. and NECOECHEA, E., *J. Amer. Chem. Soc.* **81**, 427 (1959).
[542] RINGOLD, H. J., RUELAS, J. P., BATRES, E. and DJERASSI, C., *J. Amer. Chem. Soc.* **81**, 3712 (1959).
[543] ROBINSON, C. H., FINCKENOR, L., KIRTLEY, M., GOULD, D. and OLIVETO, E. P., *J. Amer. Chem. Soc.* **81**, 2195 (1959).
[544] ROBINSON, C. H., FINCKENOR, L., OLIVETO, E. P. and GOULD, D., *J. Amer. Chem. Soc.* **81**, 2191 (1959).
[545] ROBINSON, C. H., GNOJ, O., CHARNEY, W., GILMORE, M. L. and OLIVETO, E. P., *J. Amer. Chem. Soc.* **81**, 408 (1959).
[546] ROBINSON, C. H., GNOJ, O. and OLIVETO, E. P., *J. Org. Chem.* **24**, 121 (1959).
[547] ROMO, J. and DEVIVAR, A. R., *J. Amer. Chem. Soc.* **81**, 3446 (1959).
[548] ROTHMAN, E. S. and WALL, M. E., *J. Amer. Chem. Soc.* **81**, 411 (1959).
[549] DERUGGIERI, P. and FARRARI, C., *J. Amer. Chem. Soc.* **81**, 5725 (1959).
[550] SCHAUB, R. E., ALLEN, G. R., Jr. and WEISS, M. J., *J. Amer. Chem. Soc.* **81**, 4962 (1959).
[551] SCHINDLER, O., *Helv. Chim. Acta* **42**, 1955 (1959).
[552] SCHNEIDER, W. P., LINCOLN, F. H., SPERO, G. B., MURRAY, H. C. and THOMPSON, J. L., *J. Amer. Chem. Soc.* **81**, 3167 (1959).
[553] SCHRÖTER, H., REES, R. and MEYER, K., *Helv. Chim. Acta* **42**, 1385 (1959).
[554] SENSI, P. and LANCINI, G. C., *Gazz. Chim. Ital.* **89**, 1965 (1959).
[555] SHAPIRO, E. L., STEINBERG, M., GOULD, D., GENTLES, M. J., HERZOG, H. L., GILMORE, M., CHARNEY, W., HERSHBERG, E. B. and MANDELL, L., *J. Amer. Chem. Soc.* **81**, 6483 (1959).
[556] SLATES, H. L. and WENDLER, N. L., *J. Amer. Chem. Soc.* **81**, 5472 (1959).
[557] SMITH, L. L. and HALWER, M., *J. Amer. Pharm. Ass.* **48**, 348 (1959).
[558] SOLLMAN, P. B., ELTON, R. L. and DODSON, R. M., *J. Amer. Chem. Soc.* **81**, 4435 (1959).
[559] SONDHEIMER, F. and BURSTEIN, S., *Proc. Chem. Soc., Lond.* 228 (1959).
[560] SONDHEIMER, F. and KLIBANSKY, Y., *Tetrahedron* **5**, 15 (1959).
[561] SONDHEIMER, F. and MECHOULAM, R., *J. Org. Chem.* **24**, 106 (1959).
[562] STICH, K., ROTZLER, G. and REICHSTEIN, T., *Helv. Chim. Acta* **42**, 1480 (1959).
[563] TAUB, D., HOFFSOMMER, R. D. and WENDLER, N. L., *J. Amer. Chem. Soc.* **81**, 3291 (1959).
[564] TURNBULL, J. H., *Chem. & Ind.* 515 (1959).
[565] TWEIT, R. C. and DODSON, R. M., *J. Org. Chem.* **24**, 277 (1959).
[566] TWEIT, R. C. and DODSON, R. M., *J. Amer. Chem. Soc.* **81**, 4409 (1959).
[567] USKOKOVIĆ, M. and GUT, M., *Helv. Chim. Acta* **42**, 2258 (1959).
[568] USKOKOVIĆ, M., GUT, M. and DORFMAN, R. I., *J. Amer. Chem. Soc.* **81**, 4561 (1959).
[569] VERLARDE, E., IRIARTE, J., RINGOLD, H. J. and DJERASSI, C., *J. Org. Chem.* **24**, 311 (1959).
[570] VILLOTTI, R., DJERASSI, C. and RINGOLD, H. J., *J. Amer. Chem. Soc.* **81**, 4566 (1959).
[571] VOLPP, G., BAUMGARTNER, G. and TAMM, CH., *Helv. Chim. Acta* **42**, 1418 (1959).
[572] VOLPP, G. and TAMM, CH., *Helv. Chim. Acta* **42**, 1408 (1959).
[573] VONWARTBURG, A. and RENZ, J., *Helv. Chim. Acta* **42**, 1643 (1959).
[574] WEISENBORN, F. L. and APPLEGATE, H. E., *J. Amer. Chem. Soc.* **81**, 1960 (1959).
[575] WENDLER, N. L., TAUB, D. and GRABER, R. P., *Tetrahedron* **7**, 173 (1959).
[576] WINTERSTEINER, O. and MOORE, M., *J. Amer. Chem. Soc.* **81**, 442 (1959).
[577] WOLFF, M. E. and KARASH, C. B., *J. Org. Chem.* **24**, 1612 (1959).
[578] ZDERIC, J. A., CARPIO, H. and DJERASSI, C., *J. Org. Chem.* **24**, 909 (1959).
[579] ZDERIC, J. A., CARPIO, H. and RINGOLD, H. J., *J. Amer. Chem. Soc.* **81**, 432 (1959).
[580] ZDERIC, J. A. and LIMON, D. C., *J. Amer. Chem. Soc.* **81**, 4570 (1959).
[581] ZDERIC, J. A., LIMON, D. C., RINGOLD, H. J. and DJERASSI, C., *J. Amer. Chem. Soc.* **81**, 3120 (1959).

FLUORESCENCE SPECTRA

JOSEPH W. GOLDZIEHER

From the Department of Endocrinology, Southwest Foundation for Research and Education, San Antonio, Texas

I. INTRODUCTION

SOLUTIONS of steroids can be made to fluoresce under a variety of circumstances, and this property has been widely used both for analytical and quantitative operations. Since the phenomenon of fluorescence is not only quite different, but also a great deal more complex than the property of absorbance, which is used in the same general manner, it is essential to have an understanding of its energy mechanism. Without this background, the development or application of fluorescence techniques will be frustrated by endless pitfalls, many of them quite unlike anything encountered in absorbance work. Moreover, the precise nomenclature of molecular physics has often been misused by those unfamiliar with the process of fluorescence emission and much confusion in terminology has resulted.

Excellent texts, both elementary[14, 52] and advanced[40] are available for an introduction into the field of fluorescence. The over-simplified, non-mathematical discussion of the subject in the following paragraphs will serve merely to introduce its application to problems of steroid chemistry.

Radiant energy (limited for our purposes to the ultraviolet and visible ranges) impinging on a solution may be absorbed either by the solvent or the solute molecules. In the former instance, a subsequent transfer of energy from the solvent to the solute molecules may take place. In the case of ultraviolet radiation directed at a solution of steroid in strong mineral acid, it is most probable that the solute molecules trap the energy directly, since their absorbance is generally far greater than that of the solvent. The absorption of a quantum of energy by a molecule takes place in an interval of the order of 10^{-15} sec. There follows a transition from the ground state of the molecule to a higher electronic energy level, and this process is usually accompanied by changes in the rotational and vibrational energy of the molecule as well. Such an excited molecule will return to the ground state after an average life of 10^{-8}–10^{-9} sec. First, the acquired rotational and vibrational energy is lost by collisional removal and then, from this lowest vibrational state, the excited molecule may make the transition from the higher electronic level to the ground state in a variety of ways. The absorbed quantum of energy may have been so large as to cause actual rupture of some of the intramolecular bonds. Dissipation of the absorbed energy by such a process is known as *predissociation.* The other mechanisms for the transition from the excited singlet state to the electronic ground state are (1) resonance radiation (in certain gases), (2) *internal conversion* or *internal quenching*—i.e., a radiationless transition to a second excited state, with conversion of electronic energy into vibrational energy, (3) collisional deactivation, also referred to as *external conversion, quenching,* or "*true*" *quenching,* (4) chemical reaction or (5) fluorescence. Thus, emission of fluorescence follows the removal of vibrational energy by collisions with other (e.g. solvent) molecules ; the transition from the higher electronic level to the ground state always occurs from the lowest vibrational state of the molecule and as a consequence the fluorescence emission is independent of the frequency of the absorbed energy within certain limits. Moreover, the energy of the emitted radiation is lower than that of the absorbed quantum under most conditions ; this is the Stokes effect. The intensity of fluorescence is therefore a function of the number of absorbed light quanta, irrespective of their wave length, and the energy distribution of fluorescence (fluorescence spectrum) is also independent of the excitation wave length. In those instances where various excitation wave lengths produce different fluorescence spectra, it is likely that several molecular species are present. A common error, however, is to irradiate a solution with a wave length which overlaps the true fluorescence spectrum of the solution ; by virtue of the Stokes effect, only that portion of the fluorescence spectrum will appear which has a longer wave length than the exciting radiation. This is obviously the reason why steroid-acid solutions will fluoresce with one color (e.g. " red ") when irradiated with the 546 mμ mercury line, but will display the entire fluorescence spectrum (" green ") when excited with 436, 405 or 365 mμ radiation.

Certain of the reactions which compete with fluorescence warrant further discussion. In the case of internal conversion or internal quenching, dissipation of the energy of the excited electronic state occurs within the molecule itself. *Concentration quenching* is a form of internal conversion which can occur in the presence of molecular aggregation, polymer formation: or similar phenomena. A collisional interaction between excited and unexcited molecules of the solute, with radiationless loss of the absorbed energy, is often referred to as *self-quenching*. Occasionally, other forms of internal energy transfer occur without the disappearance of the final radiation process. In the case of europium salicylaldehyde, for example, the organic portion of the molecule absorbs the energy but the emitted fluorescence is characteristic of europium. With gadolinium salicylate, the energy absorption and transfer go in the opposite direction. *External conversion* or *true quenching* occurs when the excited molecule loses its energy by collisional deactivation with a molecule of another species, such as a solvent or contaminant molecule. Thus the definition of quenching implies that the lifetime of the excited state is shortened. Many factors such as temperature, viscosity, pH, ionic strength, etc. may affect quenching. A contaminant which reacts with a potentially fluorescent molecule to produce another nonfluorescent molecule is not causing quenching. Likewise, a contaminant which absorbs some of the excitation energy is not causing quenching. The quenching process has been discussed in detail by numerous authors.[13, 14, 40, 44]

A number of factors may alter the emitted fluorescence radiation before it can reach a detecting device. There may be refraction, dispersion and scattering within the solution. The solvent, solute or a contaminant may trap some of the emitted radiation (converting it to thermal energy) in a manner determined by the absorption spectrum of that molecular species. This is an absorption phenomenon, and when it is due to the solute molecules it is referred to as *self-absorption*, a process entirely different from self-quenching. An example of self-absorption is seen in Fig. 1, where the fluorescence spectrum of a low concentration of corticosterone in sulfuric acid has been electronically amplified and superimposed on the fluorescence spectrum of a much higher concentration of the same material. The differences in the spectra

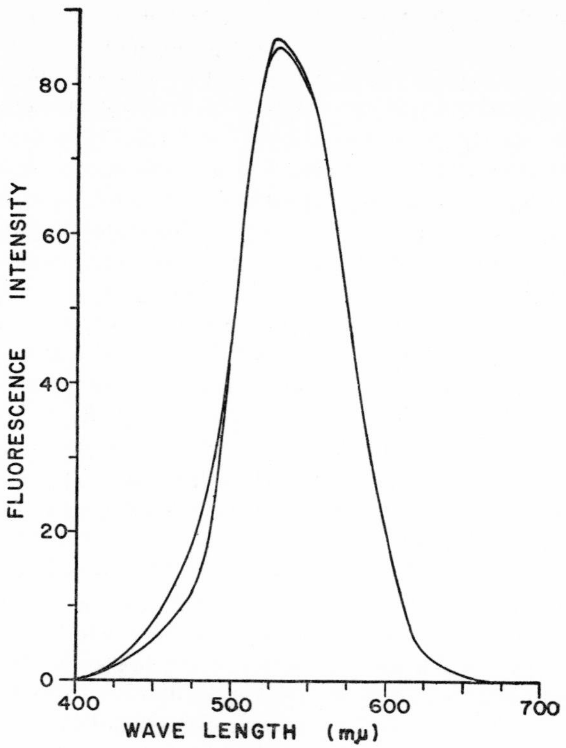

FIG. 1

Self-absorption of a solution of corticosterone in sulfuric acid. The upper curve is that of a high dilution of the steroid amplified to the peak intensity of the more concentrated solution. The lower fluorescence curve is that of the higher concentration, showing self-absorption in the 425–490 mμ region.

are confined to a narrow region corresponding to the absorption band of this solution. This is therefore a self-absorption phenomenon ; if self-quenching rather than self-absorption had occurred, the spectra would have been superimposable, but the total fluorescence emission of the two solutions would not have been in proportion to the two concentrations.

It is apparent, therefore, that the chemical and optical problems encountered in absorbance measurements are far simpler than those of fluorometry, and that the complexity of the energy exchange in fluorescence emission makes the influence of trace contaminants particularly important.

There are a number of important considerations in the instrumental applications of fluorescence. One of the major advantages of fluorometric techniques is their great sensitivity—sometimes two or three orders of magnitude higher than analogous colorimetric procedures. On the other hand, the shapes of the fluorescence spectra of steroid–acid solutions at ordinary temperatures generally vary less from one compound to another than do the absorption spectra. In most applications, therefore, instrumentation and methodology should be directed primarily at high sensitivity rather than at high resolution.

Since the fluorescence emission is proportional to the energy absorbed and is independent of the wave length of the exciting radiation (so long as the exciting wave length is shorter than the fluorescence spectrum), both the energy source and the absorption characteristics of the fluorescent molecule must be considered. In the event that the excitation source provides a uniform continuum, radiation at the wave length of maximum absorbance will give the optimum energy uptake. In using a xenon arc light source, this principle can be used as a starting guide. On the other hand, mercury vapor sources with a high yield in the 436 mμ region provide much more useful energy than is available from the xenon continuum, and from a practical point of view, the 436 mμ mercury line is the most satisfactory energy source for the excitation of steroid fluorescence, even though this wave length may not coincide with the wave length of maximum absorbance. It is also of great importance to make certain that none of the excitation spectrum overlaps the region in which fluorescence will be measured. Scattering of even a minute fraction of the exciting radiation will, if passed through the analyzing mechanism (filter, prism or grating), throw an overwhelming signal into the detector. This will vitiate entirely the inherent sensitivity advantage of the system, since sensitivity depends in part on the signal/noise ratio, and scattered exciting radiation is essentially high " noise ". Separation of the excitation wave length from the region of the fluorescence spectrum is often accomplished most easily by the use of a line spectrum such as that of mercury vapor, combined with an interference filter with high transmission at the high-energy wave length (e.g. 436 mμ) and very sharp cut-off immediately above. Often the wave lengths of maximum absorbance and peak fluorescence emission are much closer together than the selected mercury line and the wave length of peak fluorescence emission. Separation of the former pair requires a higher instrumental resolution than is usually available in commercial equipment. Another excellent method for excluding exciting radiation from the detector system (if the loss in excitation energy and sensitivity can be accepted) is to include a sheet of Polaroid in the filter system for the exciting radiation and a crossed Polaroid in front of the detector. This method has been used successfully by Slaunwhite and Engel in quantitative estrogen fluorometry. Obviously it cannot be used where the entire fluorescence spectrum is of interest, since the polarizing material has an absorption pattern of its own.

Both the total fluorescence output and the fluorescence spectrum itself are of interest in problems of steroid chemistry. For quantitative applications where maximum sensitivity is desirable, as much of the steroid fluorescence output as possible should be made available to the detector. This implies a wide-pass filter with maximum transmission at the peak fluorescence wave length, and a sharp cut-off at the lower end to exclude scattered exciting radiation. From the practical point of view, however, this may not be the ideal system. In the event that other, nonspecific fluorescence is also present and that this nonspecific fluorescence has a fairly constant intensity over the spectral range of the steroid fluorescence (as is seen with certain urinary extracts), a more selective filter system may be advisable. In a situation of this kind, the highest ratio of steroid fluorescence to nonspecific fluorescence exists at the wave length of peak steroid fluorescence emission, and a narrow-band filter such as an interference filter at this wave length will minimize the energy contribution of the nonspecific fluorescence, although at an obvious sacrifice of overall sensitivity. This is shown in Fig. 2.

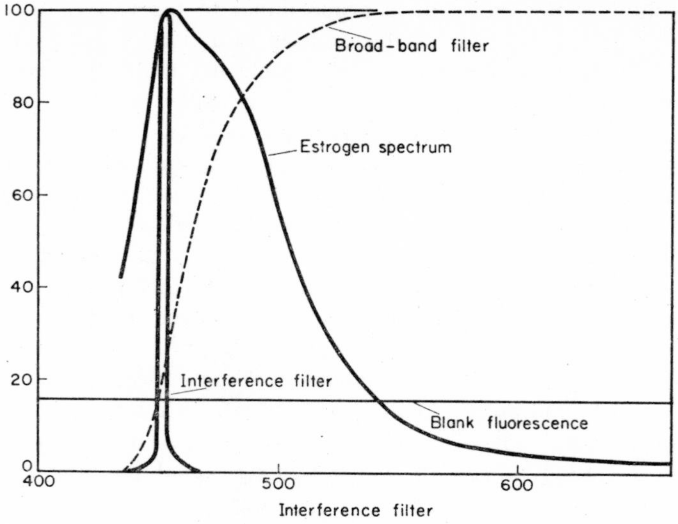

FIG. 2

The application of broad-band and interference filters to the problem of nonspecific fluorescence.

	Interference filter	Broad-band optical filter
Proportion of light due to estrogen	75 per cent	44 per cent
Ratio of estrogen fluorescence to blank fluorescence	3 : 1	0.8 : 1
Total estrogen fluorescence energy	4 units	680 units

Examination of the entire fluorescence spectrum is just as important for the development (or at times the application) of fluorometric methods as the absorption spectrum is for colorimetric procedures, and for much the same reasons. Unfortunately, commercially available spectrofluorometers are a relatively recent development, and have not attained the standards of resolution and stability at equivalent sensitivity that are available in many commercial spectrophotometers. This has prompted the development of many superb "home-made" instruments as well as modifications of commercial spectrophotometers for fluorescence work. A number of high-resolution and/or high-sensitivity recording spectrofluorometers have been designed.[1, 5, 26] The relation of the recorded fluorescence spectrum (seen through the "eye" of the instrument) to the true fluorescence spectrum presents essentially the same problems in resolution, sensitivity, detector response, recorder time-constant, etc. that are found in the recorded measurement of absorption spectra, and will not be discussed. However, the presence of scattered exciting radiation, and the need for irradiating the sample with an intense ultraviolet flux present difficult instrumental problems not encountered in absorption spectrophotometry. These questions have been discussed by Bowen and Wokes, Goldzieher *et al.*, Hercules and others.[14, 16, 26, 30]

In absorption spectrophotometry, the limit of sensitivity may be determined by the ability of an instrument to discriminate between two finite levels of light input. In fluorometry, however, it is theoretically necessary only to distinguish the finite input from zero. This means that, aside from the inherent noise of the instrument, the limiting factor to sensitivity becomes the " blank ", or nonspecific fluorescence in many instances. Needless to say, the standards of cleanliness, reagent purity, instrument care, and so forth required for fluorometric work far exceed those which are adequate for spectrophotometry, and many a " clinical " technic has foundered for neglect of these considerations. Variation of the properties of solvents and other reagents from batch to batch is very significant ; repurification is often essential, even in the case of concentrated sulfuric acid. This material can be freed of fluorescence by a simple and safe redistillation,[25] although batches may be found which have virtually no blank fluorescence. The source of manufacture may be important: Dupont sulfuric acid generally gives linear calibration curves with natural estrogens while Mallinckrodt acid generally does not.

By the same token, the best assurance for reliable results in the quantitative fluorometric determination of steroids is to have virtually pure material, thus eliminating, or at least minimizing problems of nonspecific fluorescence or quenching by contaminants. When this is impractical, various devices have been used to distinguish the steroid fluorescence from the nonspecific components. It has been shown in a few instances[8, 28] that the nonspecific fluorescence of certain urinary extracts was of approximately the same intensity in the ultraviolet and near ultraviolet regions as in the visible region where steroids fluoresce. Thus by making appropriate measurements on the recorded fluorescence spectrum, it was possible to subtract the nonspecific fluorescence from the steroid fluorescence. Whether this would be applicable to a variety of extracts (even though prepared in the same manner) is a moot question, and would require extensive experimental corroboration. Another method[6, 20, 45] which has been proposed for distinguishing steroid fluorescence from nonspecific fluorescence is based on the observation that steroids in strong acid show intense fluorescence when excited with 436 mμ radiation and much less under 365 mμ excitation, whereas the reverse is said to be true of the nonspecific fluorescence. This proposal, which appears to be questionable from the theoretical point of view, has not been supported by convincing published data. More recently, techniques have been devised for the differential quenching of steroid vs. nonspecific fluorescence. It can be shown that the fluorescence of pure steroids in strong acid solution is sensitive to the quenching action of nitrate,[37] or oxygen as in hydrogen peroxide.[31] The addition of 5 per cent by volume of 20 per cent hydrogen peroxide reduces the fluorescence of pure estrone in concentrated sulfuric acid to zero in an hour. More concentrated peroxide acts more quickly, but causes bubble formation and may increase the color of the solution. Peroxide may also produce new fluorescent species. It has been shown that the fluorescence of urinary extracts is decreased by peroxide, but to a much smaller extent than that of pure estrogen solutions. This small but significant decrease is generally ignored or attributed (without proof) to the presence of estrogen in the extract. The remaining fluorescence is then presumed to be nonsteroid. On this basis it is thought that the true steroid fluorescence can be measured by the difference in fluorescence intensity before and after the addition of such a quenching agent. It seems clear that this method, while giving some insight into the nonspecific fluorescence of a particular solution, raises new problems which in turn require further corrections.

Strickler *et al.*[46] have found that estrogen fluorescence developed in 0.1 ml 1 : 19 ethanol–toluene solvent and 0.5 ml 90 (weight) per cent sulfuric acid, heated 10 minutes at 100°, and diluted with 3.5 ml of 65 (weight) per cent sulfuric acid is less stable than estrogen fluorescence in stronger acid concentrations. On the other hand, the nonspecific fluorescence apparently remains constant over a period of 3–4 days. The logarithmic decay curve of the estrogen has been used to correct for the nonspecific fluorescence by repeated measurements of the same solution over a period of several days.

The problem of quenching has been approached in a variety of ways. One correction formula[16] is derived by analogy with the Stern–Volmer equation, and states that $R_0 = R_1 R_2 / 2(R_2 - R_1)$ where R_0 is the true fluorescence intensity and R_1 and R_2 are samples of the fluorescent solution, R_2 containing twice as much material as R_1. Another, more widely used technique is the internal standard method.[17, 32] In this procedure, known amounts of the pure steroid are added to one or more aliquots of the unknown material, and the quantity of unknown, corrected for quenching, derived by calculation or interpolation. The method assumes, of course, that there is a stoichiometric relation between the contaminant quenching and the steroid fluorescence. One additional advantage of the internal standard technique is that it corrects simultaneously for self-absorption of the solution. This method has, naturally, been combined with the quenching-by-peroxide maneuver for determination of nonspecific fluorescence in the same solution.

II. STEROID FLUORESCENCE

1. General

The conversion of a steroid into a fluorescent compound is usually brought about by reaction with a strong acid or base. A good deal is known about changes in the absorption spectrum which occur with changes in time and temperature when sulfuric or phosphoric acid are reacted with various steroids,[10, 38] and this subject is discussed in another chapter. A study of these as well as other data indicates that the formation of potentially fluorescent compounds in the steroid–acid interaction is an extremely complex phenomenon, involving among other things dehydration reactions, oxonium ion formation,[10, 36] etc. It has been shown that some of the fluorescent species produced in the reaction of corticosteroids and sulfuric acid are stable and can be isolated, whereas others dissociate upon decreasing the acid concentration.[33] The ease with which these dehydration reactions proceed has been used to distinguish stereoisomers, using either fluorometric or absorptiometric methods. Under very mild conditions, such as heating in 90 per cent formic acid, 1 μg estradiol-17α can be estimated in the presence of 100 μg estradiol-17β, and epitestosterone can be detected in an admixture with testosterone with like success.[12] Occasionally, intense ultraviolet radiation itself, at wave lengths below 313 mμ, can induce similar irreversible transformations into " lumisteroids ".[3]

The specificity of steroid fluorescence deserves some comment. It is quite true that only a limited number of steroids produce fluorescent molecular species with the reactions presently known and in use, and in this sense the fluorescence reactions have a degree of specificity. On the other hand, the fluorescence spectrum as determined by present day equipment has a far shorter spectral range than the absorption spectrum, and consequently there is less opportunity to observe individual differences between steroids. Whether the problems of self-absorption, quenching and nonspecific fluorescence, compared to the problems encountered in absorption spectrophotometry, make fluorescence more or less " specific " is a moot question.

2. Estrogens

Formic, phosphoric and sulfuric acids have been used to develop fluorescence with the C_{18} phenolic steroids. In general, formic acid is only weakly fluorogenic, and its chief advantage is in the differentiation by chromogenic as well as fluorescence reactions of stereoisomers such as estradiol-17α and -17β. Phosphoric acid has been used for the quantitative measurement of estrone (3-hydroxy $\Delta^{1,3,5(10)}$ estratriene-17-one) estradiol (3, 17β-dihydroxy $\Delta^{1,3,5(10)}$ estratriene) and estriol (3, 16α, 17β-trihydroxy $\Delta^{1,3,5(10)}$ estratriene).[15, 22, 23] It has been shown that the higher the density of the acid used, the more intense the fluorescence developed by heating the solution at 100° for 15–30 minutes. At room temperature, maximum fluorescence is reached in about two hours, but its intensity is much less than that produced by the 100° reaction. Phosphoric acid has the advantage that it does not produce chromogenic substances from the steroids or the contaminants in the solution as readily as sulfuric acid. However, the intensity of fluorescence in phosphoric acid is also less than in sulfuric acid, hence the advantage may be more apparent than real. Moreover, phosphoric acid fluorescence is influenced by moisture and sunlight.[15] A comparison of the fluorescence intensities of several natural estrogens in sulfuric and phosphoric acids has been made[28] and the figures are shown in Table I.

It is of some interest that phosphoric acid appears to be superior to sulfuric acid in the development of fluorescence with estradiol-17α, in contrast to the other three estrogens studied.

It is generally agreed that stable, optimum fluorescence of estrogens in sulfuric acid is produced by heating at 100° for 10–15 minutes. Estriol requires slightly longer—about 15–20 minutes. The fluorescence is stable for 24 hours or more with the higher concentrations of sulfuric acid, and there appears to be no particular advantage in developing fluorescence with 90 per cent acid and diluting with 65 per cent acid, as was done in the earlier studies. Estrogen fluorescence in more dilute sulfuric acid shows a logarithmic decay[46] over a period of several days.

For good reproducibility, it has been found advisable to have the steroid in solution before the addition of the acid reagent. This introduces a fluorescence-diminishing dilution factor, which should be kept to a minimum. It is also of great importance to have pure, nonfluorescing and nonquenching solvents. Most often ethanol or 1 : 19 ethanol–toluene have been used. The effect of solvent volumes is shown in the subsequent tables.

A great deal of effort has been devoted to studies of the optimum acid concentration. The reasons for discrepancies between the results of various workers have been discussed.[9] The most detailed study to date is that of Bauld and coworkers, and the data are shown in the following tables. Both absorbance and fluorescence data are given, since they are interrelated in terms of fluorescence efficiency. All fluorescence intensities are referred to a standard solution of 11.2 μg estrone (no ethanol solvent) in 3.0 ml 80 per cent v/v sulfuric acid, heated for 10 minutes in a boiling water bath. Spectra were determined in a spectro-fluorometer[26] using the optics and recording mechanism of a Beckman DK-2 spectrophotometer. The other estrogens studied were 9.6 μg estradiol-17β, 9.9 μg estriol, 9.4 μg 16-epiestriol (3, 16β, 17β trihydroxy $\Delta^{1,3,5(10)}$ estratriene), 9.6 μg 16α-hydroxyestrone (3 16α dihydroxy $\Delta^{1,3,5(10)}$ estratriene-17-one), 10.4 μg 16-ketoestradiol-17β (3, 17β-dihydroxy $\Delta^{1,3,5(10)}$ estratriene-16-one), 10.0 μg 16-ketoestrone (3-hydroxy $\Delta^{1,3,5(10)}$ estratriene-16, 17-dione), 10.0 μg 2-methoxyestrone per 3.0 ml acid. These results have been published in detail,[7] and a summary of the findings is shown in Tables II–XVII.

The most efficient conditions for production of fluorescence with each of these estrogens is shown in Table XVIII.

Of interest is the effect of various oxygen functions on the fluorescence intensity. 17-ketone, 17-hydroxyl or 16,17-diol configurations are highly fluorogenic, and under the conditions optimum for each steroid have about the same potency. A ketol configuration at the 16-17 position, however, decreases peak fluorescence tenfold, and the presence of a methoxy group to ring A virtually destroys all fluorescence. With estrone, estriol, 16-epiestriol and 16-keto estradiol-17β, an increase in acid concentration results in a reduction of the difference between the wave length of maximum absorbance and the wave length of maximum fluorescence emission.

It is to be noted that the highly fluorescent estrogens show maxima at about 480 mμ, whereas the less fluorescent ketols peak at about 530 mμ. The exception is estradiol-17β, which at high acid concentrations shows a double peak in both the absorption and the fluorescence spectra. The relative intensities of these two peaks change with changing acid concentration, and the alterations parallel each other in the absorption and fluorescence spectra. This is merely an illustration of the "mirror-image" relation of absorption and fluorescence curves.

Maximum absorbance occurs at about 455 mμ for the highly fluorescent estrogens. Theoretically, excitation at this wave length would be the most efficient, but practical considerations dictate otherwise. In the first place, available light sources which provide the ultraviolet continuum necessary for 455 mμ irradiation do not compare in intensity with those using the 436 mμ mercury line for excitation. Furthermore, complete separation of the fluorescence spectrum (from 470 mμ up) from an excitation spectrum at 455 mμ requires high resolution or a very narrow-band interference filter of unavoidably low transmission. Separation of the 436 mercury line from the fluorescence spectrum, on the other hand, can be accomplished at high efficiency with relative ease. Depending on the light source, excitation with a wave length longer than 436 mμ might have some advantage for the ketolic estrogens.

The application of fluorometry to mixtures of pure estrogens has been studied.[25] The fluorescence of estrone, estradiol-17β and estriol is additive. It can be seen from a comparison of the ordinates of Figs. 3a and 3b that 436 mμ excitation produces greater fluorescence, and that the estrone and estradiol-17β spectral curves cross at 470 mμ with 436 mμ excitation. With very careful selection of a 470 mμ interference filter, or by the use of a spectrofluorometer, these compounds can be shown to have equal and additive fluorescence. With 405 mμ excitation and measurement at 446 mμ (Fig. 3b) estrone and estradiol have very different fluorescence intensities, and estradiol-17β can be measured in a mixture with estrone and estriol with virtually no interference from the last two substances. This is illustrated by actual calibration curves in Fig. 4.

A variety of other estrogens have been examined for their fluorescence properties in sulfuric acid. The fluorescence intensities, measured with a 525 mμ filter after sulfuric acid development are shown in comparison to the major estrogens in Table XIX, col. A.[42,43] Several qualitative observations in an acetic acid–phosphoric acid reagent are shown in col. B.[11]

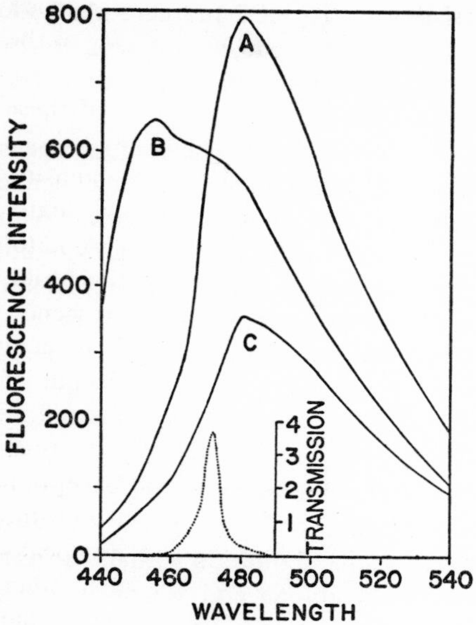

FIG. 3a

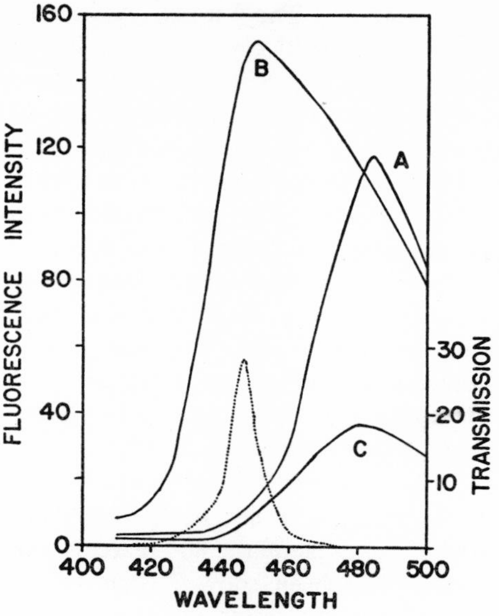

FIG. 3b

Fluorescence spectra of estrone (A), estradiol-17β (B) and estriol (C). At left is excitation with 436 mμ mercury line. Note equivalence of estrone and estradiol-17β fluorescence at 470 mμ. At right is excitation with 405 mμ mercury line. Note difference at 446 mμ of spectral intensity of estradiol-17β as compared to estrone and estriol. Dotted curves and right-hand ordinate indicate transmission curve of an appropriate interference filter for quantitative fluorometry.

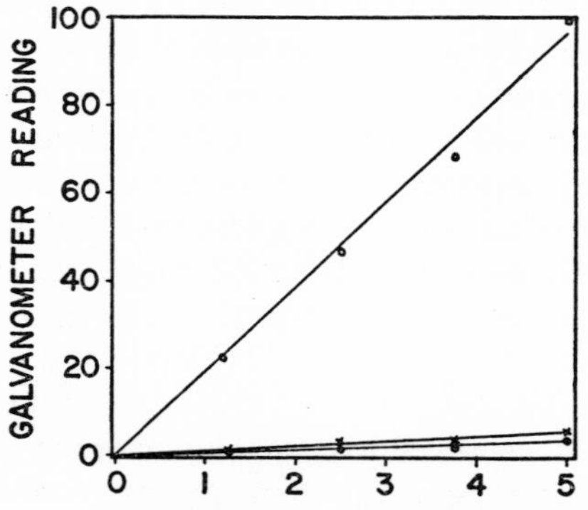

FIG. 4

Calibration curves of pure estrogens measured at 446 mμ with 405 mμ excitation. Estrone is indicated by X, estradiol by O and estriol by 0.

Recently, Touchstone *et al.*[49] have shown that $POCl_3$ (30 ml redistilled $POCl_3$ + 70 ml 88 per cent v/v sulfuric acid, heated with the estrogen for 30 minutes at 65°) produced a threefold increase of estrone and estradiol-17β fluorescence, and a twofold increase in estriol fluorescence. I_{max} for estrone and estriol was at 480 mμ and for estradiol at 490 mμ. Linear calibration curves could be obtained over the range 0.001 to 0.05 μg/ml. The method has not been applied to biological extracts.

Levine and Tao[35] noted that a reagent consisting of 0.5 ml 2 per cent alcoholic thiophene, 0.5 ml glacial acetic acid and 4 ml concentrated phosphoric acid, when reacted with the major estrogens produced maximal fluorescence with estriol, less with estradiol, and least with estrone—the reverse of the usual order.

Garst *et al.*[24] have shown that the phthaleins of the naturally occurring estrogens fluoresce when dissolved in (a) methanol acidified with HCl or (b) 9 : 1 glacial acetic acid/methanol. The fluorescence disappears fairly rapidly, even in the dark. With the more sensitive acetic acid–methanol system, 4.5 μg of estriol or 2.5 μg estradiol had the same fluorescence intensity as a standard 0.035 μg sodium fluoresceinate solution. It was noted that androsterone, dehydroisoandrosterone and cholesterol showed about 1/5 the fluorescence of estrone, while pregnanolone, cortisol or phenol showed little or no fluorescence.

3. C_{19} Compounds

The neutral C_{19} steroids show relatively low fluorescence intensities in concentrated (99 per cent) formic acid or 85 per cent phosphoric acid. With sulfuric acid, using the 80° reaction with 90 per cent acid and dilution with 65 per cent acid, it has been shown[29] that androsterone, etiocholanolone and isoandrosterone have the same order of fluorescence intensity as quinine in dilute sulfuric acid. Even so, these 17-ketosteroids showed far lower fluorescence intensities than the common estrogens, as seen in Table XX.

It would appear from an examination of these few steroids that the 3-hydroxy 17-keto compounds are much more fluorogenic than the 3-keto 17-hydroxyl or the 3,17 diketo types.

Levine and Tao[35] found that dehydroepiandrosterone fluoresced with a magenta color, while 11-hydroxy etiocholanolone fluoresced with a light green in their thiophene–glacial acetic acid–phosphoric acid reagent. No mention is made of the sensitivity of the reaction, and other compounds such as ergosterol, cortisone and hydrocortisone were also observed to fluoresce.

Clark and Haskell[19] noted that a 38 per cent solution of antimony trichloride in acetic anhydride–benzene produced a red fluorescence with testosterone, but none with dehydroepiandrosterone, Δ^4-androstenedione, or androsterone.

4. C_{21} Steroids

Of all the C_{21} steroids examined to date, only hydrocortisone, corticosterone, and one or two closely related compounds show fluorescence intensities which compare with those of androsterone and isoandrosterone; none approach one-tenth the intensity of optimum estrogen fluorescence. In one group of studies,[29] various compounds were heated with 90 per cent sulfuric acid, diluted with 65 per cent sulfuric acid, subjected to 436 mμ excitation, and examined spectrofluorometrically. The data are shown in Table 21.

In another study[47] the steroids were reacted with concentrated sulfuric acid at room temperature for 20 minutes, and the fluorescence intensity maxima found to lie between 530 and 545 mμ. The relative fluorescence intensities are shown in Table XXII.

Enhancement of the sulfuric acid fluorescence of steroids other than the estrogens has been described in a preliminary report.[48] 30 per cent $POCl_3$ in concentrated sulfuric acid was reacted with various steroids at room temperature or at 110° for

30 minutes. The room temperature reaction showed no increase in the fluorescence intensity of hydrocortisone or cortisone over sulfuric acid alone; corticosterone showed a slight improvement, but a loss of fluorescence with heating. Little change in the fluorescence spectrum appears to occur as a result of the addition of the $POCl_3$; it is stated that 436 mμ excitation did not appear to give optimum excitation for all the steroids tested, but this may have been a function of the light source used. The data are shown in Table XXIII. The increased fluorescence of Reichstein's compound S (17α, 21-dihydroxy Δ^4-pregnene-3, 20 dione), "S-glycol" (17α, 20, 21-trihydroxy Δ^4-pregnene-3-one), and aldosterone (11β-21-dihydroxy 18-aldo Δ^4-pregnene-3, 20-dione) are noteworthy.

The relatively high fluorescence intensity of certain of the corticosteroids has been noted by several workers.[21, 33, 39, 41, 47] Of interest is the fact that aldosterone has no fluorescence in "100 per cent" phosphoric acid heated to 100° for five minutes.[33, 34] The absorption and fluorescence spectra of hydrocortisone, corticosterone, cortisone and the tetrahydro derivatives of hydrocortisone and cortisone have been studied in polyphosphoric ("100 per cent") and 85 per cent phosphoric acids and in the 90+65 per cent sulfuric acid system.[27, 28] After demonstrating that the 436 mμ mercury line was the most effective excitation wave length from a xenon-mercury source, the fluorescence spectra were examined for maximum intensity. The results are shown in Table XXIV.

It is clear that sulfuric acid is the most satisfactory reagent except in the case of corticosterone, where polyphosphoric acid is seen to be superior. However, the practical difficulties of working with this highly viscous reagent cannot be ignored. Sulfuric acid has been investigated at various concentrations, and for two reaction conditions which are summarized in Table XXV.

It appears from these data that 70–80 per cent (v+v) sulfuric acid used at room temperature generally produced maximum fluorescence. For corticosterone, reaction for two hours at room temperature with 70 per cent acid represents the optimum conditions while for hydrocortisone, 80 per cent acid under the same conditions appears to be best. There seems to be no combination which will produce approximately equal fluorescence for corticosterone, hydrocortisone and the tetrahydro derivatives of hydrocortisone and cortisone. On the other hand, conditions can be developed where the two major adrenal secretory products, hydrocortisone and corticosterone, display about the same fluorescence intensity. The data are shown in Table XXVI and by projection it can be seen that reaction at 45° for 20 minutes produces the desired result. However, a considerable sacrifice of fluorescence intensity must be made, for under these conditions the fluorescence intensity of either steroid is about 60 (arbitrary) units, compared to 955 for corticosterone and 248 for hydrocortisone by the optimum individual procedures.

Peterson[39] has adapted the sulfuric acid fluorescence reaction for use in the measurement of corticosterone. Part of the problem is solved by extracting the steroid from biological material with 1:1 dichloromethane–carbon tetrachloride; this fairly selective solvent leaves a number of potentially fluorescent materials behind. The steroid is then extracted directly from pure dichloromethane into sulfuric acid, and fluorescence is allowed to develop at room temperature. Time studies of 9:1, 7:3 and 6:4 sulfuric acid–ethanol mixtures show that the 9:1 mixture develops a low but constant fluorescence level within an hour; 7:3 acid reaches $4\frac{1}{2}$ times as high a fluorescence intensity almost immediately but begins to fade rapidly after $1\frac{1}{2}$ hours ; 6:4 acid reaches a maximum fluorescence intensity in 6 hours, and begins to fade in almost linear fashion after 8 hours. Its peak intensity is somewhat higher than that of the 7:3 sulfuric acid–ethanol solution. It is stated that " no other steroids have been found that fluoresce under these conditions and also give the same time-intensity curves."

Silber *et al.*[41] used 30 N (about 84 per cent) sulfuric acid for the determination of corticosterone or hydrocortisone in plasma or rodent adrenal tissue. It is stated that 36 N acid yields no corticosterone fluorescence, but still develops the fluorescence due to nonspecific materials found in the plasma of adrenalectomized-hypophysectomized animals. Thus, the difference between aliquots developed with 30 N and 36 N acid is said to represent the fluorescence due to corticosterone alone.

Compared to 2 μg/ml of corticosterone, the following compounds showed essentially no fluorescence: cortisone, DOC, Compounds A, S and Reichstein's U (17α, 20β, 21-trihydroxy Δ^4-pregnene-11-one), tetrahydrocortisone and hydrocortisone, allodihydro-hydrocortisone (11β, 17α, 21-trihydroxy-allopregnane-3, 20-dione), 9α-fluoro hydrocortisone, prednisone (17α, 21-dihydroxy-$\Delta^{1,4}$ pregnadiene-3, 11, 20-trione) and prednisolone, (11β, 17α, 21-trihydroxy-$\Delta^{1,4}$ pregnadiene-3 20-dione), 9α fluoro-prednisolone, progesterone, 11β-hydroxy progesterone, testosterone and allodihydrotestosterone (17β-hydroxy etiocholane-3-one). Estradiol gave 32 per cent and estrone 10 per cent of the fluorescence of corticosterone.

5. Δ^4-3-ketosteroids

In 1952 Bush noted that paper chromatograms sprayed with sodium hydroxide showed a yellowish steroid fluorescence under ultraviolet (365 mμ) irradiation.[18] This reaction was specific for Δ^4-3-ketones in that no fluorescence was observed with Δ^1-3-ketones, Δ^8-7-ketones, Δ^{16}-20-ketones, $\Delta^{4,6}$-diene 3-ketones, $\Delta^{1,4}$-diene 3-ketones, $\Delta^{1,4,6}$-triene 3-ketones, Δ^5-7-ketones and $\Delta^{9(11)}$-12-ketones. Subsequently, Abelson and Bondy[2] found that 0.1–0.3 N potassium tert-butoxide could produce the alkaline fluorescence reaction in the liquid state in a satisfactory manner. In their reaction, 0.5 ml of the alkali reagent was allowed to stand for 1 hour at room temperature with the steroid. The solution was excited with 365 mμ radiation and the fluorescence measured at 580 mμ. The method was found applicable to testosterone, progesterone, and the biologically active corticosteroids, with a sensitivity of about 0.01 μg.

The fluorescence intensity at 580 mμ referred to a hydrocortisone standard and corrected for self-absorption and phototube response is shown in Table XXVII.

The following compounds showed no fluorescence in this system: cholesterol, tetrahydrocortisone, 11-hydroxy etiocholanolone, pregnanolone, dehydroepiandrosterone, Δ^1-3-ketones, $\Delta^{9(11)}$-12-ketones, $\Delta^{1,4}$- 3-ketones, estrone, estradiol, estriol, and pregnanediol.

A spray reagent for paper chromatography consisting of isonicotinic acid hydrazide in acid alcohol[51] has also been described as being specific for the Δ^4-3-keto configuration. There have been no reports to date of the adaptation of this reagent to fluorescence in solution.

6. Fluorescence on Solid Surfaces

Ultraviolet radiation is widely used for the localization and identification of steroid spots or zones on paper chromatograms. In some instances, the absorption of ultraviolet radiation by the steroid zone is of interest, in others the excitation of fluorescence. The latter phenomenon is frequently produced by applying strong acids or bases to the paper itself, and observing the result at room temperature or after heat treatment. In these respects the production of fluorescence is basically the same as that developed in solution, but there are many additional features to be taken into account when dealing with fluorescence on a surface. The paper itself, as well as its surface properties, have a considerable effect on the elicitation of fluorescence. The steroid spot or zone, moreover, represents a high concentration of steroid—usually far more than the quantities examined in fluorescent solutions. Self-absorption phenomena are consequently of great importance in the determining of the final " color ". Finally, chemical reactions between the paper and such corrosive reagents as fuming sulfuric acid introduce additional complexities. For these reasons fluorescence reactions on paper possess unique advantages and disadvantages. The color of fluorescence produced as the end-result of fluorescence + self-absorption + chromogens from the paper, etc. is quite characteristic and may readily distinguish steroids whose fluorescence spectra in solution are qualitatively identical. While on the one hand these factors are of value in qualitative applications, the quantitation of a reaction which depends on such variables as the surface texture of the paper, the chromogens and quenchers produced by sulfuric acid charring, etc. is not likely to extend far beyond estimation of the size and intensity of the spot. Devices have, however, been developed for the quantitation of alkali fluorescence on paper in the case of Δ^4-3-ketosteroids.[4]

TABLE I. RELATIVE ESTROGEN FLUORESCENCE INTENSITIES

	Observed fluorescence λ_{max}, in mμ	Observed I_{max}, rel. units	Relative phototube response, per cent	Corrected I_{max}	Corrected relative intensity, per cent
		SULFURIC ACID			
Estrone	480	800	73	1096	100*
Estradiol-17α	490	135	60	225	20.6
Estradiol-17β	455	645	96	672	61.3
Estriol	480	355	73	486	44.4
		PHOSPHORIC ACID			
Estrone	500	53	70	76	6.9
Estradiol-17α	493	315	76	414	37.8
Estradiol-17β	499	76	70	108	9.9
Estriol	520	13	61	21	1.9

Comparison of the fluorescence produced by the reaction of estrogens with sulfuric or phosphoric acid. Five micrograms of each estrogen, dissolved in 0.2 ml absolute ethanol, was reacted with (1) 5 ml 85 per cent phosphoric acid at 80°C for 10 minutes or (2) 1 ml 90 per cent (v/v) sulfuric acid at 80°C for 10 minutes, followed by dilution with 4 ml 65 per cent (v/v) sulfuric acid. Exciting wavelength was 436 mμ. The entire fluorescence spectrum was recorded and studied.

* This solution taken as the arbitrary intensity standard, = 100 units.

TABLE II. ESTRONE

Acid Concn. % v/v	Volume ethanol (ml) per 3 ml acid									
	0.0		0.05		0.1		0.2		0.4	
	λ_{max}	O.D.	λ_{max}	O.D.	λ_{max}	O.D.	λ_{max}	O.D.	λ_{max}	O.D.
50	—	—	—	—	—	—	—	—	—	—
60	458	0.110	458	0.225	458	0.221	460	0.157	460	0.083
70	455	0.221	456	0.509	457	0.490	457	0.195	458	0.270
75	455	0.533	455	0.238	457	0.531	456	0.215	457	0.355
80	454	0.513	454	0.234	456	0.469	454	0.215	456	0.210
88	451	0.371	452	0.171	452	0.182	453	0.405	453	0.220

Absorption characteristics of estrone in various concentrations of sulfuric acid, and various volumes of absolute ethanol as solvent. Wavelength of maximum absorption is indicated by λ_{max} and absorption by the symbol O.D.

TABLE III. ESTRADIOL-17β

Acid Concn. % v/v	Volume ethanol (ml) per 3 ml acid									
	0.0		0.05		0.1		0.2		0.4	
	λ_{max}	O.D.	λ_{max}	O.D.	λ_{max}	O.D.	λ_{max}	O.D.	λ_{max}	O.D.
50	462	0.019	—	—	463	0.008	459	0.004	—	—
60	458	0.146	458	0.148	458	0.160	459	0.123	460	0.098
70	456	0.205	456	0.204	456	0.205	457	0.184	458	0.150
75	455	0.202	455	0.211	455	0.222	456	0.198	457	0.156
80	454	0.184	454	0.213	455	0.188	454	0.201	456	0.175
88	454	0.086	454	0.099	454	0.118	454	0.121	454	0.127
88	428	0.182	428	0.181	428	0.171	428	0.182	430	0.143

Absorption characteristics of estradiol-17β in various concentrations of sulfuric acid, and with various volumes of absolute ethanol as solvent. Wavelength of maximum absorption is indicated by λ_{max} and absorption by the symbol O.D.

TABLE IV. ESTRIOL

Acid Concn. % v/v	Volume ethanol (ml) per 3 ml acid									
	0.0		0.05		0.1		0.2		0.4	
	λ_{max}	O.D.	λ_{max}	O.D.	λ_{max}	O.D.	λ_{max}	O.D.	λ_{max}	O.D.
50	—	—	—	—	—	—	—	—	—	—
60	448	0.041	~453	0.036	455	0.033	456	0.018	—	—
70	454	0.090	455	0.116	454	0.072	454	0.068	456	0.027
75	453	0.114	454	0.186	454	0.113	454	0.115	455	0.062
80	453	0.125	455	0.182	455	0.187	454	0.164	455	0.125
88	452	0.166	452	0.164	453	0.176	453	0.178	453	0.152

Absorption characteristics of estriol in various concentrations of sulfuric acid, and with various volumes of absolute ethanol as solvent. Wavelength of maximum absorption is indicated by λ_{max} and absorption by the symbol O.D.

TABLE V. EPIESTRIOL

Acid Concn. % v/v	Volume ethanol (ml) per 3 ml acid									
	0.0		0.05		0.1		0.2		0.4	
	λ_{max}	O.D.	λ_{max}	O.D.	λ_{max}	O.D.	λ_{max}	O.D.	λ_{max}	O.D.
50	—	—	—	—	—	—	—	—	—	—
60	458	0.068	457	0.069	459	0.068	458	0.049	460	0.024
70	454	0.206	455	0.240	456	0.220	456	0.215	457	0.122
75	454	0.240	455	0.261	454	0.218	455	0.224	457	0.157
80	453	0.290	454	0.229	454	0.294	454	0.279	457	0.198
88	451	0.163	452	0.188	451	0.208	453	0.197	453	0.201

Absorption characteristics of epiestriol in various concentrations of sulfuric acid, and with various volumes of ethanol as solvent. Wavelength of maximum absorption is indicated by λ_{max} and absorption by the symbol O.D.

TABLE VI. 16α-HYDROXYESTRONE

Acid Concn. % v/v	Volume ethanol (ml) per 3 ml acid: 0.0		0.05		0.1		0.2		0.4	
	λ_{max}	O.D.	λ_{max}	O.D.	λ_{max}	O.D.	λ_{max}	O.D.	λ_{max}	O.D.
50	Indef.	0.006	510	0.009					518	0.013
60	511	0.144	498	0.036					517	0.099
70	504	0.165	501	0.073					513	0.147
75	505	0.190	503	0.120	509	0.139	510	0.146	511	0.136
80	502	0.105	501	0.150					509	0.144
88	496	0.208	497	0.140					503	0.149

Absorption characteristics of 16α-hydroxyestrone in various concentrations of sulfuric acid, and with various volumes of absolute ethanol as solvent. Wavelength of maximum absorption is indicated by λ_{max} and absorption by the symbol O.D.

TABLE VII. 16-KETOESTRONE

Acid Concn. % v/v	Volume ethanol (ml) per 3 ml acid: 0.0		0.05		0.1		0.2		0.4	
	λ_{max}	O.D.	λ_{max}	O.D.	λ_{max}	O.D.	λ_{max}	O.D.	λ_{max}	O.D.
50	Indef.	0.004								
60	456	0.022	Indef.	0.020	Indef.	0.019	Indef.	0.018	Indef.	0.013
70	~456	0.019								
75	~460	0.022								
80	~460	0.019								
88	Indef.	0.021								

Absorption characteristics of 16-ketoestrone in various concentrations of sulfuric acid, and with various volumes of ethanol as solvent. Wavelength of maximum absorption is indicated by λ_{max} and absorption by the symbol O.D.

TABLE VIII. 16-KETOESTRADIOL-17β

Acid Concn. % v/v	Volume ethanol (ml) per 3 ml acid									
	0.0		0.05		0.1		0.2		0.4	
	λ_{max}	O.D.	λ_{max}	O.D.	λ_{max}	O.D.	λ_{max}	O.D.	λ_{max}	O.D.
50	~485	0.012	~485	0.009					—	—
60	488	0.082	494	0.069					498	0.040
70	485	0.110	503	0.113					510	0.053
75	495	0.134	503	0.147					507	0.074
80	499	0.140	502	0.172	504	0.173	505	0.141	507	0.091
88	495	0.146							502	0.160

Absorption characteristics of 16-ketoestradiol in various concentrations of sulfuric acid, and with various volumes of absolute ethanol as solvent. Wavelength of maximum absorption is indicated by λ_{max} and absorption by the letters O.D.

TABLE IX. 2-METHOXYESTRONE

Acid Concn. % v/v	Volume ethanol (ml) per 3 ml acid									
	0.0		0.05		0.1		0.2		0.4	
	λ_{max}	O.D.	λ_{max}	O.D.	λ_{max}	O.D.	λ_{max}	O.D.	λ_{max}	O.D.
50	Indef.	0.004								
60	492	0.084								
70	492	0.110								
75	488	0.103	490	0.116	491	0.111	492	0.109	493	0.086
80	488	0.104								
88	488	0.054								

Absorption characteristics of 2-methoxyestrone in various concentrations of sulfuric acid, and with various volumes of absolute ethanol as solvent. Wavelength of maximum absorption is indicated by λ_{max} and absorption by the symbol O.D.

TABLE X. ESTRONE

Sulfuric acid reagent			Volume of ethanol (in ml) per 3 ml acid									
Concn. % (v/v)	M	Sp.gr.	0.0		0.05		0.1		0.2		0.4	
			λ_{max}	I	λ_{max}	I	λ_{max}	I	λ_{max}	I	λ_{max}	I
50	7.44	1.398	—	—	—	—	—	—	—	—	—	—
60	10.91	1.569	488	39	488	59	485	55	490	42	490	23
70	12.85	1.656	483	88	484	117	485	106	485	69	485	66
75	13.66	1.686	483	105	483	100	485	113	485	77	485	95
80	14.17	1.720	481	100*	482	103	484	99	482	95	484	88
88	16.42	1.798	475	93	475	111	475	104	478	119	478	117

Characteristics of fluorescence spectrum of estrone in various concentrations of sulfuric acid, and with various volumes of absolute ethanol as solvent. Peak fluorescence wavelength indicated by λ_{max}, peak intensity (same wavelength) by I.

* This solution taken as the arbitrary intensity standard, = 100 units.

TABLE XI. ESTRADIOL-17β

Acid Concn. % (v/v)	Volume ethanol (ml) per 3 ml acid									
	0.0		0.05		0.1		0.2		0.4	
	λ_{max}	I	λ_{max}	I	λ_{max}	I	λ_{max}	I	λ_{max}	I
50	507	2	—	—	503	2	—	—	—	—
60	489	28	490	31	488	33	495	24.5	496	18
70	482	58	483	53	485	52	486	40.5	491	27
75	482	56	481	59	485	65	485	49	486	36
80	478	51	481	58	480	88	482	57	485	38
88	465	78	470	75	470	98	472	94	475	74

Characteristics of fluorescence spectrum of estradiol-17β in various concentrations of sulfuric acid, and with various volumes of absolute ethanol as solvent. Peak fluorescence wavelength is indicated by λ_{max} and peak intensity (same wavelength) by I.

TABLE XII. ESTRIOL

Acid Conc. % (v/v)	Volume of ethanol (ml) per 3 ml acid									
	0.0		0.05		0.1		0.2		0.4	
	λ_{max}	I	λ_{max}	I	λ_{max}	I	λ_{max}	I	λ_{max}	I
50	—	—	—	—	—	—	—	—	—	—
60	490	2	490	2	490	2	490	2	—	—
70	482	10	480	53.5	481	32	480	35	481	15
75	478	31	480	95.5	480	51.5	480	70	481	42
80	478	34	482	69	483	77	482	92	483	51.5
88	475	56.5	475	57	478	62	477	89	479	85

Characteristics of fluorescence spectrum of estriol in various concentrations of sulfuric acid, and with various volumes of absolute ethanol as solvent. Peak fluorescence wavelength is indicated by λ_{max} and peak intensity (same wavelength) by I.

TABLE XIII. EPIESTRIOL

Acid Concn. % (v/v)	Volume ethanol (ml) per 3 ml acid									
	0.0		0.05		0.1		0.2		0.4	
	λ_{max}	I	λ_{max}	I	λ_{max}	I	λ_{max}	I	λ_{max}	I
50	—	—	—	—	—	—	—	—	—	—
60	487	14	488	15	487	16	488	11	489	3
70	481	82	483	77	482	81	483	72.5	484	47
75	480	83	483	95.5	482	94	482	74	483	55
80	480	102	482	104	482	106	482	114	482	90
88	474	75	475	82	475	96	476	91	479	116

Characteristics of fluorescence spectrum of epiestriol in various concentrations of sulfuric acid, and with various volumes of absolute ethanol as solvent. Peak fluorescence wavelength is indicated by λ_{max} and peak intensity (same wavelength) by I.

TABLE XIV. 16α-HYDROXYESTRONE

Acid Concn. % (v/v)	Volume ethanol (ml) per 3 ml acid									
	0.0		0.05		0.1		0.2		0.4	
	λ_{max}	I	λ_{max}	I	λ_{max}	I	λ_{max}	I	λ_{max}	I
50	539	3	535	2					—	—
60	537	12.5	534	6					538	3
70	529	9.5	530	8					540	5
75	528	13	529	9	531	5	536	5	537	5
80	528	8	529	9					535	5
88	529	6	528	6.5					529	3

Characteristics of fluorescence spectrum of 16α-hydroxyestrone in various concentrations of sulfuric acid, and with various volumes of absolute ethanol as solvent. Peak fluorescence wavelength is indicated by λ_{max} and peak intensity by (same wavelength) I.

TABLE XV. 16-KETOESTRONE

Acid Concn. % (v/v)	Volume ethanol (ml) per 3 ml acid									
	0.0		0.05		0.1		0.2		0.4	
	λ_{max}	I	λ_{max}	I	λ_{max}	I	λ_{max}	I	λ_{max}	I
50	—	1								
60	518	7.5	520	6	521	6	522	5.5	522	4
70	—	2								
75	509	1.5								
80	510	1								
88	—	0								

Characteristics of fluorescence spectrum of 16-ketoestrone in various concentrations of sulfuric acid, and with various volumes of absolute ethanol as solvent. Peak fluorescence wavelength is indicated by λ_{max} and peak intensity (same wavelength) by I.

TABLE XVI. 16-KETOESTRADIOL-17β

Acid Concn. % (v/v)	Volume ethanol (ml) per 3 ml acid									
	0.0		0.05		0.1		0.2		0.4	
	λ_{max}	I	λ_{max}	I	λ_{max}	I	λ_{max}	I	λ_{max}	I
50	542	3	542	3	—	—	—	—	—	—
60	535	16	539	9	—	—	—	—	539	3
70	527	18	530	9	—	—	—	—	531	4
75	528	18	539	15	—	—	—	—	531	4
88	528	23.5	530	13	530	11.5	530	7	532	4
80	528	14							530	11

Characteristics of fluorescence spectrum of 16-ketoestradiol in various concentrations of sulfuric acid, and with various volumes of absolute ethanol as solvent. Peak fluorescence wavelength is indicated by λ_{max} and peak intensity (same wavelength) by I.

TABLE XVII. 2-METHOXYESTRONE

Acid Concn. % (v/v)	Volume ethanol (ml) per 3 ml acid									
	0.0		0.05		0.1		0.2		0.4	
	λ_{max}	I	λ_{max}	I	λ_{max}	I	λ_{max}	I	λ_{max}	I
50	—	1								
60	—	1								
70	—	1	—	0	—	0	—	0		0
75	—	1								
88	—	1								
80	—	1								

Characteristics of fluorescence spectrum of 2-methoxyestrone in various concentrations of sulfuric acid, and with various volumes of absolute ethanol as solvent. Peak fluorescence wavelength is indicated by λ_{max} and peak intensity (same wavelength) by I.

TABLE XVIII. THE RELATIVE FLUORESCENCE INTENSITIES OF 8 NATURAL ESTROGENS UNDER OPTIMAL ACID AND ETHANOL CONCENTRATIONS

Estrogen	Maximum fluorescence intensity	Peak wavelength $m\mu$	H_2SO_4 concn. % (v/v)	Amount ethanol, ml
Estrone	100	478	88	0.20
Estradiol-17β	117	470	88	0.10
Estriol	105	480	75	0.05
Epiestriol	139	479	88	0.40
16-Ketoestradiol	26	528	80	0.0
16α-Hydroxyestrone	14	528	75	0.0
16-Ketoestrone	9	518	60	0.0
2-Methoxyestrone	1	579	50	0.0

All solutions prepared by heating in a boiling water bath for 10 or 15 minutes. Excitation was with 436 $m\mu$ radiation. All values determined from measurements of recorded fluorescence spectrum, not by filter photometry. No correction for detector response was made.

TABLE XIX. FLUORESCENCE OF VARIOUS ESTROGENS

	A	B
Estrone	100	
Estradiol-17α	69	
Estradiol-17β	62	
Estriol	85	
3-Hydroxy-1,3,5(10)-estratriene (17-Desoxyestrone)	4	
3-Hydroxy-1,3,5(10)-estratrien-16-one (Estrone-16)	8	
3-Hydroxy-1,3,5(10)-estratriene-6,17-dione (6-Ketoestrone)	0	
3-Hydroxy-1,3,5(10)-estratriene-7,17-dione (7-Ketoestrone)	3	
16-Ketoestrone	8	
3,17β-Dihydroxy-1,3,5(10)-estratrien-6-one (6-Ketoestradiol-17β)	0	
16-Ketoestradiol-17β	17	
3-Methylestradiol-4,17	0	
17α-Ethinyl-3,17β-dihydroxy-1,3,5(10)-estratriene* (Ethinylestradiol)	9	orange
3-Hydroxy-1,3,5(10),7-estratetraen-17-one (Equilin)	14	pink
3-Hydroxy-1,3,5(10),6,8-estrapentaen-17-one* (Equilenin)	15	
3,17β-Dihydroxy-1,3,5(10),6,8-estrapentaen (17-Dihydroequilenin)	6	
3-Hydroxy-1,3,5(10),6,8-estrapentaen-16,17-dion	—	yellow-green
3-Hydroxy-1,3,5(10),6,8,14(15)-estrahexaen-16,17-dione	—	yellow-green

Fluorescence of various C_{18} steroids. Series A were prepared by heating 0.2 ml alcohol-toluene solution containing the steroid with 1 ml 90 per cent (v+v) sulfuric acid, and diluting with 6 ml 65 per cent (v+v) sulfuric acid. The final solutions contained 3-9 micrograms/ml steroid. Excitation was with 436 mμ radiation and fluorescence intensity was measured with a 525 mμ filter except for the steroids marked with an asterisk. Of the latter compounds, equilenin showed an I_{max} at 563 mμ, ethinylestradiol at 566 mμ. The steroids in series B were dissolved in 0.2 ml glacial acetic acid, to which was added 1.8 ml 88 per cent w/w phosphoric acid. Reaction proceeded at room temperature for one hour, after which the material was diluted with 3 ml acetic acid.

TABLE XX. FLUORESCENCE CHARACTERISTICS OF SOME C_{19} STEROIDS AND THEIR DERIVATIVES IN SULFURIC ACID

	Wavelength at peak intensity, mμ	I_{max} in relative units per μg
Reference 1: quinine	460	8.1
Reference 2: estrone	480	160
3α-Hydroxyandrostan-17-one (Androsterone)	485	8.1
3α-Hydroxyetiocholan-17-one (Etiocholanolone)	500	4.8
3β-Hydroxyandrostan-17-one (Isoandrosterone)	490	6.0
3β-Hydroxy-5-androsten-17-one (Dehydroisoandrosterone)	500	1.9
Androstane-3,17-dione	490	0.13
Etiocholane-3,17-dione	478	0.26
4-Androstene-3,17-dione	475	1.0
17β-Hydroxy-4-androsten-3-one (Testosterone)	500	0.47
17α-Hydroxy-4-androsten-3-one (Epitestosterone)	505	0.38
17α-Methyl-17β-hydroxy-4-androsten-3-one (Methyltestosterone)	520	0.54
17α-Methyl-3β,17β-dihydroxy-5-androstene (Methylandrostenediol)	530	1.1

TABLE XXI. FLUORESCENCE CHARACTERISTICS OF SOME C_{21} STEROIDS IN SULFURIC ACID

Compound	Wavelength at peak intensity, mμ	I_{max} in relative units per μg
Reference 1: quinine	460	8.1
Reference 2: estrone	480	160
Pregnane-3α,20α-diol	510	3.3
3β-Hydroxyallopregnan-20-one	500	2.3
3β-Hydroxy-5-pregnen-20-one (Pregnenolone)	500	2.1
Pregnane-3,20-dione	510	0.30
Allopregnane-3,20-dione	510	0.11
17α-Hydroxy-4-pregnene-3,20-dione (17-Hydroxyprogesterone)	520	0.048
17α,20ξ-Dihydroxy-4-pregnen-3-one	520	0.80
21-Hydroxy-4-pregnen-3,20-dione (DOC)	520	1.1
17α,20,21-Trihydroxy-4-pregnen-3-one	520	1.4
17α,21-Dihydroxy-4-pregnene-3,20-dione	520	0.48
21-hydroxy-4-pregnene-3,11,20-trione (Compound A)	558	0.80
11,21-Dihydroxy-4-pregnene-3,20-dione (Corticosterone)	470	10.0
17α,21-Dihydroxy-4-pregnene-3,11,20-trione (Cortisone)	550	0.44
11β,17α,21-trihydroxy-4-pregnene-3,20-dione (Hydrocortisone)	490	6.0

TABLE XXII. FLUORESCENCE CHARACTERISTICS OF C_{21} STEROIDS IN SULFURIC ACID

Compound	I_{max}
Reference 1: estrone	31
Reference 2: estradiol	106
Reference 3: testosterone	0.5
Reference 4: 4-Androstene-3-17-dione	1.6
Progesterone	0.8
Pregnane-3α,20α-diol	4.5
11-Hydroxy-4-pregnene-3,20-dione	4.1
17α-Hydroxy-4-pregnene-3,20-dione	0.6
21-acetoxyallopregnane-3,20-dione	0.5
3α,21-Diacetoxyallopregnan-3-one	7.5
12-Hydroxy-21-acetoxy-4-pregnene-3,20-dione	15
12-Hydroxy-21-acetoxypregnane-3,20-dione	32
21-Hydroxy-4-pregnene-3,20-dione (DOC)	4.5
21-Hydroxy-4-pregnene-3,11,20-trione (Compound A)	0.8
11β,21-Dihydroxy-4-pregnene-3,20-dione (Corticosterone)	87
11α,21-Dihydroxy-4-pregnene-3,20-dione	88
3α,11β-Dihydroxy-21-acetoxy-pregnan-20-one (Tetrahydro-B-acetate)	14.6
17α,21-Dihydroxy-4-pregnene-3,11,20-trione (Cortisone)	7.0
17α,21-Dihydroxy-4-pregnene-3,20-dione (Compound S)	12.5
11β,17α,21-Trihydroxy-4-pregnene-3,20-dione (Hydrocortisone)	100
11α,17α,21-Trihydroxy-4-pregnene-3,20-dione	100
11β,17α,21-Trihydroxypregnane-3,20-dione	5.0
3α,11β,17α,21-Tetrahydroxypregnan-20-one (Tetrahydro F)	14.3
11β,17α,20β,21-Tetrahydroxy-4-pregnen-3-one	80
17α,-hydroxy-20β,21-diacetoxy-4-pregnen-3-one	3.2

TABLE XXIII. PHOSPHORYL CHLORIDE ENHANCEMENT OF SULFURIC ACID FLUORESCENCE

Compound	Excitation wavelength, mμ	Wavelength of maximum fluorescence,	Intensity, arbitrary units/μg	Intensity, for con. H_2SO_4 without $POCl_3$
	Room temperature reaction			
17α,21-Hydroxy 4-pregnene-3,20-dione	460	510	7.2	0.88
17α,20β,21-Hydroxy-4-pregnen-3-one	450	500	8.0	1.6
dl-Aldosterone	450	510	11.2	8.0
Corticosterone	460	510	21.6	16.0
Cortisone	410	480	1.5	4.0
Hydrocortisone	460	510	32.0	48.0
	Heated at 110°C for 30 minutes			
Estrone	440	480	150	80
Androsterone	450	490	8.0	2.2
Progesterone	460	520	3.0	2.0
Testosterone	460	515	2.7	2.4
Digitoxin	460	510	120	6.4

TABLE XXIV. FLUORESCENCE EFFICIENCY OF VARIOUS ACIDS WITH BIOLOGICALLY IMPORTANT CORTICOSTEROIDS

Compound	Sulfuric acid (90% + 65%)	Polyphosphoric acid	85% phosphoric acid
Corticosterone	100*	135	80
Hydrocortisone	100*	88	69
Cortisone	100*	42	12
Tetrahydro-hydrocortisone	100*	61	62
Tetrahydrocortisone	100*	21	8

Table XXIV. Steroids dissolved in 0.2 ml ethanol. One group heated with 1 ml 90 per cent sulfuric acid at 80°C for 20 minutes, cooled and diluted with 4 ml 65 per cent sulfuric acid. Other groups were heated for the same interval with 5 ml aliquots of concentrated (85 per cent) phosphoric acid or polyphosphoric acid (79 gm phosphorus pentoxide in 100 ml concentrated phosphoric acid). Intensities were determined at peak fluorescence wavelength by spectrofluorometry.

* Arbitrary intensity setting for each steroid.

TABLE XXV. FLUORESCENCE EFFICIENCY OF VARIOUS CONCENTRATIONS OF SULFURIC ACID

Compound	Acid Concentration							
	90% (v. + v.)		80%		70%		60%	
	Intensity, arbitrary units	Wave length, mμ	Intensity	Wave length, mμ	Intensity	Wave length, mμ	Intensity	Wave length, mμ
A. Development in sulfuric acid at 23° C for 120 minutes								
Corticosterone	258	525	535	525	955	525	60	525
Hydrocortisone	210	532	248	530	210	526	34	—
Cortisone	8	—	5	—	2	—	2	—
Tetrahydro-hydrocortisone	74	525	58	525	38	525	19	—
Tetrahydrocortisone	25	525	6	—	2	—	1	—
B. Development in sulfuric acid at 100° C for 20 minutes								
Corticosterone	41	540	40	537	50	530	121	530
Hydrocortisone	100*	537	76	530	28	525	69	526
Cortisone	10	545	5	—	3	—	2	—
Tetrahydro-hydrocortisone	46	525	44	525	32	525	28	525
Tetrahydrocortisone	47	525	33	525	20	525	14	525

* Arbitrary intensity standard, identical for A and B.

TABLE XXVI. RELATIVE FLUORESCENCE INTENSITY OF HYDROCORTISONE AND CORTICOSTERONE IN 80 PER CENT SULFURIC ACID UNDER VARIOUS CONDITIONS OF REACTION TIME AND TEMPERATURE

	23° C for 120 min.		40° C for 20 min.		60° C for 20 min.		80° C for 20 min.		100° C for 20 min.	
Compound	I_{max}	mμ	I	mμ	I	mμ	I	mμ	I	mμ
Corticosterone	100*	525	77	525	21	525	12	525	12	530
Hydrocortisone	58	528	55	530	32	530	29	525	24	537

* Arbitrary intensity standard.

TABLE XXVII. FLUORESCENCE OF Δ^4-3-KETOSTEROIDS IN POTASSIUM-BUTOXIDE REAGENT

Compound	I_{max}
Reference 1: quinine 0.1 μg/ml.	28.3
Reference 2: hydrocortisone	100 (arbitrary standard)
Testosterone	60.1
Progesterone	54.1
11-Desoxycorticosterone (DOC)	62.8
11-Dehydrocorticosterone	74.8
Corticosterone	62.8
Cortisone	66.1
Cortisone acetate	57.3

Other steroids showing the same order of fluorescence intensity, but exact values not determined:
4-Androstenedione
17α,20β,21-Trihydroxy-4-pregnen-3-one
17α,21-Diacetoxy-4-pregnene-3,20-dione
11-Desoxycorticosterone acetate
Aldosterone

Compounds showing 10–30 per cent of the fluorescence intensity of cortisone:
3β-Acetoxy-5-cholesten-7-one
3-Hydroxy-8(9)-22-ergostadien-7-one

Compounds showing 1–3 per cent of the fluorescence intensity of cortisone:
Androstan-3-17-dione
3α-Hydroxyetiocholane-11,17-dione
Dihydrocortisone

Note added in proof

Since the completion of this chapter, a number of interesting and important developments in steroid fluorescence have taken place. It has been shown[53] that the sensitivity and specificity of the Kober reaction for estrogens can be greatly improved by extracting the chromogen with a halogenated hydrocarbon solvent (chloroform, tetrachloroethane, tetrabromoethane) containing 2 per cent (w/v) *p*-nitrophenol. This procedure has proved useful for both colorimetric and fluorometric techniques. *p*-Nitrophenol in tetrabromoethane[54] containing 1 per cent ethanol produces the highest fluorescence intensity of any of the halogenated solvents tested ; it also extracts less chromogenic background material than any of the chlorinated solvents. The absorbance maximum of these solutions is in the region of 530–545 mμ ; as a consequence, excitation wavelengths in this region (for example, the 547 mμ mercury line) have been used. There are no published data on the practicality (as differentiated from the efficiency) of excitation with lower wavelengths. Studies of the excitation spectrum in this region have shown similar curves for estrone, estradiol-17β, estriol, 16-epiestriol, 16-ketoestradiol-17β, 2-methoxyestrone, and the 3-methyl ether of estrone. Peak excitation wavelengths from 537 mμ to "slightly over" 540 mμ have been reported by various workers.[54,55,56] The fluorescence spectra are also quite similar, with peak intensities at 549–551 mμ for all the estrogens mentioned above.[55] Others[56] have found a peak at 560 mμ for estrone and estradiol-17β, and at 555 mμ for estriol. It is quite apparent that the excitation and fluorescence maxima are so close together that serious instrumental problems are likely to arise if measurements are made at the theoretical optima. Various compromises in filter choice and fluorometric techniques have been made to circumvent this problem. There are few published data regarding the relative fluorescence intensities of the various estrogens. Estrone appears to yield somewhat higher values than estradiol-17β and estriol, which are about equal. Of considerable interest is the report[56] that 2-methoxyestrone has the same order of fluorescence intensity as the other estrogens by this method, in contrast to its poor intensity in classical sulfuric or phosphoric acid preparations. There is no consistency in the available reports as to the relative advantages of chloroform vs. tetrabromoethane with regard to the stability of the fluorescence. However, it is generally agreed that the fluorescence is both more stable and more intense at 0–4° C than at room temperature. The intensity lost during warming can be restored by re-cooling the sample. Ittrich[54] and Stoa[56] found no loss of fluorescence intensity for periods of 15–60 minutes with tetrabromoethane in the dark and under refrigeration, while Strickler *et al.*[55] found irreversible losses which were worse with tetrabromoethane than with chloroform. The various modifications of this solvent-extraction procedure have increased the sensitivity of the colorimetric Kober reaction 11–14 times with pure steroids and about half as much with urine extracts.[57] Fluorometric measurement of the *p*-nitrophenol-solvent extract increases the sensitivity about tenfold over colorimetry, and quantities of 0.025 μg of estriol in a urinary extract have been measured with an error of $\pm$13 per cent.[56]

The phenomenon of alkali fluorescence has been used in a novel way to increase the fluorescence of certain steroids. Pretreatment with 2N methanolic potassium hydroxide at 60° C for 30 minutes, followed by the usual sulfuric acid reaction to produce fluorescence, has been shown to increase the normally low fluorescence intensity of progesterone approximately 4 times, that of 17α-hydroxyprogesterone

5 times, testosterone twofold, and androstane-3, 17-dione (*sic*) 30 times. Other compounds tested, such as various estrogens, progesterone metabolites and corticosteroids were unfavorably affected by this treatment.[58]

Another method of correcting for nonspecific fluorescence has been proposed.[59] In the determination of corticosterone in tissue or plasma, fluorescence has been shown to be a linear function of the amount of extract used. A line drawn through values for several aliquots of different size may be extrapolated to the ordinate of the plot, and the value of the intercept used as a measure of blank fluorescence (cf. also p 300, Silber *et al.*[41]).

III. REFERENCES

1 AITKEN, E. H. and PREEDY, J. R. K., *J. Endocrin.* **9**, 251 (1953).
2 ABELSON, D. and BONDY, P. K., *Arch. Biochem. Biophys.* **57**, 208 (1955).
3 ARRHENIUS, S., *Acta Chem. Scand.* **10**, 154 (1956).
4 AYRES, P. J., SIMPSON, S. and TAIT, J. F., *Biochem. J.* **65**, 647 (1957).
5 BARTHOLOMEW, R. J., DALGLEISH, C. E. and WOOTTON, O. P., *Biochem. J.* **65**, 27P (1957).
6 BATES, R. W. and COHEN, H., *Endocrinology* **47**, 166 (1950).
7 BAULD, W. S., GIVNER, M., ENGEL, L. L. and GOLDZIEHER, J. W., *Canad. J. Biochem. and Physiol.* **38**, 213 (1960).
8 BAULD, W. S. and GOLDZIEHER, J. W. (unpublished studies).
9 BAULD, W. S. and GREENWAY, R. M., *Methods of Biochemical Analysis* Vol. 5, p. 337. Interscience, New York (1957).
10 BERNSTEIN, S. and LENHARD, R. H., *J. Org. Chem.* **18**, 1146 (1953).
11 BOSCOTT, R. J., *Nature, Lond.* **162**, 577 (1948).
12 BOSCOTT, R. J., *Nature, Lond.* **164**, 140 (1949).
13 BOWEN, E. J., *Quart. Rev. Chem. Soc., Lond.* **1**, 1 (1947).
14 BOWEN, E. J. and WOKES, F., *Fluorescence of solutions.* Longmans & Green, New York (1953).
15 BRAUNSBERG, H., *J. Endocrin.* **8**, 11 (1952).
16 BRAUNSBERG, H. and OSBORN S. B., *Anal. Chim. Acta* **6**, 84 (1951).
17 BRAUNSBERG, H., OSBORN, S. B. and STERN, M. I., *J. Endocrin.* **11**, 177 (1954).
18 BUSH, I. E., *Biochem. J.* **50**, 370 (1952).
19 CLARK, L. C. and HASKELL, T., *Science* **107**, 429 (1948).
20 FINKELSTEIN, M., *Nature, Lond.* **168**, 830 (1951).
21 FINKELSTEIN, M., *Nature, Lond.* **169**, 929 (1952).
22 FINKELSTEIN, M., *Acta Endocr.* **10**, 149 (1952).
23 FINKELSTEIN, M., HESTRIN, S. and KOCH, W., *Proc. Soc. Exp. Biol. Med.* **64**, 64 (1947).
24 GARST, J. B., NYC, J. F., MARON, D. M. and FRIEDGOOD, H. B., *J. Biol. Chem.* **186**, 119 (1950).
25 GOLDZIEHER, J. W., *Endocrinology* **53**, 527 (1953).
26 GOLDZIEHER, J. W., BAULD, W. S., ENGEL, L. L. and GIVNER, M., *Canad. J. Biochem. and Physiol,* **38**, 233 (1960).
27 GOLDZIEHER, J. W. and BESCH, P. K., *Analyt. Chem.* **30**, 962 (1958).
28 GOLDZIEHER, J. W., BODENCHUK, J. M. and NOLAN, P., *J. Biol. Chem.* **199**, 621 (1952).
29 GOLDZIEHER, J. W., BODENCHUK, J. M. and NOLAN, P., *Analyt. Chem.* **26**, 853 (1954).
30 HERCULES, D. M., *Science* **21**, 1242 (1957).
31 HEUSGHEM, C., *Nature, Lond.* **173**, 1043 (1954).
32 HEUSGHEM, C. and LEJEUNE, G., *Ann. Endocr.* **13**, 479 (1952).
33 KALANT, H., *Biochem. J.* **69**, 79 (1958).
34 KALANT, H., *Biochem. J.* **69**, 93 (1958).
35 LEVINE, V. E. and TAO, A. H., *Federation Proc.* **12**, 238 (1953).
36 LINFORD, J. H., *Canad. J. Biochem. and Physiol.* **35**, 299 (1957).
37 MCANALLY, J. S. and HAUSMAN, E. R., *J. Lab. Clin. Med.* **44**, 647 (1954).
38 NOWACZYNSKI, W. J. and STEYERMARK, P. R., *Arch. Biochem. Biophys.* **58**, 453 (1955).
39 PETERSON, R. E., *J. Biol. Chem.* **225**, 25 (1957).
40 PRINGSHEIM, P., *Trans. Faraday Soc.* **35**, 28 (1939).
41 SILBER, R. H., BUSCH, R. D. and OSLAPAS, R., *Clin. Chem.* **4**, 278 (1958).
42 SLAUNWHITE, W. R., ENGEL, L. L., OLMSTED, P. C. and CARTER, P. C., *J. Biol. Chem.* **191**, 627 (1951).
43 SLAUNWHITE, W. R., ENGEL, L. L., SCOTT, J. F. and HAM, C. L., *J. Biol. Chem.* **201**, 615 (1953).
44 STEVENS, B., *Chem. Revs.* **57**, 439 (1957).

[45] STRICKLER, H., GRAUER, R. C. and CAUGHEY, M. R., *Arch. Biochem. Biophys.* **64**, 88 (1956).
[46] STRICKLER, H. S., GRAUER, R. C. and CAUGHEY, M. R., *Analyt. Chem.* **28**, 1240 (1956).
[47] SWEAT, M. L., *Analyt. Chem.* **26**, 773 (1954).
[48] TOUCHSTONE, J. C., KEISMAN, R. A., MARCANTONIO, A. F. and GREENE, J. W., *Analyt. Chem.* **30**, 1707 (1958).
[49] TOUCHSTONE, J. C., GREENE, J. W., and KUKOVETZ, W. R., *Analyt. Chem.* **31**, 1693 (1959).
[50] UMBERGER, E. J. and CURTIS, J. M., *J. Biol. Chem.* **178**, 275 (1949).
[51] WEICHSELBAUM, T. E. and MARGRAF, H., *J. Clin. Endocrin. and Metab.* **17**, 959 (1957).
[52] WEST, W., *Techniques of Organic Chemistry* Vol. 9, Ch. 6. Interscience, New York (1956).
[53] ITTRICH, G., *Ztschr. Physiol. Chem.* **321**, 1 (1958).
[54] ITTRICH, G., *Acta Endocrinol.* **35**, 34 (1960).
[55] STRICKLER, H. S., WILSON, G. A. and GRAUER, R. C., *Anal. Biochem.* **2**, 486 (1961).
[56] STOA, K. F. and THORSEN, T., *Acta Endocrinol.* **41**, 481 (1962).
[57] SALOKANGAS, R. A. and BULBROOK, R. D., *J. Endocrinol.* **22**, 47 (1961).
[58] TOUCHSTONE, J. C. and MURAWEC, T., *Analyt. Chem.* **32**, 822 (1960).
[59] MONCLOA, F., PERON, F. G. and DORFMAN, R. I., *Endocrinol.* **65**, 717 (1959).

ABSORPTION SPECTRA IN CONCENTRATED SULFURIC ACID

LELAND L. SMITH AND SEYMOUR BERNSTEIN

From the Lederle Laboratories, A Division of American Cyanamid Co., Pearl River, N.Y.

I. INTRODUCTION

THE use of strong acids to obtain coloration and fluorescence with a variety of types of steroids dates back many years, and several recent papers cover certain review aspects of the field.[53, 69, 74] Use of strong acids in the study of selective absorption spectra of steroids is a more recent development. Current interest in the study of selective absorption spectra of steroids in concentrated sulfuric acid finds its origin in the initial work of Zaffaroni[137] published in 1950. In the past decade absorption spectra in concentrated sulfuric acid of over four hundred steroids have been recorded, and the technique is well established in the laboratories of steroid biochemists.

The present review will deal exclusively with selective absorption spectra of steroids in concentrated sulfuric acid without heating. The many variants of technique requiring addition of excess sulfur trioxide,[3] thiophen,[71] diphenylamine,[35] thiol compounds,[19] anthrone,[55] phosphorus pentoxide,[124] phosphoryl chloride,[131] dilution with water or alcohols,[69, 73–76] etc., combined with special heating and timing procedures will not be covered. For certain classes of steroids these procedures have become of special importance, to the exclusion of use of concentrated sulfuric acid; thus 65 per cent sulfuric acid has become of great use in the bile acid area[43, 112] as has diluted acid and heat for certain estrogens,[113] and special heat treatment and dilution for steroidal sapogenins.[37, 134] Other strong acids such as "100 per cent" phosphoric acid,[68, 92, 93] perchloric acid,[101, 126] formic acid,[74] etc., have been of use in the steroid field but to a lesser extent, and will not be reviewed except where a useful correlation or contrast can be made.

The use of selective absorption spectra of steroids in concentrated sulfuric acid centers about two major areas: (1) identification and characterization of unknown steroids by their spectra, and (2) recognition of certain structural features of the steroid molecule based on the character of the spectra. Two lesser areas include: (3) steroid homogeneity and purity, and (4) quantitative analytical procedures for mixtures of steroids. By far the most frequent use of the technique is for the identification of minute amounts of steroids isolated from biological sources, this aspect of use being fully exploited by biochemical and endocrinological investigators. The present review will attempt to elucidate the other items of information which may be derived from spectra in concentrated sulfuric acid.

II. TECHNIQUE

The experimental procedures to be followed have been outlined by several investigators.[13, 43, 69, 138] Generally the pure steroid or evaporated residue containing steroid is dissolved in concentrated reagent purity sulfuric acid so as to make a final steroid concentration within the range 5–50 μg/ml, depending on the class of steroid involved and the intensity of absorption to be observed. The use of a single selected batch of acid is recommended.[13] The steroid solutions are allowed to stand at room temperature (20–25°) for varying lengths of time. A standard two hour period has been recommended by Zaffaroni,[137] and this has been the basis of most of the data in the literature, although for certain types of observations (mainly related to structural correlations) different time periods are required.

It has been recommended that the two hour period of standing be in the dark,[69] but most investigators do not make mention of this point (Axelrod[3] also recommends standing in the dark for the use of fuming sulfuric acid). After the specified time interval the spectra are recorded over the 220–600 mμ range using a suitable spectrophotometer, with concentrated sulfuric acid being used as the reference liquid. Many types of spectrophotometers have been used, and for occasional operations any type is of use. For extended studies self-recording spectrophotometers are advisable. The 220–600 mμ range usually studied is also limited by the instrument used ; no studies in the 185–220 mμ range or in ranges above 600 mμ have been reported.

Methods of reporting spectral data generally employ wave length measured in millimicrons (although one laboratory persists in using wave numbers)[73–76] and absorption intensity reported as optical density, $E_{1\,cm}^{1\%}$ values, or logarithm of molecular extinction[61] values. Ratios of optical densities have also been reported in lieu of specific measurements at each maximum. The data of this review are uniformly reported in millimicrons (wave length) and $E_{1\,cm}^{1\%}$ extinction coefficients. These units will thus be of use for characterization of unknown steroids whose molecular weights have not been determined.

III. PROPERTIES OF SPECTRA

Sulfuric acid spectra of steroids in general consist of several well defined maxima and minima, together with frequent inflections, etc. While some steroids are devoid of marked selective absorption within the 220–600 mμ ranges covered (5β-androstane-

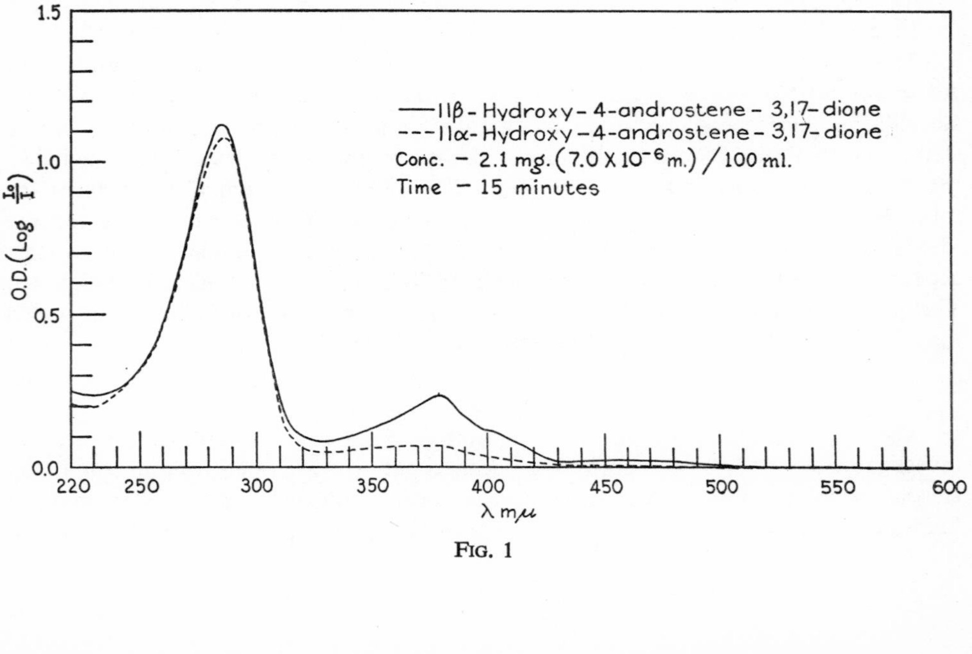

FIG. 1

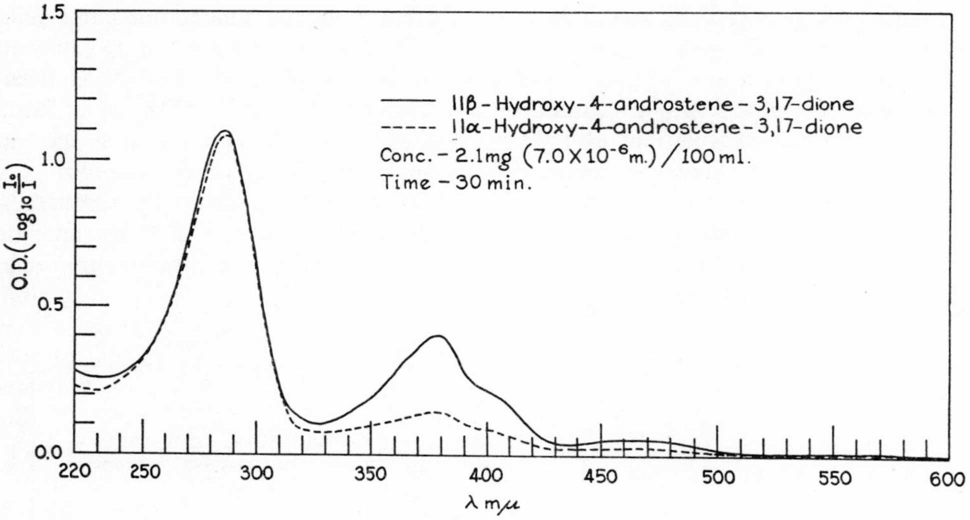

FIG. 2

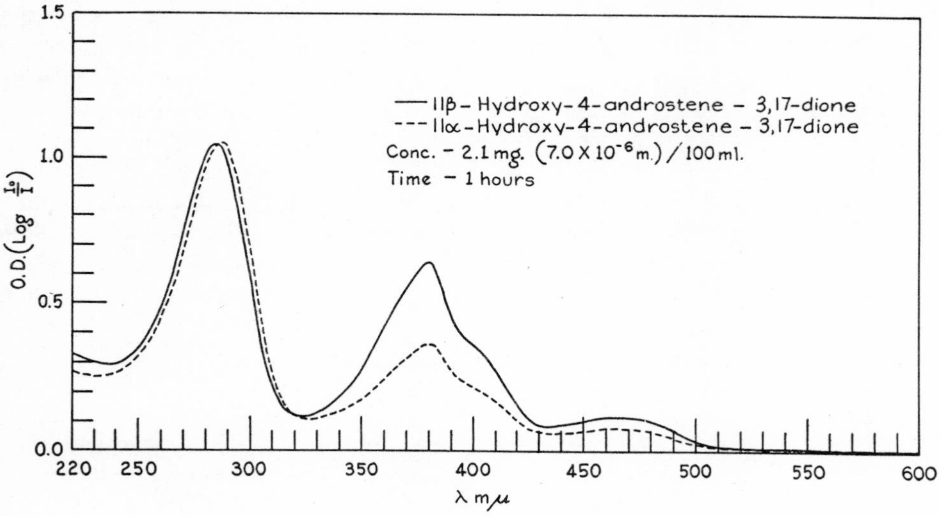

FIG. 3

3,11,17-trione, No. 22 ; dehydrocholic acid, No. 249 ; cholanic acid, No. 265), others frequently so reported as devoid of selective absorption (5α-androstane-3,11,17-trione, No. 21)[2, 74, 137] do in fact show weak selective absorption when critically observed.[13] While it cannot be categorically stated that all steroids exhibit selective absorption, it must be recalled that the majority of spectra recorded in the literature do not cover any time longer than two hours, and that consequently certain possibilities of absorption phenomena have been overlooked.

A disturbing property of steroid spectra in concentrated sulfuric acid is the unpredictable lack of stability of absorption with regard to time. Certain steroids exhibit remarkably stable spectra over twenty hours or more, the only variation recorded being most likely due to the error inherent in the instrumentation employed. Other steroids undergo rapid, drastic alteration in absorption to such an extent that spectra recorded a few minutes after solution are completely distinguished from spectra of the same solution recorded several hours after solution. The use of heat, or perhaps of special dilutions with alcohol or water, may lead to more stable spectra in select situations ; however, the problem of stable spectra has yet to be solved.

The time alteration of spectra in certain cases may be turned to advantage, however, in the identification of test samples with authentic steroids and in differentiation between steroids of very similar structures, as for example, epimeric pairs of hydroxy steroids.

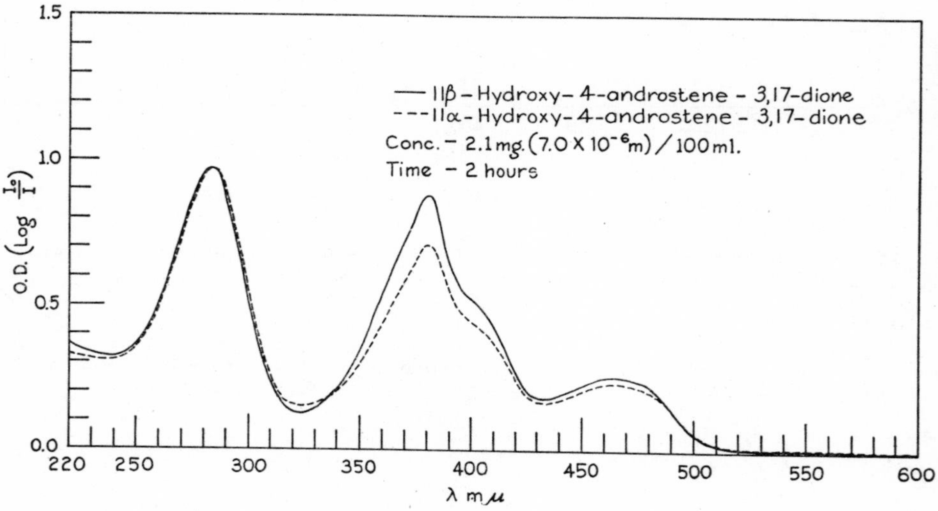

FIG. 4

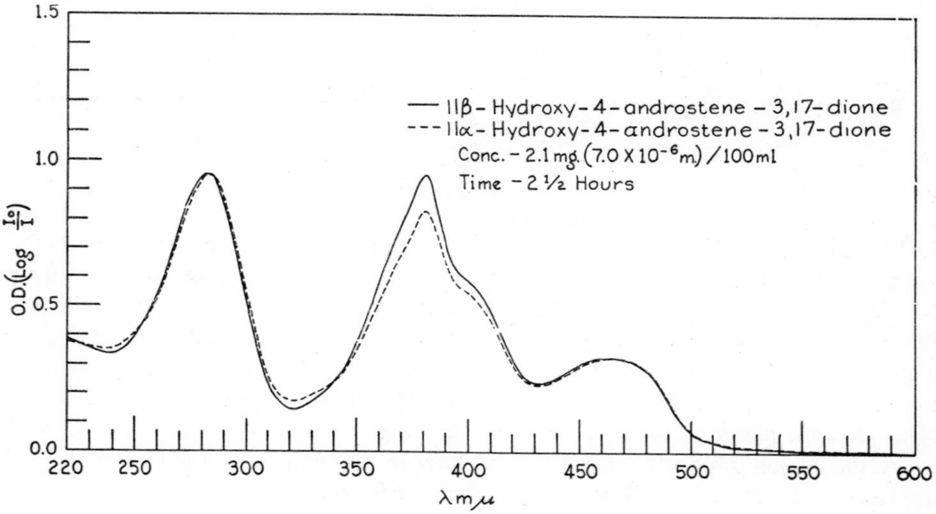

FIG. 5

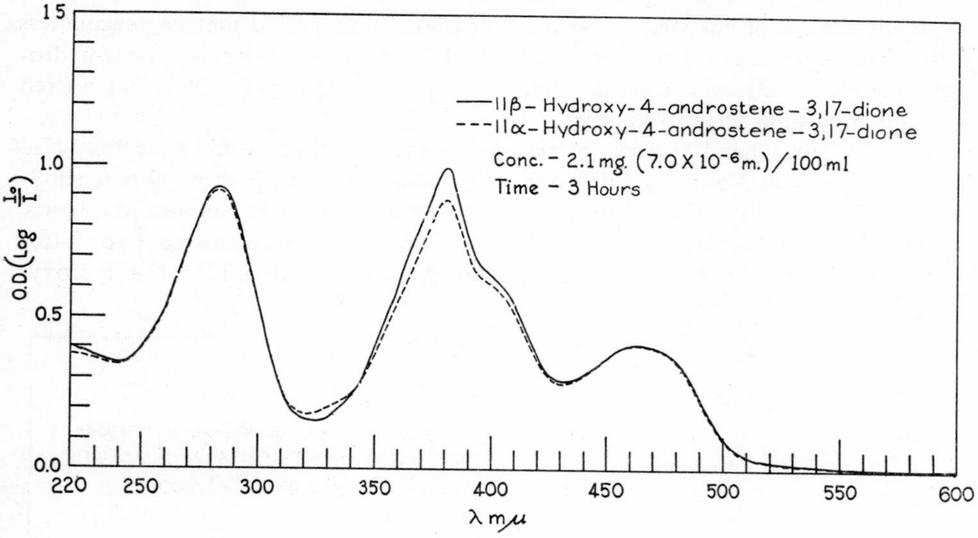

FIG. 6

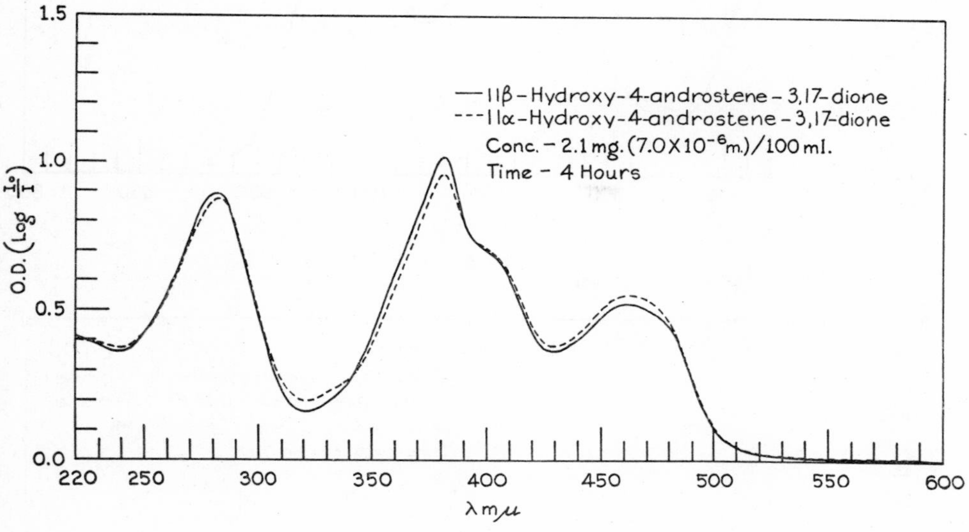

FIG. 7

Bernstein and Lenhard[16] have made an extensive study of the behavior with time of the spectra in concentrated sulfuric acid of a large number of steroids. Their data are included in the tables. These investigators were also concerned with the behavior of epimeric compounds under these conditions. In this connection the spectra of 11β-hydroxy-4-androstene-3,17-dione (No. 26) and its 11α-epimer (No. 25) were compared over a period of 15 minutes to 24 hours (Figs 1–9).[18] The 15 minutes, 30 minutes and 1 hour spectra are dissimilar. However, it was observed that starting with the 2 hour spectra the behavior of the two compounds approached similarity with eventual identity at about 4 hours. These time studies demonstrated decisively the major changes in spectra over a long time period that one encounters with certain steroids. This is in contrast, e.g., to the behavior of 11-*epi*-hydrocortisone (No. 145) over a similar time period where the spectrum is not altered very much by time after 15 minutes.

On the other hand it was interesting to observe that 20β,21-diacetoxy-17α-hydroxy-4-pregnen-3-one (No. 302) and 20α,21-diacetoxy-17α-hydroxy-4-pregnen-3-one (No. 301) exhibit different spectra over the time period of 15 minutes to 6 hours.

The following epimeric pairs were also studied: hydrocortisone (No. 146)–11-*epi*-hydrocortisone (No. 145); 11β-hydroxy-progesterone (No. 125)–11α-hydroxy-

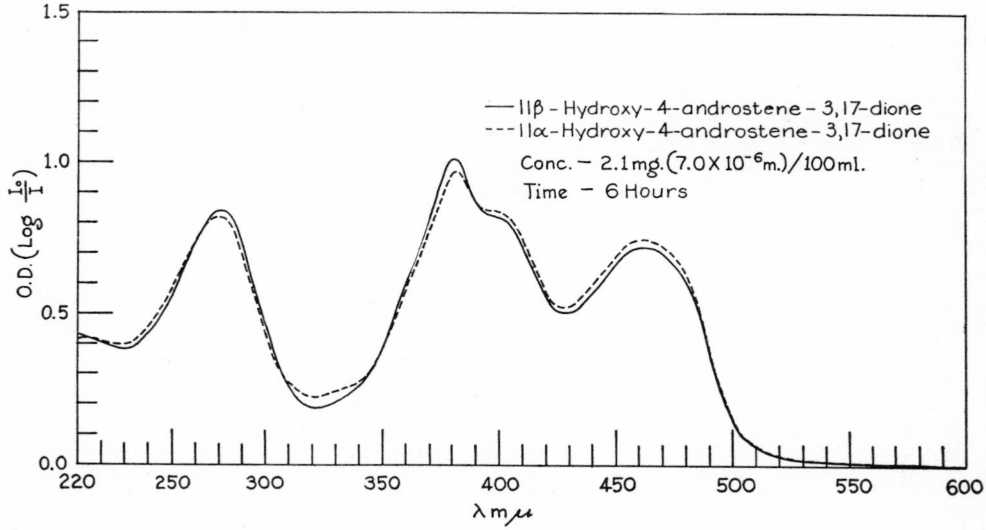

FIG. 8

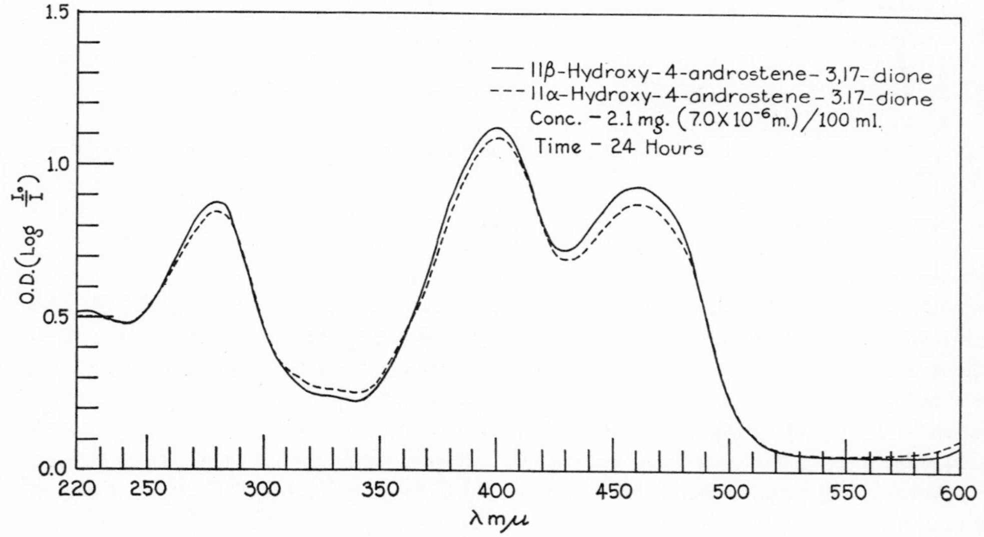

FIG. 9A

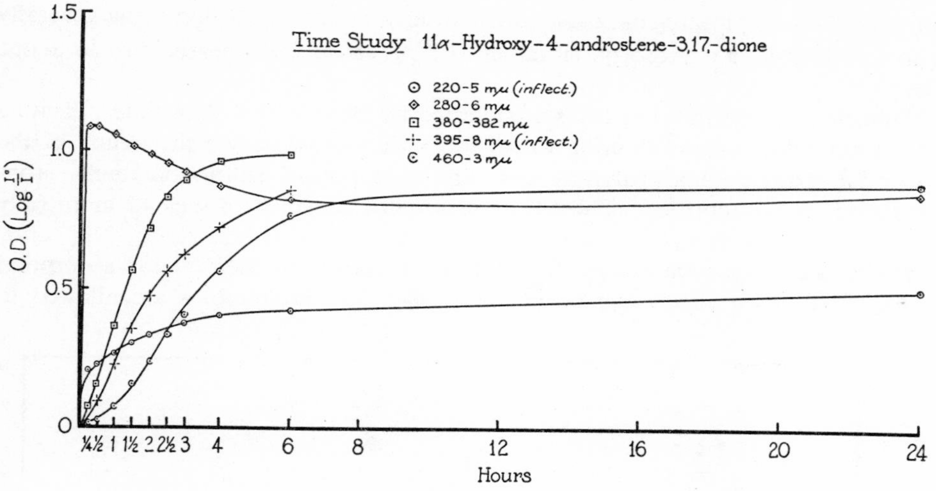

FIG. 9B

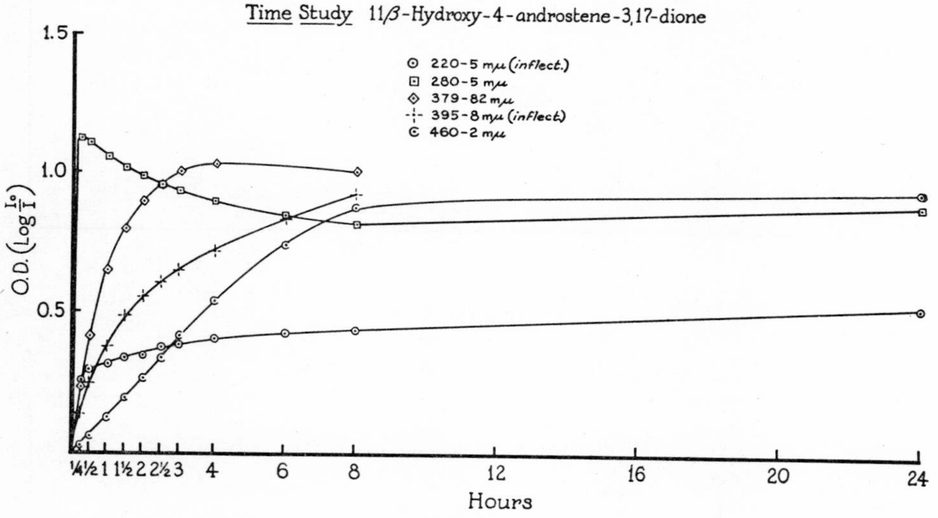

FIG. 9C

FIGS. 1–9. Spectra of 11α- and 11β-Hydroxy-4-androstene-3,17-dione at different times.

progesterone (No. 124); 11β-hydroxy-testosterone (No. 45)–11α-hydroxy-testosterone (No. 44); pregnane-3α,20β-diol (No. 191)–pregnane-3α,20α,-diol (No. 190); and 5-androstene-3β,17β-diol (No. 55)–5-androstene-3β,17α-diol (No. 54). See Figs. 10–12.

Generally it has been found that the behavior of epimeric steroids in concentrated sulfuric acid with time is diverse within the range from complete identity to dissimilarity.[5, 69, 138]

Whereas absorption bands may be observed throughout the 220–600 mμ region usually studied, bands much below 240 mμ or above 550 mμ are rare, and are thus all the more distinctive when observed. The majority of bands with high extinction fall in the 240–400 mμ region, most bands in the 400–550 mμ region being generally of lower absorption. Absorption values ($E^{1\%}_{1\,cm}$) range from nearly zero to about 900.

Sulfuric acid spectra of steroids are affected by factors other than time. Heating the steroid solutions and diluting with hydroxylic solvents alters the nature of the absorption patterns markedly, as does the presence of sulfur-containing, iron-containing, etc., impurities. The effects of impurities will be discussed more fully later.

While steroid spectra follow Beer's Law in regard to their major absorption bands,[13, 43] dilution effects can be detected when steroid solutions are allowed to

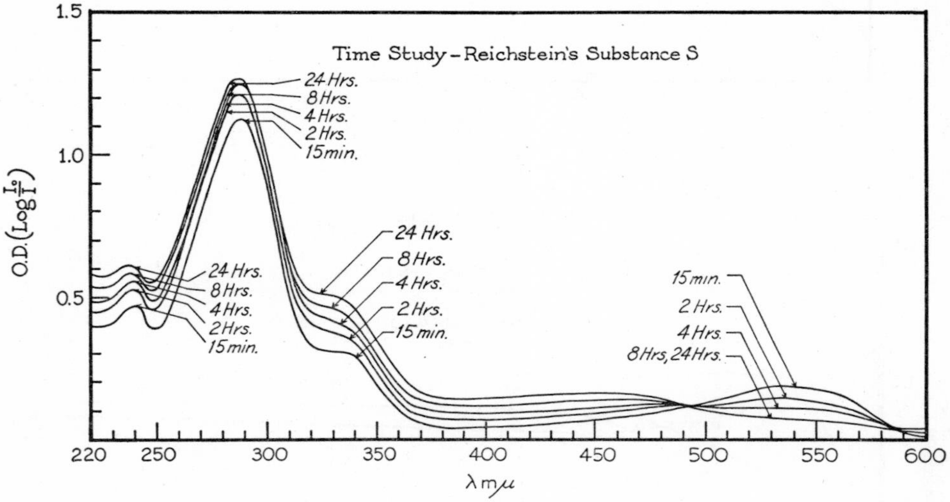

FIG. 10

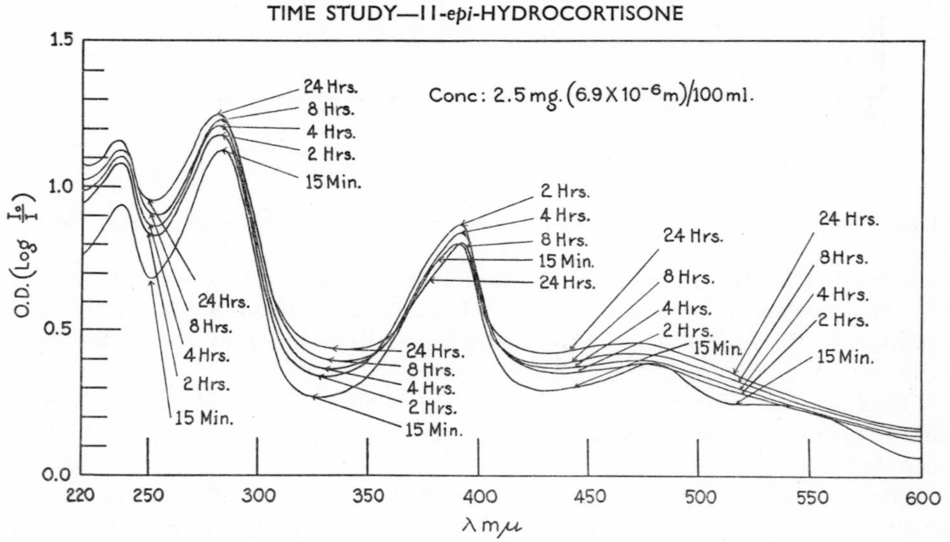

FIG. 11A

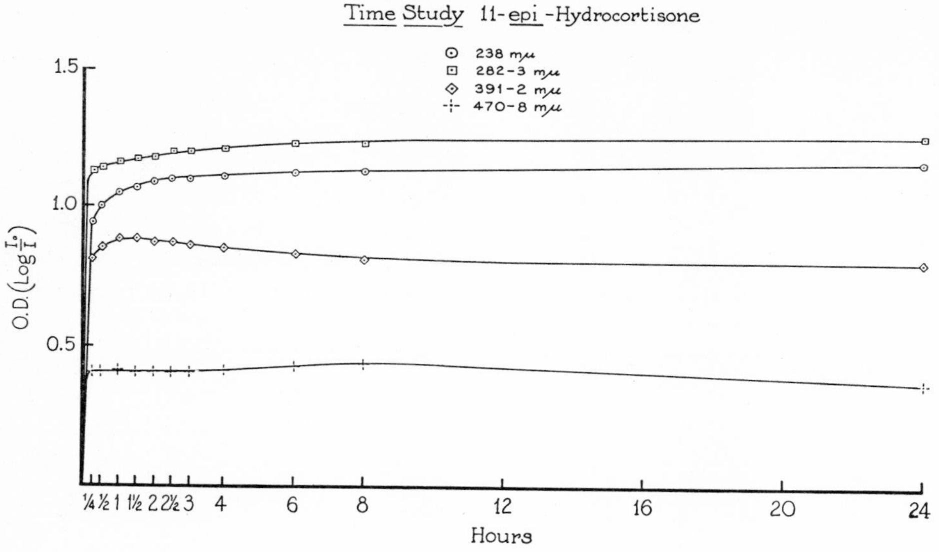

FIG. 11B

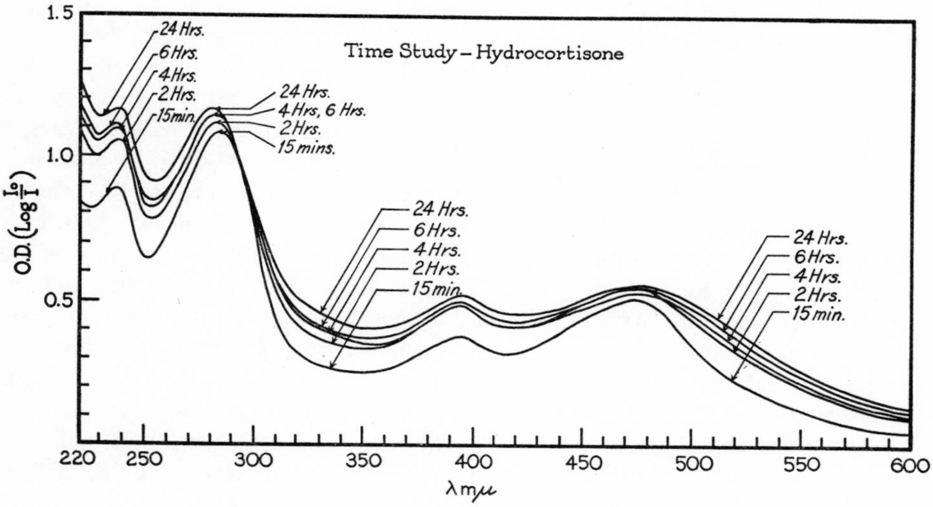

FIG. 12A

stand at one concentration and then diluted prior to final recording of spectra.[69] For this reason any studies based on different steroid concentrations must be made using separately weighed samples of the steroid in question.

While differing in many specific points, spectra of steroids in concentrated sulfuric acid are generally similar to spectra in " 100 per cent " phosphoric acid,[92, 93] fuming sulfuric acid,[3] etc. In the few published cases where direct comparisons between spectra in these acids can be made[2, 69, 117, 119] no advantage generally obtains in the use of the experimentally more involved " 100 per cent " phosphoric or fuming sulfuric acids. An exception obtains in the case of aldosterone (No. 100) where

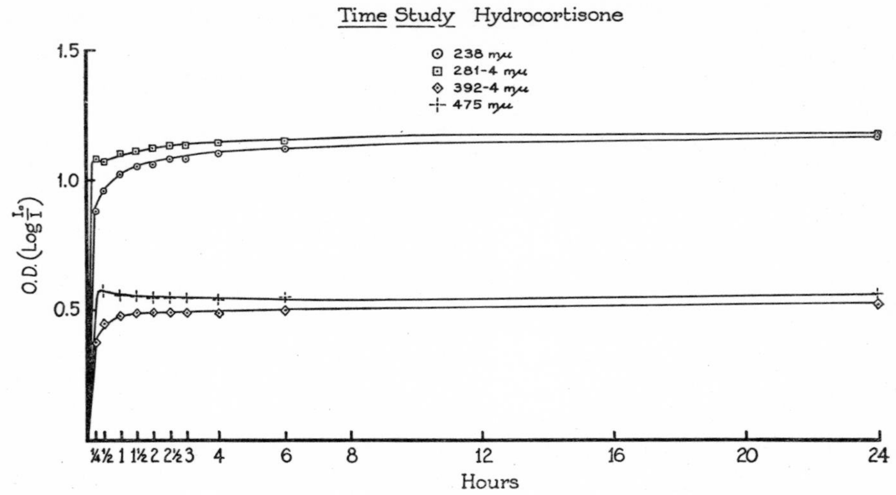

FIG. 12B

FIGS. 10–12. Time course of alteration of three steroids.

spectra in concentrated sulfuric acid contain but one maximum, but spectra in fuming sulfuric acid have several peaks (at 250 mμ, 280 mμ, 340 mμ, 470 mμ, etc.). Aldosterone is distinguished also by spectral changes in ordinary concentrated sulfuric acid after specific heating periods.[31, 34]

The effects of heating sulfuric acid solutions of steroids may be quite variable and presently unpredictable. Solutions of hydrocortisone (No. 146) allowed to stand for one hour at room temperature (20°) then heated for ten minutes at 100° showed parallel shifts in extinction but otherwise no wave length changes. Spectra of cortisone (No. 103) on the other hand changed markedly by this treatment. Initially (one hour at 20°) the spectra consisted of bands at 345 mμ, 410 mμ, 420 mμ (inflection), and 480 mμ, with minima at 370 mμ and 460 mμ ; this solution heated at 100° for ten minutes then showed bands at 380 mμ, 390 mμ (inflections) and 460 mμ, with minima at 345 mμ and 440 mμ. Absorption values at the maxima were also affected.[67] Aldosterone spectra (No. 100) after 2–3 hours at room temperature are undistinguished, showing only one band at 288 mμ, but by heating these solutions for an additional hour at 90° distinctive spectra are obtained, with λ_{max} 247 mμ, 285 mμ, 342 mμ, and 460 mμ.[31, 111]

Other similar effects of heating are displayed graphically by Kalant.[69]

IV. USES OF SPECTRA

1. Identification and Characterization

Absorption spectra in concentrated sulfuric acid afford a ready means for identification of many steroids ; a catalog of over four hundreds steroids is included here (Tables I–XVI) for this purpose. An examination of the tables indicates that only a few steroids are not distinguished from one another in some way. Even where similar spectra are recorded, as for steroid alcohols and their respective acetates,[16] steroid acids and their methyl esters,[43] etc., when pure samples are critically examined slight differences in absorption maxima, absorbance at various wave lengths, ratios of absorbance at two or more maxima and minima, etc., become apparent. In actual practice those instances where parent steroid and derivative might be confused would not be of concern since other physical and chemical evidence would be available for auxiliary differentiation.

The problem of identification of sub-milligram samples of steroids isolated *via* chromatography, countercurrent distribution, fractional crystallization, etc., may best be faced by recourse to infrared absorption spectra in a suitable medium. Where sample size, nature of sample, or lack of adequate infrared instrumentation precludes proper use of infrared spectra for identification, the use of selective absorption in sulfuric acid becomes the next best procedure for most purposes. Suitable quartz spectrophotometers are generally more widely available than are infrared spectrophotometers, and the amounts of steroid sample needed are usually less. Although fewer absorption bands are present in the 220–600 mμ range usually studied with the sulfuric acid technique, the study of characteristic time-course of alteration of spectra permits an approach to the specificity inherent in the infrared technique.

Reliance on sulfuric acid spectra alone for complete identification of an unknown with a known steroid, while possible in certain instances, is unwise. Usually chromatographic and partition data, color test behavior, etc., are available to support an assigned identity, and in actual use small differences between spectra of the pure known standard and the supposed steroid require full use of supporting evidence for identification.

The inclusion of absorption spectra as a standard means of characterization of new steroids prepared in the course of other work has not been widely practised by organic chemists. For this reason a more full catalog of spectral data is unavailable. Sulfuric acid spectra have become a standard means of characterization of the many unknown steroids isolated during the course of metabolic studies in biological systems.[65, 135, 136]

While spectra in sulfuric acid of unidentified steroids afford a very acceptable means of identification with known steroids, spectra obtained on natural products in general cannot be safely used to suggest the steroid nature of the material isolated. Thus spectra of the cevine alkaloids are similar in certain properties with steroid spectra,[13] and the similarity between spectra of ubiquinone (λ_{max} 315 mμ),[36] while differing from 3,5-cholestadien-7-one (No. 326), could be confused with a number of ketosteroids having a single absorption band in this region.

Inclusion of other properties with sulfuric acid spectra may not be enough for the presumed recognition of an unknown as a steroid. Thus the probable sesquiterpenoid X_6 of Gray, *et al.*,[63] Compound III of Nowaczynski, *et al.*,[91] etc., tentatively given the partial structure I, has papergram mobility and color test

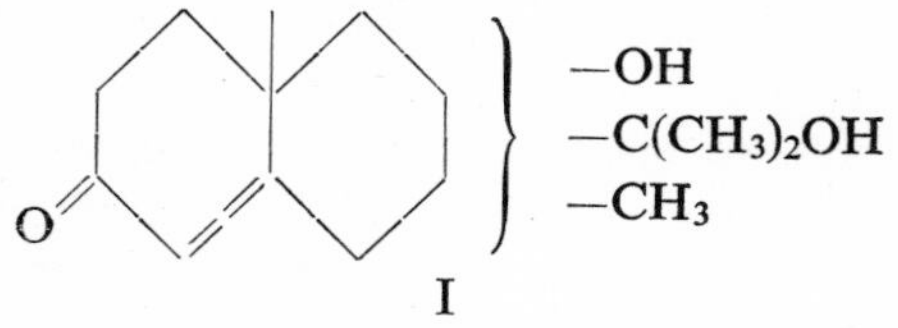

I

behavior, as well as sulfuric acid and " 100 per cent " phosphoric acid spectra resembling α,β-unsaturated 3-ketosteroids. In sulfuric acid the compound absorbs λ_{max} 288 mμ, 385 mμ, 450 mμ, with λ_{min} 240 mμ and 370 mμ.[62, 91, 132]

In order to consider in detail the reliance which can be placed on a given identification based on sulfuric acid spectra it is necessary to examine the reproducibility of the spectra of a single sample, and of different samples of a given steroid. In our hands pure known steroids have always given excellent reproducibility as regards wave length of absorption and shape of curve, although some variation in absorption values has been noted. An error of ± 1 mμ in position of the absorption band is generally acceptable. For samples of lower (or dubious) purity disagreement in band position may be as much as 5 mμ.

For those steroids most often studied, as corticosterone (No. 135), hydrocortisone (No. 146), and cortisone (No. 103), several entries have been made in the tables. These data include many different laboratories, and many determinations from the same laboratory. Usually the reliable data are in agreement within 5 mμ ; however, certain sets of data show differences as great as 10–15 mμ. Other such examples abound in the tables.

In certain cases an important band is not recorded by some investigators. Thus for hydrocortisone the short wave length band near 240 mμ is omitted by some and the 475 mμ band by the same and others, and neither band is of low absorption. Were these bands inflections or shoulders on rapidly changing curves such omission might be better understood.

These problems of reproducibility are presumably derived from spectra recorded of pure steroids. Where steroids are isolated in impure state for identification, or samples of doubtful identity and purity are taken, these problems become serious for reliable identification. The use of different spectrophotometers (Beckman DU, DK, Cary, etc.) may cause some of the disagreement in spectra, as may different dilutions, temperature of recording spectra, etc. More likely the major causes of such problems lie in the make or quality of sulfuric acid used, the inherent instability of the spectra during the period of recording, that is, poor comparison times, and most probably, in the purity of the steroid used.

The first of the difficulties may be overcome by careful choice of the batch of sulfuric acid to be employed in a given series of studies.[13] The time alteration of spectra may be quite serious in certain cases, and of no consequence in others. Usually with the modern recording spectrophotometers no time lapse of consequence is involved between starting and completing the spectra.

Purity of steroid is the most important factor in assuring satisfactory spectra for identification and characterization. Small amounts of impurities eluted from paper chromatograms (to be discussed later), minute amounts of iron present in the sample (metal spatulas?),[43] and the presence of wholly unanticipated impurities may lead to spurious spectra. Thus the 350 mμ absorption band reported for estrone (No. 5) has been shown to be probably due to equilin,[60] and an unidentified steroidal impurity has been cited as the cause of the major absorption reported for cholanic acid (No. 265).[13, 43]

Most of the identifications made using biological samples are presented in the literature in the form of figures showing both the sample and the pure standard spectra. A study of a few of these figures indicates the nature of the differences in spectra to be expected. Such data range from absolute identity (superposition) through doubtful or uncertain (impurities present), to incorrect identification.[2, 9, 41, 12, 70, 89, 98, 100, 103, 120, 122, 136, etc.]

In certain instances poor agreement between spectra obtained on a given sample and the standard may not be sufficiently impressive for negation of the proposed identity. Thus Dohan, *et al.*[38] identified tetrahydrocortisone (No. 171) from biological samples despite a 15 mμ differential between spectra of their sample and that of authentic tetrahydrocortisone.

Questionable identifications may result in certain cases. It has been suggested that 11-*epi*-corticosterone (11α,21-dihydroxy-4-pregnene-3,20-dione) (No. 145) is present in steroid fractions isolated from rat adrenals.[42] This suggestion is based on an identity assigned on the basis of sulfuric acid spectra obtained on an eluate of the corticosterone zone of a papergram. This identification has been criticized on paper chromatographic mobility considerations.[30]

Most frequently sulfuric acid spectral identifications have been made in connection with paper chromatographic separations. Spectra of the eluted steroid are read against a blank prepared from a piece of filter paper (not bearing steroid) of the same area as that of the sample, cut from the chromatogram, eluted, etc.[2, 6, 9, 98, 127] Otherwise an intermediate purification procedure of the steroid eluates by chromatography on alumina[120] may be used for satisfactory spectra. Although Kalant[69] has reported that paper blanks are unnecessary it is the predominant experience of others that paper blanks are required, and that their omission may lead to poor spectra or to spurious maxima in the regions of interest.

The effects of non-specific impurities on the spectra of steroids isolated from chromatographic systems may be disturbing. Thus spectra of cortisone and hydrocortisone eluted from Zaffaroni-type paper chromatographic systems have been reported as not agreeing well with spectra of the pure standards while corticosterone eluted from the same chromatograms did give satisfactory identity with the standard.[20] Others have reported satisfactory identification of cortisone and hydrocortisone by sulfuric acid spectra however. Corticosterone is one of the steroids most frequently identified by sulfuric acid spectra, after repeated chromatography,[140] after a single chromatography (read versus paper blank),[98, 103] etc., and in one instance identification by sulfuric acid spectra was acceptable although infrared studies on the same eluted sample did not afford a convincing identification with pure material.[59]

It has long been recognized that steroids eluted from papergrams are not sufficiently pure for ultraviolet measurements (in alcohol) without use of papergram blanks or multi-point absorption measurements. Chromatographic washing or extraction of the filter paper is not sufficient to remove all of the "dirt" present, spurious absorption in the 230 mμ and 257 mμ regions persisting after these treatments.[29] Similarly, for sulfuric acid spectra, elution of Whatman No. 1 filter paper, chromatographically washed with methanol or not, in the usual manner results in eluted material giving rise to sulfuric acid spectra with a characteristic absorption maximum in the 310–313 mμ region. Chromatographic washing with ethanol reduces the absorption to about one-third the levels of unwashed paper.[5, 115]

This interference is especially important where the steroid of interest exhibits selective absorption in the 310 mμ region. Such steroids as $\Delta^{1,4}$-3-ketones[119] are affected adversely. Elution of triamcinolone 16α,17α-acetonide (No. 246) from papergrams run in typical Bush-type chromatographic systems led to sulfuric acid spectra (no paper blank was used) with poor correspondence of characteristics in the 310 mμ region with pure standard material. The actual maximum developed by the eluted sample shifted as high as 318 mμ over 20 hours at room temperature,

	Sulfuric Acid Spectra		
Paper Treatment	Time	λ_{max}	Absorbance/cm²
Washed	15 min	310 mμ	3.8×10^{-4}
	2 hr	310 mμ	5.3×10^{-4}
	20 hr	313 mμ	7.8×10^{-4}
Unwashed	15 min	310 mμ	11.7×10^{-4}
	2 hr	310 mμ	15.8×10^{-4}
	20 hr	313 mμ	22.8×10^{-4}

and the absorbance value increased to about twice that of the pure acetonide not chromatographed. Identity of the steroid based on absorption at 260 mμ and 375 mμ was very satisfactory, and infrared absorption spectra of the sample (in micro potassium bromide disks) were superimposable over spectra of pure triamcinolone acetonide. Correction of the absorbance in the 310–318 mμ region for absorbance of the paper blank afforded spectra with acceptable wave length (310 mμ) and absorbance.[115]

Some indication that steroid-free zones of paper chromatograms give rise to serious absorption in the 310–320 mμ region is recorded in the case of 5β-pregnane-3α,17α,20α-triol.[23] Absorption in this region was found on eluates taken immediately on either side of the 5β-pregnane-3α,17α,20α-triol zone.

2. Homogeneity and Purity

Sulfuric acid spectra may be used for purity arguments, both from a total steroid content aspect and from steroid homogeneity aspects. Identical spectra obtained on a steroid subjected to repeated chromatography has been used for homogeneity determination,[2] while another test involves dividing the steroid zone on a paper chromatogram into three sub-zones (front, center, and rear) and examination of spectra obtained on each sub-zone.[138] Both procedures require use of appropriate paper blanks. A more rigorous use of sulfuric acid spectra for identity and homogeneity involves its use on both the steroid alcohol and on an ester derivative.[139]

Total steroid content as determined by use of sulfuric acid spectra of a given steroid sample obviously depends on absence of other absorbing impurities or of a suitable means to correct for their presence. Where steroids of high purity are at hand sulfuric acid spectra may be of some use as a measure of total steroid content; however, for routine analyses, quality control purposes, etc., there is too little stability of spectra (2 hours, room temperature), and no such use has found favor in the literature.

For identity and quality control the spectra of twenty separate batches of triamcinolone 16α, 21-diacetate (No. 279) were examined.[116] Identity was established in all cases, and the wave lengths of maximum and minimum absorption were identical in all cases. The absorbance at either of the major absorption maxima did not correlate with the purity of the samples determined by more well established means as ultraviolet spectra in ethanol, polarography, etc. Although each sample was greater than 95 per cent pure triamcinolone diacetate absorbance varied over a wide range. Triamcinolone diacetate absorbs: 261 mμ ($E_{1\,cm}^{1\%}$ 297), 308 mμ ($E_{1\,cm}^{1\%}$ 136), 380 mμ ($E_{1\,cm}^{1\%}$ 35), while the spectra of the twenty samples averaged 261 mμ ($E_{1\,cm}^{1\%}$ 283, range 249–302), 308 mμ ($E_{1\,cm}^{1\%}$ 127, range 111–140), 380 mμ ($E_{1\,cm}^{1\%}$ 28, range 21–35), thus barring such spectra for strict purity determination.

3. Quantitative Analysis and Reaction Kinetics

Use of concentrated sulfuric acid spectra for quantitative analysis of certain mixtures of steroids obtained in biological extracts has been reported, *sans* chromatographic separation.[21] Also mention of its use in connection with paper chromatography of extracts from biological sources has been made.[95] No great use of the technique has otherwise been made, probably because of the difficulties with reproducing absorption at maxima. More success is to be expected in such ventures when diluted acid, heated acid, or use of fluorescence in such systems is utilized.

As a very minor use, the course of certain chemical reactions has been followed by sulfuric acid spectral changes,[77] as has the course of microbiological 11α-hydroxylation of Reichstein's Substance S (No. 136)[16] to 11-*epi*-hydrocortisone (No. 145)[16] and the microbiological dehydrogenation of 9α-fluoro-16α-hydroxyhydrocortisone (No. 112) to triamcinolone (No. 85).[115] Where decided spectral differences between reactant and product exist, kinetic studies using sulfuric acid spectra for analysis may be of value.

4. Structural Correlations

A number of investigators[14, 15, 74, 75, 119, 138] have examined the possibilities of formulating structural correlations for the spectra of steroids in concentrated sulfuric acid. The most extensive work in this area has been published by Bernstein and

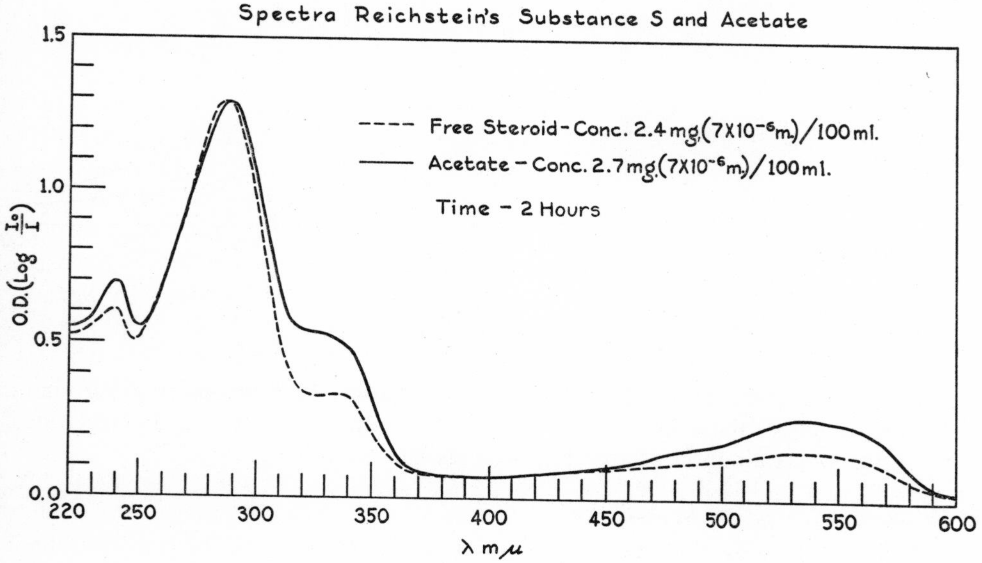

FIG. 13

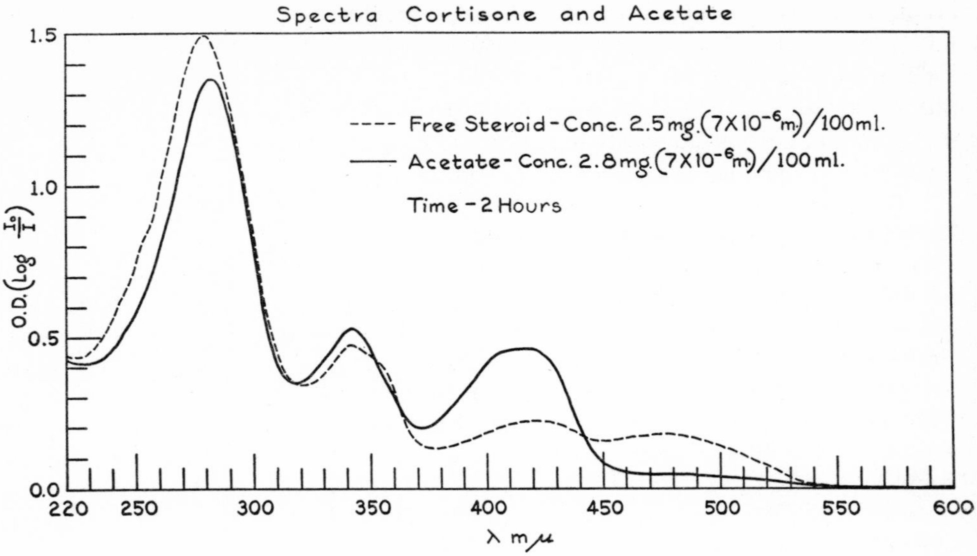

FIG. 14

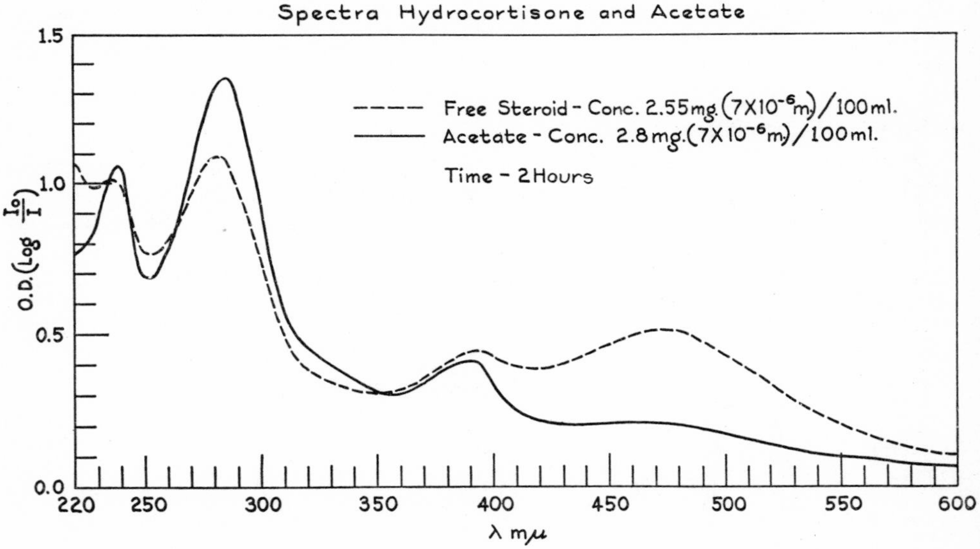

FIG. 15

FIGS. 13–15. Spectra of steroid esters and alcohols.

Lenhard.[14] On the basis of analysis of 177 steroids (2 hour spectra) (aromatic steroids excluded) these investigators proposed a number of structural correlations. No systemic examination of aromatic steroids has been made.

Absorption spectra of free steroids vs. esters

It has been observed that for all practical purposes free steroids and their acetates may be considered " equivalent " for the purpose of structural analysis. It is not implied, however, that their absorption spectra were always identical in all respects. This point may be neatly demonstrated by an examination of the spectrograms of Reichstein's Substance S (No. 136), cortisone (No. 103) and hydrocortisone (No. 146) and their respective acetates (Nos. 228, 218, 230) (Figs. 13–15).

Hydroxyl group

It has been proposed that hydroxylated steroids will generally exhibit selective absorption in the 220–278 mμ and 300–600 mμ regions.[14, 15, 74, 75] 3α- or 3β-Hydroxylated steroids will probably possess a maximum in the 300–350 mμ region. It was also observed that with increasing number of hydroxyl groups the spectrograms of steroids become increasingly more complicated in the 300–549 mμ region with a definite trend toward increasing absorption at the higher wave lengths. These correlations were based on the analysis of 146 steroids containing one to five hydroxyl groups.

The absorption spectra of epimeric steroids

Bernstein and Lenhard[16] and Zaffaroni[138] have examined the spectra of hydroxy steroids epimeric at C_3, C_{11}, C_{17}, and C_{20} in concentrated sulfuric acid for purposes of possible structural differentiation.

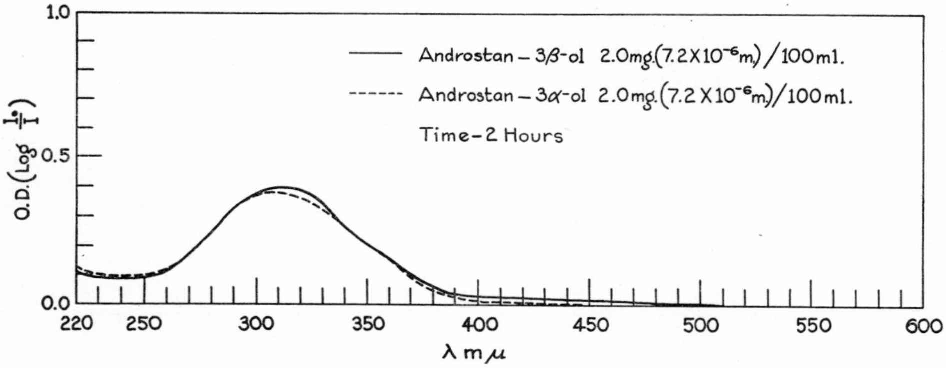

FIG. 16

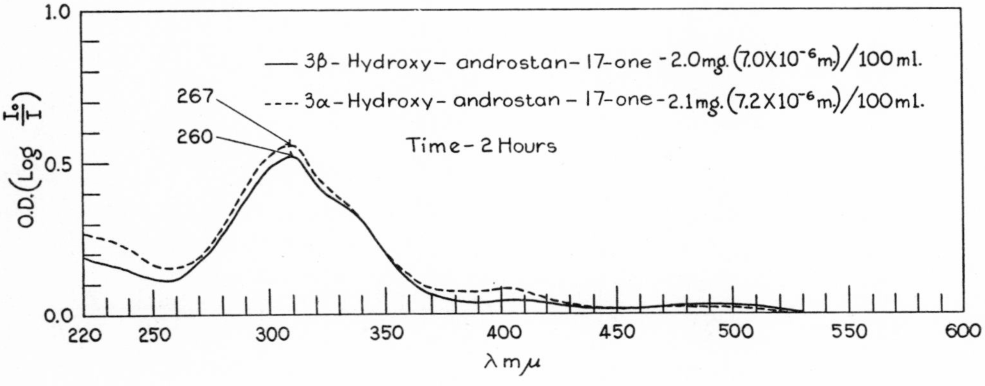

FIG. 17

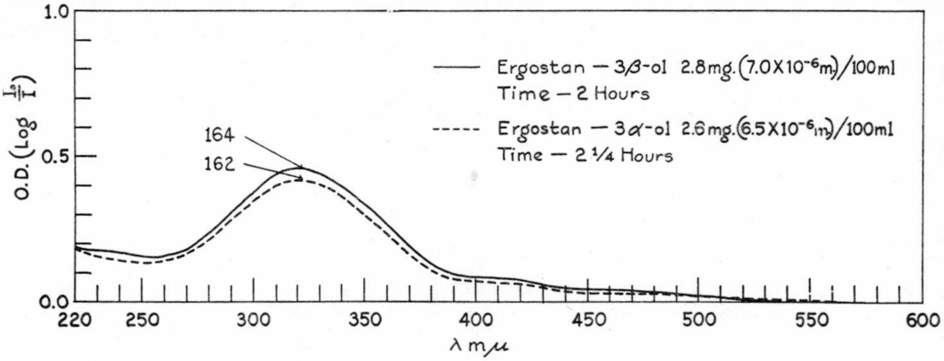

FIG. 18

FIGS. 16–18. Spectra of C_3-epimers.

C_3-Epimers

In Fig. 16 are given the spectra of ergostan-3β-ol (No. 366) and its 3α-epimer (No. 365). The numbers recorded at the principal maxima are the $E_{1\,cm}^{1\%}$ values included since the solutions had different concentrations. On the basis of this and a comparison of the spectra of androstan-3β-ol (No. 61) and its 3α-epimer (No. 60) (Fig. 17), and 3β-hydroxy androstan-17-one (No. 49) and its 3α-epimer (No. 48) (Fig. 18) Bernstein and Lenhard[16] concluded that 2 hour spectra in concentrated sulfuric acid do not differentiate C_3-epimeric steroids.

C_6-Epimers

Zaffaroni[138] mentions that 6α- and 6β-hydroxy epimers can be differentiated in concentrated sulfuric acid; however, no data were given. Figures presented for the epimeric 6α- and 6β-hydroxy-4-androstene-3,17-diones[2] support the concept.

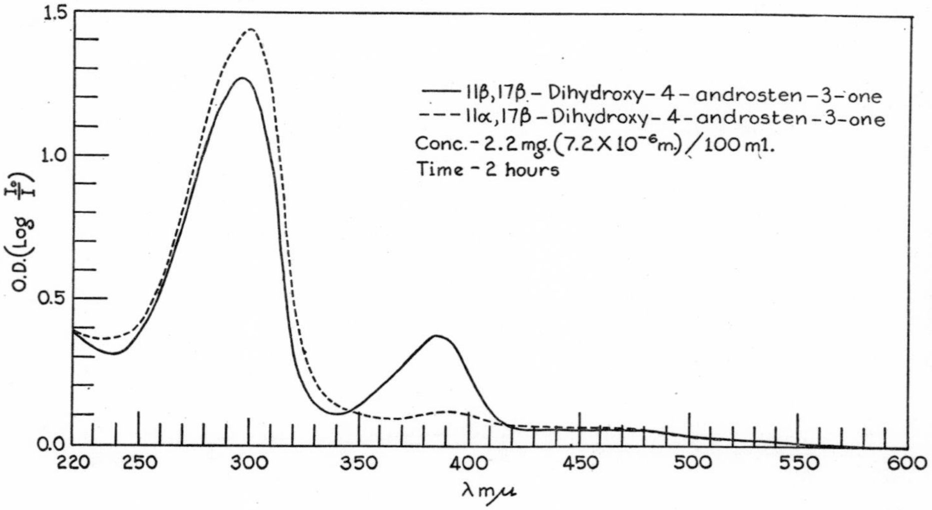

FIG. 19

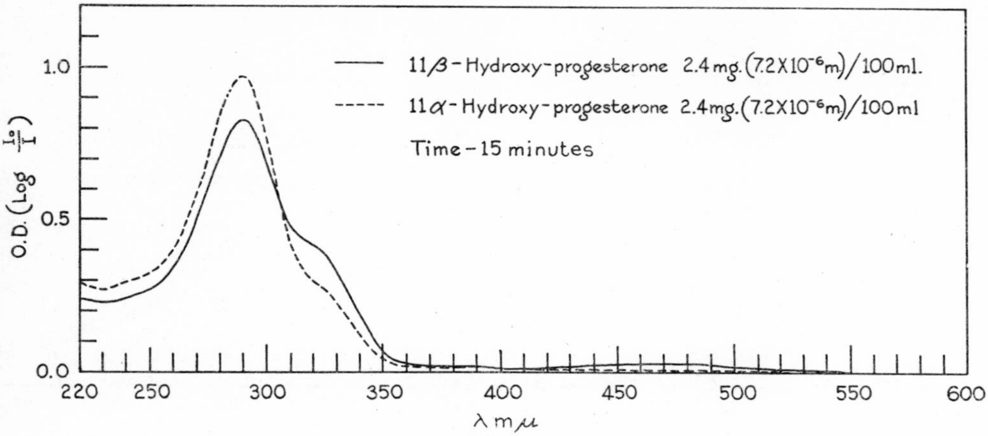

FIG. 20

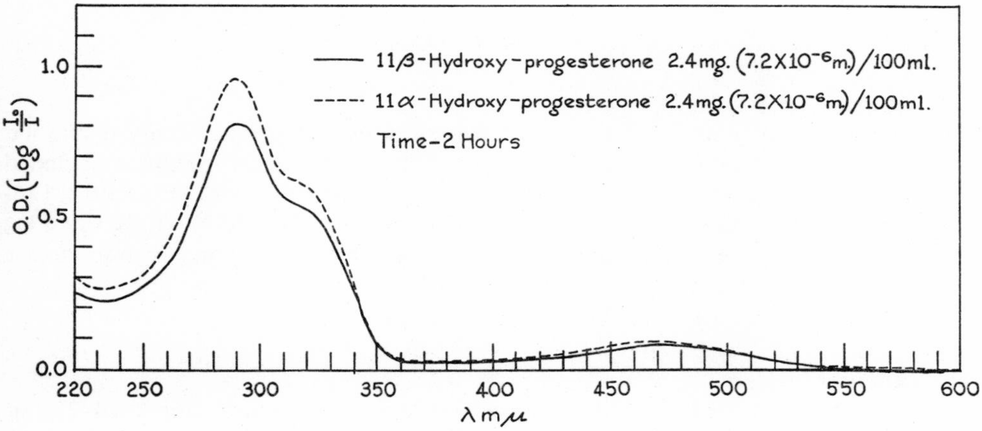

FIG. 21

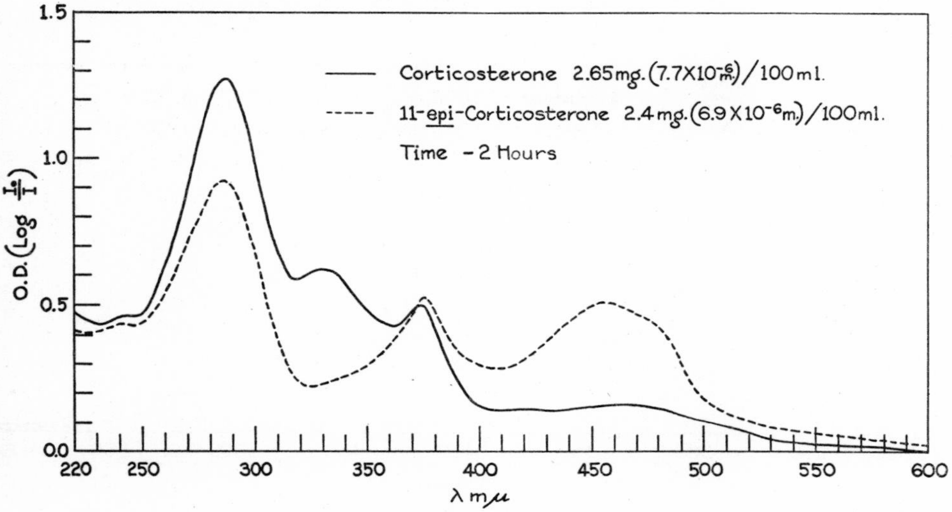

FIG. 22

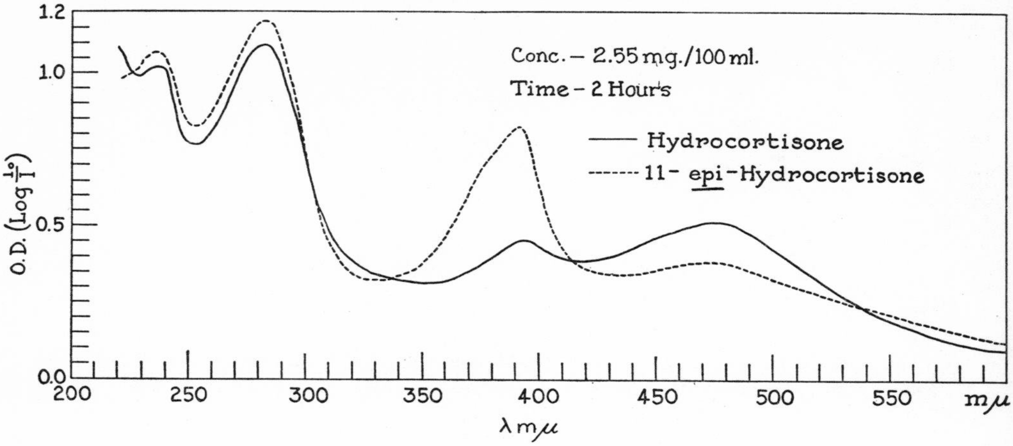

FIG. 23

FIGS. 19–23. Spectra of C_{11}-epimers.

C_{11}-*Epimers*

Bernstein and Lenhard[16] have noted that sulfuric acid spectral analysis may be used to differentiate C_{11}-epimeric steroids. The compounds examined included 11β-hydroxy-testosterone (No. 45) and its 11α-epimer (No. 44) (Fig. 19); 11β-hydroxy-progesterone (No. 125) and its 11α-epimer (No. 124) (Figs. 20–21); corticosterone (No. 135) and its 11α-epimer (No. 134) (Fig. 22) and hydrocortisone (No. 146) and its 11α-epimer (No. 145) (Fig. 23).

A similar observation has been made by Zaffaroni.[138]

C_{17}-*Epimers*

Bernstein and Lenhard[16] have observed that the spectra (Figs. 24–25) of 5-androstene-3β,17β-diol (No. 55) and 5-androstene-3β,17α-diol (No. 54) at 15 minutes and 2 hours, while similar, do allow some differentiation.

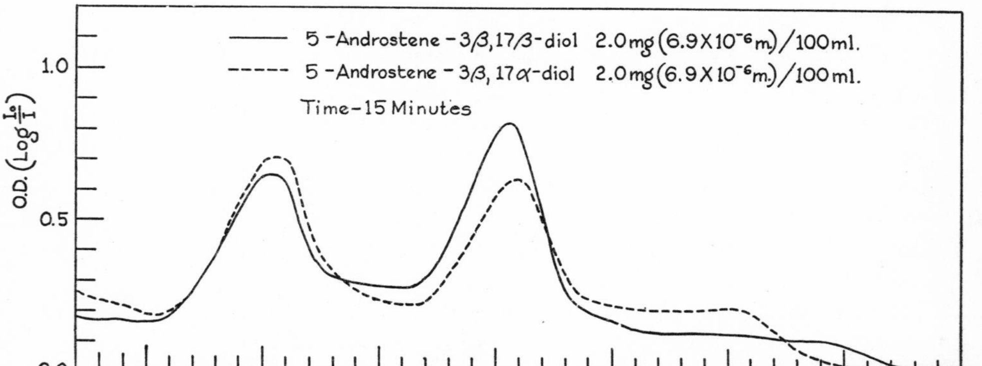

FIG. 24

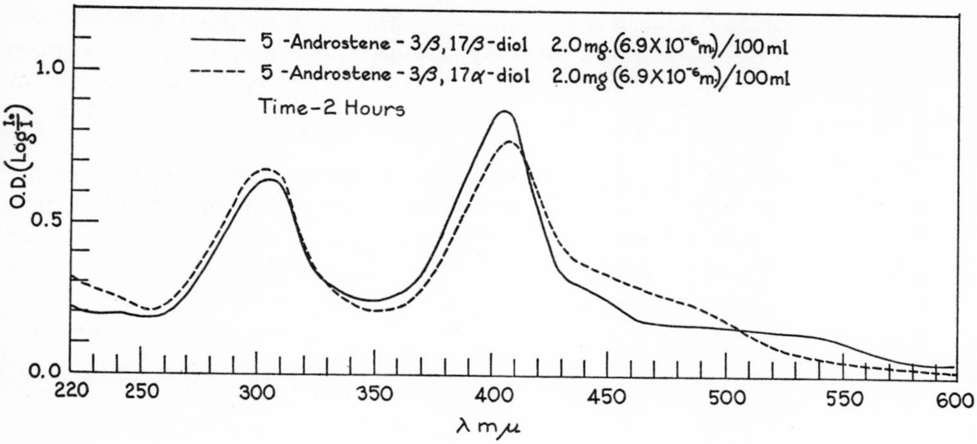

FIG. 25

FIGS. 24–25. Spectra of C_{17}-epimers.

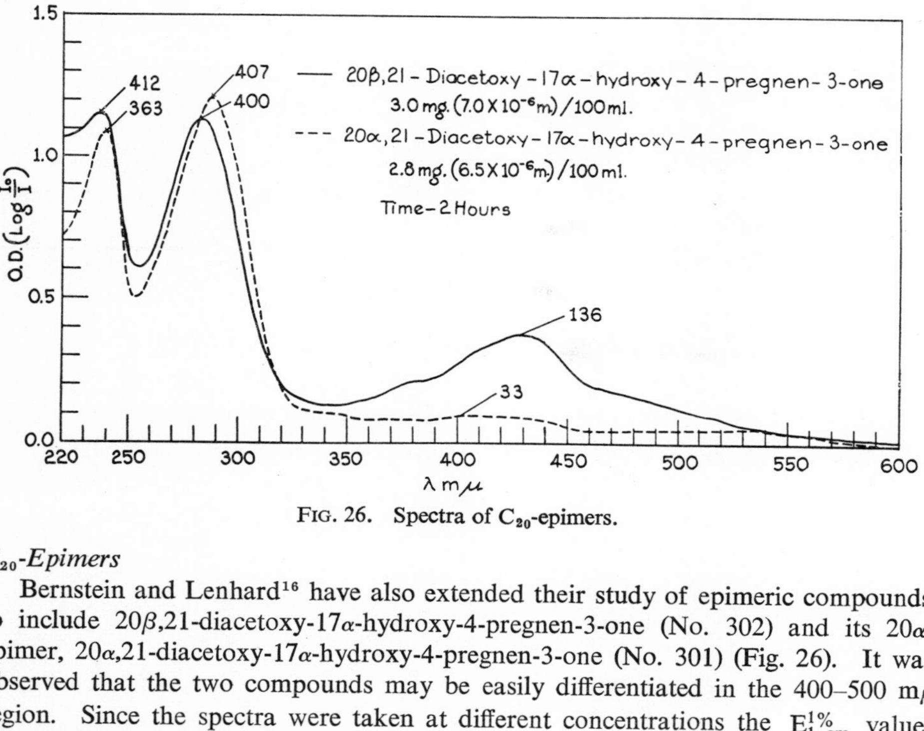

FIG. 26. Spectra of C_{20}-epimers.

C_{20}-Epimers

Bernstein and Lenhard[16] have also extended their study of epimeric compounds to include 20β,21-diacetoxy-17α-hydroxy-4-pregnen-3-one (No. 302) and its 20α-epimer, 20α,21-diacetoxy-17α-hydroxy-4-pregnen-3-one (No. 301) (Fig. 26). It was observed that the two compounds may be easily differentiated in the 400–500 mμ region. Since the spectra were taken at different concentrations the $E^{1\%}_{1\,cm}$ values are given at the various maxima.

The spectra of 20α- and 20β-dihydrohydrocortisone (Nos. 171, 172) are also differentiated one from the other (see reference 106 for Figs.).

Isolated double bonds

On the basis of an analysis of 67 steroids containing isolated (i.e., non-conjugated to a ketone group) double bonds (mono-, di-, tri- and tetra-enes) Bernstein and

Lenhard[14] concluded that such compounds show selective absorption in the 400–449 mμ region. As discussed above, hydroxyl groups also show selective absorption in this region. It is therefore suggested that both types of compounds in concentrated sulfuric acid give rise to a common species, such as an alkyl hydrogen sulfate, etc.[51]

In order to obtain additional evidence for this operation Bernstein and Lenhard[16] have compared the absorption spectra of 11β-hydroxy-4-androstene-3,17-dione (No. 26), its 11α-epimer (No. 25) and 4,9(11)-androstadiene-3,17-dione (No. 13). It was found that the spectra are equivalent (Fig. 27). This result supports the possibility

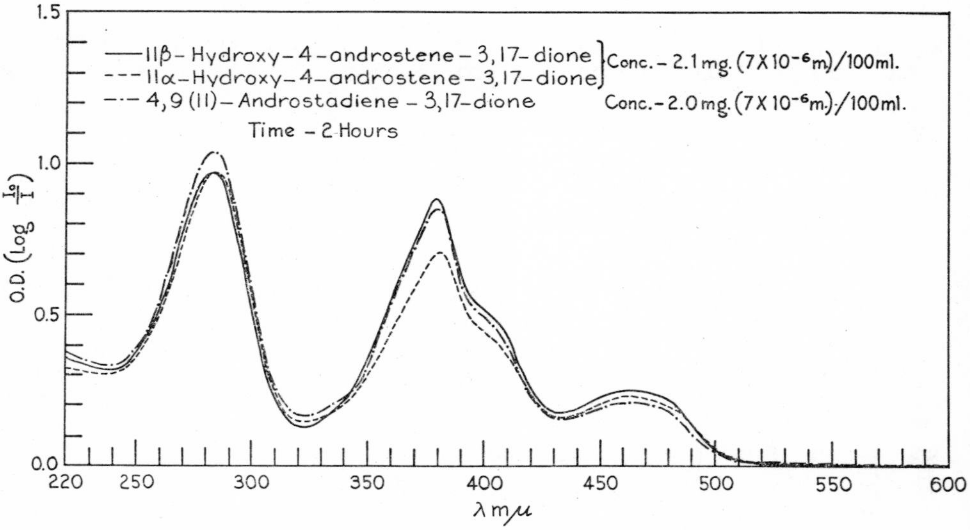

FIG. 27. Equivalent spectra of 11-hydroxy steroids and $\Delta^{9(11)}$-steroids.

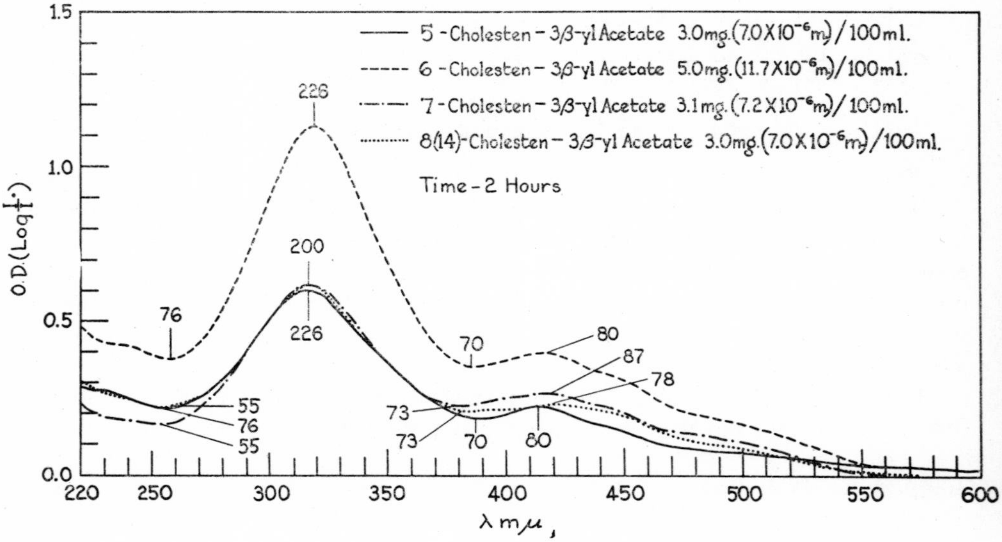

FIG. 28

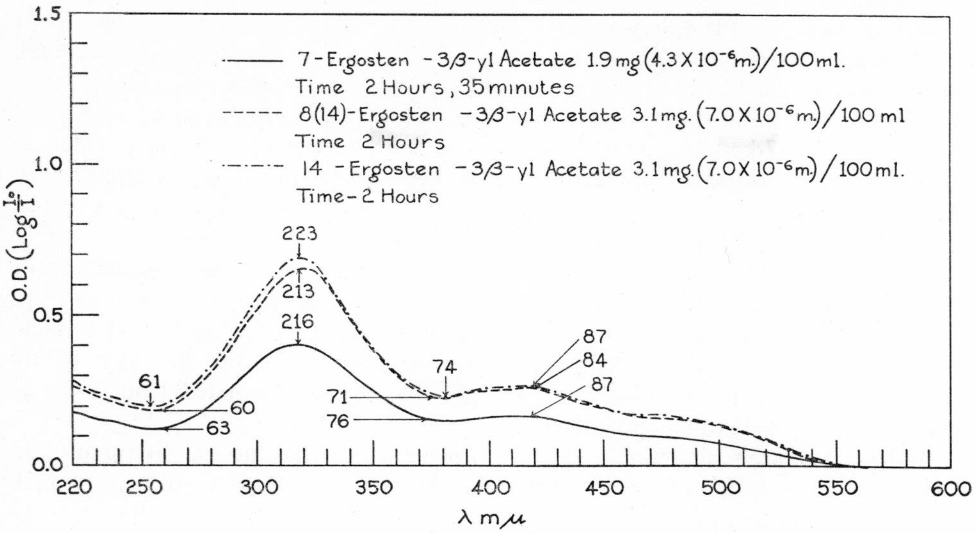

FIGS. 28–29. Equivalence of spectra of double bond isomers.

of a common species from a double bond and a hydroxyl group. In this respect, Zaffaroni has announced the isolation of a $\Delta^{9(11)}$-steroid from the solution of an 11β-hydroxy steroid in concentrated sulfuric acid.[138]

Bernstein and Lenhard[16] have made a study of the spectra in concentrated sulfuric acid of steroids which differ solely by the location of a double bond.

In Fig. 28 are shown the 2 hour spectrograms of 5-cholesten-3β-ol acetate (No. 386), its Δ^{6}- (No. 387), Δ^{7}- (No. 388) and $\Delta^{8(14)}$- (No. 389) isomers. Since the spectra of the compounds were determined at different concentrations the $E^{1\%}_{1\,cm}$ values for the maxima and minima are indicated. It was concluded that for all practical purposes the four compounds exhibit identical spectra.

The same conclusion was reached for 7-ergosten-3β-ol acetate (No. 396), its $\Delta^{8(14)}$- (No. 397) and Δ^{14}- (No. 398) isomers (Fig. 29). Parenthetically, it should be noted that the spectrum for 7-ergosten-3β-ol acetate was recorded at 2 hours 35 minutes rather than at 2 hours.

Isolated (non-conjugated) ketone

Bernstein and Lenhard[15] have pointed out that an isolated or non-conjugated ketone group will generally exhibit selective absorption in the 220–278 mμ and 300–399 mμ regions. In regard to the latter region selective absorption will be exhibited especially between 300–325 mμ.

It has been observed that if the non-conjugated ketone displays selective absorption in both of the designated ketone regions, the band at the longer wave length invariably possesses the higher extinction coefficient. Therefore, it is believed that the region at approximately 300–325 mμ most likely represents the major ketone absorption band. In conventional absorption spectroscopy, a non-conjugated ketone will exhibit selective absorption in the 170–200 mμ and 280–300 mμ regions.[39, 50] Thus, one also finds in " sulfuric acid spectroscopy " two ketone absorption regions which apparently have resulted by reason of a bathochromic effect on the sulfuric acid solvent.

α,β-Unsaturated ketone grouping

Bernstein and Lenhard[14] on the basis of an analysis of 49 α,β-unsaturated ketosteroids concluded that generally an α,β-unsaturated ketosteroid will exhibit a pronounced maximum between 279–302 mμ. This analysis included Δ^{1}-3-ketones, Δ^{4}-3-ketones, Δ^{5}-7-ketones, $\Delta^{9(11)}$-12-ketones and Δ^{16}-20-ketones. Similar observations have been made by Zaffaroni[138] and Linford.[74] The possible application of this generalization to other types of α,β-unsaturated ketones such as a $\Delta^{8(9)}$-11-ketone has not been investigated.

Bernstein and Lenhard[14] have also made a number of other observations in regard to the absorption of an α,β-unsaturated ketosteroid in concentrated sulfuric acid. It was noted that certain Δ^{4}-3-ketosteroids may be differentiated from each other not only by the wave length of the absorption maximum but also by its extinction coefficient. Testosterone (No. 38) may be differentiated from its C_{17}-epimer (No. 37) by extinction coefficient.

It has also been observed that a C_{11}-ketone group produces a hypsochromic effect on the absorption of the Δ^{4}-3-ketone parallel to that observed in conventional ultraviolet spectroscopy.[1, 39] Generally it was concluded that an 11-keto-Δ^{4}-3-ketosteroid will exhibit an absorption maximum in the 279–302 mμ region which will be at a shorter wave length (hypsochromic effect of 5–13 mμ) than the maximum of the parent Δ^{4}-3-ketosteroid unsubstituted in the C_{11}-position. The effect of a C_{11}-hydroxyl group (α- or β- configuration) is variable, and no definite conclusions may be stated.

Bernstein and Lenhard[14] compared the spectrum of progesterone (No. 116) (λ_{max} 291 mμ, $E_{1\,cm}^{1\%}$ 504) with that of 4,16-pregnadiene-3,20-dione (No. 87) (λ_{max} 302 mμ, $E_{1\,cm}^{1\%}$ 773), and concluded that the extinction coefficient of the latter indicates

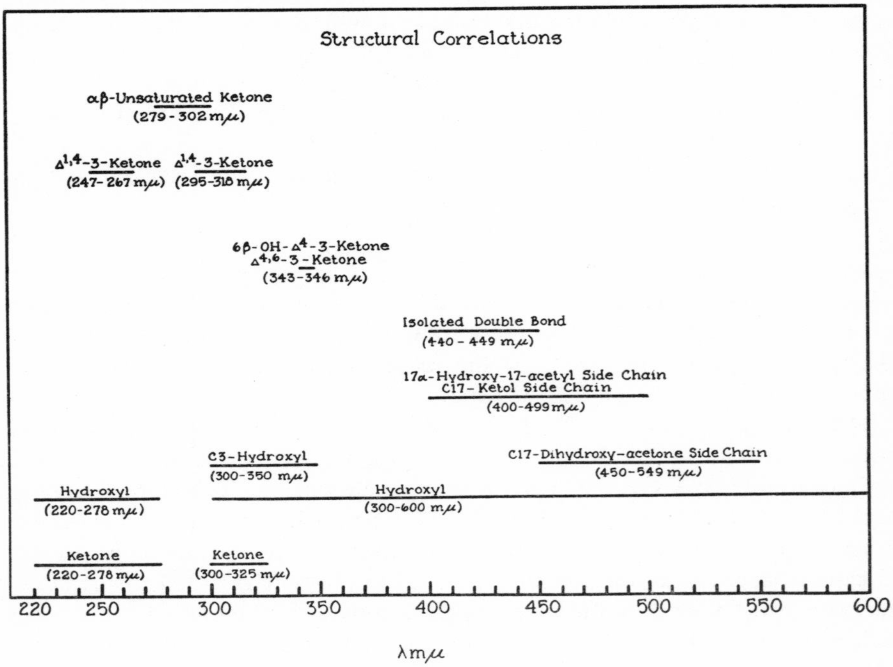

FIG. 30

a more or less additivity of the extinction coefficients of the two isolated α,β-unsaturated ketone chromophores. In conformity with this conclusion, the spectra of jervine (λ_{max} 282 mμ, $E_{1\,cm}^{1\%}$ 203) and Δ[4]-jervone (λ_{max} 281 mμ, $E_{1\,cm}^{1\%}$ 471) were cited.[14]

Δ[1,4]-3-Ketone groupings

Smith and Muller[119] have suggested that the combination of selective absorption in the 247–267 mμ region and in the 295–318 mμ region is characteristic of the $\Delta^{1,4}$-3-ketone grouping in the corticoid series.[125] Moreover in this respect Bernstein and Lenhard[14] have recorded the spectrum of 17β-hydroxy-1,4-androstadien-3-one (No. 17) which exhibits a prominent maximum at 327 mμ. This latter finding may be ascribable to the time at which the spectrum was determined. A time study on this compound has not been carried out.

A similar correlation between absorption in the 260 mμ region in " 100 per cent " phosphoric acid[93] and the $\Delta^{1,4}$-3-ketone structure has been suggested.

Other structural correlations

Bernstein and Lenhard[14] have determined the absorption spectrum of 4-pregnene-3,6,20-trione (No. 92) which exhibits a single maximum at 348 mμ. It was proposed that this selective absorption may be diagnostic for the Δ^{4}-3,6-diketone grouping.

Bernstein and Lenhard[14] have expressed the opinion that the absorption analysis of steroids in concentrated sulfuric acid may find an important use, among others, in the formation of a new chromophore *in situ,* which should offer valuable structural information. It appears that an hydroxyl group either in the α- or β- carbon position to an unsaturated ketone will give " rise " to a new chromophore, e.g., 6β-hydroxy-Δ^{4}-3-ketones yielding $\Delta^{4,6}$-3-ketones,[14] 7ξ-hydroxy-Δ^{4}-3-ketones giving also $\Delta^{4,6}$-3-ketones,[12] and 3β-hydroxy-Δ^{5}-7-ketones giving $\Delta^{3,5}$-7-ketones.[14] Bernstein and Lenhard observed that the 6β-hydroxy-Δ^{4}-3-ketone grouping exhibits two characteristic maxima, namely, at about 286–290 mμ and 343–346 mμ. The latter has the higher extinction coefficient. The 286–290 mμ maxima are of lower extinction coefficients than those found with the parent 6-deoxy compounds. The appearance of the 343–346 mμ maximum was conveniently explained by assuming the removal of the C_6-hydroxyl group to give the equivalent species of a $\Delta^{4,6}$-3-ketone in concentrated sulfuric acid. It is not implied, however, that the spectrum of a 6β-hydroxy-Δ^{4}-3-ketosteroid will be identical in all aspects with that of its corresponding $\Delta^{4,6}$-3-ketosteroid. On this basis 6β-hydroxy-4-pregnene-3,20-dione (No. 121) was found to be easily differentiated from either 11α-hydroxy- or 11β-hydroxy-4-pregnene-3,20-dione (Nos. 124, 125). No definite data have been published on the influence of a 6α-hydroxyl group on the Δ^{4}-3-ketone grouping. In this regard the work of Axelrod[2] and Zaffaroni[138] should be consulted.

Bernstein and Lenhard[14] have determined the spectrum of 7-keto-5-cholestene-3β-ol acetate (No. 378) and found, among others, maxima at 285 mμ (ascribable to the α, β-unsaturated ketone group) and at 355 mμ. The latter is the principal maximum and was ascribed to the $\Delta^{3,5}$-7-ketone group which would result from the removal of the C_3-hydroxyl group.

Little information is available in regard to a hydroxyl group on an adjacent carbon (either α or β) to a non-conjugated ketone. However, it has been observed that 17α-hydroxy-progesterone (No. 126) did not give rise to a spectrum " equivalent " to that of 4,16-pregnadiene-3,20-dione (No. 87). Also it has been observed that the 2 hour spectra of hydrocortisone (No. 146) and 5α,11β,17α,21-tetrahydroxy-pregnane-3,20-dione (No. 173) are not identical.

17-*Acetyl side-chain*

In the Bernstein–Lenhard catalog[13] there are seven steroids (Nos. 126, 133, 159, 177, 179, 182, 183)* with the 17α-hydroxy-17-acetyl side chain. Also there are three steroids (Nos. 127, 134, 135)* which contain an α-ketol side-chain at C_{17}. All ten compounds showed selective absorption in the 400–499 mμ region.

Also in the Bernstein–Lenhard catalog[13] there are twelve steroids (Nos. 103, 136, 140, 143, 145, 146, 217, 229, 239, 303, 310)* which contain the dihydroxy-acetone side-chain at C_{17}. All twelve showed selective absorption (maximum or inflection, $E^{1\%}_{1\,cm}$ 11–204) between 474–535 mμ. Of these twelve compounds eleven (one exception, No. 310, 3α,21-diacetoxy-11β,17α-dihydroxy-5β-pregnan-20-one, λ_{max} 506 mμ) show selective absorption between 474–490 mμ ($E^{1\%}_{1\,cm}$ 11–204). It was also observed that eight of twelve of the above compounds also show selective absorption in the 338–343 mμ region ($E^{1\%}_{1\,cm}$ 93–450) and nine out of twelve show selective absorption in the 233–271 mμ region ($E^{1\%}_{1\,cm}$ 109–420).

In this connection, Smith and Muller[119] have recorded the spectra in concentrated sulfuric acid (at 15 minutes, 2 hours and 20 hours) of twenty-six 1-dehydro-corticosteroids (with a dihydroxy-acetone side-chain). Of this number eighteen contain in addition to the $\Delta^{1,4}$-3-ketone grouping a 16α-hydroxy or acetoxy group. Of the eight corticosteroids which do not contain a 16-oxygenated function, 3/8 (15 minutes), 5/8 (2 hours) and 7/8 (20 hours) show selective absorption in the 450–549 mμ region. Of the eighteen corticosteroids which contain a 16-oxygenated function 1/18 (15 minutes), 2/18 (2 hours) and 8/18 (20 hours) show selective absorption in the 450–549 mμ region.

Carboxyl group

An isolated carboxyl group in the steroid (bile acid) molecule does not give rise to selective absorption spectra in concentrated sulfuric acid.[43] Esterification of the carboxyl group does not generally affect the spectra of the bile acid, and no specific effects are reported where the carboxyl group is converted to a secondary amide (conjugated bile acids).[44]

The selective absorption of bile acids is thus due to the hydroxyl and ketone groups and to carbon–carbon double bonds present in the molecule, and the spectral properties generally are in accord with the structural arguments already developed.[14, 15]

In the Chart there is given the absorption bands of the principal groups discussed. An examination of this chart reveals that there are many overlapping absorption bands for the various structural groups. As a consequence of this it may be stated that structural interpretation of an absorption curve of an unknown steroid will be difficult and highly tentative. It should be emphasized that these structural correlations must be used cautiously and with proper respect for the complexities involved.

* The numbers in parentheses refer to the numbering of Tables I–XVI of this review and not to the original numbering of the Bernstein–Lenhard catalog.

Theory of spectra

A limited amount of work has been done in developing a unified theory of the origins of selective absorption spectra in concentrated sulfuric acid. The review by Gillespie and Leisten[51] discusses the general approaches, and the studies of Linford[53, 74] afford a basis for further work. To date, no definitive theory has been proposed which accounts for the many intricacies of steroid spectra in sulfuric (indeed any) acid.

Linford[74] proposes that protonated species are formed in the strong acid, and that these ionic species give rise to the observed spectra. That so simple an expedient is inadequate to explain the complex time, heating and dilution effects has been pointed out by Kalant.[69] The proposals of Bernstein and Lenhard[14] relative to the formation of new chromophores *in situ* already discussed in this review are pertinent also.

It is beyond the scope of the present review to delve further into theoretical treatment of spectra.

V. FIGURES

INDIVIDUAL SPECTRA OF SELECTED STEROIDS

2

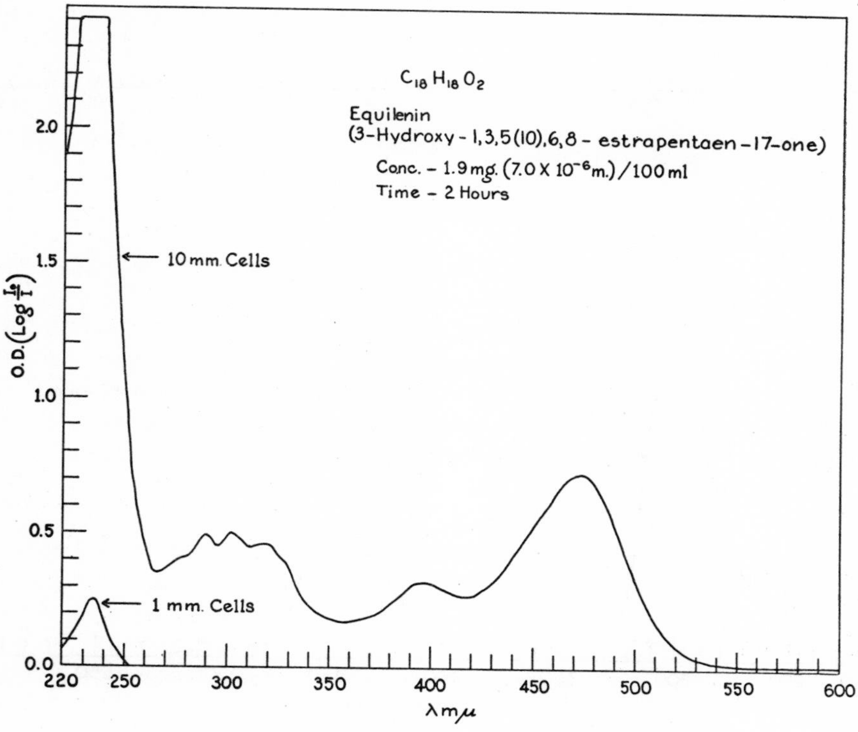

4

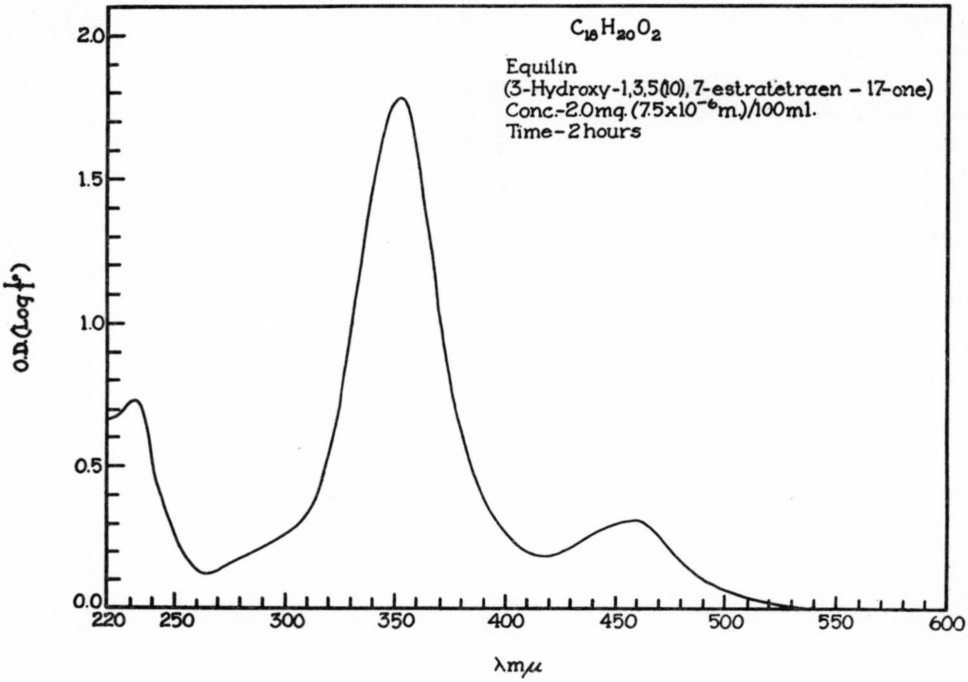

C18H20O2
Equilin
(3-Hydroxy-1,3,5(10), 7-estratetraen - 17-one)
Conc.-2.0mg. (7.5x10⁻⁶m.)/100ml.
Time-2 hours
O.D.(Log I₀/I)
λmμ

5

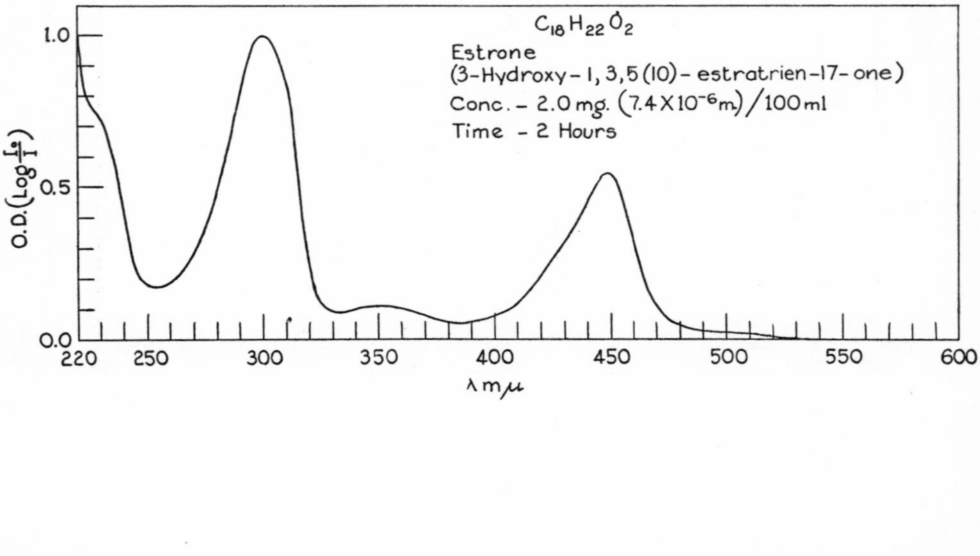

C18H22O2
Estrone
(3-Hydroxy-1, 3,5 (10)- estratrien-17- one)
Conc. - 2.0 mg. (7.4X10⁻⁶m.)/100 ml
Time - 2 Hours
O.D.(Log I₀/I)
λmμ

8

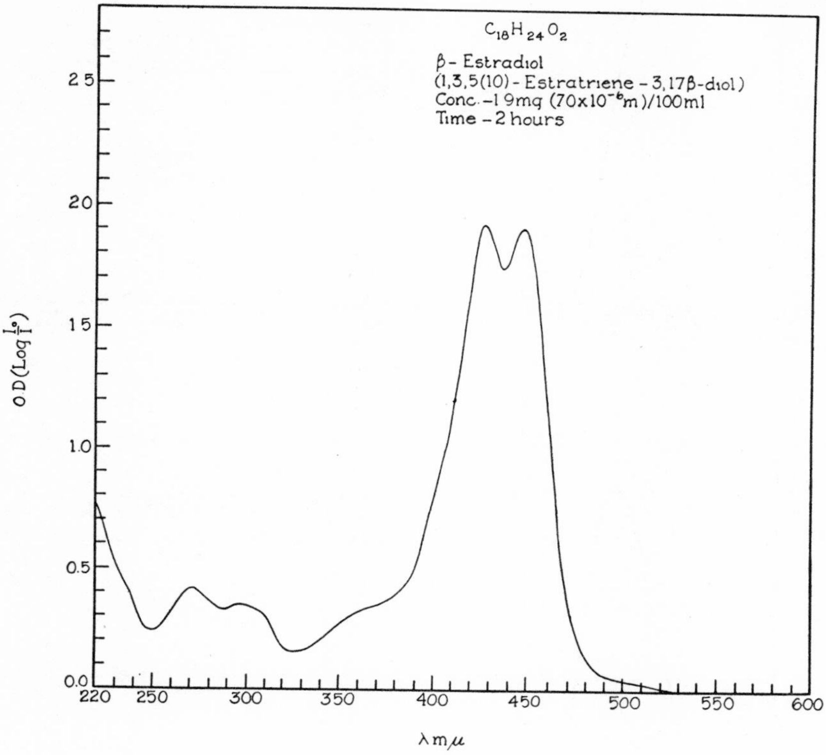
$C_{18}H_{24}O_2$
β- Estradiol
(1,3,5(10)- Estratriene - 3,17β-diol)
Conc.-1.9mg (7.0x10⁻⁶m)/100ml
Time - 2 hours
O.D (Log I₀/I)
0.0
0.5
1.0
1.5
2.0
2.5
220
250
300
350
400
450
500
550
600
λ mμ

10

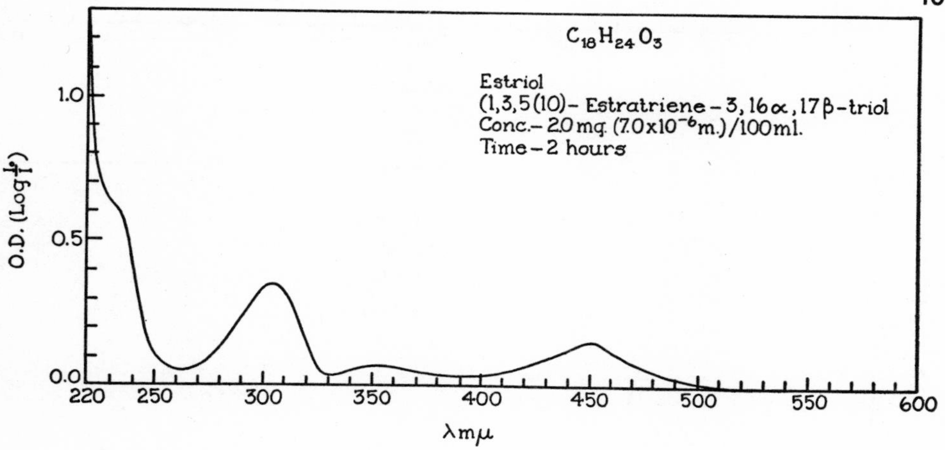
$C_{18}H_{24}O_3$
Estriol
(1,3,5(10)- Estratriene - 3, 16α, 17β-triol
Conc.- 2.0 mg. (7.0x10⁻⁶m.)/100ml.
Time - 2 hours
O.D. (Log I₀/I)
0.0
0.5
1.0
220
250
300
350
400
450
500
550
600
λmμ

14

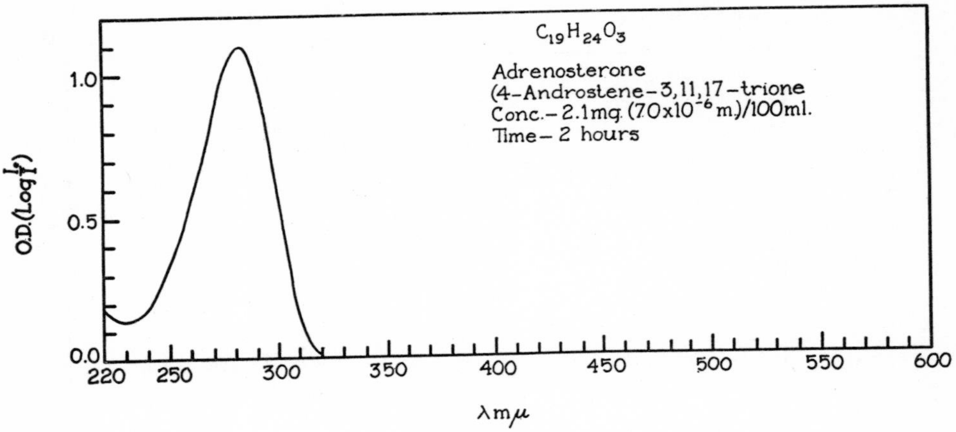
$C_{19}H_{24}O_3$
Adrenosterone
(4-Androstene-3,11,17-trione
Conc.-2.1mg. (7.0x10^{-6} m.)/100ml.
Time- 2 hours
O.D.(Log I₀/I)
1.0
0.5
0.0
220
250
300
350
400
450
500
550
600
λ mμ

19

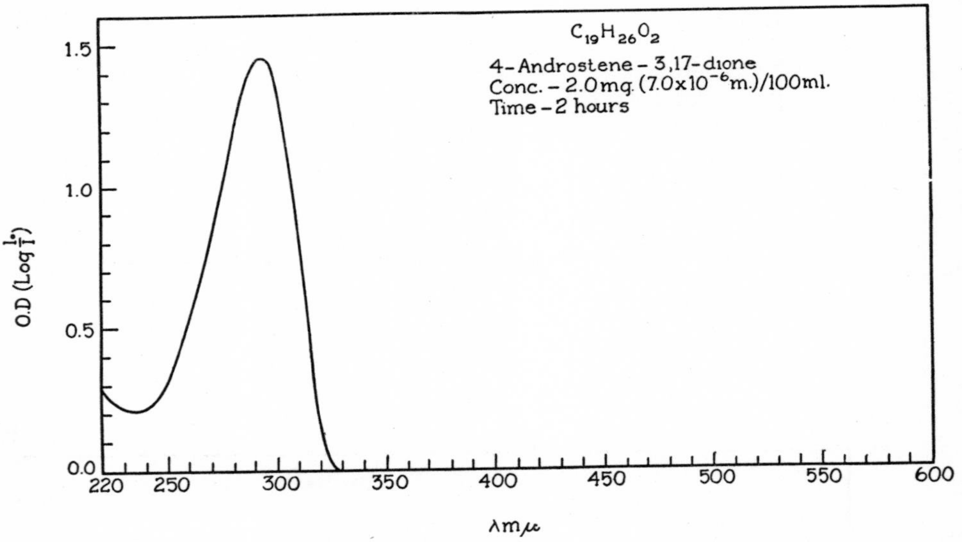
$C_{19}H_{26}O_2$
4-Androstene-3,17-dione
Conc. - 2.0mg. (7.0x10^{-6}m.)/100ml.
Time-2 hours
O.D (Log I₀/I)
1.5
1.0
0.5
0.0
220
250
300
350
400
450
500
550
600
λ mμ

30

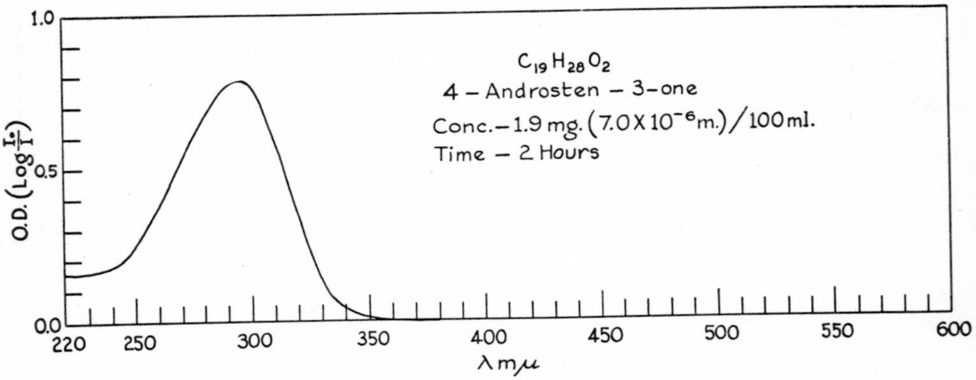
$C_{19}H_{28}O_2$
4 - Androsten - 3-one
Conc.-1.9 mg. (7.0X10^{-6}m.)/100ml.
Time - 2 Hours
O.D. (Log I₀/I)
1.0
0.5
0.0
220
250
300
350
400
450
500
550
600
λ mμ

32

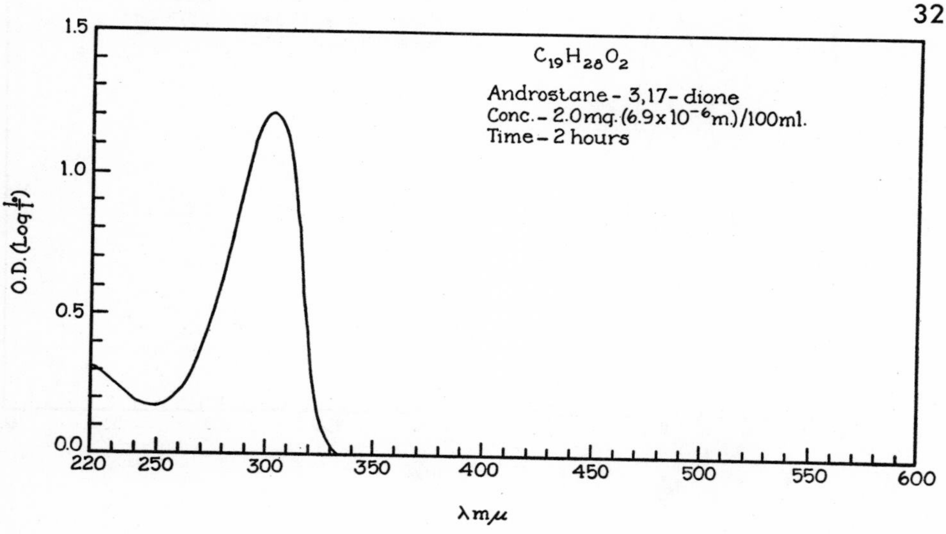
$C_{19}H_{28}O_2$
Androstane - 3,17- dione
Conc. - 2.0 mg. (6.9 x 10^{-6}m.)/100ml.
Time - 2 hours
O.D. (Log $\frac{I_0}{I}$)
1.5
1.0
0.5
0.0
220
250
300
350
400
450
500
550
600
λ mμ

33

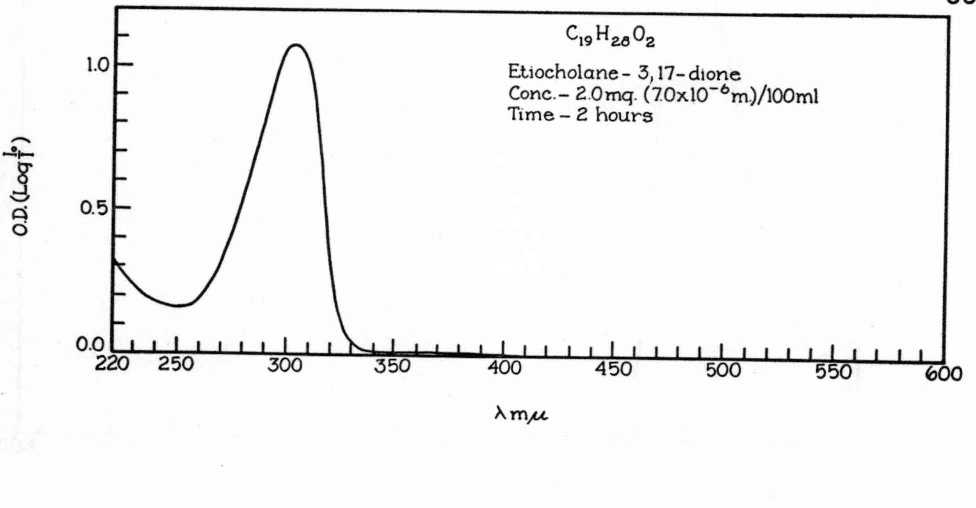
$C_{19}H_{28}O_2$
Etiocholane - 3,17- dione
Conc. - 2.0 mg. (7.0x10^{-6}m.)/100ml
Time - 2 hours
O.D. (Log $\frac{I_0}{I}$)
1.0
0.5
0.0
220
250
300
350
400
450
500
550
600
λ mμ

37

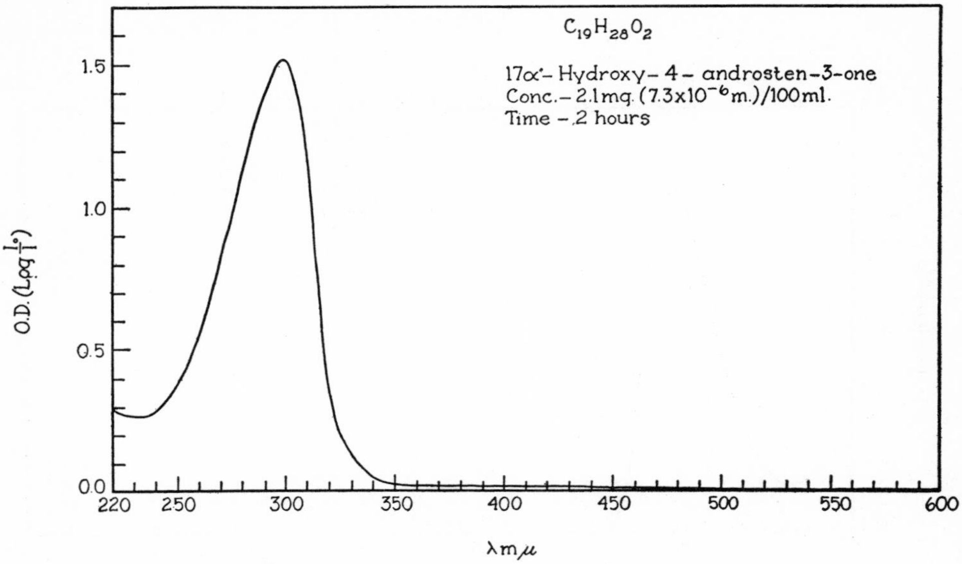
$C_{19}H_{28}O_2$
17α-Hydroxy-4-androsten-3-one
Conc.-2.1mg. (7.3×10^{-6}m.)/100ml.
Time-2 hours
O.D. (Log $\frac{I_0}{I}$)
λmμ

38

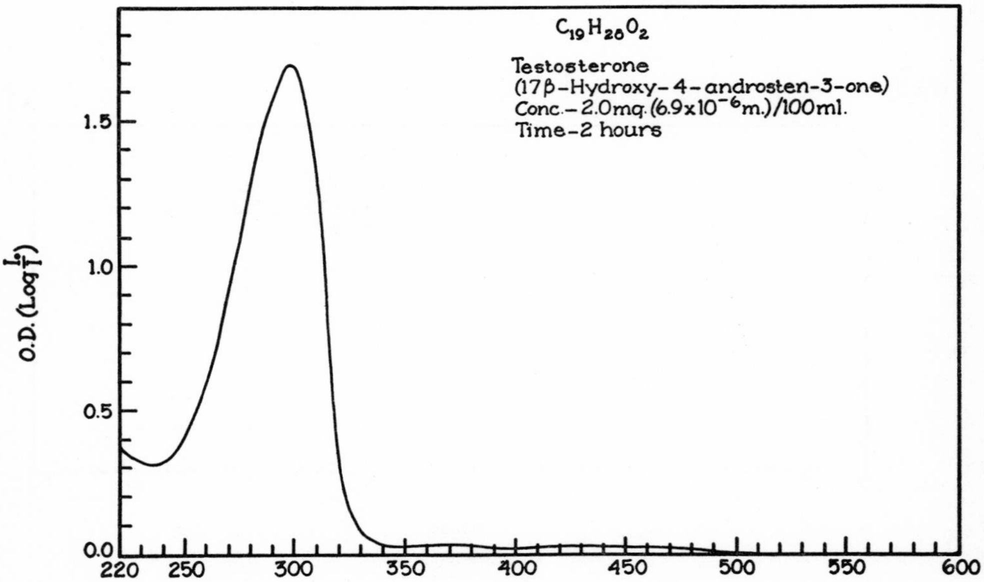
$C_{19}H_{28}O_2$
Testosterone
(17β-Hydroxy-4-androsten-3-one)
Conc.-2.0mg. (6.9×10^{-6}m.)/100ml.
Time-2 hours
O.D. (Log $\frac{I_0}{I}$)
λmμ

39

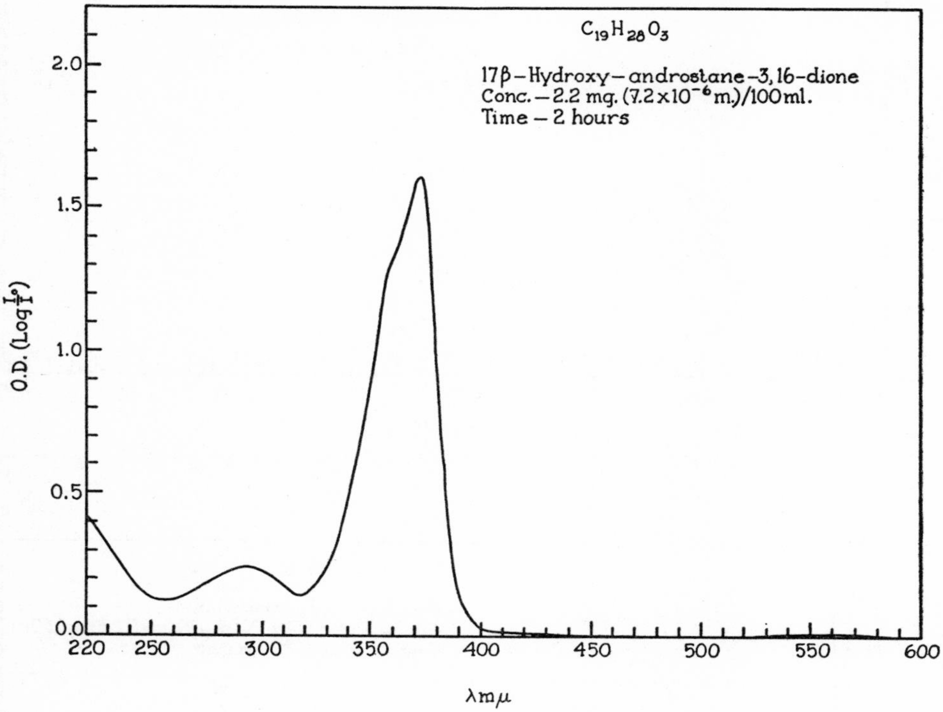
C19H28O3
17β-Hydroxy-androstane-3,16-dione
Conc.-2.2 mg. (7.2x10⁻⁶ m.)/100ml.
Time - 2 hours
O.D. (Log I₀/I)
2.0
1.5
1.0
0.5
0.0
220
250
300
350
400
450
500
550
600
λmμ

40

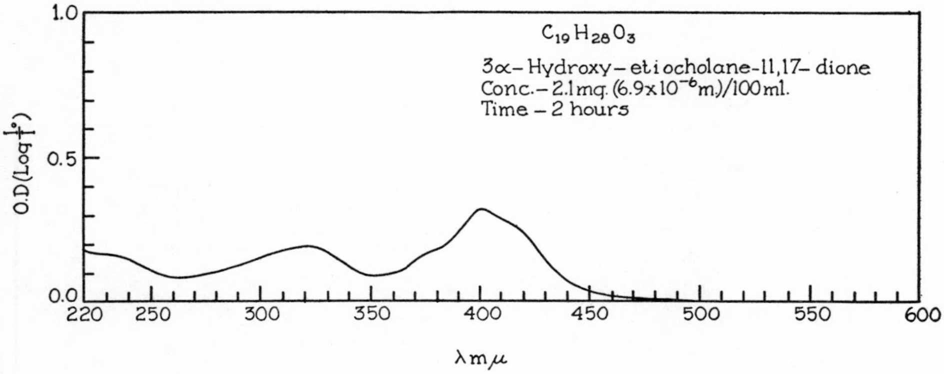
C19H28O3
3α-Hydroxy-etiocholane-11,17-dione
Conc.-2.1mg. (6.9x10⁻⁶m.)/100ml.
Time - 2 hours
O.D (Log I₀/I)
1.0
0.5
0.0
220
250
300
350
400
450
500
550
600
λmμ

47

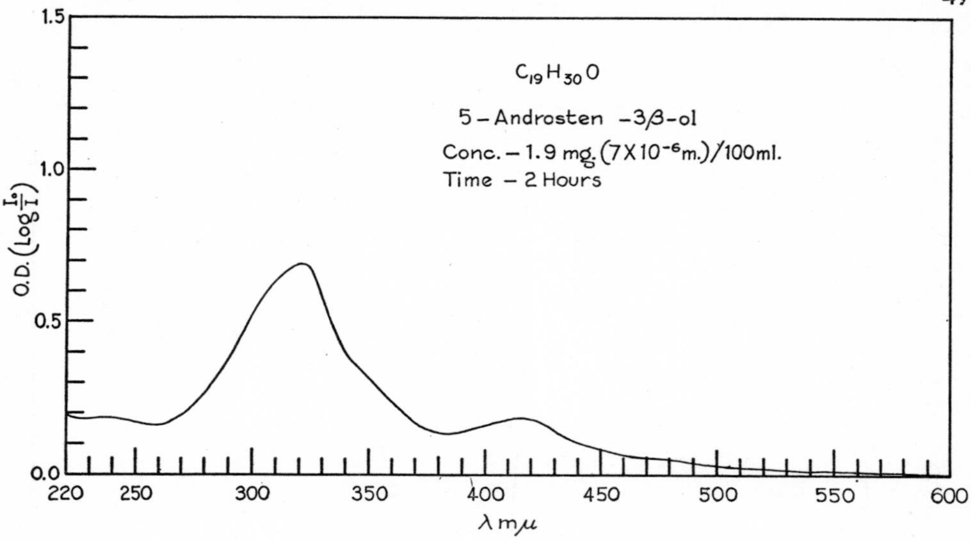
$C_{19}H_{30}O$
5-Androsten-3β-ol
Conc.—1.9 mg. (7×10⁻⁶m.)/100 ml.
Time — 2 Hours
O.D. (Log I₀/I)
λ mμ

50

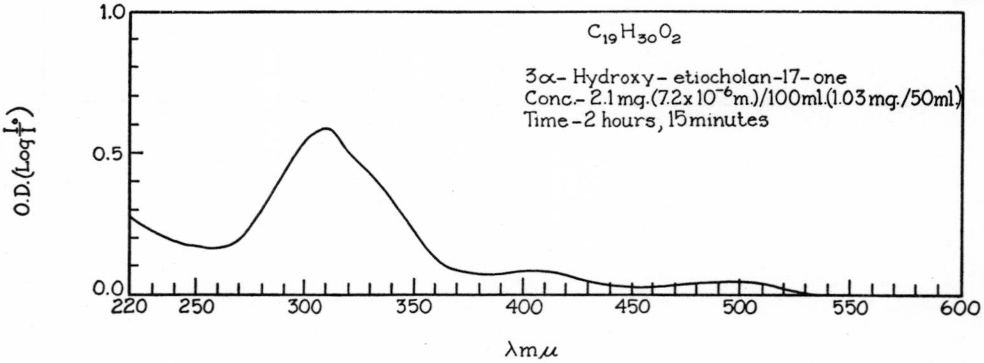
$C_{19}H_{30}O_2$
3α-Hydroxy-etiocholan-17-one
Conc.—2.1 mg. (7.2×10⁻⁶m.)/100 ml. (1.03 mg./50 ml.)
Time—2 hours, 15 minutes
O.D. (Log I₀/I)
λ mμ

51

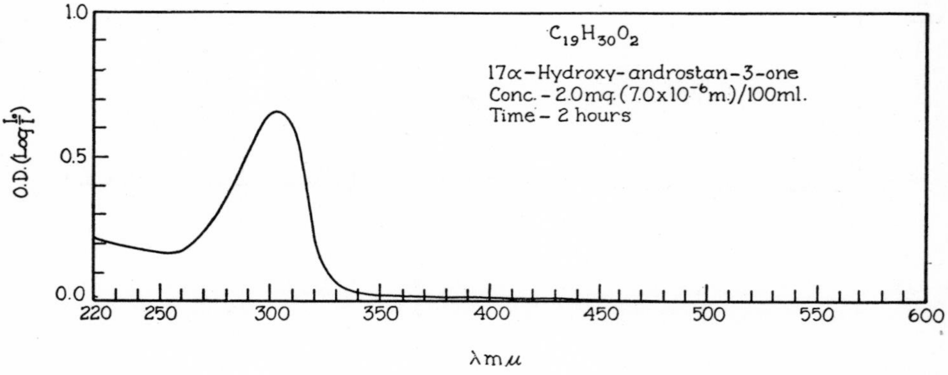
$C_{19}H_{30}O_2$
17α-Hydroxy-androstan-3-one
Conc.—2.0 mg. (7.0×10⁻⁶m.)/100 ml.
Time — 2 hours
O.D. (Log I₀/I)
λ mμ

52

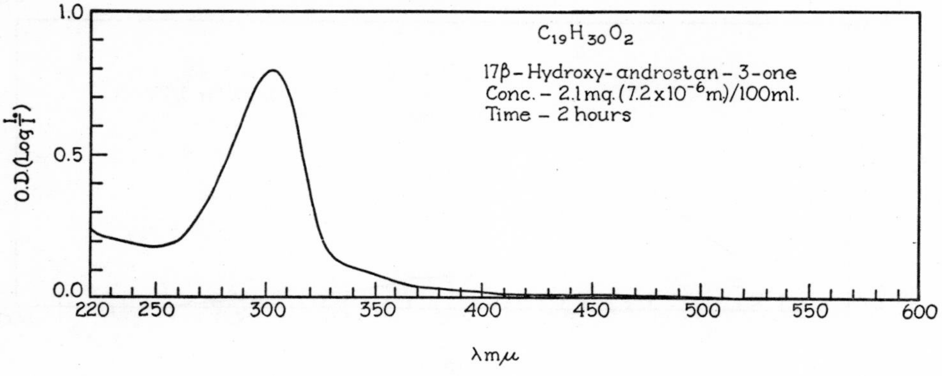
$C_{19}H_{30}O_2$
17β-Hydroxy-androstan-3-one
Conc. - 2.1 mg. (7.2 x 10⁻⁶ m)/100 ml.
Time - 2 hours
O.D. (Log I₀/I)
1.0
0.5
0.0
220
250
300
350
400
450
500
550
600
λ mμ

53

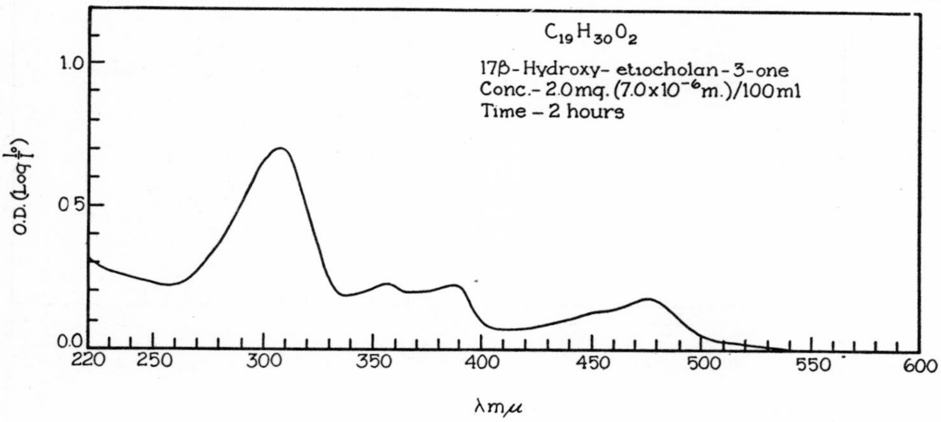
$C_{19}H_{30}O_2$
17β-Hydroxy-etiocholan-3-one
Conc.- 2.0 mg. (7.0 x 10⁻⁶ m.)/100 ml
Time - 2 hours
O.D. (Log I₀/I)
1.0
0.5
0.0
220
250
300
350
400
450
500
550
600
λ mμ

58

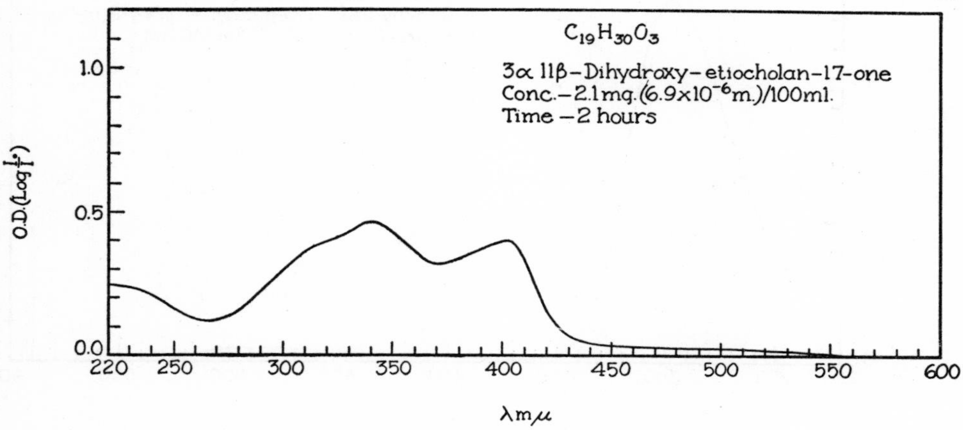
$C_{19}H_{30}O_3$
3α 11β-Dihydroxy-etiocholan-17-one
Conc.-2.1 mg. (6.9 x 10⁻⁶ m.)/100 ml.
Time - 2 hours
O.D. (Log I₀/I)
1.0
0.5
0.0
220
250
300
350
400
450
500
550
600
λ mμ

63

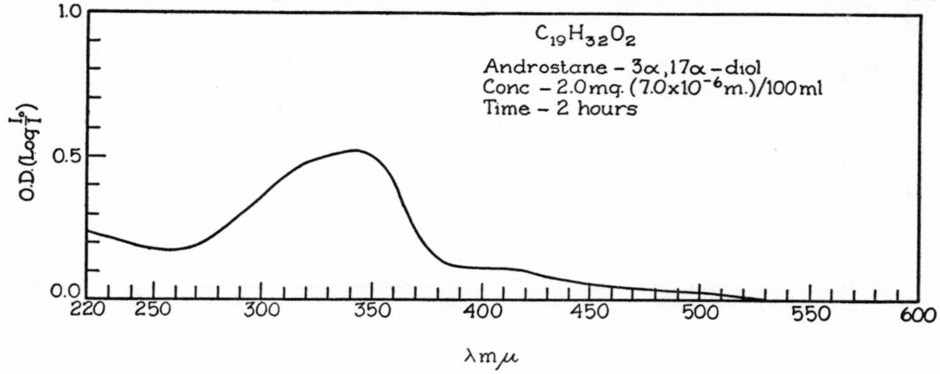

$C_{19}H_{32}O_2$
Androstane - 3α,17α - diol
Conc - 2.0mg. (7.0x10^{-6}m.)/100ml
Time - 2 hours
O.D. (Log $\frac{I_o}{I}$)
1.0
0.5
0.0
220
250
300
350
400
450
500
550
600
λmμ

66

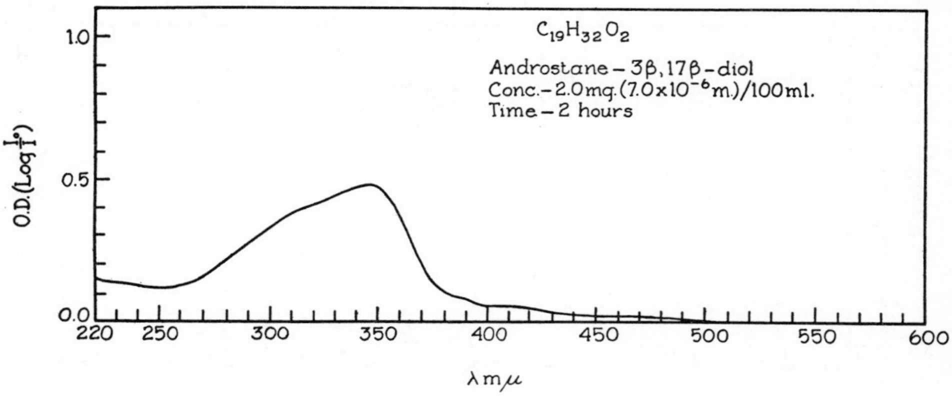

$C_{19}H_{32}O_2$
Androstane - 3β, 17β - diol
Conc. - 2.0mg. (7.0x10^{-6}m.)/100ml.
Time - 2 hours
O.D. (Log $\frac{I_o}{I}$)
1.0
0.5
0.0
220
250
300
350
400
450
500
550
600
λmμ

72

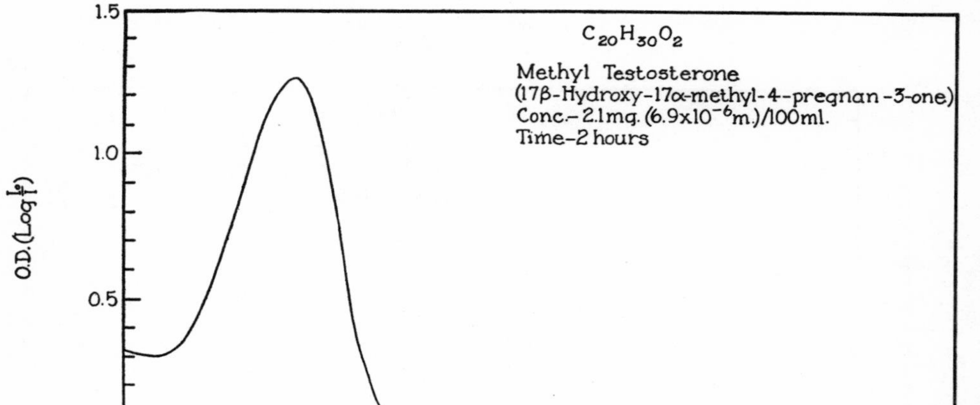

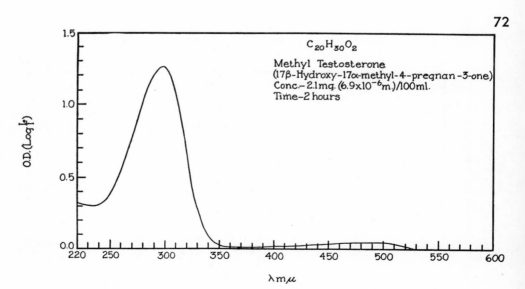

$C_{20}H_{30}O_2$
Methyl Testosterone
(17β-Hydroxy-17α-methyl-4--pregnan-3-one)
Conc.- 2.1mg. (6.9x10^{-6}m.)/100ml.
Time-2 hours
O.D. (Log $\frac{I_o}{I}$)
1.5
1.0
0.5
0.0
220
250
300
350
400
450
500
550
600
λmμ

75

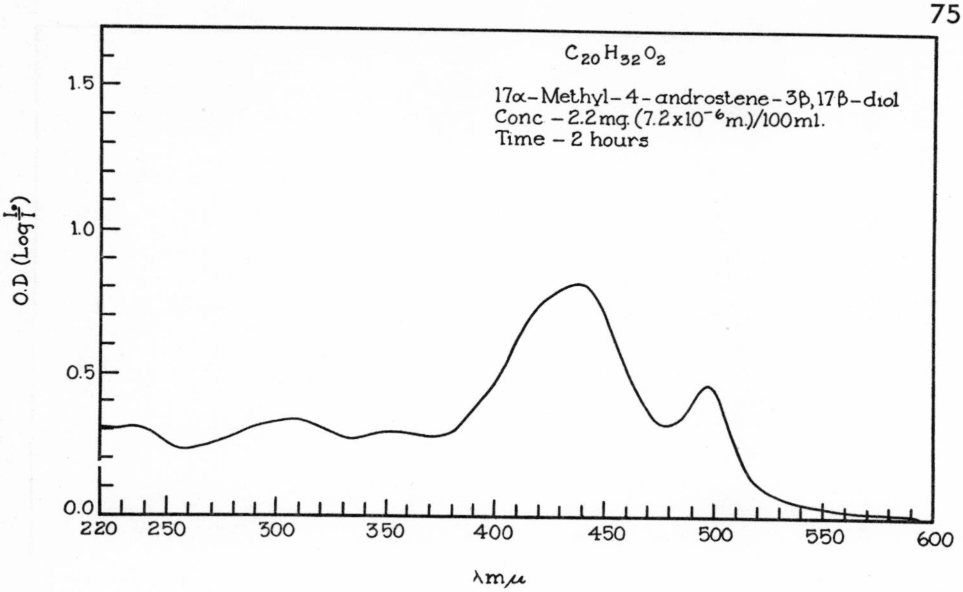
$C_{20}H_{32}O_2$
17α-Methyl-4-androstene-3β,17β-diol
Conc – 2.2 mg. (7.2x10⁻⁶m.)/100 ml.
Time – 2 hours
O.D (Log I₀/I)
λmμ

80

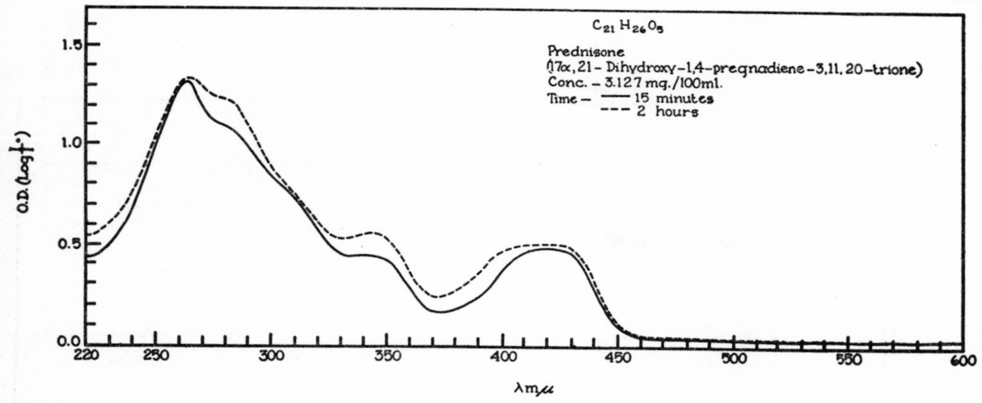
$C_{21}H_{26}O_5$
Prednisone
(17α, 21-Dihydroxy-1,4-pregnadiene-3,11,20-trione)
Conc. – 3.127 mg./100ml.
Time – —— 15 minutes
- - - 2 hours
O.D. (Log I₀/I)
λmμ

85

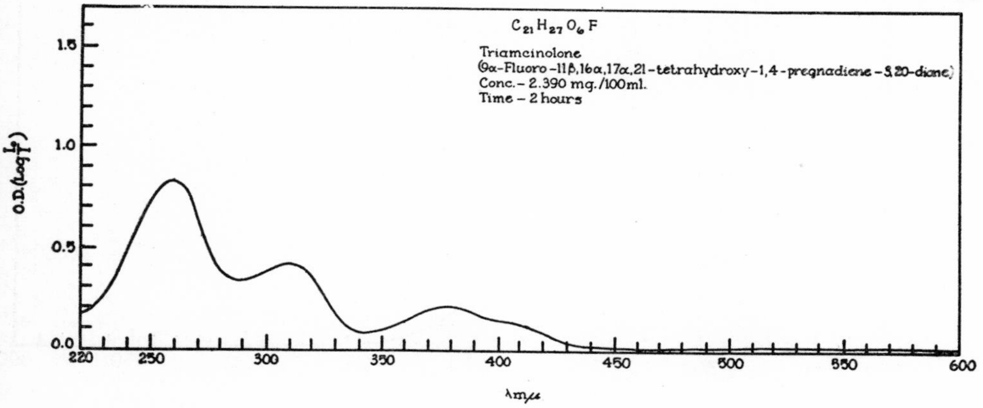
$C_{21}H_{27}O_6F$
Triamcinolone
(9α-Fluoro-11β,16α,17α,21-tetrahydroxy-1,4-pregnadiene-3,20-dione)
Conc. – 2.390 mg./100ml.
Time – 2 hours
O.D. (Log I₀/I)
λmμ

87

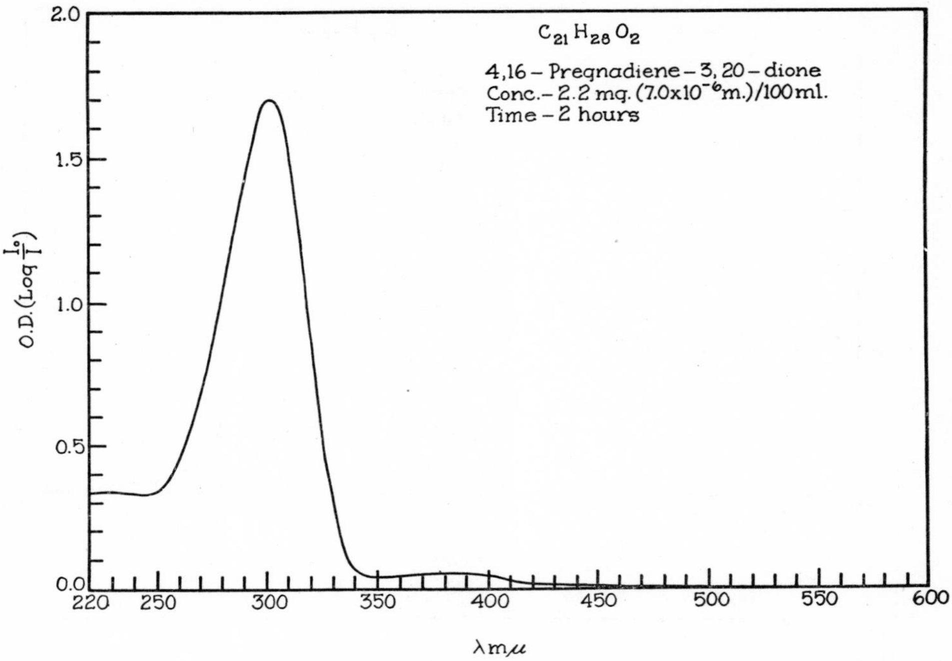
$C_{21}H_{28}O_2$
4,16 – Pregnadiene – 3, 20 – dione
Conc.– 2.2 mg. (7.0x10⁻⁶m.)/100 ml.
Time – 2 hours
O.D. (Log I₀/I)
2.0
1.5
1.0
0.5
0.0
220
250
300
350
400
450
500
550
600
λ mμ

92

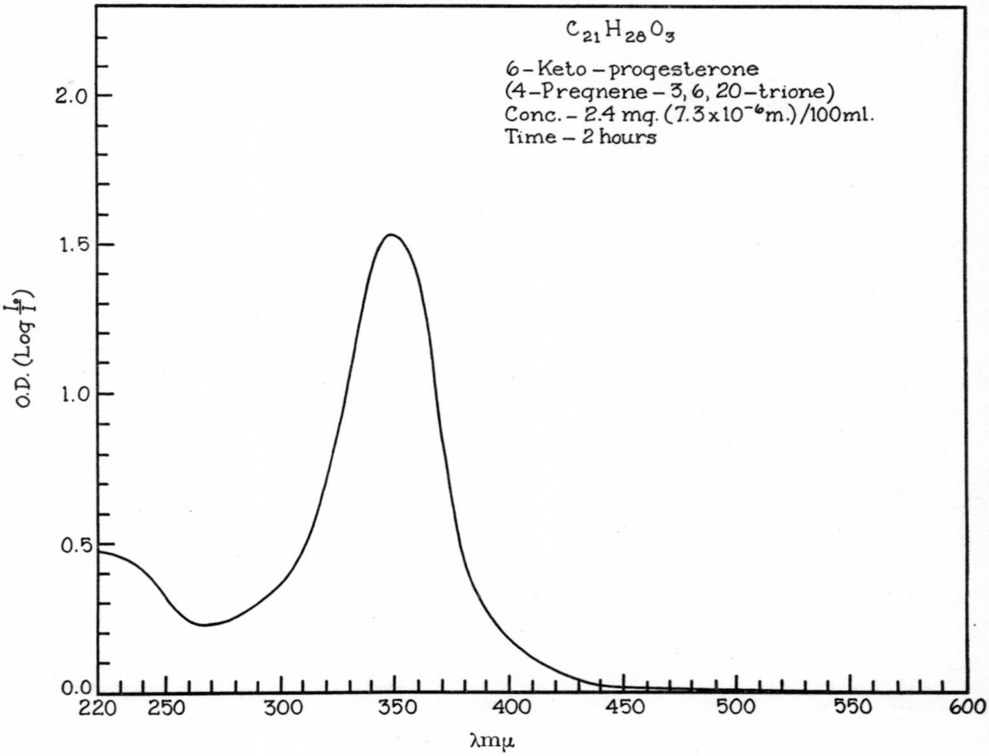
$C_{21}H_{28}O_3$
6 – Keto – progesterone
(4 – Pregnene – 3, 6, 20 – trione)
Conc. – 2.4 mg. (7.3 x 10⁻⁶m.)/100 ml.
Time – 2 hours
O.D. (Log I₀/I)
2.0
1.5
1.0
0.5
0.0
220
250
300
350
400
450
500
550
600
λmμ

93

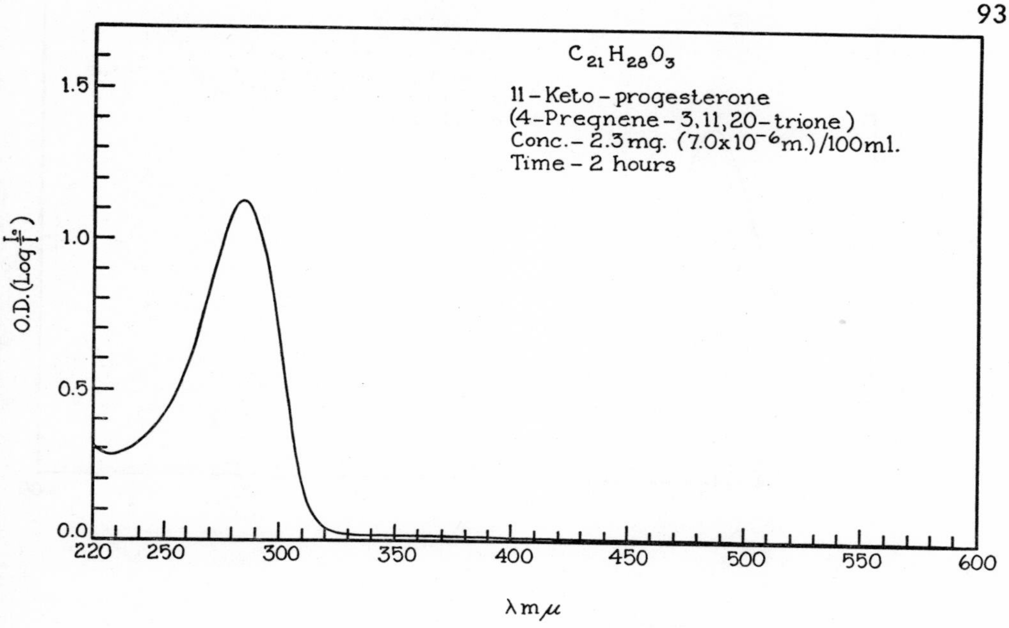
C21 H28 O3
11 - Keto - progesterone
(4-Pregnene - 3,11,20 - trione)
Conc. - 2.3 mg. (7.0x10-6 m.)/100 ml.
Time - 2 hours
O.D. (Log I0/I)
1.5
1.0
0.5
0.0
220
250
300
350
400
450
500
550
600
λ mμ

99

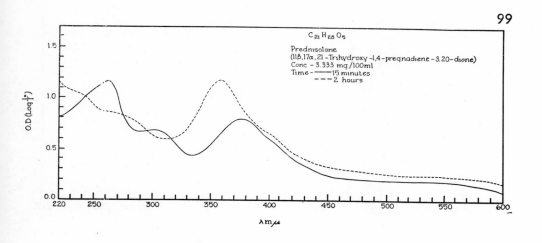

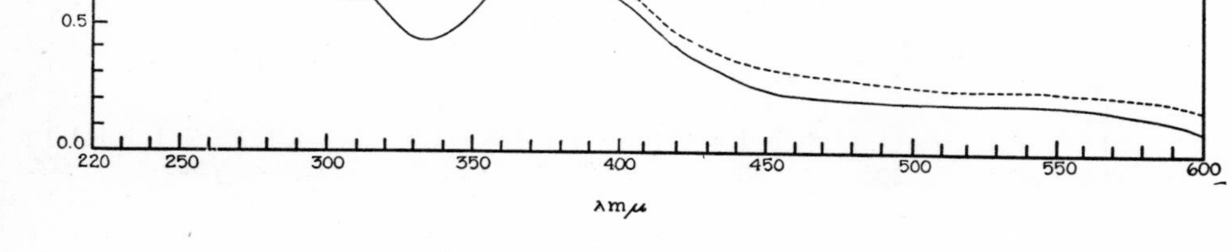
C21 H28 O5
Prednisolone
(11β,17α, 21 - Trihydroxy -1,4 - pregnadiene - 3,20 - dione)
Conc - 3.333 mg/100ml
Time - —— 15 minutes
- - - 2 hours
O.D (Log I0/I)
1.5
1.0
0.5
0.0
220
250
300
350
400
450
500
550
600
λ mμ

113

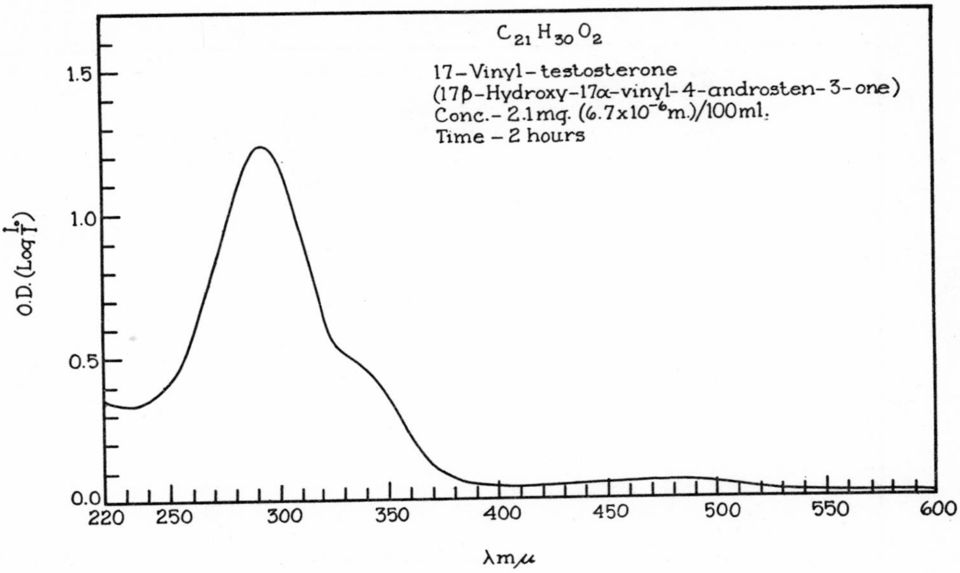
$C_{21}H_{30}O_2$
17-Vinyl-testosterone
(17β-Hydroxy-17α-vinyl-4-androsten-3-one)
Conc.- 2.1mg. (6.7x10⁻⁶m.)/100ml.
Time - 2 hours
O.D. (Log I₀/I)
1.5
1.0
0.5
0.0
220
250
300
350
400
450
500
550
600
λmμ

116

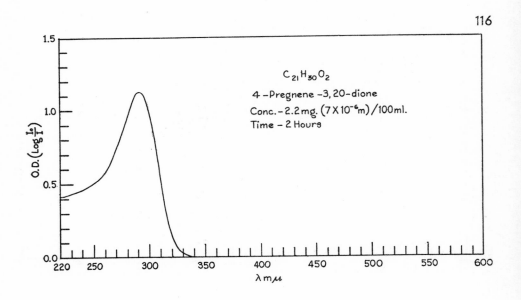

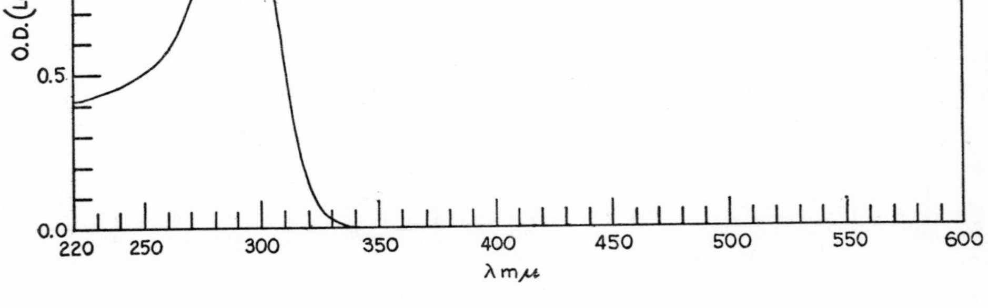
$C_{21}H_{30}O_2$
4-Pregnene-3,20-dione
Conc.-2.2mg. (7X10⁻⁶m)/100ml.
Time - 2 Hours
O.D. (Log I₀/I)
1.5
1.0
0.5
0.0
220
250
300
350
400
450
500
550
600
λmμ

119

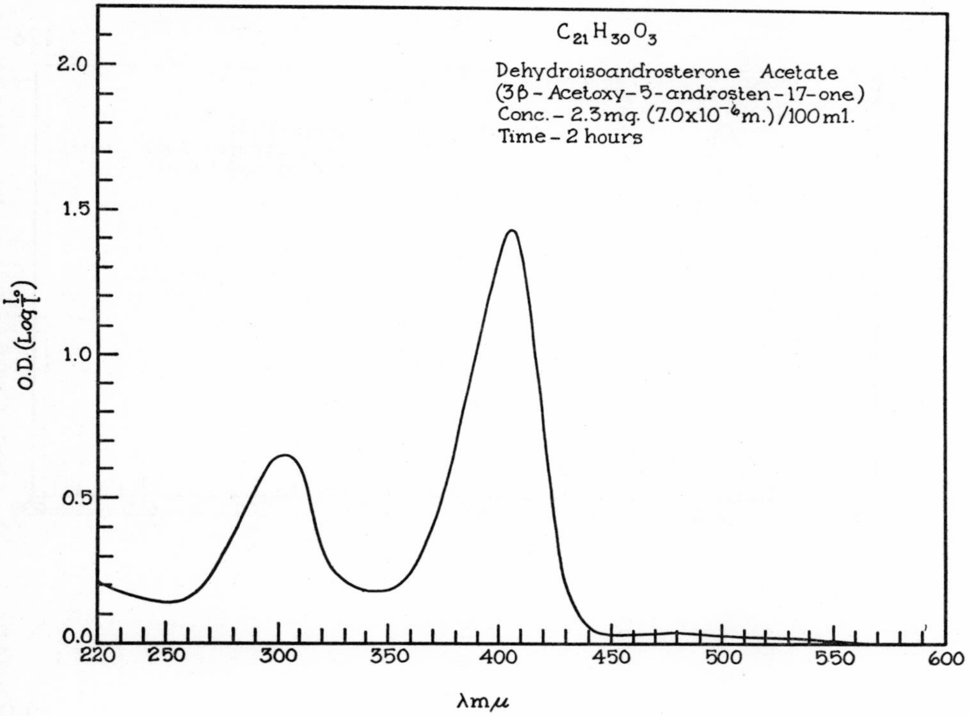
$C_{21}H_{30}O_3$
Dehydroisoandrosterone Acetate
(3β-Acetoxy-5-androsten-17-one)
Conc. - 2.3 mg. (7.0x10⁻⁶m.)/100 ml.
Time - 2 hours
O.D. (Log I₀/I)
2.0
1.5
1.0
0.5
0.0
220
250
300
350
400
450
500
550
600
λmμ

121

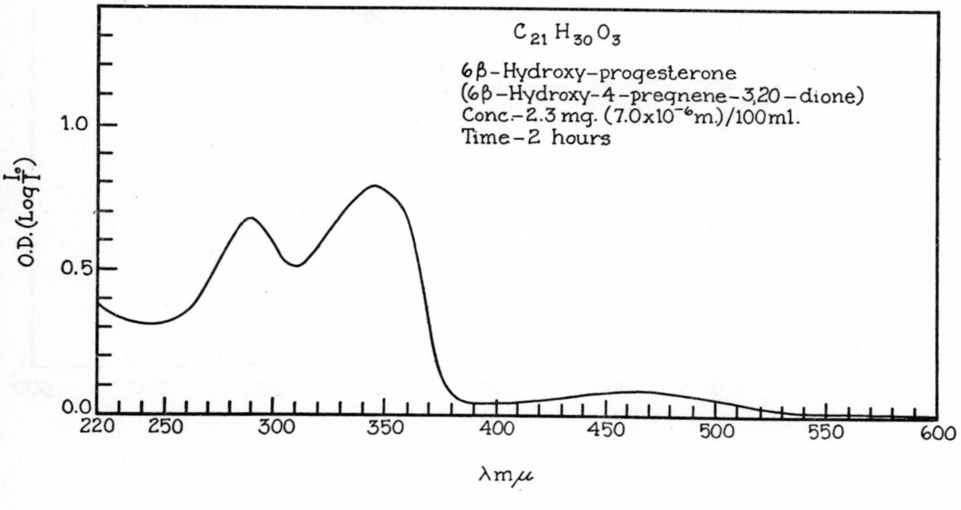
$C_{21}H_{30}O_3$
6β-Hydroxy-progesterone
(6β-Hydroxy-4-pregnene-3,20-dione)
Conc.-2.3 mg. (7.0x10⁻⁶m.)/100 ml.
Time-2 hours
O.D. (Log I₀/I)
1.0
0.5
0.0
220
250
300
350
400
450
500
550
600
λmμ

126

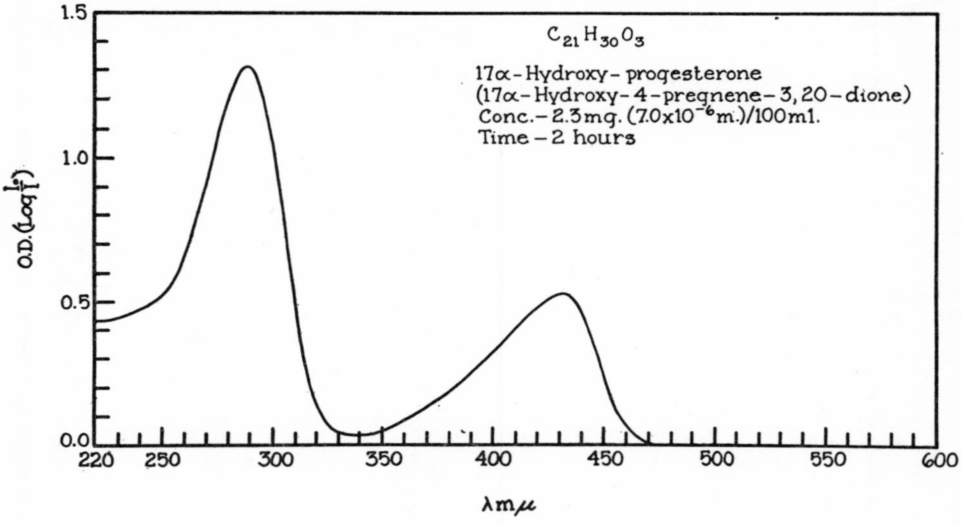
$C_{21}H_{30}O_3$
17α-Hydroxy-progesterone
(17α-Hydroxy-4-pregnene-3,20-dione)
Conc.-2.3mg. (7.0x10⁻⁶m.)/100ml.
Time-2 hours
O.D.(Log I₀/I)
1.5
1.0
0.5
0.0
220
250
300
350
400
450
500
550
600
λmμ

127

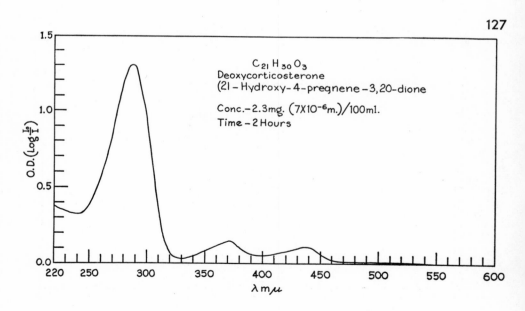

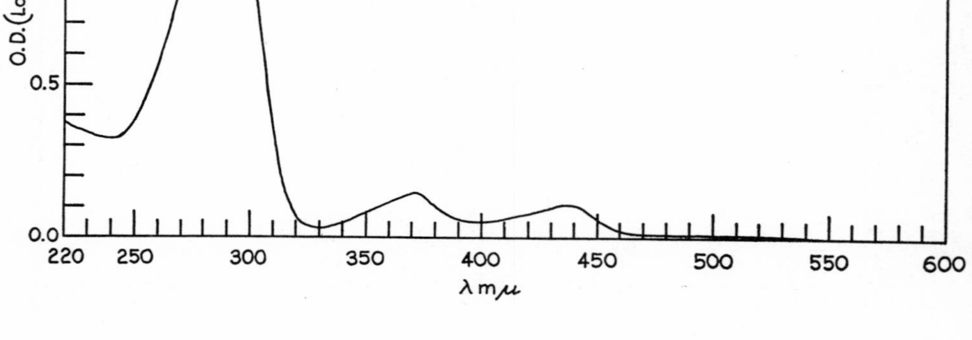
$C_{21}H_{30}O_3$
Deoxycorticosterone
(21-Hydroxy-4-pregnene-3,20-dione
Conc.-2.3mg. (7X10⁻⁶m.)/100ml.
Time-2 Hours
O.D.(Log I₀/I)
1.5
1.0
0.5
0.0
220
250
300
350
400
450
500
550
600
λmμ

140

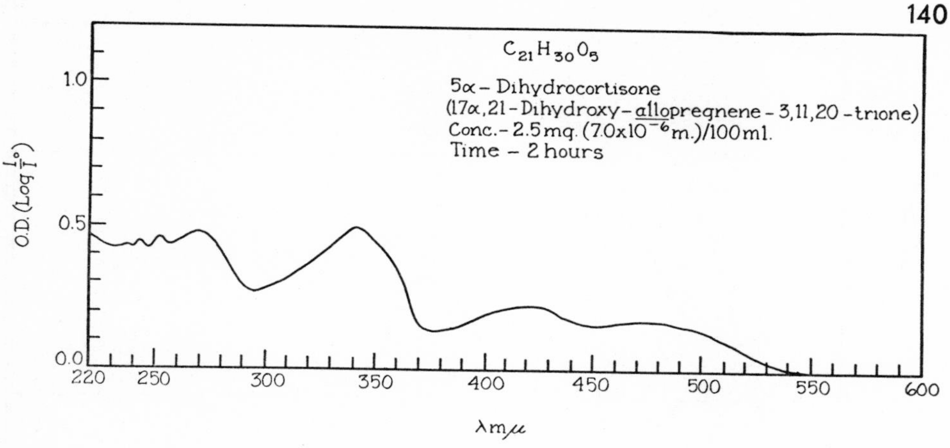
$C_{21}H_{30}O_5$
5α – Dihydrocortisone
(17α,21-Dihydroxy-allopregnene-3,11,20-trione)
Conc.- 2.5 mg. (7.0x10⁻⁶m.)/100 ml.
Time – 2 hours
O.D. (Log I₀/I)
1.0
0.5
0.0
220 250 300 350 400 450 500 550 600
λmμ

143

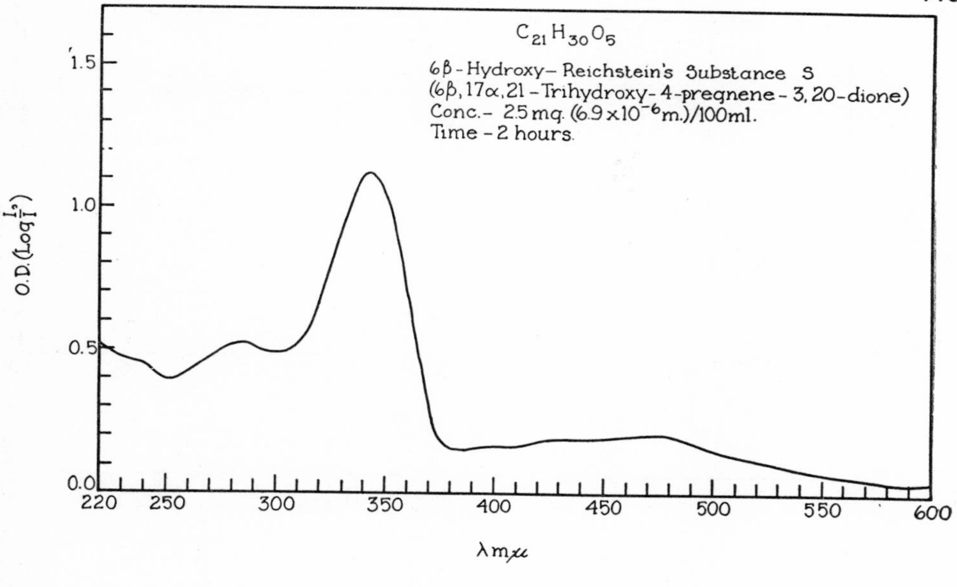
$C_{21}H_{30}O_5$
6β-Hydroxy-Reichstein's Substance S
(6β,17α,21-Trihydroxy-4-pregnene-3,20-dione)
Conc.- 2.5 mg. (6.9x10⁻⁶m.)/100ml.
Time - 2 hours.
O.D. (Log I₀/I)
1.5
1.0
0.5
0.0
220 250 300 350 400 450 500 550 600
λmμ

154

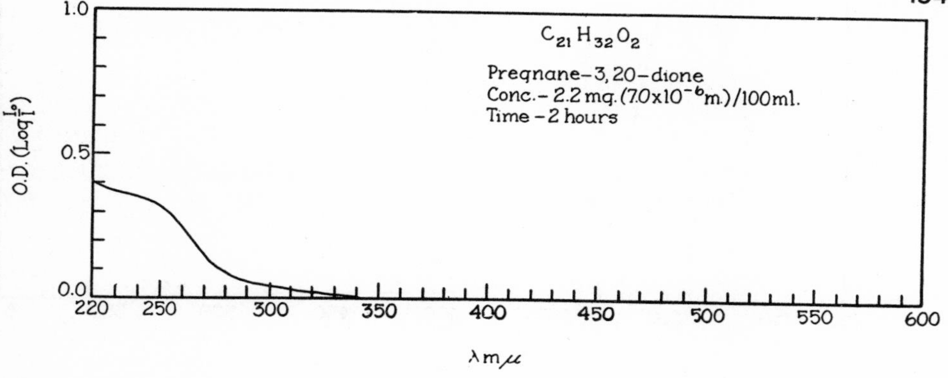
$C_{21}H_{32}O_2$
Pregnane-3,20-dione
Conc.- 2.2 mg. (7.0x10⁻⁶m.)/100ml.
Time - 2 hours
O.D. (Log I₀/I)
1.0
0.5
0.0
220 250 300 350 400 450 500 550 600
λmμ

156

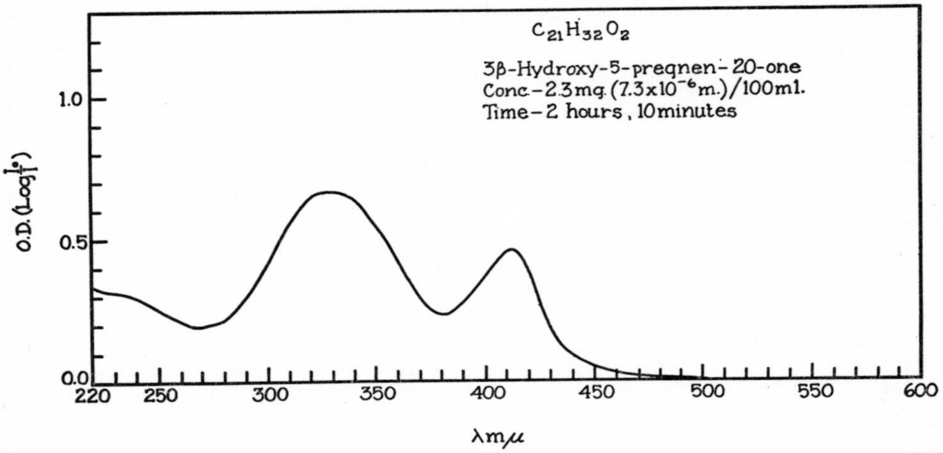
$C_{21}H_{32}O_2$
3β-Hydroxy-5-pregnen-20-one
Conc.-2.3mg.(7.3x10⁻⁶m.)/100ml.
Time-2 hours, 10 minutes
O.D. (Log I₀/I)
1.0
0.5
0.0
220 250 300 350 400 450 500 550 600
λmμ

159

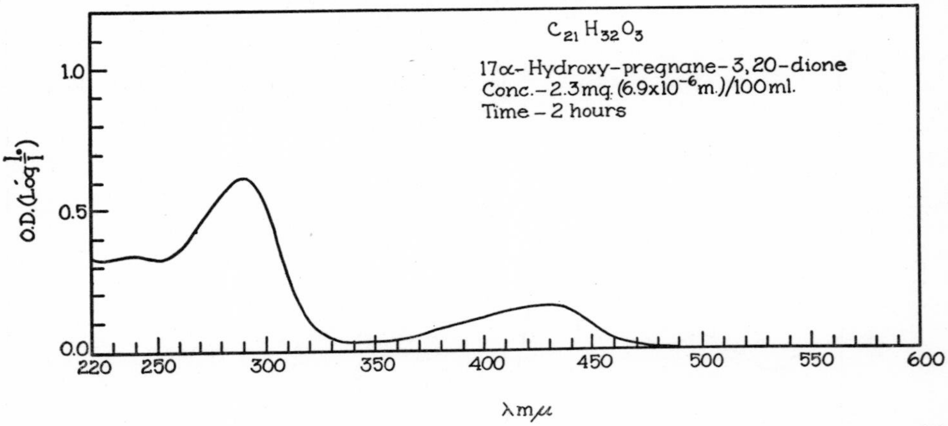
$C_{21}H_{32}O_3$
17α-Hydroxy-pregnane-3,20-dione
Conc.-2.3mg.(6.9x10⁻⁶m.)/100ml.
Time - 2 hours
O.D. (Log I₀/I)
1.0
0.5
0.0
220 250 300 350 400 450 500 550 600
λmμ

160

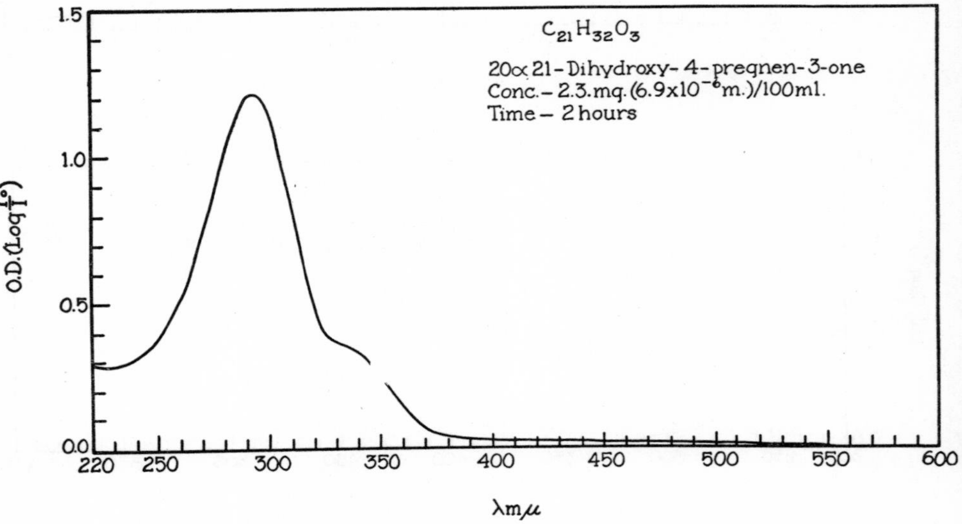
$C_{21}H_{32}O_3$
20α 21-Dihydroxy-4-pregnen-3-one
Conc.-2.3.mg.(6.9x10⁻⁶m.)/100ml.
Time - 2 hours
O.D. (Log I₀/I)
1.5
1.0
0.5
0.0
220 250 300 350 400 450 500 550 600
λmμ

198

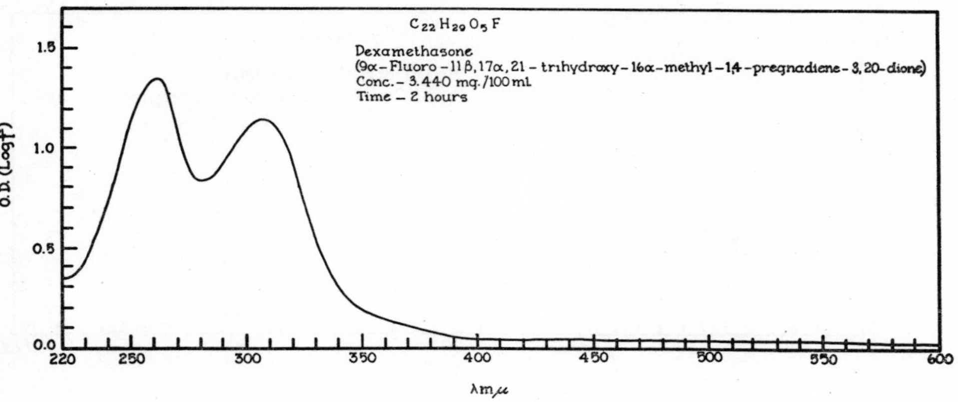
$C_{22}H_{29}O_5F$
Dexamethasone
(9α-Fluoro-11β, 17α, 21-trihydroxy-16α-methyl-1,4-pregnadiene-3, 20-dione)
Conc.-3.440 mg./100 ml.
Time - 2 hours
O.D. (Log I₀/I)
1.5
1.0
0.5
0.0
220
250
300
350
400
450
500
550
600
λmμ

175

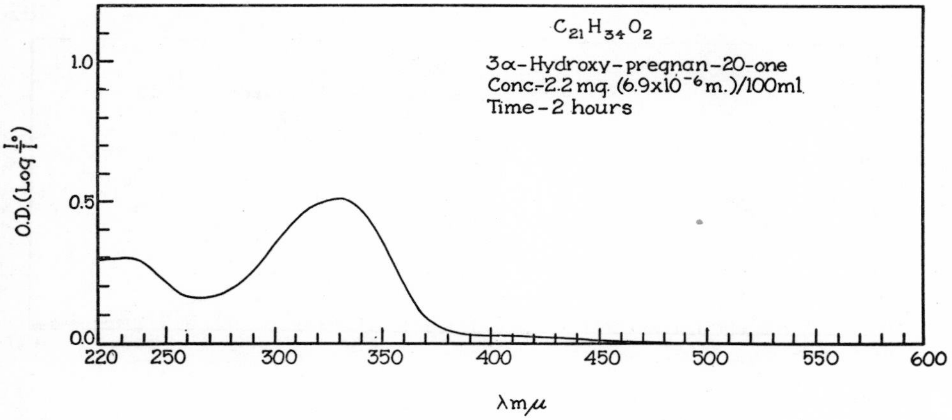
$C_{21}H_{34}O_2$
3α-Hydroxy-pregnan-20-one
Conc.-2.2 mg. (6.9x10⁻⁶m.)/100ml.
Time - 2 hours
O.D. (Log I₀/I)
1.0
0.5
0.0
220
250
300
350
400
450
500
550
600
λmμ

176

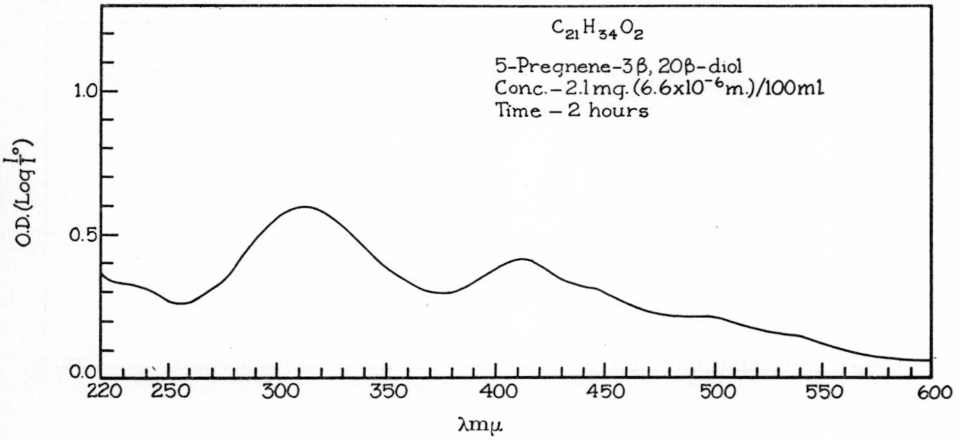
$C_{21}H_{34}O_2$
5-Pregnene-3β, 20β-diol
Conc.-2.1 mg. (6.6x10⁻⁶m.)/100ml.
Time - 2 hours
O.D. (Log I₀/I)
1.0
0.5
0.0
220
250
300
350
400
450
500
550
600
λmμ

177

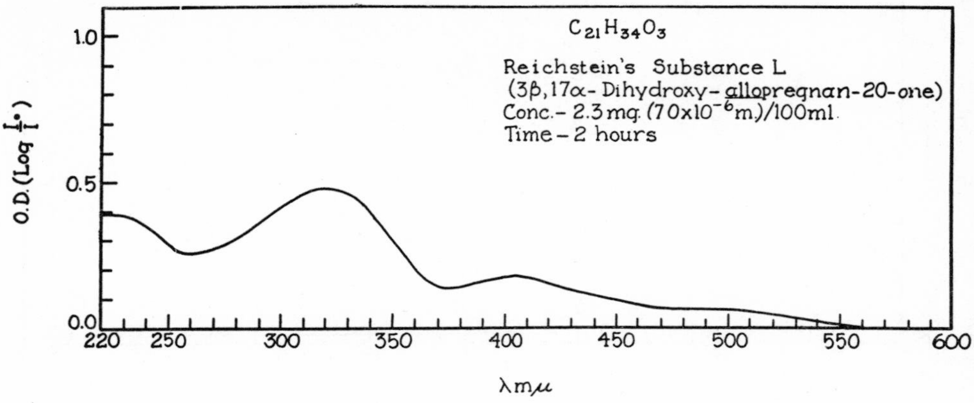
$C_{21}H_{34}O_3$
Reichstein's Substance L
(3β,17α-Dihydroxy-allopregnan-20-one)
Conc.-2.3 mg. (7.0×10⁻⁶ m.)/100 ml.
Time-2 hours
O.D. (Log I₀/I)
1.0
0.5
0.0
220 250 300 350 400 450 500 550 600
λmμ

182

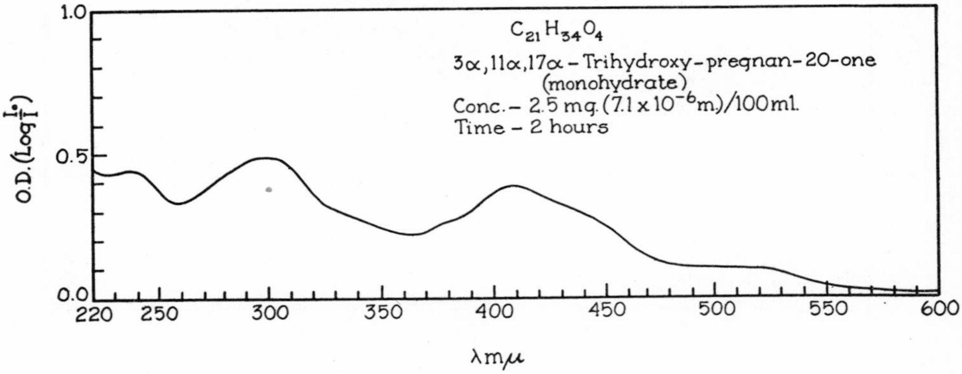
$C_{21}H_{34}O_4$
3α,11α,17α-Trihydroxy-pregnan-20-one
(monohydrate)
Conc.-2.5 mg. (7.1×10⁻⁶ m.)/100 ml.
Time-2 hours
O.D. (Log I₀/I)
1.0
0.5
0.0
220 250 300 350 400 450 500 550 600
λmμ

183

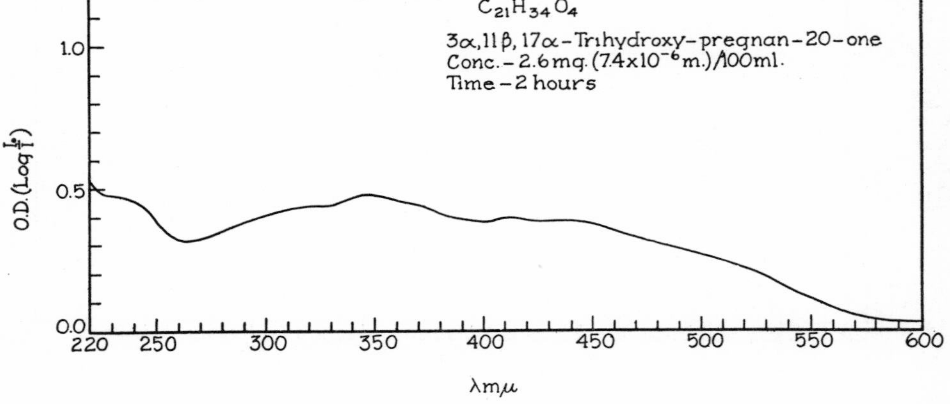
$C_{21}H_{34}O_4$
3α,11β,17α-Trihydroxy-pregnan-20-one
Conc.-2.6 mg. (7.4×10⁻⁶ m.)/100 ml.
Time-2 hours
O.D. (Log I₀/I)
1.0
0.5
0.0
220 250 300 350 400 450 500 550 600
λmμ

189

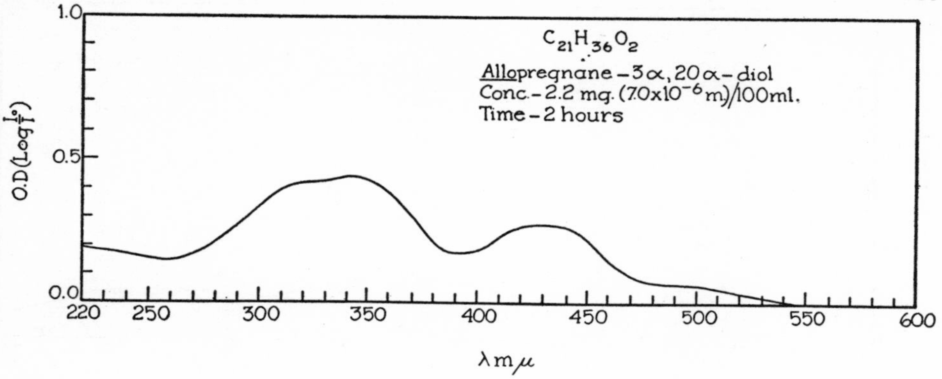
$C_{21}H_{36}O_2$
Allopregnane-3α, 20α-diol
Conc.-2.2 mg. (7.0x10⁻⁶ m)/100ml.
Time-2 hours
O.D (Log I₀/I)
1.0
0.5
0.0
220
250
300
350
400
450
500
550
600
λ mμ

193

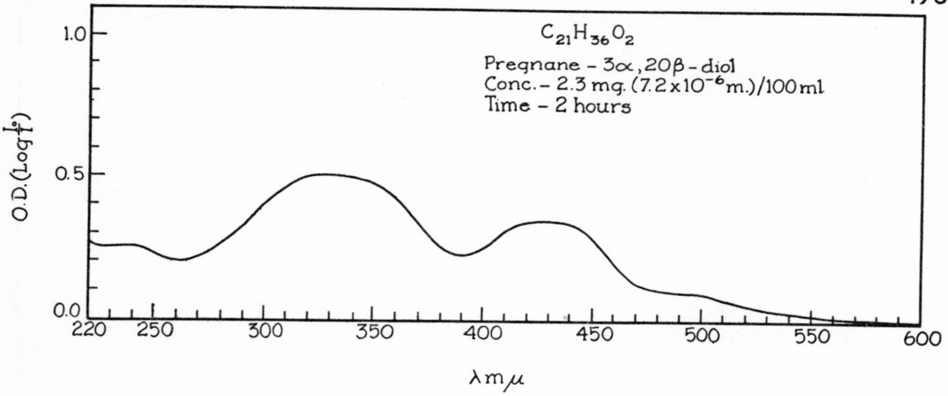
$C_{21}H_{36}O_2$
Pregnane-3α, 20β-diol
Conc.-2.3 mg. (7.2x10⁻⁶ m.)/100 ml
Time-2 hours
O.D. (Log I₀/I)
1.0
0.5
0.0
220
250
300
350
400
450
500
550
600
λ mμ

196

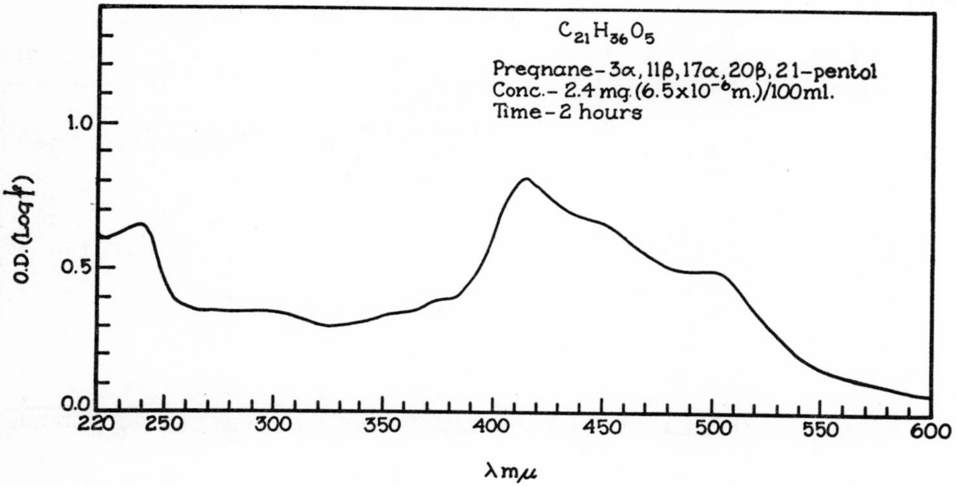
$C_{21}H_{36}O_5$
Pregnane-3α, 11β, 17α, 20β, 21-pentol
Conc.-2.4 mg. (6.5x10⁻⁶ m.)/100 ml.
Time-2 hours
O.D. (Log I₀/I)
1.0
0.5
0.0
220
250
300
350
400
450
500
550
600
λ mμ

199

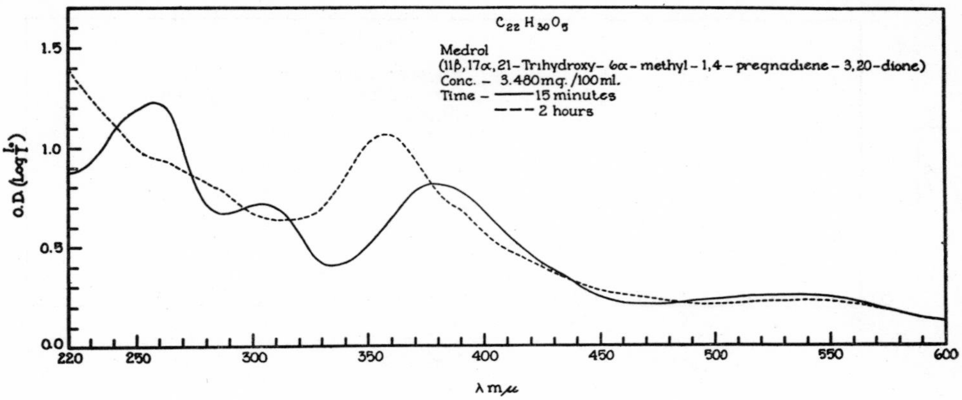
$C_{22}H_{30}O_5$
Medrol
(11β,17α,21-Trihydroxy-6α-methyl-1,4-pregnadiene-3,20-dione)
Conc. – 3.480 mg./100 ml.
Time – 15 minutes
– – – 2 hours
O.D. (Log $\frac{I_0}{I}$)
λ mμ

214

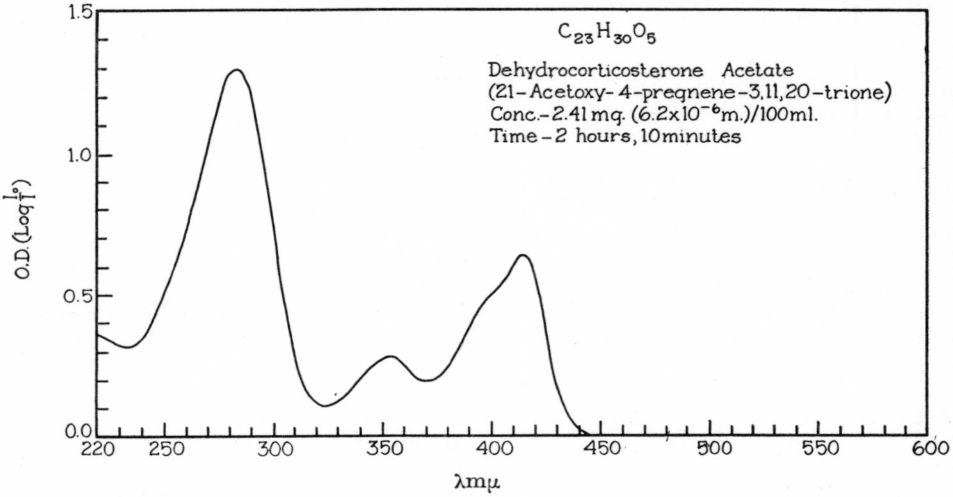
$C_{23}H_{30}O_5$
Dehydrocorticosterone Acetate
(21-Acetoxy-4-pregnene-3,11,20-trione)
Conc.-2.41 mg. (6.2x10⁻⁶m.)/100ml.
Time-2 hours, 10 minutes
O.D. (Log $\frac{I_0}{I}$)
λmμ

218A

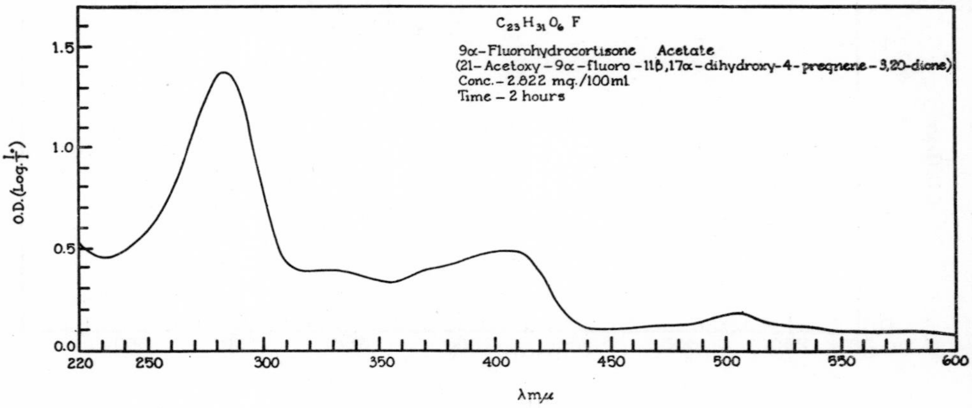
$C_{23}H_{31}O_6F$
9α-Fluorohydrocortisone Acetate
(21-Acetoxy-9α-fluoro-11β,17α-dihydroxy-4-pregnene-3,20-dione)
Conc.-2.822 mg./100ml
Time – 2 hours
O.D. (Log. $\frac{I_0}{I}$)
λmμ

219

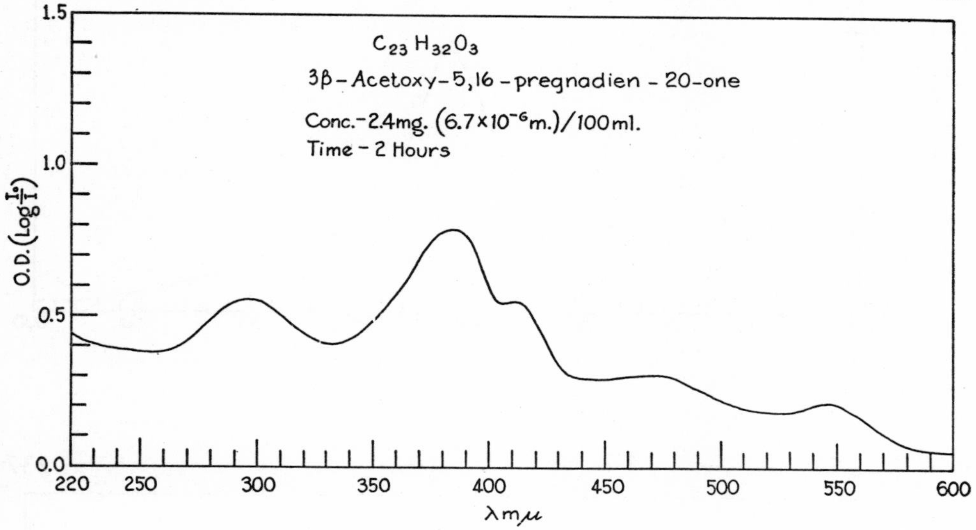

$C_{23}H_{32}O_3$
3β-Acetoxy-5,16-pregnadien-20-one
Conc.-2.4mg. (6.7×10⁻⁶m.)/100ml.
Time - 2 Hours
1.5
1.0
0.5
0.0
O.D. (Log I₀/I)
220
250
300
350
400
450
500
550
600
λ mμ

229

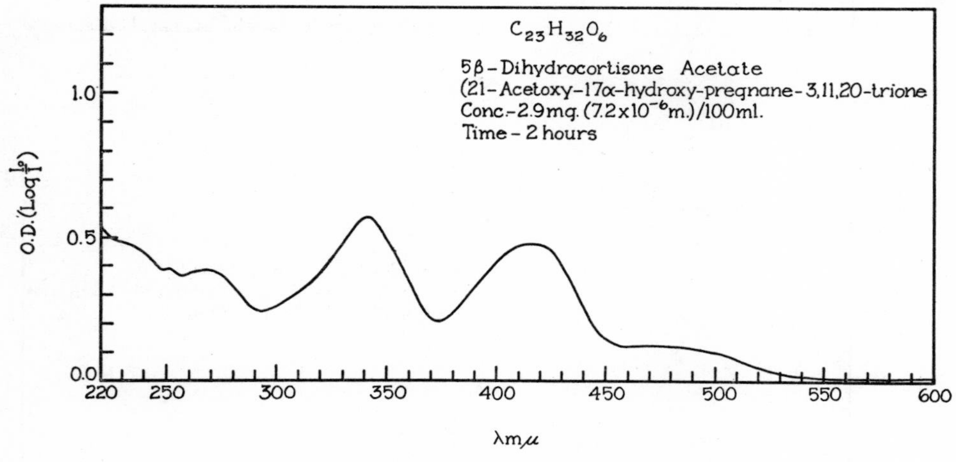

$C_{23}H_{32}O_6$
5β-Dihydrocortisone Acetate
(21-Acetoxy-17α-hydroxy-pregnane-3,11,20-trione
Conc.-2.9mg. (7.2x10⁻⁶m.)/100ml.
Time - 2 hours
1.0
0.5
0.0
O.D. (Log I₀/I)
220
250
300
350
400
450
500
550
600
λ mμ

233

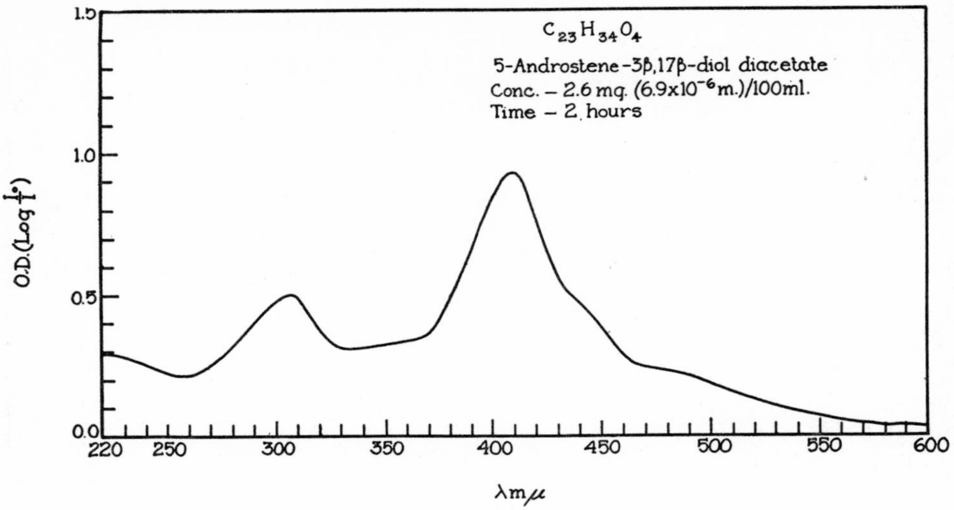
C23H34O4
5-Androstene-3β,17β-diol diacetate
Conc. – 2.6 mg. (6.9x10⁻⁶m.)/100ml.
Time – 2 hours
O.D.(Log I₀/I)
λmμ

237

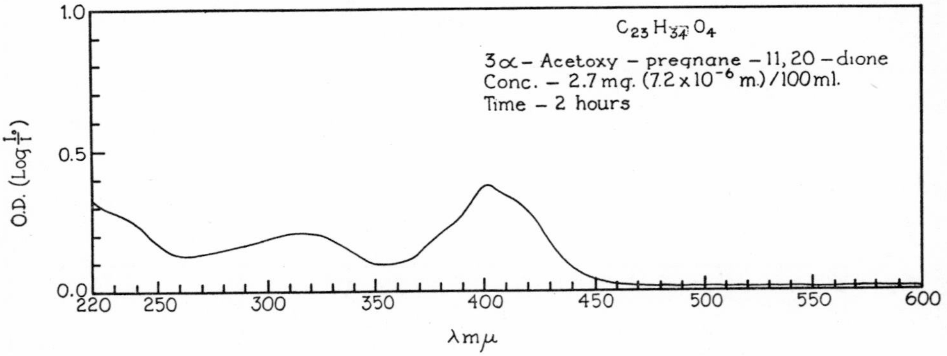
C23H34O4
3α – Acetoxy – pregnane – 11, 20 – dione
Conc. – 2.7 mg. (7.2 x 10⁻⁶ m.)/100ml.
Time – 2 hours
O.D. (Log I₀/I)
λmμ

239

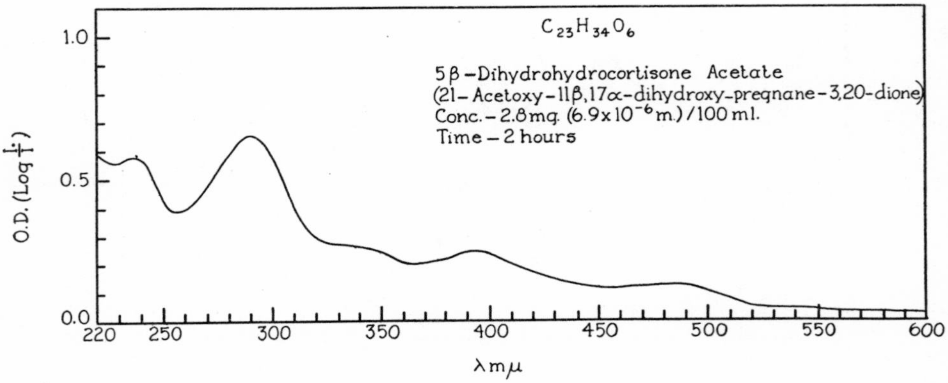
C23H34O6
5β –Dihydrohydrocortisone Acetate
(21– Acetoxy–11β,17α–dihydroxy–pregnane–3,20-dione)
Conc.–2.8mg. (6.9x10⁻⁶m.)/100 ml.
Time – 2 hours
O.D. (Log I₀/I)
λmμ

240

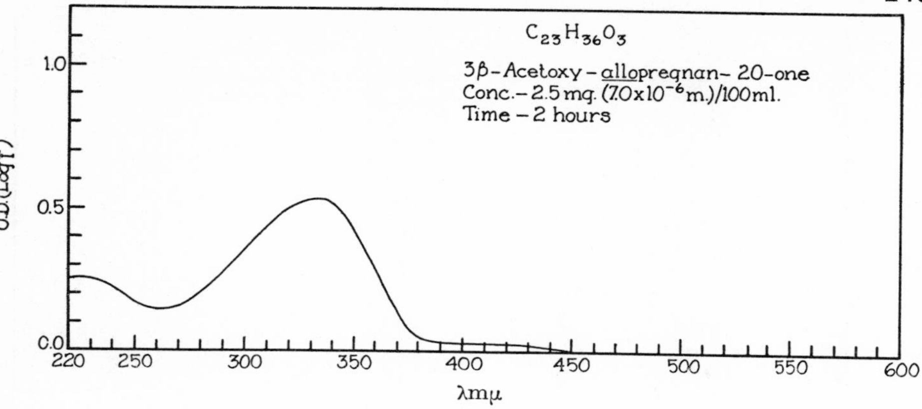
$C_{23}H_{36}O_3$
3β-Acetoxy-allopregnan-20-one
Conc.-2.5 mg. (7.0x10^{-6}m.)/100ml.
Time-2 hours
O.D. (Log $\frac{I_0}{I}$)
1.0
0.5
0.0
220 250 300 350 400 450 500 550 600
λmμ

295

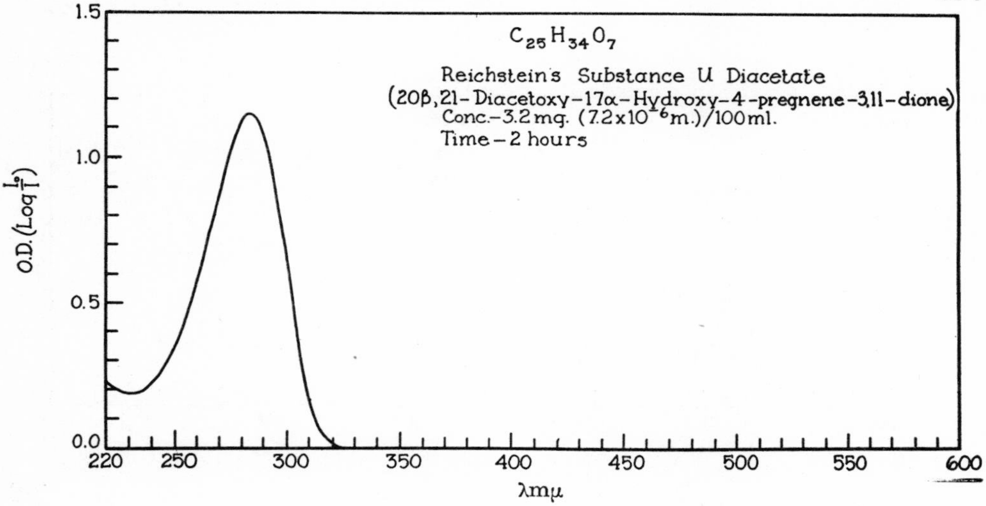
$C_{25}H_{34}O_7$
Reichstein's Substance U Diacetate
(20β,21-Diacetoxy-17α-Hydroxy-4-pregnene-3,11-dione)
Conc.-3.2 mg. (7.2x10^{-6}m.)/100ml.
Time-2 hours
O.D. (Log $\frac{I_0}{I}$)
1.5
1.0
0.5
0.0
220 250 300 350 400 450 500 550 600
λmμ

300

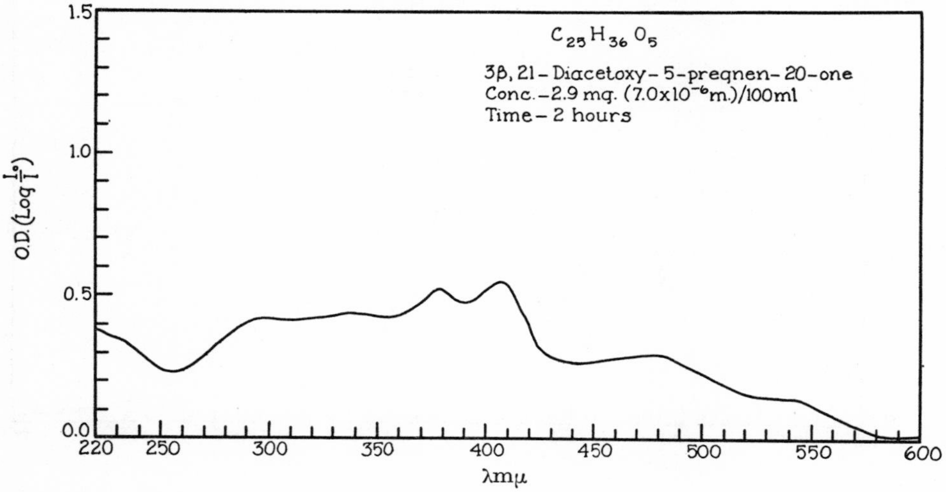
$C_{25}H_{36}O_5$
3β, 21-Diacetoxy-5-pregnen-20-one
Conc.-2.9 mg. (7.0x10^{-6}m.)/100ml
Time-2 hours
O.D. (Log $\frac{I_0}{I}$)
1.5
1.0
0.5
0.0
220 250 300 350 400 450 500 550 600
λmμ

303

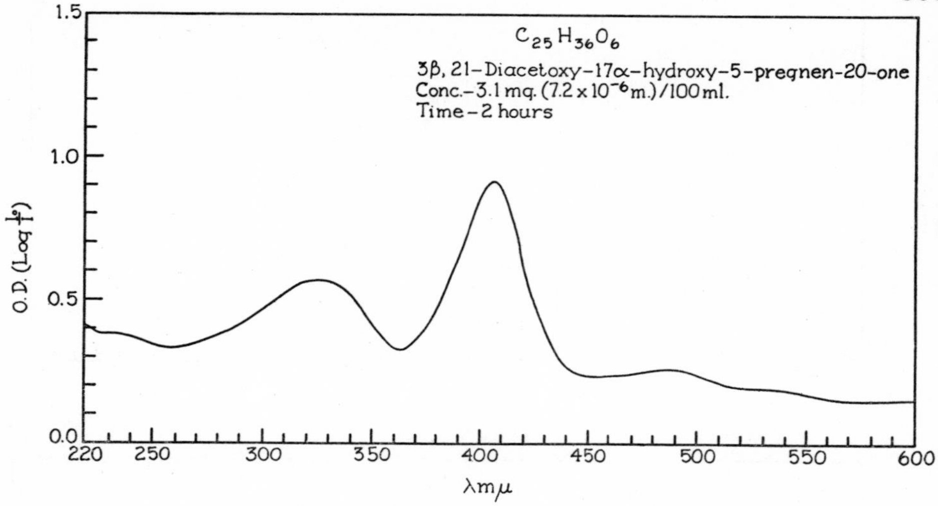
C25 H36 O6
3β, 21-Diacetoxy-17α-hydroxy-5-pregnen-20-one
Conc.-3.1 mg. (7.2 x 10⁻⁶ m.)/100 ml.
Time-2 hours
O.D. (Log I₀/I)
λmμ

304

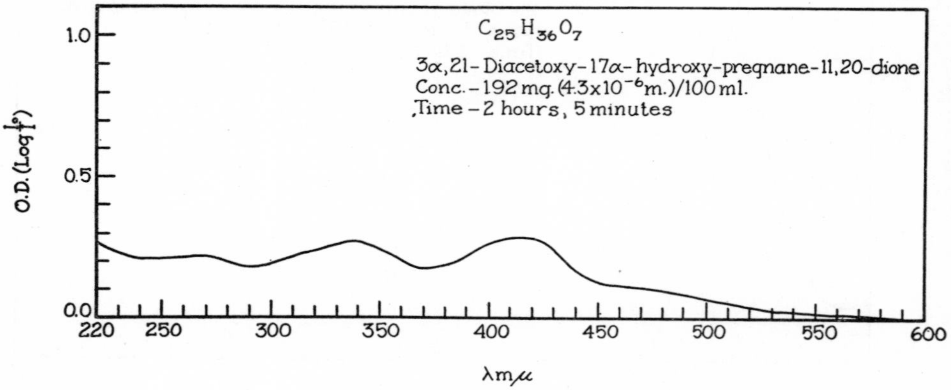
C25 H36 O7
3α,21-Diacetoxy-17α-hydroxy-pregnane-11,20-dione
Conc.-192 mg. (4.3x10⁻⁶ m.)/100 ml.
Time-2 hours, 5 minutes
O.D. (Log I₀/I)
λmμ

310

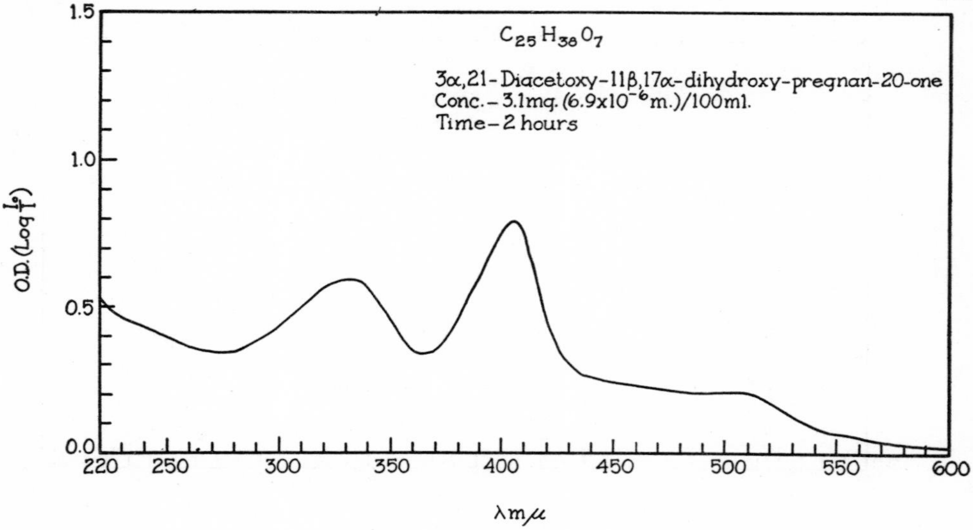
C25 H38 O7
3α,21-Diacetoxy-11β,17α-dihydroxy-pregnan-20-one
Conc.-3.1 mg. (6.9x10⁻⁶ m.)/100 ml.
Time-2 hours
O.D. (Log I₀/I)
λmμ

345

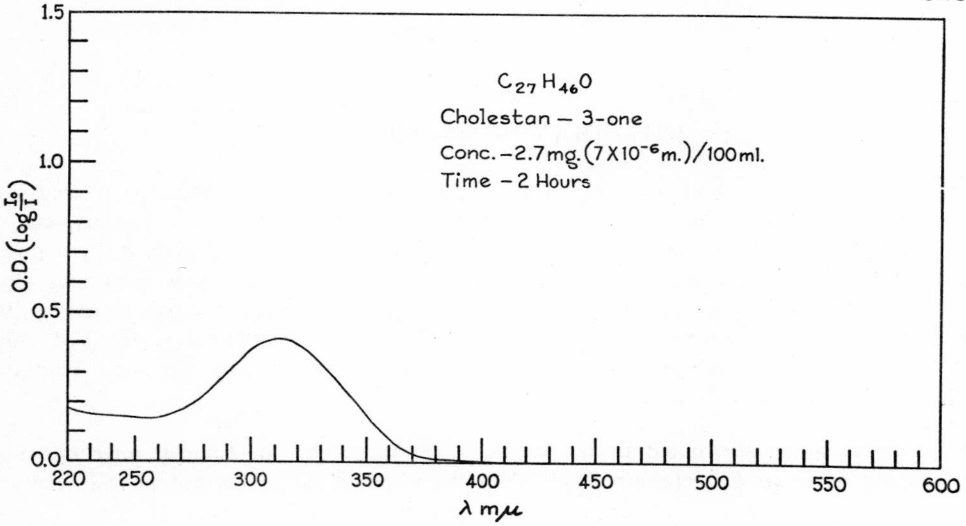
$C_{27}H_{46}O$
Cholestan – 3-one
Conc. –2.7 mg. (7 X 10^{-6} m.)/100 ml.
Time – 2 Hours
O.D. $\left(\text{Log}\frac{I_0}{I}\right)$
1.5
1.0
0.5
0.0
220
250
300
350
400
450
500
550
600
λ mμ

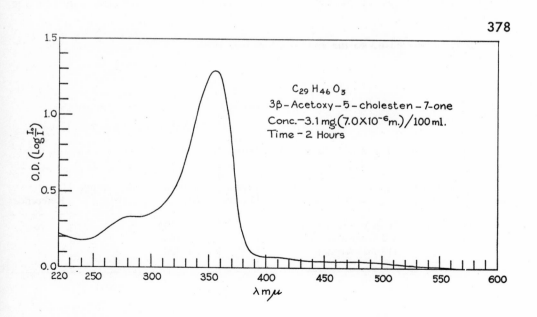

378

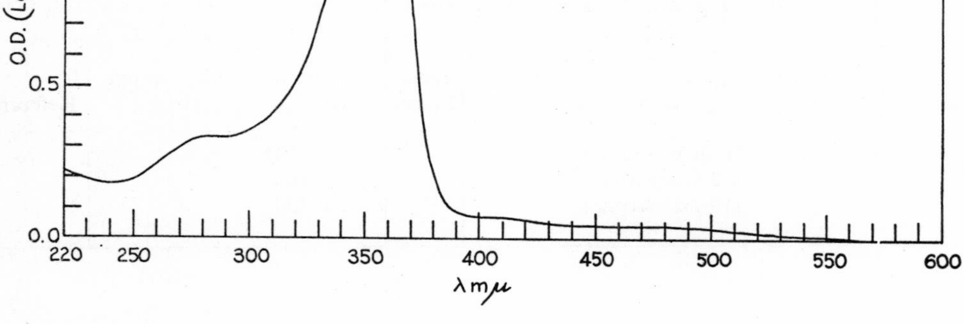
$C_{29}H_{46}O_3$
3β-Acetoxy-5-cholesten-7-one
Conc. –3.1 mg. (7.0 X 10^{-6} m.)/100 ml.
Time – 2 Hours
O.D. $\left(\text{Log}\frac{I_0}{I}\right)$
1.5
1.0
0.5
0.0
220
250
300
350
400
450
500
550
600
λ mμ

VI. TABLES

INTRODUCTION TO THE TABLES

The data of Tables I–XVI were taken from published sources as cited, from charts and curves published but without specific mention as to accurately measured maxima, etc. and from certain unpublished sources as mentioned. All steroids are catalogued by empirical formula, and within the same empirical formula groupings, by alphabet according to the fundamental hydrocarbon nucleus as derived from the latest International Union of Pure and Applied Chemistry nomenclature practices. Where further ordering is required, alphabetical order of prefixes and lowest numbers of prefix were used. Common names are included in parenthesis in certain cases.

All data not specifically noted to the contrary are supposedly determined after two hours of standing at room temperature. Many data from the literature do not provide the exact time employed, however, and no entry is made in the Time column in these instances. Wavelengths marked by an asterisk were interpolated from charts or graphs and are thus less exact. Optical density data were converted to $E_{1\,cm}^{1\%}$ values wherever possible. Where no extinction data are included, either none was given, or lack of precise concentration, etc. obviated meaningful calculation. Those data followed by the letter "I" are either inflection points, plateaus, or shoulders, without specification as to the exact nature of the selective absorption.

The literature is covered up to the end of December, 1959.

TABLE I. ABSORPTION SPECTRA OF C_{17} STEROIDS.

No.	Empirical Formula	Compound	Time, hours	λ_{max} in mμ ($E_{1\,cm}^{1\%}$)	λ_{min} in mμ ($E_{1\,cm}^{1\%}$)	Reference
1	$C_{17}H_{20}O_2$	3-Hydroxy-18-norestra-1,3,5(10)-trien-17-one (18-norestrone)	2	*ca.* 310* *ca.* 360 *ca.* 400	—	78

TABLE II. ABSORPTION SPECTRA OF C_{18} STEROIDS.

No.	Empirical Formula	Compound	Time, hours	λ_{max} in mμ ($E^{1\%}_{1\,cm}$)	λ_{min} in mμ ($E^{1\%}_{1\,cm}$)	Reference
2	$C_{18}H_{18}O_2$	3-Hydroxy-1,3,5(10),6,8-estrapentaen-17-one (equilenin)	2	234(1315) 280(216) I 289(263) 301(268) 319(247) 395(168) 472(384)	265(184) 295(237) 311(232) 355(84) 416(142)	13
			—	230 300 320 400 472	—	109
3	$C_{18}H_{20}O_2$	3-Hydroxy-1,3,5(10),6-estratetraen-17-one	—	295 370 430 460	—	109
4	$C_{18}H_{20}O_2$	3-Hydroxy-1,3,5(10),7-estratetraen-17-one (equilin)	2	232(370) 353(895) 459(155)	264(60) 419(90)	13
5	$C_{18}H_{22}O_2$	3-Hydroxy-1,3,5(10)-estratrien-17-one (estrone)	2	228(375) I 300(500) 352(55) 448(275)	253(85) 332(45) 385(25)	4,13,60
6	$C_{18}H_{22}O_3$	3,18-Dihydroxy-1,3,5(10)-estratrien-17-one (18-hydroxyestrone)	2	*ca.* 310* *ca.* 360 *ca.* 460		78
7	$C_{18}H_{24}O_2$	1,3,5(10)-Estratriene-3,17α-diol (estradiol-17α)	2	300 I* 365 400 I 454 500 I	270* 420	4
8	$C_{18}H_{24}O_2$	1,3,5(10)-Estratriene-3,17β-diol (estradiol-17β)	2	272(216) 298(184) 360(168) I 428(1015) 449(1010)	250(121) 288(169) 326(79) 438(910)	13
			2	308* 455	350	4
9	$C_{18}H_{24}O_2$	1-Estrene-3,17-dione	—	297	225	72
10	$C_{18}H_{24}O_3$	1,3,5(10)-Estratriene-3,16α,17β-triol (estriol)	2	230(320) I 305(180) 355(35) 450(80)	262(25) 330(15) 388(15)	13
				306* 452	400*	4

TABLE III. ABSORPTION SPECTRA OF C_{19} STEROIDS.

No.	Empirical Formula	Compound	Time, hours	λ_{max} in mμ ($E^{1\%}_{1\,cm}$)	λ_{min} in mμ ($E^{1\%}_{1\,cm}$)	Reference
11	$C_{19}H_{22}O_3$	1,4-Androstadiene-3,11,17-trione	—	258(505) 306(260)	224(94) 280(182)	56
12	$C_{19}H_{24}O_2$	1,4-Androstadiene-3,17-dione	—	265 305 390	288 350	72
13	$C_{19}H_{24}O_2$	4,9(11)-Androstadiene-3,17-dione	2	285(521) 382(421) 400(250) I 463(115)	240(220) 323(88) 435(88)	16
14	$C_{19}H_{24}O_3$	4-Androstene-3,11,17-trione (adrenosterone)	2	283(524)	230(62)	13,18
			—	285	—	49
			2	280(540)	—	2,6,137
			2	280–282	—	79
15	$C_{19}H_{24}O_3$	14β-Androst-4-ene-3,15,17-trione	2	277(826)	none	16
16	$C_{19}H_{24}O_3$	11β-Hydroxy-1,4-androstadiene-3,17-dione	—	355(567)	275(112)	56
17	$C_{19}H_{26}O_2$	17β-Hydroxy-1,4-androstadien-3-one	2	232(250) I 327(500) 395(65) 487(80)	251(110) 359(30) 428(35)	13
18	$C_{19}H_{26}O_2$	1-Androstene-3,17-dione	2	299(653)	230(182)	13
19	$C_{19}H_{26}O_2$	4-Androstene-3,17-dione	2	294(730)	235(105)	13
			2	295	—	5
			—	295	—	8
20	$C_{19}H_{26}O_3$	5α-Androstane-3,6,17-trione	2	265* 305 400	—	2
21	$C_{19}H_{26}O_3$	5α-Androstane-3,11,17-trione	2	321(18) 400(18)	300(9) 352(0)	13
			2	none	—	2,137
22	$C_{19}H_{26}O_3$	5β-Androstane-3,11,17-trione	2	none	none	13
23	$C_{19}H_{26}O_3$	6α-Hydroxy-4-androstene-3,17-dione	2	285* 350 465	—	2
24	$C_{19}H_{26}O_3$	6β-Hydroxy-4-androstene-3,17-dione	2	290 345–350 450–465	—	2,7,8
25	$C_{19}H_{26}O_3$	11α-Hydroxy-4-androstene-3,17-dione	2	284(466) 381(340) 400(214) I 465(110)	235(148) 322(71) 433(76)	13,18
			0.25	286(514) 377(33) 394(24) I 461(5) I	229(91) 326(24)	16

TABLE III—*continued*

No.	Empirical Formula	Compound	Time, hours	λ_{max} in mμ ($E^{1\%}_{1\ cm}$)	λ_{min} in mμ ($E^{1\%}_{1\ cm}$)	Reference
25 cont.	$C_{19}H_{26}O_3$	11α-Hydroxy-4-androstene-3,17-dione	0.50	286(514) 379(71) 395(43) I 463(10) I	230(100) 327(33)	16
			1.0	285(500) 380(171) 397(105) I 462(33)	230(114) 324(48) 434(24)	16
			1.5	285(481) 381(267) 397(167) I 462(71)	232(133) 323(62) 434(48)	16
			2	283(466) 381(338) 398(219) I 462(110)	235(148) 322(71) 433(76)	16
			2.5	283(452) 381(395) 396(267) I 462(157)	239(162) 322(81) 432(110)	16
			3	283(438) 381(423) 396(295) I 462(190)	239(162) 322(81) 431(133)	16
			4	282(414) 381(457) 396(343) I 462(267)	240(171) 321(90) 430(181)	16
			6	281(391) 381(467) 394(405) I 461(362)	239(186) 321(105) 429(248)	16
			24	280(405) 330(129) I 400(519) 460(419)	240(224) 340(119) 430(329)	16
26	$C_{19}H_{26}O_3$	11β-Hydroxy-4-androstene-3,17-dione	2	283(467) 380(443) 402(257) I 460(129)	241(157) 322(62) 433(95)	13,18
			0.25	285(533) 380(110) 396(62) I 463(10)	231(110) 327(43) 438(5)	16
			0.50	285(523) 379(195) 395(114) I 462(24)	232(124) 325(48) 435(14)	16

TABLE III—*continued*

No.	Empirical Formula	Compound	Time, hours	λ_{max} in mμ ($E^{1\%}_{1\,cm}$)	λ_{min} in mμ ($E^{1\%}_{1\,cm}$)	Reference
26 cont.	$C_{19}H_{26}O_3$	11β-Hydroxy-4-androstene-3,17-dione	1.0	284(500) 380(305) 398(176) I 462(57)	237(138) 323(52) 434(38)	16
			1.5	283(481) 380(376) 397(229) I 462(91)	238(148) 322(57) 433(62)	16
			2	282(467) 380(423) 397(262) I 462(124)	239(152) 322(62) 433(86)	16
			2.5	282(452) 380(452) 398(286) I 462(157)	239(162) 321(67) 432(110)	16
			3	282(443) 380(476) 399(305) I 462(195)	240(167) 322(71) 430(133)	16
			4	282(423) 381(486) 397(338) I 462(252)	240(172) 322(81) 430(172)	16
			6	281(400) 381(486) 396(395) I 462(348)	240(181) 321(91) 429(238)	16
			8	280(386) 382(476) 395(438) I 461(414)	240(191) 321(95) 428(286)	16
			24	225(248) 280(419) 331(114) I 400(533) 460(442)	241(224) 340(105) 429(338)	16
			—	285 380 400 I 460	—	80,82
			—	280 380 400 460	—	130
			—	285 380 465	—	49

TABLE III—*continued*

No.	Empirical Formula	Compound	Time, hours	λ_{max} in mμ ($E^{1\%}_{1\,cm}$)	λ_{min} in mμ ($E^{1\%}_{1\,cm}$)	Reference
26 cont.	$C_{19}H_{26}O_3$	11β-Hydroxy-4-androstene-3,17-dione	—	283 380 410 I 465 560	—	103
			—	285* 380 405 I 465	—	2
27	$C_{19}H_{26}O_3$	17β-Hydroxy-4-androstene-3,11-dione	2	285(563) 350(41)	230(105) 330(36)	13,18
			2	285(600) 355(27)	—	6
28	$C_{19}H_{26}O_3$	15α-Hydroxy-4-androstene-3,17-dione	2	285(653) 378(40) 460(36)	326(19) 400(14)	16
29	$C_{19}H_{26}O_3$	15β-Hydroxy-4-androstene-3,17-dione	2	285(600) 356(110) 375(78) I 460(59)	311(52) 396(24)	16
30	$C_{19}H_{28}O$	4-Androsten-3-one	2	296(416)	none	13
31	$C_{19}H_{28}O_2$	5,7-Androstadiene-3β,17β-diol	2	414(380) 466(455) 505(195) I	320(125) 432(345)	13
32	$C_{19}H_{28}O_2$	5α-Androstane-3,17-dione	2	302(595)	251(119)	13
			2	302(566)	250(76)	13
33	$C_{19}H_{28}O_2$	5β-Androstane-3,17-dione (etiocholane-3,17-dione)	2	302(540)	250(75)	13
			2	305*	—	5
34	$C_{19}H_{28}O_2$	3α-Hydroxy-5α-androst-9(11)-en-17-one	2	310 348	—	21
			—	340* 420 I	—	52
35	$C_{19}H_{28}O_2$	3α-Hydroxy-5β-androst-9(11)-en-17-one	2	312 342	—	21
36	$C_{19}H_{28}O_2$	3β-Hydroxy-5-androsten-17-one(dehydroiso-androsterone)	2	305* 412 485	—	5
			—	305* 405*	—	96
			—	305 410	—	82
37	$C_{19}H_{28}O_2$	17α-Hydroxy-4-androsten-3-one(*cis*-testosterone)	—	295	—	8
			2	299(724)	232(124)	13
38	$C_{19}H_{28}O_2$	17β-Hydroxy-4-androsten-3-one(testosterone)	2	298(850)	236(150)	13
			2	299(837)	235(150)	13
			2	297*	—	5

TABLE III—*continued*

No.	Empirical Formula	Compound	Time, hours	λ_{max} in mμ ($E^{1\%}_{1\,cm}$)	λ_{min} in mμ ($E^{1\%}_{1\,cm}$)	Reference
39	$C_{19}H_{28}O_3$	17β-Hydroxy-5α-androstane-3,16-dione	2	294(109) 372(736)	258(55) 318(64)	13
40	$C_{19}H_{28}O_3$	3α-Hydroxy-5β-androstane-11,17-dione (3α-hydroxy-etiocholane-11,17-dione)	2	238(71) I 321(91) 380(86) I 401(152) 412(129) I	265(40) 353(40)	13
			2	315 400–405	—	79
			2	273* 318 405	—	2
			—	320* 380 I 400 410 I	—	52
41	$C_{19}H_{28}O_3$	2α,17β-Dihydroxy-4-androsten-3-one	0.25	300(750) 480(25)	350(12)	115
			2	299(652) 370(59) 463(75)	340(50) 400(41)	115
			20	295(407) 403(266) 440(310)	240(191) 340(91) 412(264)	115
42	$C_{19}H_{28}O_3$	2β,17β-Dihydroxy-4-androsten-3-one	—	295 340	—	8
43	$C_{19}H_{28}O_3$	6β,17β-Dihydroxy-4-androsten-3-one	—	300 350	—	8
44	$C_{19}H_{28}O_3$	11α,17β-Dihydroxy-4-androsten-3-one	2	300(659) 390(55) 470(27) I	238(164) 367(43)	13,18
			2	295(600) 385(95)	—	2,6
			0.25	297(623) 350(109) 490(9) I	230(155) 333(100)	16
			0.50	299(655) 351(86) 480(18) I	232(159) 342(82)	16
			1	299(659) 350(64) I 388(50) I 470(23) I	235(164) 371(45)	16
			1.5	299(659) 389(55) 470(27) I	235(164) 368(45)	16
			2	300(659) 389(55) 470(27) I	237(164) 367(45)	16

TABLE III—*continued*

No.	Empirical Formula	Compound	Time, hours	λ_{max} in mμ ($E^{1\%}_{1\,cm}$)	λ_{min} in mμ ($E^{1\%}_{1\,cm}$)	Reference
44 cont.	$C_{19}H_{28}O_3$	11α,17β-Dihydroxy-4-androsten-3-one	2.5	299(659) 389(55) 472(32) I	236(164) 366(45)	16
			3	299(659) 389(55) 470(32) I	235(168) 365(41)	16
			4	300(654) 390(59) 470(32) I	236(168) 365(45)	16
			6	299(654) 389(59) 470(32) I	235(173) 365(45)	16
45	$C_{19}H_{28}O_3$	11β,17β-Dihydroxy-4-androsten-3-one	2	295(582) 385(177)	236(141) 340(50)	13,18
			0.25	298(619) 384(129) 478(19) I	233(148) 337(71)	16
			0.50	298(619) 385(157) 474(19) I	233(148) 338(62)	16
			1	297(614) 385(172) 470(19) I	234(148) 339(57)	16
			1.5	297(614) 385(176) 465(24) I	233(153) 339(57)	16
			2	296(619) 385(176) 465(24) I	235(153) 339(57)	16
			2.5	298(614) 385(176) 465(24) I	234(153) 340(57)	16
			3	298(619) 385(176) 474(24) I	235(153) 340(57)	16
			4	298(619) 384(181) 471(29)	235(157) 340(62) 435(24)	16
			6	298(619) 384(181) 472(29)	235(162) 341(62) 432(24)	16
46	$C_{19}H_{28}O_3$	16α,17β-Dihydroxy-4-androsten-3-one	—	295	—	8
47	$C_{19}H_{30}O$	5-Androsten-3β-ol	2	236(97) 321(368) 416(100)	229(92) 258(84) 384(68)	13
48	$C_{19}H_{30}O_2$	3α-Hydroxy-5α-androstan-17-one (androsterone)	2	310(267) 331(186) I 402(43) 480(14)	258(71) 385(33) 455(10)	13

TABLE III—*continued*

No.	Empirical Formula	Compound	Time, hours	λ_{max} in mμ ($E^{1\%}_{1\,cm}$)	λ_{min} in mμ ($E^{1\%}_{1\,cm}$)	Reference
48 cont.	$C_{19}H_{30}O_2$	3α-Hydroxy-5α-androstan-17-one (androsterone)	2	305* 410 490	—	5
			—	310* 330 I 410 480	—	52
			—	310	—	21
49	$C_{19}H_{30}O_2$	3β-Hydroxy-5α-androstan-17-one (iso-androsterone)	2	310(260) 331(185) I 407(25) 490(15)	252(55) 389(20) 450(5)	13
			—	312	—	21
			2	310* 410 490	—	5
50	$C_{19}H_{30}O_2$	3α-Hydroxy-5β-androstan-17-one (etiocholanolone)	2	311(281) I 332(195) I 409(38) 500(24)	259(76) 389(33) 452(14)	13
			—	310 335 I 410 480	—	52
			—	312	—	21
51	$C_{19}H_{30}O_2$	17α-Hydroxy-5α-androstan-3-one	2	302(330)	253(85)	13
52	$C_{19}H_{30}O_2$	17β-Hydroxy-5α-androstan-3-one	2	302(381)	252(86)	13
			2	302*	—	5
53	$C_{19}H_{30}O_2$	17β-Hydroxy-5β-androstan-3-one (17β-hydroxyetiocholan-3-one)	2	240(125) I 307(355) 356(115) 387(115) 450(65) I 475(90)	255(105) 336(90) 366(100) 412(35)	13
54	$C_{19}H_{30}O_2$	5-Androstene-3β,17α-diol	2	302(300) 408(360) 449(160) I 509(70) I	252(80) 351(95)	13
			2	305* 410	—	5
			0.25	237(110) I 304(355) 407(325) 479(110) 500(115)	252(90) 361(115) 467(105) 486(105)	16

TABLE III—*continued*

No.	Empirical Formula	Compound	Time, hours	λ_{max} in mμ ($E^{1\%}_{1\,cm}$)	λ_{min} in mμ ($E^{1\%}_{1\,cm}$)	Reference
54 cont.	$C_{19}H_{30}O_2$	5-Androstene-3β,17α-diol	0.50	234(120) I 303(350) 407(350) 451(135) I 483(120) I	253(95) 355(110)	16
			1	234(135) I 303(355) 408(370) 450(155) I 476(125) I	253(110) 355(110)	16
			1.5	235(130) I 303(340) 406(380) 450(165) I 489(115) I	253(105) 352(105)	16
			2	240(130) I 303(340) 407(390) 451(170) I 488(120) I	253(105) 351(105)	16
			2.5	240(135) I 303(335) 407(390) 450(175) I 489(120) I	254(110) 352(105)	16
			3	240(135) I 303(335) 407(395) 450(180) I 488(120) I	254(110) 351(105)	16
			4	238(140) I 302(335) 406(400) 450(185) I 486(125) I	253(110) 352(105)	16
			6	240(145) I 303(335) 407(405) 452(190) I 490(120) I	255(115) 351(105)	16
55	$C_{19}H_{30}O_2$	5-Androstene-3β,17β-diol	2	240(100) 307(320) 404(438) 440(145) I 482(90) 540(70) I	233(95) 255(90) 348(120) 472(87)	13
			0.25	239(90) 304(330) 406(415) 491(75) 533(60) I	232(85) 249(85) 360(145) 472(70)	16

TABLE III—*continued*

No.	Empirical Formula	Compound	Time, hours	λ_{max} in mμ ($E^{1\%}_{1\,cm}$)	λ_{min} in mμ ($E^{1\%}_{1\,cm}$)	Reference
55 cont.	$C_{19}H_{30}O_2$	5-Androstene-3β,17β-diol	0.50	239(90) 304(325) 405(430) 445(115) I 491(80) 526(70) I	232(85) 251(80) 350(135) 471(75)	16
			1	240(95) 304(325) 404(435) 443(130) I 489(85) 534(70) I	232(90) 253(85) 348(125) 470(80)	16
			1.5	233(95) I 304(320) 404(435) 442(135) I 484(90) 533(70) I	252(85) 348(125) 471(85)	16
			2	240(100) 305(320) 404(435) 440(145) I 482(90) 530(70) I	232(95) 254(90) 348(120) 472(85)	16
			2.5	240(110) 305(325) 403(435) 440(150) I 480(90) I 530(70) I	232(105) 254(95) 350(120)	16
			3	240(110) 304(320) 404(435) 440(155) I 478(90) I 530(70) I	232(105) 254(95) 346(120)	16
			4	240(215) 304(320) 404(435) 440(155) I 480(90) I 526(70) I	233(110) 255(95) 348(120)	16
			6	239(125) 304(320) 404(430) 441(160) I 481(95) I 522(75) I	233(120) 254(110) 348(120)	16
56	$C_{19}H_{30}O_2$	6β-Hydroxy-3,5-cyclo-androstan-17-one (*i*-androsterone)	2	*ca.* 310* 410	350*	52

TABLE III—*continued*

No.	Empirical Formula	Compound	Time, hours	λ_{max} in mμ ($E^{1\%}_{1\,cm}$)	λ_{min} in mμ ($E^{1\%}_{1\,cm}$)	Reference
57	$C_{19}H_{30}O_3$	3α,11β-Dihydroxy-5α-androstan-17-one	—	305* 380 405	—	52
			2	300* 380 405	—	2
58	$C_{19}H_{30}O_3$	3α,11β-Dihydroxy-5β-androstan-17-one (3α,11β-Dihydroxyetiocholan-17-one)	2	230(114) I 322(190) I 341(224) 402(191)	266(57) 371(152)	13
			2	310 I* 340 400	—	2
			2	340 395–405 I	—	79
59	$C_{19}H_{30}O_3$	5-Androstene-3β,16α,17β-triol	2	273 I* 318 I 380 415 470 500 I	—	2
60	$C_{19}H_{32}O$	5α-Androstan-3α-ol	2	308(190)	242(45)	13
61	$C_{19}H_{32}O$	5α-Androstan-3β-ol	2	312(200)	242(40)	13
62	$C_{19}H_{32}O$	5α-Androstan-17β-ol	2	240(82) 310(229)	225(71) 255(71)	13
63	$C_{19}H_{32}O_2$	5α-Androstane-3α,17α-diol	2	343(260) 410(55) I	257(85)	13
			2	350*	—	5
64	$C_{19}H_{32}O_2$	5α-Androstane-3α,17β-diol	2	314(200) I 345(245) 390(45) I 410(30) I	250(60)	13
65	$C_{19}H_{32}O_2$	5α,14β-Androstane-3β,17α-diol	2	235(105) I 305(280) 391(115) 412(85) I 445(60) I	252(90) 378(100)	13
66	$C_{19}H_{32}O_3$	5β-Androstane-3α,11β,17β-triol	2	270* 310 375 400 I	—	2

TABLE IV. ABSORPTION SPECTRA OF C_{20} STEROIDS.

No.	Empirical Formula	Compound	Time, hours	λ_{max} in mμ ($E^{1\%}_{1\,cm}$)	λ_{min} in mμ ($E^{1\%}_{1\,cm}$)	Reference
67	$C_{20}H_{24}O_2$	17α-Ethinyl-1,3,5(10)-estratriene-3,17β-diol (17α-ethinylestradiol)	2	276* 360 466 523	*ca.* 270* *ca.* 320 *ca.* 420 *ca.* 480	4
68	$C_{20}H_{26}O_5$	17α,21-Dihydroxy-19-norpregn-4-ene-3,11,20-trione(19-norcortisone)	—	280 340 415 490	—	141
69	$C_{20}H_{28}O_4$	11β,21-Dihydroxy-19-norpregn-4-ene-3,20-dione	—	285 390 475	—	141
70	$C_{20}H_{28}O_4$	3α,9α-Epoxy-11-oxo-5β-androstan-17β-carboxylic acid	2	290 405	—	137
71	$C_{20}H_{28}O_5$	11β,17α,21-Trihydroxy-19-norpregn-4-ene-3,20-dione(19-norhydrocortisone)	—	240 282 385 470	—	141
72	$C_{20}H_{30}O_2$	17β-Hydroxy-17α-methyl-4-androsten-3-one(17α-methyl testosterone)	2	298(605) 497(24)	235(143) 365(5)	13
73	$C_{20}H_{30}O_3$	3β-Hydroxy-5-androstene-17β-carboxylic acid	2	240(105) 319(241) 342(255) 412(182)	230(100) 265(77) 328(227) 381(105)	13
74	$C_{20}H_{30}O_4$	3α-Hydroxy-11-oxo-5β-androstane-17β-carboxylic acid	2	235(78) I 320(100) 401(178)	261(48) 352(39)	13
			2	320 405	—	137
75	$C_{20}H_{32}O_2$	17α-Methyl-5-androstene-3β,17β-diol	2	235(141) 309(155) 355(136) 390(168) I 438(373) 497(209)	226(136) 258(105) 335(123) 372(123) 478(145)	13
76	$C_{20}H_{34}O$	17α-Methyl-5α-androstan-17β-ol	2	241(75) 318(230)	255(70)	13

TABLE V. ABSORPTION SPECTRA OF C_{21} STEROIDS.

No.	Empirical Formula	Compound	Time, hours	λ_{max} in mμ ($E^{1\%}_{1\,cm}$)	λ_{min} in mμ ($E^{1\%}_{1\,cm}$)	Reference
77	$C_{21}H_{26}O_3$	3β-Acetoxy-5,7,9(11)-androstatrien-17-one	2	292(200) 349(250) 412(508)	270(167) 317(175) 368(208)	13

TABLE V—*continued*

No.	Empirical Formula	Compound	Time, hours	λ_{max} in mμ ($E^{1\%}_{1\,cm}$)	λ_{min} in mμ ($E^{1\%}_{1\,cm}$)	Reference
78	$C_{21}H_{26}O_4$	17α,21-Dihydroxy-1,4,9(11)-pregnatriene-3,20-dione	0.25	265(344) 280(256) I 308(190) I 359(259)	235(292) 325(178)	119
			2	267(275) I 278(289) 358(480)	260(257) 305(177)	119
			20	242(482) I 278(377) 285(364) I 354(311) 460(134)	262(358) 311(243) 430(128)	119
79	$C_{21}H_{26}O_5$	16α,17α-Epoxy-11α,21-dihydroxy-1,4-pregnadiene-3,20-dione	0.25	268(415) 306(190) 395(49)	222(113) 298(186) 342(39)	115
			2	270(472) 310(171) I 359(125) 390(92) I 450(162) I	225(159) 332(92)	115
			20	273(442) 311(158) I 358(172) 450(94) I	230(235) 330(125)	115
80	$C_{21}H_{26}O_5$	17α,21-Dihydroxy-1,4-pregnadiene-3,11,20-trione (prednisone)	0.25	264(419) 283(345) I 310(234) I 332–345 (141) I 410–428(153)	220(142) 372(51)	119
			2	265(428) 280(393) I 310(243) I 345(179) 410–428(158)	220(173) 330(170) 371(77)	119
			20	265(430) 280(400) I 347(192) 410(200) I 425(205)	220(222) 330(176) 370(108)	119
			—	275(445) 348(220) 420(255)	—	56
			—	263 340 I 420	—	114
			—	265 345 420	325 372	133

TABLE V—*continued*

No.	Empirical Formula	Compound	Time, hours	λ_{max} in mμ ($E^{1\%}_{1 cm}$)	λ_{min} in mμ ($E^{1\%}_{1 cm}$)	Reference
81	$C_{21}H_{27}O_5F$	9α-Fluoro-11β,16α,17α-trihydroxy-1,4-pregnadiene-3,20-dione	0.25	258(263) 309(142)	215(35) 285(94)	115
			2	259(270) 306(186)	215(43) 283(130)	115
			20	262(303) 303(340)	215(54) 278(206)	115
82	$C_{21}H_{27}O_5F$	9α-Fluoro-11β,17α,21-trihydroxy-1,4-pregnadiene-3,20-dione (9α-fluoro-prednisolone)	0.25	263(364) 308(223) I 375(115) 451(123)	228(241) 350(106) 400(89)	119
			2	262(341) 308(233) I 372(92) I 451(141)	237(279) 400(85)	119
			20	263(359) 308(259) I 450(167)	240(311) 385(97)	119
83	$C_{21}H_{27}O_6Cl$	9α-Chloro-11β,16α,17α,21-tetrahydroxy-1,4-pregnadiene-3,20-dione	0.25	258(244) 262(242) I 315(105) 395(36)	220(59) 286(58) 350(13)	119
			2	258–262(250) 315(110) 381(65)	220(82) 289(73) 345(29)	119
			20	258(270) I 264(276) 312(118) 375(82)	220(123) 298(107) 345(49)	119
84	$C_{21}H_{27}O_6F$	9α-Fluoro-11β,16α,17aα-trihydroxy,17aβ-hydroxymethyl-1,4-D-homo-androstadiene-3,17-dione(triamcinolone isomer)	0.25	259(311) 310(159)	—	118
			2	260(317) 310(164)	—	118
			20	262(365) 310(175)	—	118
85	$C_{21}H_{27}O_6F$	9α-Fluoro-11β,16α,17α,21-tetrahydroxy-1,4-pregnadiene-3,20-dione(triamcinolone)	0.25	260(334) 310(172) 390(42)	220(63) 287(128) 345(16)	117,119
			2	260(346) 310(176) 380(86)	218(71) 288(142) 342(34)	117,119

TABLE V—*continued*

No.	Empirical Formula	Compound	Time, hours	λ_{max} in mμ ($E^{1\%}_{1\,cm}$)	λ_{min} in mμ ($E^{1\%}_{1\,cm}$)	Reference
85 cont.	$C_{21}H_{27}O_6F$	9α-Fluoro-11β,16α,17α, 21-tetrahydroxy-1,4-pregnadiene-3,20-dione(triamcinolone)	20	263(386) 310(176) 375(94)	220(80) 300(166) 340(40)	117,119
86	$C_{21}H_{28}O_2$	4,11-Pregnadiene-3,20-dione	2	290(526) 318(265) I 473(39)	231(135) 400(17)	13
87	$C_{21}H_{28}O_2$	4,16-Pregnadiene-3,20-dione	2	302(773) 376(23)	245(145) 352(18)	13
88	$C_{21}H_{28}O_2$	3β-Hydroxy-5,7,9(11)-pregnatrien-20-one	2	306(227) 363(491) 377(513) 412(100) I 470(82)	282(195) 326(191) 368(482) 435(73)	13
89	$C_{21}H_{28}O_3$	21-Hydroxy-4,6-pregnadiene-3,20-dione	2	290(387) 355(505) 373(330) I 455(185) 540(57) I	235(122) 319(217) 395(83)	16
90	$C_{21}H_{28}O_3$	21-Hydroxy-4,7-pregnadiene-3,20-dione	0.25	215(324) I 265(393) 395(162) 475(282)	250(255) 340(90) 405(159)	16
91	$C_{21}H_{28}O_3$	21-Hydroxy-4,9(11)-pregnadiene-3,20-dione	2	285* 330 370 460	—	138
92	$C_{21}H_{28}O_3$	4-Pregnene-3,6,20-trione	2	348(637)	268(92)	13
			—	294	—	57
93	$C_{21}H_{28}O_3$	4-Pregnene-3,11,20-trione	2	283(491)	229(122)	13
94	$C_{21}H_{28}O_4$	17β-Acetoxy-4-androstene-3,11-dione	2	285(496) 360(16) I	229(84)	13
95	$C_{21}H_{28}O_4$	17α,21-Dihydroxy-1,4-pregnadiene-3,20-dione	0.25	267(305) 276(286) I 305(239) 345(121) I 426(94)	225(202) 292(235) 373(57)	119
			2	234(271) I 267(376) 275(370) I 298–307 (268) I 343(129) I 385(81) I 420(99) 520(62)	221(255) 370(66) 465(58)	119

TABLE V—*continued*

No.	Empirical Formula	Compound	Time, hours	λ_{max} in mμ ($E^{1\%}_{1\,cm}$)	λ_{min} in mμ ($E^{1\%}_{1\,cm}$)	Reference
95 cont.	$C_{21}H_{28}O_4$	17α,21-Dihydroxy-1,4-pregnadiene-3,20-dione	20	233(317) I 267–274(418) 285(370) I 308(304) I 342(169) I 385(103) 395–415(97) I 500(69)	221(306) 372(88) 460(66)	119
96	$C_{21}H_{28}O_4$	17α,21-Dihydroxy-4,15-pregnadiene-3,20-dione	2	239(446) 280(406) 396(154) 470(233)	252(312) 350(113) 405(150)	16
97	$C_{21}H_{28}O_4$	17α-Hydroxy-4-pregnene-3,11,20-trione	2	285* 350 415	—	133
98	$C_{21}H_{28}O_4$	21-Hydroxy-4-pregnene-3,11,20-trione (Kendall's Compound A)	—	280 355 415	—	40
			—	288 350 410	—	128
			2	280 355 415	—	137,138,139
			—	284 354 416	—	103
			2	280 360 420	—	11
99	$C_{21}H_{28}O_5$	11β,17α,21-Trihydroxy-1,4-pregnadiene-3,20-dione (prednisolone)	0.25	240(298) I 262(348) 303(204) 375(239)	222(250) 289(210) 333(129)	119
			2	240(312) I 265(263) 278(250) 359(353) 390(222) I 470(89)	310(183)	119
			20	240(424) I 270–278(300) 355(254) 390(195) I 470(132)	321(210)	119

TABLE V—*continued*

No.	Empirical Formula	Compound	Time, hours	λ_{max} in mμ ($E^{1\%}_{1\,cm}$)	λ_{min} in mμ ($E^{1\%}_{1\,cm}$)	Reference
99 cont.	$C_{21}H_{28}O_5$	11β,17α,21-Trihydroxy-1,4-pregnadiene-3,20-dione (prednisolone)	1–2 min.	240 I	225(308)	34
				263(366)	285(221)	
				306(244)	340(128)	
				379(215)		
				ca. 530		
			1	240 I	330(198)	34
				263 I		
				315 I		
				361(337)		
			—	242(380)	—	56
				370(295)		
			—	267	—	114
				359		
			—	242	—	133
				370		
100	$C_{21}H_{28}O_5$	11β,21-Dihydroxy-3,20-dioxo-4-pregnen-18-al (aldosterone)	2	288(615)	—	111
			3	288(615)	—	111
			—	290	—	54
			—	287	—	85
				390 I		
			—	288	234	90,94
			—	287	235	58
				420		
				450		
			2	288	—	31
101	$C_{21}H_{28}O_5$	16α,17α-Epoxy-11α,21-dihydroxy-4-pregnene-3,20-dione	20	283(500)	230(177)	115
				479(186)		
102	$C_{21}H_{28}O_5$	17α,21-Dihydroxy-5β-pregn-1-ene-3,11,20-trione	1–2 min.	273(228)	242(181)	34
				350(59)	375(18)	
				408(23)		
			1	273 I	242	34
				297(328)	375	
				350(129)		
				408(70)		
			2	265(340)	242	34
				302(362)	375	
				350(140)		
				408(76)		
103	$C_{21}H_{28}O_5$	17α,21-Dihydroxy-4-pregnene-3,11,20-trione (cortisone)	2	283(532)	231(154)	13
				342(215)	318(142)	
				413(185) I	371(81)	
				419(188)		
				480(21) I		

TABLE V—*continued*

No.	Empirical Formula	Compound	Time, hours	λ_{max} in mμ ($E^{1\%}_{1\,cm}$)	λ_{min} in mμ ($E^{1\%}_{1\,cm}$)	Reference
103 cont.	$C_{21}H_{28}O_5$	17α,21-Dihydroxy-4-pregnene-3,11,20-trione (cortisone)	2	283(527) 343(219) 413(170) I 420(173) 480(19) I	232(181) 318(148) 373(85)	13
			—	285 343 415	—	40
			—	283 340 415	—	49
			—	283 345 415	—	87
			2	284 343 420	—	66
			0.25	283(510) 341(184)	230(151)	115
			2	283(520) 341(213) 408–420(194)	230(165) 318(151) 368(90)	115
			20	283(546) 341(203) 408–420(194)	228(176) 318(153) 368(104)	115
			2	280–285 340–345 415	—	137,138,139
			2	285 340 415	—	11
			—	280 340 410–415	—	105
			—	280 340 415	—	38
			1	345* 410 420 I 480	370* 460	67
104	$C_{21}H_{28}O_5$	17α,21-Dihydroxy-14β-pregn-4-ene-3,15,20-trione	2	286(452) 366(536) 450(80) I 500(36) I	236(156) 318(129)	16

TABLE V—*continued*

No.	Empirical Formula	Compound	Time, hours	λ_{max} in mμ ($E^{1\%}_{1\,cm}$)	λ_{min} in mμ ($E^{1\%}_{1\,cm}$)	Reference
105	$C_{21}H_{28}O_6$	11β,16α,17α,21-Tetrahydroxy-1,4-pregnadiene-3,20-dione	0.25	262(184) 288(124) I 358(256)	227(107) 317(92)	119
			2	235(163) I 244(152) I 280(143) 359(404)	258(133) 308(83)	119
			20	241(308) I 268(272) I 280(260) I 359(285) 500(85) I	310(157)	119
106	$C_{21}H_{29}O_4F$	9α-Fluoro-11β,21-dihydroxy-4-pregnene-3,20-dione	0.25	220(137) 380(510) 372(212)	237(118) 314(20)	115
			2	223(223) 281(553) 371(524)	242(154) 315(35)	115
			20	230(271) I 282(578) 372(302) 460(87) 500(65) I 527(61) I	247(240) 321(107)	115
107	$C_{21}H_{29}O_5F$	9α-Fluoro-11β,17α,20β,21-tetrahydroxy-1,4-pregnadien-3-one	0.25	227(301) I 236(342) 262(430) 287(230) I 308(247)	219(271) 243(333) 393(227)	115
			2	227(321) I 238(335) 262(435) 288(246) 305(244) 355–380(47) I	219(291) 243(338) 283(244) 295(235)	115
			20	228(334) I 236(350) 255(417) I 262(434) 288(234) 305(230) 380(44) I 490(338)	219(304) 243(340) 282(232) 295(221) 450(321)	115
108	$C_{21}H_{29}O_5F$	9α-Fluoro-11β,17α,21-trihydroxy-4-pregnene-3,20-dione (9α-fluorohydrocortisone)	0.25	283(478) 319–332 (110) I 400(163) I 408(170) 503(68)	231(158) 353(96) 450(35)	119

TABLE V—*continued*

No.	Empirical Formula	Compound	Time, hours	λ_{max} in mμ ($E^{1\%}_{1\,cm}$)	λ_{min} in mμ ($E^{1\%}_{1\,cm}$)	Reference
108 cont.	$C_{21}H_{29}O_5F$	9α-Fluoro-11β,17α,21-trihydroxy-4-pregnene-3,20-dione (9α-fluorohydro-cortisone)	2	283(488) 318–333 (138) I 370(139) I 400(167) I 408(174) 503(63)	231(162) 352(117) 450(39)	119
			20	283(493) 333(147) I 370(147) I 400(181) I 408(184) 502(55) 530(53)	230(173) 353(123) 450(42) 517(50)	119
109	$C_{21}H_{29}O_6F$	9α-Fluoro-11β,16α,17aα-trihydroxy-17aβ-hydroxymethyl-4-D-homoandro-stene-3,17-dione (hemihydrate)	0.25	283(400)	—	118
			2	283(420)	—	118
			20	283(530)	—	118
110	$C_{21}H_{29}O_6F$	9α-Fluoro-11β,16α,17α,20β,21-pentahydroxy-1,4-pregnadien-3-one (20β-dihydrotriamcin-olone)	0.25	259(318) 310(160)	215(37) 287(107)	116
			2	259(320) 309(165)	215(42) 285(109)	116
			20	259(332) 308(172) 350(25) I 470(28)	218(121) 285(126) 390(14)	116
111	$C_{21}H_{29}O_6F$	9α-Fluoro-1ξ,11β,17α,21-tetrahydroxy-4-pregnene-3,20-dione	0.25	278(392) 385–405(188) 498(322) 550(17)	227(142) 314(73) 455(22) 525(16)	115
			2	278(473) 330(113) I 385–405(216) 498(48) 568(32)	227(180) 314(97) 450(34) 530(31)	115
			20	279(495) 380(196) 500(54) I	228(246) 320(145)	115
112	$C_{21}H_{29}O_6F$	9α-Fluoro-11β,16α,17α,21-tetrahydroxy-4-pregnene-3,20-dione	0.25	284(440) 390(57)	227(59) 330(10)	119
			2	283(462) 380(78)	228(65) 325(16)	119

TABLE V—*continued*

No.	Empirical Formula	Compound	Time, hours	λ_{max} in mμ ($E^{1\%}_{1\,cm}$)	λ_{min} in mμ ($E^{1\%}_{1\,cm}$)	Reference
112 cont.	$C_{21}H_{29}O_6F$	9α-Fluoro-11β,16α,17α,21-tetrahydroxy-4-pregnene-3,20-dione	20	283(565) 375(78)	227(76) 325(25)	119
113	$C_{21}H_{30}O_2$	17β-Hydroxy-17α-pregna-4,20-dien-3-one	2	292(590) 335(229) I 475(29)	230(157) 410(19)	13
114	$C_{21}H_{30}O_2$	3β-Hydroxy-5,7-pregnadien-20-one	2	238(244) 323(161) 405(730)	231(239) 282(117) 339(144)	13
115	$C_{21}H_{30}O_2$	5α-Pregn-7-ene-3,20-dione	2	289(132) I 322(209)	255(59)	13
116	$C_{21}H_{30}O_2$	4-Pregnene-3,20-dione (progesterone)	2	291(504)	229(174)	13
			2	292(513)	none	13
			2	295*	—	5
117	$C_{21}H_{30}O_3$	3-Ethylenedioxy-5,7-androstadien-17β-ol	2	302(735) 386(117) 495(48)	235(144) 344(65) 436(30)	13
118	$C_{21}H_{30}O_3$	17β-Acetoxy-4-androsten-3-one	2	296(558)	231(96)	13
119	$C_{21}H_{30}O_3$	3β-Acetoxy-5-androsten-17-one	2	304(283) 404(626) 482(17)	250(57) 344(74) 456(13)	13
			—	305 406 460–470	—	9
120	$C_{21}H_{30}O_3$	Methyl 3-oxo-4-androstene-17β-carboxylate	2	292(513)	236(127)	13
121	$C_{21}H_{30}O_3$	6β-Hydroxy-4-pregnene-3,20-dione	2	290(296) 344(343) 465(38)	245(133) 309(222) 397(17)	13
122	$C_{21}H_{30}O_3$	7α-Hydroxy-4-pregnene-3,20-dione	2	287.5(505) 315(314) I	234(122)	86
123	$C_{21}H_{30}O_3$	7β-Hydroxy-4-pregnene-3,20-dione	2	287.5(473) 317(265) I 357(60) I	233(126)	86
124	$C_{21}H_{30}O_3$	11α-Hydroxy-4-pregnene-3,20-dione	2	290(404) 318(254) I 473(38)	232(108) 380(13)	13
			0.25	289(408) 321(125) I	228(113)	16
			0.50	289(408) 321(217) I 470(17)	231(108) 409(4)	16
			1	291(408) 320(250) I 472(29)	231(108) 397(8)	16
			1.5	290(404) 319(254) I 473(33)	231(108) 386(13)	16

TABLE V—*continued*

No.	Empirical Formula	Compound	Time, hours	λ_{max} in mμ ($E^{1\%}_{1\,cm}$)	λ_{min} in mμ ($E^{1\%}_{1\,cm}$)	Reference
124 cont.	$C_{21}H_{30}O_3$	11α-Hydroxy-4-pregnene-3,20-dione	2	290(404) 319(254) I 472(38)	231(108) 385(13)	16
			2.5	289(404) 318(254) I 472(38)	231(108) 380(13)	16
			3	291(404) 319(258) I 470(38)	232(113) 382(13)	16
			4	290(404) 319(254) I 470(38)	230(113) 380(13)	16
			6	289(404) 318(254) I 470(42)	231(121) 380(17)	16
125	$C_{21}H_{30}O_3$	11β-Hydroxy-4-pregnene-3,20-dione	2	290(337) 318(221) I 474(29)	231(92) 380(8)	13
			0.25	290(346) 319(175) I 470(13)	230(92) 412(4)	16
			0.50	290(346) 318(204) I 472(17)	230(92) 405(8)	16
			1	290(342) 317(221) I 473(25)	229(92) 392(8)	16
			1.5	290(342) 318(221) I 472(29)	230(92) 390(8)	16
			2	290(338) 318(221) I 472(29)	231(92) 380(8)	16
			2.5	290(338) 316(225) I 471(33)	230(96) 379(8)	16
			3	290(338) 317(221) I 470(33)	230(96) 376(13)	16
			4	290(338) 317(221) I 470(33)	230(96) 380(13)	16
			6	290(338) 316(221) I 470(37)	231(100) 380(13)	16
126	$C_{21}H_{30}O_3$	17α-Hydroxy-4-pregnene-3,20-dione (17α-hydroxy-progesterone)	2	289(570) 431(230)	337(13)	13
			2	290 430	—	5,80,81

TABLE V—*continued*

No.	Empirical Formula	Compound	Time, hours	λ_{max} in mμ ($E^{1\%}_{1\,cm}$)	λ_{min} in mμ ($E^{1\%}_{1\,cm}$)	Reference
127	$C_{21}H_{30}O_3$	21-Hydroxy-4-pregnene-3,20-dione (cortexone, deoxycorticosterone)	2	288(570) 372(65) 438(48)	239(139) 330(13) 395(22)	13
			—	285 370 440	—	105
			2	285 370 440	—	137,138
128	$C_{21}H_{30}O_4$	3β-Acetoxy-14α-hydroxy-5-androsten-17-one	2	240(246) 317(129) 402(517) 500(125)	227(217) 272(100) 342(117) 452(88)	13
129	$C_{21}H_{30}O_4$	5α,21-Dihydroxy-5α-pregnane-3,20-dione	0.25	290(318) 320(179) 370(37) I 470(15) I	240(88)	16
			2	287(368) 330(108) I 375(92) 438(33) 480(25)	240(104) 355(83) 420(31) 465(23)	16
130	$C_{21}H_{30}O_4$	17α-Hydroxy-5β-pregnane-3,11,20-trione	2	280* 350 410	—	138
131	$C_{21}H_{30}O_4$	6β,11α-Dihydroxy-4-pregnene-3,20-dione	2	288(174) 346(532) 470(96)	255(125) 300(160) 406(56)	13
132	$C_{21}H_{30}O_4$	6β,21-Dihydroxy-4-pregnene-3,20-dione	—	285 350 455	—	7,87
133	$C_{21}H_{30}O_4$	11α,17α-Dihydroxy-4-pregnene-3,20-dione	2	242(214) I 286(504) 375(154) 449(112)	230(202) 333(82) 415(102)	13
134	$C_{21}H_{30}O_4$	11α,21-Dihydroxy-4-pregnene-3,20-dione	2	241(183) 287(383) 377(221) 456(212) 473(190) I	225(167) 247(179) 324(94) 409(117)	13
			0.25	242(133) I 287(433) 347(88) I 361(100) I 374(133) 452(71) 511(167) I	231(125) 324(75) 410(38)	16

TABLE V—*continued*

No.	Empirical Formula	Compound	Time, hours	λ_{max} in mμ ($E^{1\%}_{1\,cm}$)	λ_{min} in mμ ($E^{1\%}_{1\,cm}$)	Reference
134 cont.	$C_{21}H_{30}O_4$	11α,21-Dihydroxy-4-pregnene-3,20-dione	0.50	243(142) I	231(133)	16
				288(425)	324(75)	
				343(96) I	411(46)	
				361(121) I		
				374(167)		
				451(79)		
				471(67) I		
				511(25) I		
			1	244(154) I	228(146)	16
				288(412)	324(83)	
				343(104) I	409(71)	
				360(142) I		
				374(200)		
				452(129)		
				471(113) I		
				512(33) I		
			1.5	242(171)	225(158)	16
				287(396)	246(167)	
				343(108) I	323(88)	
				361(154) I	409(96)	
				375(217)		
				453(175)		
				471(158) I		
			2	241(183)	225(167)	16
				286(383)	246(179)	
				347(117) I	323(96)	
				363(163) I	408(117)	
				376(221)		
				456(213)		
				473(192) I		
			2.5	241(192)	225(175)	16
				285(375)	247(188)	
				343(113) I	323(96)	
				361(154) I	407(133)	
				375(221)		
				456(242)		
				469(225) I		
			3	242(200)	225(183)	16
				285(371)	248(196)	
				342(108) I	323(96)	
				362(163)	405(146)	
				375(217)		
				456(263)		
				472(238) I		
			4	241(212)	226(196)	16
				285(363)	248(204)	
				340(104) I	325(100)	
				361(150) I	403(163)	
				376(208)		
				456(287)		
				471(267) I		

TABLE V—*continued*

No.	Empirical Formula	Compound	Time, hours	λ_{max} in mμ ($E^{1\%}_{1\,cm}$)	λ_{min} in mμ ($E^{1\%}_{1\,cm}$)	Reference
134 cont.	$C_{21}H_{30}O_4$	11α,21-Dihydroxy-4-pregnene-3,20-dione	6	242(225) 284(362) 337(104) 378(200) 384(196) I 456(304)	227(208) 249(217) 325(100) 342(100) 402(171)	16
135	$C_{21}H_{30}O_4$	11β,21-Dihydroxy-4-pregnene-3,20-dione (corticosterone)	2	241(177) 287(479) 331(238) 374(192) 418(57) 460(64)	230(162) 247(174) 318(223) 362(162) 407(53) 432(53)	13
			—	285 330 375 455	—	40
			—	288 328 373 454	—	121
			—	284 330 375 440	—	128
			—	288* 325 375 456	—	103
			2	285 330 373–375 455	—	137,138,139
			—	280 320 370 445	—	38
			—	284 320 375 450	—	105
			2	287 330 I 375 455	—	31
			—	285 330 373 455	—	80,82

TABLE V—*continued*

No.	Empirical Formula	Compound	Time, hours	λ_{max} in mμ ($E^{1\%}_{1\,cm}$)	λ_{min} in mμ ($E^{1\%}_{1\,cm}$)	Reference
136	$C_{21}H_{30}O_4$	17α,21-Dihydroxy-4-pregnene-3,20-dione (Reichstein's Substance S)	2	240(254) 288(537) 338(142) 486(50) I 535(67)	249(208) 327(138) 390(29)	13
			2	241(235) 289(530) 330(165) I 490(52) I 534(65)	248(196) 392(30)	13
			2	285 535	—	137
			—	290 340 535	—	40
			2	240* 295 535	—	138
			0.25	241(204) 288(491) 332(135) I 532(83)	248(170) 390(17)	16
			0.50	241(213) 288(500) 330(144) I 532(78)	248(174) 390(20)	16
			1.0	241(222) 288(508) 332(148) I 488(52)I 533(74)	248(183) 390(22)	16
			1.5	240(230) 288(521) 332(157) I 488(52) I 531(70)	247(191) 394(26)	16
			2	241(235) 288(530) 334(161) I 487(52) I 531(65)	248(196) 292(30)	16
			2.5	240(239) 288(535) 332(170) I 480(52) I 532(61)	248(204) 395(30)	16
			3	240(239) 288(539) 332(174) I 482(52) I 531(57)	248(209) 395(35)	16

TABLE V—*continued*

No.	Empirical Formula	Compound	Time, hours	λ_{max} in mμ ($E^{1\%}_{1\,cm}$)	λ_{min} in mμ ($E^{1\%}_{1\,cm}$)	Reference
136 cont.	$C_{21}H_{30}O_4$	17α,21-Dihydroxy-4-pregnene-3,20-dione (Reichstein's Substance S)	4	240(243) 288(543) 332(183) I 480(52) 530(52)	248(213) 400(39) 507(48)	16
			6	240(248) 288(543) 332(191) I 475(57)	248(217) 398(44)	16
			8	239(252) 288(547) 330(204) I 463(61)	248(226) 399(52)	16
			24	238(269) 287(552) 331(217) I 445(70)	247(239) 396(61)	16
			—	240 290 340 I 535	—	82
137	$C_{21}H_{30}O_5$	11β,17α,20β,21-Tetrahydroxy-1,4-pregnadien-3-one (20-dihydro-prednisolone)	—	240 280 390	260 360	133
138	$C_{21}H_{30}O_5$	3α,17α,21-Trihydroxy-5α-pregnane-11,20-dione	—	335 410	—	87
139	$C_{21}H_{30}O_5$	3β,17α,21-Trihydroxy-5α-pregnane-11,20-dione (Reichstein's Substance D)	—	270 333 410	—	87
140	$C_{21}H_{30}O_5$	17α,21-Dihydroxy-5α-pregnane-3,11,20-trione	2	242(280) 252(188) 270(192) 341(200) 424(92) 474(72)	229(168) 246(168) 256(172) 295(108) 378(52) 450(64)	13
			—	270 342 417	—	87
141	$C_{21}H_{30}O_5$	17α,21-Dihydroxy-5β-pregnane-3,11,20-trione	2	270 340 415	—	137
			0.25	340(158) 410–420(158)	373(50)	115
			2	232(142) I 250–270(101) 341(206) 410–420(158)	290(83) 370(78)	115

TABLE V—*continued*

No.	Empirical Formula	Compound	Time, hours	λ_{max} in mμ ($E^{1\%}_{1\,cm}$)	λ_{min} in mμ ($E^{1\%}_{1\,cm}$)	Reference
141 cont.	$C_{21}H_{30}O_5$	17α,21-Dihydroxy-5β-pregnane-3,11,20-trione	20	250–270(119) 340(186) 410–420(142) 475(37) I	290(87) 370(87)	115
142	$C_{21}H_{30}O_5$	17α,20β,21-Trihydroxy-4-pregnene-3,11-dione (Reichstein's Substance U)	—	280 370 410	—	79
143	$C_{21}H_{30}O_5$	6β,17α,21-Trihydroxy-4-pregnene-3,20-dione	2	237(182) I 286(208) 343(450) 398(65) 430(76) 475(84)	252(156) 302(192) 383(60) 403(64) 438(74)	13
144	$C_{21}H_{30}O_5$	7α,17α,21-Trihydroxy-4-pregnene-3,20-dione	0.25	215(240) 281(442) 337(356) 380(45) I 470(75)	240(183) 308(161) 410(41)	115
			2	215(277) 239(219) I 279(443) 338(373) 380(69) I 470(97)	245(214) 308(168) 410(64)	115
			20	240(240) 278(431) 336(398) 385(86) I 465(118)	230(236) 245(236) 307(183) 410(94)	115
145	$C_{21}H_{30}O_5$	11α,17α,21-Trihydroxy-4-pregnene-3,20-dione (11-*epi*-hydrocortisone)	2	237(420) 282(462) 391(325) 475(153)	252(326) 330(130) 435(137)	1,13
			0.25	238(376) 283(452) 391(324) 478(160) 528(100) I	252(272) 328(108) 433(120)	16
			0.50	238(400) 282(456) 392(340) 478(160) 528(108) I	252(296) 329(120) 437(128)	16
			1.0	237(420) 282(464) 391(352) 477(164) 535(104) I	252(316) 330(128) 435(136)	16

TABLE V—*continued*

No.	Empirical Formula	Compound	Time, hours	λ_{max} in mμ ($E^{1\%}_{1\,cm}$)	λ_{min} in mμ ($E^{1\%}_{1\,cm}$)	Reference
145 cont.	$C_{21}H_{30}O_5$	11α,17α,21-Trihydroxy-4-pregnene-3,20-dione (11-*epi*-hydrocortisone)	1.5	237(428) 282(468) 391(352) 475(160)	252(324) 331(132) 437(140)	16
			2	237(436) 282(472) 391(348) 475(160)	252(328) 332(136) 439(144)	16
			2.5	237(440) 282(480) 391(348) 474(160)	252(336) 332(144) 438(144)	16
			3	237(440) 282(480) 392(344) 474(160)	252(340) 333(144) 437(148)	16
			4	238(444) 282(484) 392(340) 474(164)	252(344) 335(148) 436(148)	16
			6	238(448) 282(492) 392(332) 473(168)	252(352) 336(156) 433(152)	16
			8	238(452) 282(492) 392(324) 473(172)	252(356) 339(160) 433(156)	16
			24	238(468) 282(504) 392(320) 470(184)	252(380) 340(172) 431(168)	16
			2	240* 285 390 470 540	—	138
146	$C_{21}H_{30}O_5$	11β,17α,21-Trihydroxy-4-pregnene-3,20-dione (cortisol, hydrocortisone)	2	237(400) 282(431) 393(180) 475(204)	229(388) 252(302) 352(122) 417(153)	1,13
			2	238–240 280 395 475	—	102,137,139
			—	282 392 474	—	46
			—	285 380–395	—	40

TABLE V—*continued*

No.	Empirical Formula	Compound	Time, hours	λ_{max} in mμ ($E^{1\%}_{1\,cm}$)	λ_{min} in mμ ($E^{1\%}_{1\,cm}$)	Reference
146 cont.	$C_{21}H_{30}O_5$	11β,17α,21-Trihydroxy-4-pregnene-3,20-dione (cortisol, hydrocortisone)	—	240 280 395 470	—	49
			—	240 280 395 475	—	87
			2	237 282 395 478	—	66
			2	240* 280 390 475	—	138
			—	240 280 390 475	—	33
			0.5 min.	239(894) 285(157) 390(253) 475(480)	—	88
			2	239(600) 280(580) 390(272) 480(396)	—	88
			—	238–240 278–285 390–395 475	—	79,80,81, 82,83
			—	240 280 395 470	—	11
			—	240 280 390 475	—	38,105
			1	390* 480	420*	67
			0.25	238(352) 284(432) 393(152) 475(204)	226(320) 251(256) 348(100) 414(128)	16
			0.50	238(384) 283(428) 394(180) 475(232)	228(356) 251(280) 346(116) 416(156)	16

TABLE V—*continued*

No.	Empirical Formula	Compound	Time, hours	λ_{max} in mμ ($E^{1\%}_{1\,cm}$)	λ_{min} in mμ ($E^{1\%}_{1\,cm}$)	Reference
146 cont.	$C_{21}H_{30}O_5$	11β,17α,21-Trihydroxy-4-pregnene-3,20-dione (cortisol, hydrocortisone)	1.0	238(408) 282(440) 394(192) 474(224)	228(384) 252(300) 348(128) 417(160)	16
			1.5	238(420) 282(444) 393(196) 474(224)	228(392) 252(304) 348(132) 417(164)	16
			2	238(424) 282(448) 394(196) 475(220)	228(400) 252(312) 350(132) 418(164)	16
			2.5	238(432) 282(452) 394(196) 475(220)	228(404) 252(316) 351(136) 419(164)	16
			3	238(432) 282(452) 394(196) 475(220)	229(408) 253(316) 352(136) 419(164)	16
			4	238(440) 282(456) 394(196) 475(216)	229(420) 253(328) 356(140) 420(164)	16
			6	238(448) 282(460) 394(200) 475(220)	229(424) 253(332) 355(144) 420(172)	16
			24	238(463) 281(468) 394(208) 475(224)	229(452) 253(360) 355(160) 421(180)	16
147	$C_{21}H_{30}O_5$	15α,17α,21-Trihydroxy-4-pregnene-3,20-dione	2	230(364) 284(416) 393(421) 475(208)	250(276) 332(108) 420(150)	16
148	$C_{21}H_{30}O_5$	15β,17α,21-Trihydroxy-4-pregnene-3,20-dione	2	235(384) 280(400) 375(192) I 394(236) 455(228) I 472(236)	250(296) 337(124) 414(164)	16
149	$C_{21}H_{30}O_6$	2α,11β,17α,21-Tetrahydroxy-4-pregnene-3,20-dione	0.5 min.	239(282) 292(360) 383(114) 500(168)	—	24,37
			2	240(330) 289(294) 330(222) I 390(234) 485(132)	—	24,37

TABLE V—*continued*

No.	Empirical Formula	Compound	Time, hours	λ_{max} in mμ ($E^{1\%}_{1\ cm}$)	λ_{min} in mμ ($E^{1\%}_{1\ cm}$)	Reference
150	$C_{21}H_{30}O_6$	9α,11β,17α,21-Tetrahydroxy-4-pregnene-3,20-dione	2	238(397) 282(503) 332(164) I 407(239) 505(111)	253(337) 350(143) 458(105)	16
151	$C_{21}H_{31}O_5F$	9α-Fluoro-11β,17α,20β,21-tetrahydroxy-4-pregnen-3-one	0.25	228(242) I 235(250) 283(49) 390(28)	218(219) 249(162) 350(21)	115
			2	227(267) I 235(279) 282(49) 385(32)	218(240) 249(172) 350(25)	115
			20	227(307) I 235(328) 281(49) 390(32)	218(274) 250(186) 350(25)	115
152	$C_{21}H_{31}O_6F$	9α-Fluoro-11β,16α,17α,20β,21-pentahydroxy-4-pregnen-3-one (dihydrate)	0.25	283(346)	none	116
			2	283(346)	none	116
			20	283(360) 370(36)	335(24)	116
153	$C_{21}H_{32}O$	4-Pregnen-3-one	2	294(409)	none	13
154	$C_{21}H_{32}O_2$	5β-Pregnane-3,20-dione	2	237(159) I	none	13
155	$C_{21}H_{32}O_2$	20α-Hydroxy-4-pregnen-3-one (20α-dihydroprogesterone)	—	290	—	10
156	$C_{21}H_{32}O_2$	3β-Hydroxy-5-pregnen-20-one(pregnenolone)	2	239(130) I 330(287) 412(200)	270(83) 381(100)	13
			2	330* 412	—	5
157	$C_{21}H_{32}O_3$	11α-Hydroxy-5α-pregnane-3,20-dione	2	228(200) I 320(213)	259(76)	13
158	$C_{21}H_{32}O_3$	21-Hydroxy-5α-pregnane-3,20-dione	2	295* 375 440	—	5
159	$C_{21}H_{32}O_3$	17α-Hydroxy-5β-pregnane-3,20-dione	2	240(148) 290(270) 432(65)	228(139) 252(139) 342(13)	13
160	$C_{21}H_{32}O_3$	20α,21-Dihydroxy-4-pregnen-3-one	2	292(526) 337(144) I	230(122)	13
161	$C_{21}H_{32}O_3$	3β,17α-Dihydroxy-5-pregnen-20-one	2	310* 410 495	—	5
			—	325* 350 I 420 450 I 490	—	32

TABLE V—*continued*

No.	Empirical Formula	Compound	Time, hours	λ_{max} in mμ ($E^{1\%}_{1\,cm}$)	λ_{min} in mμ ($E^{1\%}_{1\,cm}$)	Reference
162	$C_{21}H_{32}O_3$	3β,21-Dihydroxy-5-pregnen-20-one	2	300 I* 340 380 405 440 I	—	5
163	$C_{21}H_{32}O_3$	5-Pregnene-3β,16α,20α-triol	2	390(200) 475(194) 235(50) I 320(120) I 355(155) I 510(111) I 540(60) I	265(40) 452(104)	47
			24	310(130) 385(188) 475(212) 530(79) I	260(50) 335(92) 430(139)	47
164	$C_{21}H_{32}O_4$	3β,21-Dihydroxy-5α-pregnane-11,20-dione (Reichstein's Substance N)	2	290 350 415	—	139
165	$C_{21}H_{32}O_4$	3α,17α-Dihydroxy-5β-pregnane-11,20-dione	2	280* 350 415	—	138
166	$C_{21}H_{32}O_4$	3α,21-Dihydroxy-5β-pregnane-11,20-dione	—	280 350 415	—	40
			—	290 350 415	—	38,105
167	$C_{21}H_{32}O_4$	11β,20α,21-Trihydroxy-4-pregnen-3-one (20α-dihydrocorticosterone)	—	285 380	—	121
			—	285 340	—	123
168	$C_{21}H_{32}O_4$	11β,20β,21-Trihydroxy-4-pregnen-3-one (20β-dihydrocorticosterone)	—	285 380	—	104,121
169	$C_{21}H_{32}O_5$	3β,17α,21-Trihydroxy-5α-pregnane-11,20-dione(Reichstein's Substance D)	2	333 410	—	137
			2	270 335 410	—	139

TABLE V—*continued*

No.	Empirical Formula	Compound	Time, hours	λ_{max} in mμ ($E^{1\%}_{1\,cm}$)	λ_{min} in mμ ($E^{1\%}_{1\,cm}$)	Reference
170	$C_{21}H_{32}O_5$	3α,17α,21-Trihydroxy-5β-pregnane-11,20-dione (tetrahydrocortisone)	—	340 412	—	28
			—	330–335 405–410	—	40
			—	310 400–405	—	79
			—	310–330 410–415	—	107
			—	315 410	290 370	133
			—	270–272 330–335 410	—	38,105
171	$C_{21}H_{32}O_5$	11β,17α,20α,21-Tetrahydroxy-4-pregnen-3-one	—	236 284 320 380 460 520	—	129
			0.5 min.	240* 285 338 360 375 400 490 525	—	26
			2	240* 285 335 375 400 525	—	26
172	$C_{21}H_{32}O_5$	11β,17α,20β,21-Tetrahydroxy-4-pregnen-3-one (monohydrate) (Reichstein's Substance E)	2	240(538) 283(446) 330(139) I 405(119) 468(112) 505(85) I	256(289) 359(88) 443(106)	13
			—	240 280–285 320 460	—	49,129

TABLE V—*continued*

No.	Empirical Formula	Compound	Time, hours	λ_{max} in mμ ($E^{1\%}_{1\,cm}$)	λ_{min} in mμ ($E^{1\%}_{1\,cm}$)	Reference
172 cont.	$C_{21}H_{32}O_5$	11β,17α,20β,21-Tetrahydroxy-4-pregnen-3-one (monohydrate) (Reichstein's Substance E)	0.5 min.	240* 285 338 360 375 400 450 I 525	—	26
			2	240* 285 330 400 460	—	26
173	$C_{21}H_{32}O_6$	5α,11β,17α,21-Tetrahydroxy-5α-pregnane-3,20-dione	0.25	235(204) 288(248) 394(204) 488(222) I 520(313)	253(159) 337(106) 442(135)	16
			2	235(289) 285(270) 390(209) 485(188) I 520(303)	254(205) 340(130) 440(145)	16
174	$C_{21}H_{34}O$	5-Pregnen-3β-ol	2	237(119) 313(252) 418(105) 500(33) I	226(114) 256(95) 389(86)	13
175	$C_{21}H_{34}O_2$	3α-Hydroxy-5β-pregnan-20-one	2	233(130) I 331(227) 396(18) I	267(75)	13
			2	325*	—	5
			0.25	230(127) I 331(227)	266(73)	16
			0.50	230(127) I 331(227)	265(73)	16
			1	230(127) I 331(227)	266(73)	16
			1.5	231(127) I 330(227)	266(77)	16
			2	232(132) I 331(227)	266(77)	16
			2.5	232(132) I 329(227)	267(77)	16
			3	232(132) I 328(223)	266(77)	16
			4	231(136) I 328(223)	266(82)	16
			6	232(141) I 326(223)	266(82)	16

TABLE V—*continued*

No.	Empirical Formula	Compound	Time, hours	λ_{max} in mμ ($E^{1\%}_{1\,cm}$)	λ_{min} in mμ ($E^{1\%}_{1\,cm}$)	Reference
176	$C_{21}H_{34}O_2$	5-Pregnene-3β,20β-diol	2	234(152) I 312(286) 411(195) 439(148) I 490(100) I	256(124) 376(138)	13
			2	330* 425	—	5
177	$C_{21}H_{34}O_3$	3β,17α-Dihydroxy-5α-pregnan-20-one	2	229(165) I 319(209) 407(78) 489(26) I	260(113) 378(61)	13
178	$C_{21}H_{34}O_3$	3β,21-Dihydroxy-5α-pregnan-20-one	2	300* 385 440	—	5
179	$C_{21}H_{34}O_3$	3α,17α-Dihydroxy-5β-pregnan-20-one	2	238(148) 315(191) 327(183) I 410(87) 500(35) I	225(139) 258(113) 379(65)	13
			0.25	237(130) 317(183) 328(178) I 412(65) 500(30)	222(122) 259(100) 384(52) 472(22)	16
			0.50	237(135) 316(187) 329(178) I 411(70) 497(30)	223(126) 259(104) 383(57) 471(26)	16
			1	238(139) 314(187) 327(183) I 410(78) 495(35)	223(135) 258(104) 379(61) 474(30)	16
			1.5	237(148) 314(191) 325(187) I 406(78) 492(39)	225(139) 259(109) 374(61) 472(30)	16
			2	237(148) 314(191) 327(183) I 410(87) 485(35) I	224(139) 258(113) 379(65)	16
			3	237(152) 313(191) 322(183) I 409(91) 485(39) I	222(148) 259(113) 377(65)	16

TABLE V—*continued*

No.	Empirical Formula	Compound	Time, hours	λ_{max} in mμ ($E^{1\%}_{1\,cm}$)	λ_{min} in mμ ($E^{1\%}_{1\,cm}$)	Reference
179 cont.	$C_{21}H_{34}O_3$	3α,17α-Dihydroxy-5β-pregnan-20-one	4	237(161) 315(191) 323(187) I 410(96) 435(70) I 487(39) I	224(152) 259(117) 376(70)	16
			6	237(165) 313(191) 323(187) I 409(100) 431(78) I 486(44) I	225(157) 258(122) 374(70)	16
			8	237(174) 313(196) 326(183) I 410(100) 431(83) I 488(44) I	224(165) 259(122) 373(70)	16
			24	235(200) 309(187) 324(165) I 411(113) 427(104) I 486(57) I	225(191) 258(135) 371(78)	16
180	$C_{21}H_{34}O_4$	3α,11β,21-Trihydroxy-5α-pregnan-20-one	—	321* 410	—	40
			—	320 410	—	38,105
181	$C_{21}H_{34}O_4$	3β,17α,21-Trihydroxy-5α-pregnan-20-one	2	315 410	—	137
182	$C_{21}H_{34}O_4$	3α,11α,17α-Trihydroxy-5β-pregnan-20-one (hydrate)	2	239(176) 300(196) 379(106) I 408(156) 431(128) I 520(40) I	226(168) 258(132) 363(88)	13
183	$C_{21}H_{34}O_4$	3α,11β,17α-Trihydroxy-5β-pregnan-20-one	2	234(181) I 321(169) 347(185) 415(150) 440(146)	262(119) 328(165) 401(142) 429(142)	13
184	$C_{21}H_{34}O_4$	3α,11β,21-Trihydroxy-5β-pregnan-20-one (tetrahydro-corticosterone)	—	310 415	—	38,40,105
185	$C_{21}H_{34}O_4$	3α,17α,21-Trihydroxy-5β-pregnan-20-one (tetrahydro Substance S)	—	315 410	—	40,105
			—	310 410	—	38,128

TABLE V—*continued*

No.	Empirical Formula	Compound	Time, hours	λ_{max} in mμ ($E^{1\%}_{1\,cm}$)	λ_{min} in mμ ($E^{1\%}_{1\,cm}$)	Reference
186	$C_{21}H_{34}O_5$	3α,11β,17α,21-Tetrahydroxy-5α-pregnan-20-one (Reichstein's Substance C)	—	340 415 510	—	87
187	$C_{21}H_{34}O_5$	3β,11β,17α,21-Tetrahydroxy-5α-pregnan-20-one (Reichstein's Substance V)	—	330 415 510	—	28,87,137
			—	310–330 410–415 505–510	—	107
188	$C_{21}H_{34}O_5$	3α,11β,17α,21-Tetrahydroxy-5β-pregnan-20-one (tetrahydrocortisol, tetrahydro F)	—	330 415 510	—	40
			—	320(216) 405(184) 500(109)	265(138) 370(128) 480(100)	64
			2	335 408	—	11
			—	310–330 410–415 505–510	—	107
			—	330 405 505	265 365 475	133
			—	260 330 415 515	—	38,105
189	$C_{21}H_{36}O_2$	5α-Pregnane-3α,20α-diol	2	322(191) I 343(200) 430(123) 502(27) I	256(64) 391(77)	13
			2	325* 435	—	5
190	$C_{21}H_{36}O_2$	5α-Pregnane-3β,20α-diol	2	320* 420 500 I	—	5
191	$C_{21}H_{36}O_2$	5α-Pregnane-3β,20β-diol	2	235(135) 330(243) 411(30)	227(130) 267(74) 390(22)	13
192	$C_{21}H_{36}O_2$	5β-Pregnane-3α,20α-diol	2	233(86) I 323(200) I 340(204) 431(155) 497(32) I	258(73) 389(86)	13

TABLE V—*continued*

No.	Empirical Formula	Compound	Time, hours	λ_{max} in mμ ($E^{1\%}_{1\,cm}$)	λ_{min} in mμ ($E^{1\%}_{1\,cm}$)	Reference
192 cont.	$C_{21}H_{36}O_2$	5β-Pregnane-3α,20α-diol	2	325*	—	22
				425		
			—	420*	385*	120
			2	320*	—	5
				440		
			0.25	237(105)	229(100)	16
				319(182)	261(73)	
				344(195)	325(177)	
				433(164)	389(91)	
				500(45)	485(41)	
			0.50	232(105) I	260(77)	16
				318(182)	326(177)	
				345(195)	388(91)	
				433(164)		
				491(45) I		
			1	233(105) I	261(77)	16
				319(186)	326(182)	
				344(200)	389(95)	
				433(173)		
				493(45) I		
			1.5	233(109) I	261(82)	16
				319(191)	326(186)	
				344(200)	388(100)	
				432(173)		
				492(45) I		
			2	233(109) I	261(82)	16
				319(191)	327(186)	
				343(200)	388(100)	
				432(177)		
				492(45) I		
			2.5	238(114)	228(109)	16
				320(200)	261(82)	
				343(204)	327(195)	
				433(177)	388(100)	
				492(45) I		
			3	238(114)	229(109)	16
				320(200)	261(86)	
				342(204)	328(195)	
				433(177)	388(110)	
				492(45) I		
			4	238(118)	229(114)	16
				319(209)	261(91)	
				342(209)	330(204)	
				432(182)	388(100)	
				493(45) I		
			6	238(123)	228(118)	16
				320(218)	260(95)	
				336(214) I	387(105)	
				431(186)		
				494(45) I		

TABLE V—*continued*

No.	Empirical Formula	Compound	Time, hours	λ_{max} in mμ ($E^{1\%}_{1 cm}$)	λ_{min} in mμ ($E^{1\%}_{1 cm}$)	Reference
193	$C_{21}H_{36}O_2$	5β-Pregnane-3α,20β-diol	2	239(113) 323(217) 428(152) 496(39) I	228(104) 260(87) 388(96)	13
			0.25	239(100) 319(195) 337(191) I 431(145) 500(45)	226(95) 261(73) 389(82) 485(41)	16
			0.50	239(105) 319(200) 340(195) 430(150) 490(45) I	226(100) 261(77) 332(191) 388(86)	16
			1	238(105) 319(200) 341(195) 431(155) 490(45) I	228(100) 261(77) 331(191) 388(86)	16
			1.5	239(109) 319(204) 341(200) 431(155) 490(45) I	228(105) 260(77) 333(195) 387(91)	16
			2	237(109) 319(204) 341(200) 431(159) 491(45) I	228(105) 260(77) 331(195) 387(91)	16
			2.5	238(114) 319(200) 342(200) 432(164) 492(45) I	229(109) 260(82) 330(195) 387(91)	16
			3	232(114) I 319(200) 343(195) 431(164) 492(45) I	260(82) 329(191) 387(91)	16
			4	233(114) I 318(195) 343(195) 431(164) 494(45) I	260(82) 329(186) 386(95)	16
			6	233(118) I 315(191) 343(195) 431(168) 490(50) I	259(86) 327(182) 386(95)	16

TABLE V—*continued*

No.	Empirical Formula	Compound	Time, hours	λ_{max} in mμ ($E^{1\%}_{1\ cm}$)	λ_{min} in mμ ($E^{1\%}_{1\ cm}$)	Reference
194	$C_{21}H_{36}O_3$	5α-Pregnane-3β,20β?, 21-triol	2	314(163) 339(154) 418(221) 435(184) I 498(46) I	256(75) 334(150) 374(121)	13
195	$C_{21}H_{36}O_3$	5β-Pregnane-3α,17α, 20α-triol	—	440	—	23
			—	315	—	22
196	$C_{21}H_{36}O_5$	5β-Pregnane-3α,11β, 17α,20β,21-pentaol (β-cortol)	2	239(273) 290(146) I 360(146) I 378(165) I 414(340) 446(279) I 500(208)	225(250) 323(125) 489(204)	13

TABLE VI. ABSORPTION SPECTRA OF C_{22} STEROIDS.

No.	Empirical Formula	Compound	Time, hours	λ_{max} in mμ ($E^{1\%}_{1\ cm}$)	λ_{min} in mμ ($E^{1\%}_{1\ cm}$)	Reference
197	$C_{22}H_{26}O_5$	3,16α-Diacetoxy-1,3,5(10)-estratrien-17-one	—	290* 370 490	—	84
198	$C_{22}H_{29}O_5F$	9α-Fluoro-11β,17α,21-trihydroxy-16α-methyl-1,4-pregnadiene-3,20-dione (dexamethasone)	0.25	260(374) 308(338) 372(27) I	280(214)	115
			2	261(402) 307(348) 370(33) I	280(252)	115
			20	261(423) 303(322) 420(46)	280(278) 377(45)	115
199	$C_{22}H_{30}O_5$	11β,17α,21-Trihydroxy-6α-methyl-1,4-pregnadiene-3,20-dione(medrol)	0.25	258(354) 304(205) 377(235) 540(69)	285(193) 335(118) 475(60)	115
			2	240(322) I 262(267) I 357(305) 385(198) I 540(65)	314(181) 495(60)	115
			20	268(319) I 350(241) 466(144) I 535(115) I	324(224)	115
200	$C_{22}H_{34}O_2$	3β-Methoxy-5-pregnen-20-one	2	239(152) 322(300) 413(222)	227(148) 270(96) 380(113)	13
201	$C_{22}H_{34}O_3$	3α-Hydroxy-11-bisnorcholenic acid	2	234(88) 339(267)	225(83) 252(58)	13
202	$C_{22}H_{36}O_5$	3α,7α,12α-Trihydroxy-5β-bisnorcholanic acid	2	306(136) 390(490) 443(112)	260(64) 333(107) 437(110)	43

TABLE VII. ABSORPTION SPECTRA OF C_{23} STEROIDS.

No.	Empirical Formula	Compound	Time, hours	λ_{max} in mμ ($E^{1\%}_{1\,cm}$)	λ_{min} in mμ ($E^{1\%}_{1\,cm}$)	Reference
203	$C_{23}H_{26}O_4$	21-Acetoxy-1,4,9(11), 16-pregnatetraene-3,20-dione	0.25	265(457) 297(440) 357(540) 390(226) I	225(235) 280(380) 327(286)	115
			2	245(354) I 290(322) 355(664) 390(394) I 520(153)	265(301) 312(280) 450(106)	115
			20	235(710) I 270(494) 340(334) I 387(377) 430(234) I 485(233)	261(487) 320(315) 448(205)	115
204	$C_{23}H_{26}O_5$	21-Acetoxy-1,4,16-pregnatriene-3,11,20-trione	0.25	259(544) 295(285) 355(32) I	220(126) 282(274)	115
			2	259(533) 296(277) 360(42) I	220(126) 282(270)	115
			20	259(494) 297(251) 360(121)	220(126) 282(240) 333(80)	115
205	$C_{23}H_{28}O_4$	21-Acetoxy-4,9(11),16-pregnatriene-3,20-dione	0.25	288(438) 387(648)	240(155) 326(46)	119
			2	288(419) 387(708)	240(148) 325(42)	119
			20	288(404) 385(740)	239(129) 325(29)	119
206	$C_{23}H_{28}O_4$	3β-Acetoxy-16α,17α-epoxy-5,7,9(11)-pregnatrien-20-one	2	243(441) 259(407) I 278(322) I 290(285) I 309(241) I 484(630)	225(407) 352(115)	13
207	$C_{23}H_{28}O_5$	21-Acetoxy-4,16-pregnadiene-3,11,20-trione	0.25	285(513) 380(19)	335(7)	119
			2	285(550) 380(37)	335(19)	119
			20	285(518) 364(125)	325(46)	119
208	$C_{23}H_{29}O_6F$	9α-Fluoro-11β-hydroxy-16α,17α-iso-propylidenedioxy-3-oxo-1,4-androstadien-17β-oic acid	0.25	258(267) 309(133)	—	118
			2	258(267) 309(133)	—	118

TABLE VII—*continued*

No.	Empirical Formula	Compound	Time, hours	λ_{max} in mμ ($E^{1\%}_{1\,cm}$)	λ_{min} in mμ ($E^{1\%}_{1\,cm}$)	Reference
208 cont.	$C_{23}H_{29}O_6F$	9α-Fluoro-11β-hydroxy-16α,17α-isopropylidenedioxy-3-oxo-1,4-androstadien-17β-oic acid	20	220(489) 278(277) 370(132) 468(106)	—	118
209	$C_{23}H_{29}O_6F$	21-Acetoxy-9α-fluoro-11β,17α-dihydroxy-1,4-pregnadiene-3,20-dione	0.25	263(370) 308(228) I 380(141) 410(117) I 452(148)	235(268) 350(123) 400(110)	119
			2	263(342) 290(275) I 310(247) I 373(114) I 450(171)	242(291) 390(104)	119
			20	264(345) 290(285) I 310(252) I 373(114) I 450(193)	245(304) 383(107)	119
			2	262.5 310	—	61
210	$C_{23}H_{29}O_7F$	17aβ-Acetoxymethyl-9α-fluoro-11β,16α,17aα-trihydroxy-1,4-D-homoandrostadiene-3,17-dione	0.25	258(302) 307(151)	—	118
			2	258(295) 307(146)	—	118
			20	258(288) 307(137)	—	118
211	$C_{23}H_{30}O_4$	3β-Acetoxy-16α,17α-epoxy-5,7-pregnadien-20-one	2	230(350) I 410(300) 428(273) I 475(242)	343(115) 462(235)	13
212	$C_{23}H_{30}O_5$	21-Acetoxy-17α-hydroxy-4,9(11)-pregnadiene-3,20-dione	0.25	239(273) 284(450) 328(98) I 387(89) 470(60)	250(179) 358(54)	115
			2	239(357) 284(474) 328(146) I 387(121) 450(67)	250(222) 358(88)	115
213	$C_{23}H_{30}O_5$	21-Acetoxy-16α,17α-epoxy-4-pregnene-3,20-dione	0.25	285(387) 375(126) I 389(146)	245(115) 335(31)	115

TABLE VII—*continued*

No.	Empirical Formula	Compound	Time, hours	λ_{max} in mμ ($E^{1\%}_{1\,cm}$)	λ_{min} in mμ ($E^{1\%}_{1\,cm}$)	Reference
213 cont.	$C_{23}H_{30}O_5$	21-Acetoxy-16α,17α-epoxy-4-pregnene-3,20-dione	2	225(220) 285(404) 375(390) I 389(474)	248(162) 325(51)	115
			20	225(240) 283(418) 373(428) I 389(543) 430(93) 480(103)	247(175) 320(66) 418(87) 445(87)	115
214	$C_{23}H_{30}O_5$	21-Acetoxy-4-pregnene-3,11,20-trione	2	283(540) 354(116) 401(207) I 415(266)	233(129) 323(42) 371(79)	13
215	$C_{23}H_{30}O_6$	21-Acetoxy-11β,17α-dihydroxy-1,4-pregnadiene-3,20-dione(prednisolone acetate)	—	305(235) I 375(250)	—	56
			2	235 360	—	25
216	$C_{23}H_{30}O_6$	21-Acetoxy-11β-hydroxy-3,20-dioxo-4-pregnen-18-al (aldosterone 21-acetate)	—	285 390 I	—	45
217	$C_{23}H_{30}O_6$	21-Acetoxy-17α-hydroxy-5α-pregn-1-ene-3,11,20-trione	2	279(243) 340(93) I 415(54) 480(11) I	378(29)	13
218	$C_{23}H_{30}O_6$	21-Acetoxy-17α-hydroxy-4-pregnene-3,11,20-trione (cortisone acetate)	2	283(486) 342(193) 415(164) 486(18) I	228(146) 319(125) 371(68)	13
			2	280–285 340–345 410–415	—	110
218a	$C_{23}H_{31}O_6F$	21-Acetoxy-9α-fluoro-11β,17α-dihydroxy-4-pregnene-3,20-dione	0.25	283(478) 330(107) I 407(170) 503(64)	230(158) 351(96) 450(35)	115
			2	283(487) 330(138) I 370(141) I 390(156) I 406(174) 503(64) 525(39) I 538(35) I	230(156) 353(107) 450(38)	115

TABLE VII—*continued*

No.	Empirical Formula	Compound	Time, hours	λ_{max} in mμ ($E^{1\%}_{1\,cm}$)	λ_{min} in mμ ($E^{1\%}_{1\,cm}$)	Reference
218a cont.	$C_{23}H_{31}O_6F$	21-Acetoxy-9α-fluoro-11β,17α-dihydroxy-4-pregnene-3,20-dione	20	282(495) 330(149) I 372(149) I 389(170) I 406(182) 503(55) 530(55) 575(32) I	230(173) 353(123) 450(42) 516(51)	115
219	$C_{23}H_{32}O_3$	3β-Acetoxy-5,16-pregnadien-20-one	2	296(233) 384(329) 412(229) 470(129) 547(92)	255(154) 331(171) 407(225) 442(121) 525(75)	13
220	$C_{23}H_{32}O_4$	5,7-Androstadiene-3β,17β-diol diacetate	2	231(162) I 290(127) 248(158) I 358(173) 416(285) 465(335) 497(158) I	272(123) 319(115) 367(162) 432(258)	13
221	$C_{23}H_{32}O_4$	5,14-Androstadiene-3β,17β-diol diacetate	2	271(169) 307(112) I 409(242) 480(504) I 490(527)	237(131) 337(81) 425(231)	13
222	$C_{23}H_{32}O_4$	21-Acetoxy-4-pregnene-3,20-dione	2	288(475) 371(52) 437(38)	234(111) 331(19) 395(23)	13
223	$C_{23}H_{32}O_4$	3α-Acetoxy-16-pregnene-11,20-dione	2	283(371) 328(70) I 380(74) I 400(111)	230(104) 352(33)	13
224	$C_{23}H_{32}O_4$	3β-Acetoxy-16α,17α-epoxy-5-pregnen-20-one	2	313(115) 334(114) 405(408) 471(289)	275(104) 327(112) 346(96) 436(239)	13
225	$C_{23}H_{32}O_5$	2α,17β-Diacetoxy-4-androsten-3-one	0.25	300(246)	none	115
			2	299(283) 350(100)	330(90)	115
			20	297(396) 403(90) 437(96)	235(96) 350(59) 415(85)	115
226	$C_{23}H_{32}O_5$	3,17-Bis-ethylenedioxy-5-androsten-11-one	2	293(459)	235(74)	13
227	$C_{23}H_{32}O_5$	21-Acetoxy-11β-hydroxy-4-pregnene-3,20-dione	2	285* 330 375 455	—	138

TABLE VII—*continued*

No.	Empirical Formula	Compound	Time, hours	λ_{max} in mμ ($E^{1\%}_{1\,cm}$)	λ_{min} in mμ ($E^{1\%}_{1\,cm}$)	Reference
228	$C_{23}H_{32}O_5$	21-Acetoxy-17α-hydroxy-4-pregnene-3,20-dione	2	241(259) 289(478) 328(196) I 490(63) I 535(100) 550(93) I	251(204) 385(26)	13
229	$C_{23}H_{32}O_6$	21-Acetoxy-17α-hydroxy-5β-pregnane-3,11,20-trione	2	233(164) I 242(150) I 251(136) 270(135) 342(198) 421(165) 475(43)	248(135) 257(126) 292(83) 372(72) 463(41)	13
230	$C_{23}H_{32}O_6$	21-Acetoxy-11β,17α-dihydroxy-4-pregnene-3,20-dione (hydrocortisone acetate)	2	240(382) 285(486) 392(150) 460(75)	252(243) 358(107) 434(71)	13
			0.5 min.	240(605) 285(925) 387(150) 475(300)	—	88
			2	240(1225) 285(1575) 387(450) 475(230)	—	88
			2	280–285 390–395 470–480	—	110
			—	240 285 390 465	—	122
231	$C_{23}H_{32}O_7$	21-Acetoxy-9α,11β,17α-trihydroxy-4-pregnene-3,20-dione	2	238(328) 282(426) 332(146) I 405(203) 505(89)	253(279) 355(157) 470(81)	16
232	$C_{23}H_{34}O_4$	4-Androstene-3β,17β-diol diacetate	2	240(93) I 305(215) 354(137) 408(282) 483(93) 517(70) I	252(85) 336(126) 365(130) 463(85)	13
233	$C_{23}H_{34}O_4$	5-Androstene-3β,17β-diol diacetate	2	307(192) 408(358) 440(177) I 480(85) I	257(81) 336(119)	13

TABLE VII—*continued*

No.	Empirical Formula	Compound	Time, hours	λ_{max} in mμ ($E^{1\%}_{1\,cm}$)	λ_{min} in mμ ($E^{1\%}_{1\,cm}$)	Reference
234	$C_{23}H_{34}O_4$	7-Androstene-3β,17β-diol diacetate	2	233(100) I 308(142) 411(327) 431(277) I 497(85) I	259(62) 350(96)	13
235	$C_{23}H_{34}O_4$	8(14)-Androstene-3β,17β-diol diacetate	2	233(96) I 308(139) 411(327) 432(269) I 491(89) I	259(58) 350(96)	13
236	$C_{23}H_{34}O_4$	3α,9α-Epoxy-11-oxo-5β-norcholanic acid	2	290(165) 341(58) I 412(42)	250(85) 372(27)	13
237	$C_{23}H_{34}O_4$	3α-Acetoxy-5β-pregnane-11,20-dione	2	319(48) 382(100) I 401(177) 414(131) I	262(35) 350(27)	13
			2	228(107) I 318(78) 384(85) I 402(137) 408(126) I	262(44) 354(33)	13
238	$C_{23}H_{34}O_5$	3,17-Bis-ethylenedioxy-5-androsten-11α-ol	2	296(481) 379(122) 402(48) I 462(26)	242(93) 335(41) 435(19)	13
239	$C_{23}H_{34}O_6$	21-Acetoxy-11β,17α-dihydroxy-5β-pregnane-3,20-dione	2	238(207) 291(234) 341(93) I 395(88) 490(43)	229(198) 256(136) 368(71) 452(41)	13
240	$C_{23}H_{36}O_3$	3β-Acetoxy-5α-pregnan-20-one	2	226(100) I 333(216) 412(14)	261(56) 395(12)	13
			2	234(112) 329(235) 415(15) I	228(110) 263(65)	13
241	$C_{23}H_{36}O_4$	5β-Androstane-3α,17β-diol diacetate	2	343(226) 410(37) I 470(15) I	250(59)	13
242	$C_{23}H_{38}O_3$	3β-Acetoxy-5α-pregnan-20β-ol	2	237(102) 314(188) 421(160) 430(156) I 492(52) I	227(98) 260(76) 380(96)	13
243	$C_{23}H_{38}O_5$	3α,7α,12α-Trihydroxy-5β-norcholanic acid	2	304(95) 389(458) 480(58)	254(42) 334(77) 442(43)	43

TABLE VIII. ABSORPTION SPECTRA OF C_{24} STEROIDS.

No.	Empirical Formula	Compound	Time, hours	λ_{max} in mμ ($E^{1\%}_{1\,cm}$)	λ_{min} in mμ ($E^{1\%}_{1\,cm}$)	Reference
244	$C_{24}H_{29}O_6F$	9α-Fluoro-17aβ-hydroxymethyl-16α, 17aα-iso-propylidene-dioxy-1,4-D-homo-androstadiene-3,11, 17-trione	0.25	256(339) 307(152)	—	118
			2	256(339) 307(152)	—	118
			20	256(303) 307(145)	—	118
245	$C_{24}H_{31}O_6F$	9α-Fluoro-11β-hydroxy-17aβ-hydroxymethyl-16α,17aα-iso-propylidenedioxy-1, 4-D-homoandrosta-diene-3,17-dione	0.25	258(282) 309(145)	—	118
			2	258(282) 309(145)	—	118
			20	261(304) 309(141)	—	118
246	$C_{24}H_{31}O_6F$	9α-Fluoro-11β,21-dihydroxy-16α,17α-iso-propylidenedioxy-1,4-pregnadiene-3, 20-dione (triamcinol-one acetonide)	0.25	260(474) 310(240) 390(52)	285(165) 345(14)	115
			2	259(484) 310(234) 380(120)	286(176) 340(37)	115
			20	260(570) 309(276) 374(145)	295(242) 340(61)	115
247	$C_{24}H_{33}O_6F$	9α-Fluoro-11β,21-dihydroxy-16α,17α-iso-propylidenedioxy-4-pregnene-3,20-dione	0.25	283(389) 390(47)	320(12)	115
			2	281(400) 376(83)	320(14)	115
			20	281(455) 375(87)	320(29)	115
248	$C_{24}H_{33}O_6F$	9α-Fluoro-11β,16α,17α-trihydroxy-20β,21-iso-propylidenedioxy-1,4-pregnadien-3-one	0.25	258(273) 308(163)	285(118)	116
			2	258(273) 308(163)	285(118)	116
			20	259(302) 308(153)	285(101)	116

TABLE VIII—*continued*

No.	Empirical Formula	Compound	Time, hours	λ_{max} in mμ ($E^{1\%}_{1\,cm}$)	λ_{min} in mμ ($E^{1\%}_{1\,cm}$)	Reference
249	$C_{24}H_{34}O_5$	3,7,12-Trioxo-5β-cholanic acid (dehydrocholic acid)	2	none	none	43
250	$C_{24}H_{36}O_4$	3β-Acetoxy-5-bis-norcholenic acid	2	235(37) I 339(148) 416(167)	257(30) 377(67)	13
251	$C_{24}H_{36}O_4$	3,7-Dioxo-5β-cholanic acid	2	none	none	43
252	$C_{24}H_{36}O_4$	3,12-Dioxo-5β-cholanic acid	2	none	none	43
253	$C_{24}H_{36}O_4$	3α-Hydroxy-12-oxo-5β-chol-9(11)-enic acid	2	290(169) 378(158)	255(104) 336(73)	13
254	$C_{24}H_{36}O_5$	3α-Acetoxy-11-oxo-5β-bisnorcholanic acid	2	320(82) 402(143) 414(125) I	262(39) 352(32)	13
255	$C_{24}H_{36}O_5$	3α-Hydroxy-7,12-dioxo-5β-cholanic acid	2	293(207)	255(82)	43
256	$C_{24}H_{38}O_3$	3-Oxo-5β-cholanic acid	2	310(7)	275(4)	13
257	$C_{24}H_{38}O_3$	3β-Hydroxy-5-cholenic acid	2	307(304)	250(64)	43
258	$C_{24}H_{38}O_3$	12-Oxo-5β-chol-9(11)-enic acid	2	305(268) 394(38)	240(90) 362(19)	43
259	$C_{24}H_{38}O_3$	3α-Hydroxy-5β-chol-11-enic acid	2	235(73) I 307(289) 430(27) I	255(62)	13
260	$C_{24}H_{38}O_4$	3α-Hydroxy-7-oxo-5β-cholanic acid	2	301(161)	240(69)	43
261	$C_{24}H_{38}O_4$	3α-Hydroxy-12-oxo-5β-cholanic acid	2	317(177) 390(225)	264(70) 346(85)	43
			2	231(143) I 315(168) 389(257)	263(82) 346(93)	13
262	$C_{24}H_{38}O_4$	11-Hydroxy-12-oxo-5β-cholanic acid	2	323(207)	248(45)	43
263	$C_{24}H_{38}O_4$	3α,12α-Dihydroxy-5β-chol-8(14)-enic acid (apocholic acid)	2	303(122) 390(676) 478(61)	254(56) 334(92) 435(40)	43
264	$C_{24}H_{38}O_5$	3α,7α-Dihydroxy-12-oxo-5β-cholanic acid	2	280(154) 391(221) 480(46)	251(91) 315(74) 442(35)	43
265	$C_{24}H_{40}O_2$	5β-Cholanic acid	2	none	none	43
			2	313(212)	238(27)	13
266	$C_{24}H_{40}O_3$	3α-Hydroxy-5β-cholanic acid (lithocholic acid)	2	311(200)	249(42)	13
			2	316(90)	250(26)	43
267	$C_{25}H_{40}O_3$	Methyl 12α-hydroxy-5β-chol-3-enate	2	304(207) 380(99)	252(134) 360(94)	43
268	$C_{24}H_{40}O_4$	3α,6α-Dihydroxy-5β-cholanic acid	2	305(308)	246(59)	43

TABLE VIII—*continued*

No.	Empirical Formula	Compound	Time, hours	λ_{max} in mμ ($E^{1\%}_{1\,cm}$)	λ_{min} in mμ ($E^{1\%}_{1\,cm}$)	Reference
269	$C_{24}H_{40}O_4$	3α,7α-Dihydroxy-5β-cholanic acid (chenodesoxycholic acid)	2	310(261)	250(55)	43
270	$C_{24}H_{40}O_4$	3α,12α-Dihydroxy-5β-cholanic acid (deoxycholic acid)	2	311(272) 390(54) I	253(68)	13
			2	312(268)	245(74)	43
271	$C_{24}H_{40}O_5$	3α,7α,12α-Trihydroxy-5β-cholanic acid (cholic acid)	2	304(117) 371(424) I 389(627) 454(62) I 478(76)	256(59) 335(90) 439(52)	13
			2	305(132) 389(661) 478(63)	256(69) 335(107) 439(44)	43

TABLE IX. ABSORPTION SPECTRA OF C_{25} STEROIDS.

No.	Empirical Formula	Compound	Time, hours	λ_{max} in mμ ($E^{1\%}_{1\,cm}$)	λ_{min} in mμ ($E^{1\%}_{1\,cm}$)	Reference
272	$C_{25}H_{29}O_8Cl$	16α,21-Diacetoxy-9α-chloro-17α-hydroxy-1,4-pregnadiene-3,11,20-trione	0.25	257(285) 311(98)	221(66) 280(59)	119
			2	257(283) 311(98) 390(28)	221(66) 280(61) 350(12)	119
			20	258(295) 312(107) 390(96)	220(84) 294(92) 345(30)	119
273	$C_{25}H_{29}O_8F$	16α,21-Diacetoxy-9α-fluoro-17α-hydroxy-1,4-pregnadiene-3,11,20-trione	0.25	258(354) 305(149)	220(74) 279(100)	119
			2	258(354) 305(151) 385(41)	220(74) 279(100) 345(22)	119
			20	258(354) 307(158) 381(96)	220(91) 279(144) 342(46)	119
274	$C_{25}H_{30}O_7$	16α,21-Diacetoxy-17α-hydroxy-1,4,9(11)-pregnatriene-3,20-dione	0.25	262(260) 308(115) 355(156)	310(132) 430(129)	119
			2	250(152) 283(101) I 355(423) 520(57)	238(149) 300(79) 460(52)	119
			20	241(330) I 281(183) I 355(195) 515(196)	230(103) 283(90) 325(102)	119
275	$C_{25}H_{30}O_8$	16α,21-Diacetoxy-9β,11β-epoxy-17α-hydroxy-1,4-pregnadiene-3,20-dione	0.25	230(271) I 247–253 (208) I 318(163) 415(84) 500(113) I 570(133)	290(129) 350(52) 435(81)	119
			2	220–230(305) 248–251 (259) I 319(200) 405(104) 505(129) I 568(132)	285(158) 350(81) 435(91)	119
			20	232(339) 252(317) I 316(244) 400(149) 490(149)	221(333) 290(200) 345(105) 435(123)	119

TABLE IX—*continued*

No.	Empirical Formula	Compound	Time, hours	λ_{max} in mμ ($E^{1\%}_{1\,cm}$)	λ_{min} in mμ ($E^{1\%}_{1\,cm}$)	Reference
276	$C_{25}H_{30}O_8$	16α,21-Diacetoxy-17α-hydroxy-1,4-pregnadiene-3,11,20-trione	0.25	259(310) 295(142)	221(63) 281(135)	119
			2	259(310) 295(140) 385(27)	221(67) 281(138) 345(9)	119
			20	259(312) 310(137) I 380(137)	221(104) 337(43)	119
277	$C_{25}H_{31}O_8Cl$	16α,21-Diacetoxy-9α-chloro-11β,17α-dihydroxy-1,4-pregnadiene-3,20-dione	0.25	258–261(280) 313(109)	220(66) 285(50)	119
			2	258–261(280) 313(112) 382(32)	220(73) 285(57) 345(17)	119
			20	258–261(299) 313(130) 378(143)	220(124) 289(100) 342(60)	119
278	$C_{25}H_{31}O_8F$	16α-Acetoxy-17aβ-acetoxymethyl-9α-fluoro-11β,17aα-dihydroxy-1,4-D-homoandrostadiene-3,17-dione	0.25	261(269) 310(127)	—	118
			2	261(269) 310(127)	—	118
			20	261(272) 310(129)	—	118
279	$C_{25}H_{31}O_8F$	16α,21-Diacetoxy-9α-fluoro-11β,17α-dihydroxy-1,4-pregnadiene-3,20-dione (triamcinolone diacetate)	0.25	261(297) 308(136)	220(59) 283(88)	117,119
			2	261(297) 308(136) 380(35)	220(59) 283(88) 345(17)	117,119
			20	260(302) 308(133) 375(187) 477(10) I	217(82) 285(109) 335(50)	117,119
			—	261 308 387	—	17
280	$C_{25}H_{31}O_8F$	16α,21-Diacetoxy-9α-fluoro-17α-hydroxy-4-pregnene-3,11,20-trione	0.25	280(338)	230(63)	119

TABLE IX—*continued*

No.	Empirical Formula	Compound	Time, hours	λ_{max} in mμ ($E^{1\%}_{1\ cm}$)	λ_{min} in mμ ($E^{1\%}_{1\ cm}$)	Reference
280 cont.	$C_{25}H_{31}O_8F$	16α,21-Diacetoxy-9α-fluoro-17α-hydroxy-4-pregnene-3,11,20-trione	2	280(338) 390(36)	230(63) 333(14)	119
			20	280(353) 382(90)	230(63) 323(23)	119
281	$C_{25}H_{32}O_7$	20β,21-Diacetoxy-11β,17α-dihydroxy-1,4-pregnadien-3-one	2	284 340 I 410	245 365	133
282	$C_{25}H_{32}O_7$	16α,21-Diacetoxy-17α-hydroxy-4,9(11)-pregnadiene-3,20-dione	0.25	285(320)	233(46)	119
			2	285(313) 380(23)	233(46) 340(16)	119
			20	250(132) I 284(292) 475(146)	230(91) 345(34)	119
283	$C_{25}H_{32}O_8$	16α,21-Diacetoxy-11β,17α-dihydroxy-1,4-pregnadiene-3,20-dione	0.25	263(261) 315(125) 338–355(25)	221(69) 285(100)	119
			2	261(148) 353(296)	230(109) 300(77)	119
			20	243(286) I 353(185) 520(164)	308(109) 430(108)	119
284	$C_{25}H_{32}O_8$	16α,21-Diacetoxy-9β,11β-epoxy-17α-hydroxy-4-pregnene-3,20-dione	0.25	283(317)	235(111)	119
			2	282(331) 390(44)	239(137) 350(36)	119
			20	282(350) 380(93) 483(146)	240(173) 340(62) 410(84)	119
285	$C_{25}H_{32}O_8$	16α,21-Diacetoxy-17α-hydroxy-4-pregnene-3,11,20-trione	0.25	283(336)	231(57)	119
			2	283(338) 385(30)	231(60) 333(13)	119
			20	281(345) 381(133)	233(77) 322(25)	119
286	$C_{25}H_{32}O_8$	2α,21-Diacetoxy-17-hydroxy-4-pregnene-3,11,20-trione	—	317 405 I 462	240 385 455	97
287	$C_{25}H_{32}O_8$	6β,21-Diacetoxy-17-hydroxy-4-pregnene-3,11,20-trione	0.5 min.	280* 340 420	—	26
			2	280* 340 420	—	26

TABLE IX—*continued*

No.	Empirical Formula	Compound	Time, hours	λ_{max} in mμ ($E^{1\%}_{1\,cm}$)	λ_{min} in mμ ($E^{1\%}_{1\,cm}$)	Reference
288	$C_{25}H_{33}O_8Br$	16α,21-Diacetoxy-9α-bromo-11β,17α-dihydroxy-4-pregnene-3,20-dione	0.25	289(277)	228(68)	119
			2	289(183)	239(62)	119
			20	235(151) I 288(172) 385(64) I	245(136) 345(47)	119
289	$C_{25}H_{33}O_8F$	16α-Acetoxy-17aβ-acetoxymethyl-9α-fluoro-11β,17aα-dihydroxy-4-D-homoandrostene-3,17-dione	0.25	224(162) 282(287)	—	118
			2	224(161) 282(285)	—	118
			20	224(155) 281(281) 390(83)	—	118
290	$C_{25}H_{33}O_8F$	16α,20β-Diacetoxy-9α-fluoro-11β,17α,21-trihydroxy-1,4-pregnadien-3-one	0.25	260(284) 308(131)	—	115
			2	260(284) 308(131)	—	115
			20	260(278) 308(125)	—	115
291	$C_{25}H_{33}O_8F$	16α,21-Diacetoxy-9α-fluoro-11β,17α-dihydroxy-4-pregnene-3,20-dione	0.25	283(373)	230(67)	119
			2	283(373) 380(32)	230(67) 324(12)	119
			20	281(379) 377(163)	233(79) 317(19)	119
292	$C_{25}H_{34}O_5$	3α,21-Diacetoxy-11β-hydroxy-5β-pregnan-20-one	—	310 415	255 390	63
293	$C_{25}H_{34}O_6$	21-Acetoxy-20-ethylenedioxy-17α-hydroxy-4,7-pregnadien-3-one	2	235(283) I 281(340) 395(203) 472(223)	250(253) 342(117) 410(160)	13
294	$C_{25}H_{34}O_7$	20β,21-Diacetoxy-11β,17α-dihydroxy-1,4-pregnadien-3-one	—	356(492)	278(99)	56
295	$C_{25}H_{34}O_7$	20β,21-Diacetoxy-17α-hydroxy-4-pregnene-3,11-dione	2	283(359)	230(56)	13
			2	283(344)	230(28)	13
			—	284 400	235 350	64

TABLE IX—*continued*

No.	Empirical Formula	Compound	Time, hours	λ_{max} in mμ ($E^{1\%}_{1\,cm}$)	λ_{min} in mμ ($E^{1\%}_{1\,cm}$)	Reference
296	$C_{25}H_{34}O_7$	11α,21-Diacetoxy-17α-hydroxy-4-pregnene-3,20-dione	—	240 285 390 475	—	108
297	$C_{25}H_{34}O_8$	2α,21-Diacetoxy-11β, 17α-dihydroxy-4-pregnene-3,20-dione	0.5 min.	240(280) 290(404) 380(127) 500(140)	—	26,88
			2	240(314) 285(354) 340(177) 387(177) 510(130)	—	26,88
298	$C_{25}H_{34}O_8$	6β,21-Diacetoxy-11β, 17α-dihydroxy-4-pregnene-3,20-dione	0.5 min.	240(885) 280(630) 340(270) 390(300) 480(224)	—	26,88
			2	240(915) 280(580) 340(690) 390(400) 480(364) 550(294)	—	26,88
299	$C_{25}H_{34}O_8$ (H_2O)	6β,21-Diacetoxy-11β, 17α-dihydroxy-4-pregnene-3,20-dione (monohydrate)	0.5 min.	249* 283 345 I 400 470 I	—	26,27
			2	249* 345 400 470 550 I	—	26,27
300	$C_{25}H_{36}O_5$	3β,21-Diacetoxy-5-pregnen-20-one	2	314(141) I 339(152) 378(183) 406(193) 476(103) 533(55) I	255(76) 352(145) 390(162) 437(93)	13
301	$C_{25}H_{36}O_6$	20α,21-Diacetoxy-17α-hydroxy-4-pregnen-3-one	2	237(412) 282(407) 380(75) I 430(136) 470(64) I	255(218) 347(46)	13
			0.25	235(325) 285(411) 373(104)	252(182) 331(43) 389(68)	16

TABLE IX—*continued*

No.	Empirical Formula	Compound	Time, hours	λ_{max} in mμ ($E^{1\%}_{1\,cm}$)	λ_{min} in mμ ($E^{1\%}_{1\,cm}$)	Reference
301 cont.	$C_{25}H_{36}O_6$	20α,21-Diacetoxy-17α hydroxy-4-pregnen-3-one		409(86) 423(82) I 472(46) I 520(39) I		
			0.50	234(364) 284(418) 375(75) 418(107) I 428(111) 473(57) I	253(200) 335(43) 383(71)	16
			1	234(389) 283(414) 380(75) I 416(121) I 429(136) 476(64) I	254(211) 337(43)	16
			1.5	235(403) 282(411) 380(75) I 412(121) I 429(136) 472(64) I	254(214) 341(46)	16
			2	236(411) 282(407) 381(74) I 415(121) I 430(136) 470(64) I	255(218) 346(46)	16
			2.5	237(418) 282(403) 381(75) I 414(121) I 429(136) 473(61) I	223(389) 256(222) 346(50)	16
			3	238(428) 282(403) 381(79) I 413(121) I 429(136) 472(61) I	223(393) 255(222) 347(50)	16
			4	238(439) 282(407) 381(79) I 411(121) I 428(136) 474(57) I	225(400) 255(229) 348(50)	16
			6	239(450) 282(414) 380(82) I 411(121) I 429(139)	224(407) 255(239) 350(57)	16

TABLE IX—*continued*

No.	Empirical Formula	Compound	Time, hours	λ_{max} in mμ ($E^{1\%}_{1\,cm}$)	λ_{min} in mμ ($E^{1\%}_{1\,cm}$)	Reference
302	$C_{25}H_{36}O_6$	20β,21-Diacetoxy-17α-hydroxy-4-pregnen-3-one	2	238(513) 285(427) 340(57) I 403(57) 421(50) I 530(30)	253(213) 360(47) 478(27)	13
			2	239(363) 288(400) 405(33) 530(17)	253(163) 370(27) 465(13)	13
			0.25	240(174) 290(373) 345(17) I 373(13) I 427(13) 529(20)	220(130) 251(123) 390(10) 450(10)	16
			0.50	239(260) 288(383) 344(23) I 374(20) I 415(20) 530(23)	251(147) 386(17) 462(13)	16
			1	239(383) 288(407) 342(37) I 405(37) 421(33) I 530(27)	253(177) 370(30) 470(20)	16
			1.5	239(463) 287(420) 344(47) I 405(50) 421(43) I 530(27)	253(197) 368(40) 478(23)	16
			2	238(513) 286(426) 340(57) I 403(57) 421(50) I 530(30)	253(213) 366(47) 478(27)	16
			2.5	238(543) 285(433) 341(60) I 403(63) 423(57) I 532(33)	253(223) 366(53) 484(30)	16

TABLE IX—*continued*

No.	Empirical Formula	Compound	Time, hours	λ_{max} in mμ ($E^{1\%}_{1\,cm}$)	λ_{min} in mμ ($E^{1\%}_{1\,cm}$)	Reference
302 cont.	$C_{25}H_{36}O_6$	20β,21-Diacetoxy-17α-hydroxy-4-pregnen-3-one	3	238(566) 285(437) 342(67) I 402(70) 422(60) I 534(33)	253(233) 365(57) 484(30)	16
			4	238(590) 285(440) 341(73) I 402(77) 421(63) I 538(37)	253(243) 366(63) 485(33)	16
			6	238(606) 286(443) 341(83) I 402(83) 416(73) I 538(43)	255(257) 365(70) 485(40)	16
303	$C_{25}H_{36}O_6$	3β,21-Diacetoxy-17α-hydroxy-5-pregnen-20-one	2	235(123) I 326(184) 407(297) 489(84) 525(61) I	256(106) 363(103) 455(74)	13
			2	326(186) 406(259) 489(82) 520(59) I	253(100) 365(100)	13
304	$C_{25}H_{36}O_7$	3α,21-Diacetoxy-17α-hydroxy-5β-pregnane-11,20-dione	2	271(109) 340(141) 415(151) 475(52) I	252(104) 290(91) 371(89)	13
			—	265 340 410	245 290 375	64
			2	330–340 410–420	—	110
305	$C_{25}H_{36}O_7$	20α,21-Diacetoxy-11β,17α-dihydroxy-4-pregnen-3-one	—	236 284 375 460	260 350 410	106
			2	240 283 330 I 385 465 525	250 350 420 515	99
306	$C_{25}H_{36}O_7$	20β,21-Diacetoxy-11β,17α-dihydroxy-4-pregnen-3-one	2	242(188) 282(344) 332(44) I 465(238)	247(181) 383(25)	13

TABLE IX—*continued*

No.	Empirical Formula	Compound	Time, hours	λ_{max} in mμ ($E^{1\%}_{1 cm}$)	λ_{min} in mμ ($E^{1\%}_{1 cm}$)	Reference
306 cont.	$C_{25}H_{36}O_7$	20β,21-Diacetoxy-11β, 17α-dihydroxy-4-pregnen-3-one	—	284 310 I 460	385	106
307	$C_{25}H_{36}O_7$	3,20-Bis-ethylenedioxy-17α,21-dihydroxy-5-pregnen-11-one	2	292(472) 343(169) 415(131) 486(13) I	235(134) 327(144) 374(66)	13
308	$C_{25}H_{38}O_4$	5-Pregnene-3,20-dione-3,20-bis-ethylene ketal	2	240(179) 302(458)	255(166)	13
309	$C_{25}H_{38}O_6$	3,20-Bis-ethylene-dioxy-5-pregnene-17α,21-diol	2	238(290) 295(438) 339(197) 500(97) I 540(152) 566(155)	251(184) 329(184) 405(39) 553(148)	13
310	$C_{25}H_{38}O_7$	3α,21-Diacetoxy-11β, 17α-dihydroxy-5β-pregnan-20-one	2	332(190) 405(255) 506(68)	275(110) 365(107) 488(65)	13
311	$C_{25}H_{38}O_7$	3,20-Bis-ethylenedioxy-5-pregnene-11α,17α, 21-triol	2	237(327) 291(379) 392(291) 480(158)	253(249) 335(112) 428(121)	13
312	$C_{25}H_{38}O_7$	3,20-Bis-ethylenedioxy-5-pregnene-11β,17α, 21-triol	2	237(316) 291(422) 389(209) 480(131)	225(294) 252(234) 337(106) 435(112)	13
313	$C_{25}H_{40}O_4$	Methyl 3α-hydroxy-12-oxo-5β-cholanate	2	315(125) 389(196)	265(68) 345(61)	13
314	$C_{25}H_{40}O_4$	5β-Pregnane-3α,20α-diol diacetate	2	317(157) 331(147) I 430(168) 490(43) I	258(68) 381(89)	13
			—	315* 420	—	70
315	$C_{25}H_{40}O_5$	Methyl 3α,12α-di-hydroxy-7-oxo-5β-cholanate	2	302(201) 390(100)	245(90) 347(58)	43
316	$C_{25}H_{42}O_3$	Methyl 12α-hydroxy-5β-cholanate	2	317(110)	246(26)	43
317	$C_{25}H_{42}O_5$	Methyl 3α,7α,12α-tri-hydroxy-5β-cholanate	2	302(98) 389(705) 480(60)	253(43) 331(71) 436(36)	43

TABLE X. ABSORPTION SPECTRA OF C_{26} STEROIDS.

No.	Empirical Formula	Compound	Time, hours	λ_{max} in mμ ($E^{1\%}_{1\,cm}$)	λ_{min} in mμ ($E^{1\%}_{1\,cm}$)	Reference
318	$C_{26}H_{31}O_7F$	17aβ-Acetoxymethyl-9α-fluoro-16α,17aα-iso-propylidenedioxy-1,4-D-homo-androstadiene-3,11,17-trione	0.25	256(317) 305(140)	—	118
			2	256(317) 305(140)	—	118
			20	256(302) 305(127)	—	118
319	$C_{26}H_{33}O_7F$	17aβ-Acetoxymethyl-9α-fluoro-11β-hydroxy-16α,17aα-iso-propylidenedioxy-1,4-D-homoandro-stadiene-3,17-dione	0.25	258(273) 309(135)	—	118
			2	258(273) 309(135)	—	118
			20	258(269) 309(130)	—	118
320	$C_{26}H_{35}O_7F$	16α-Acetoxy-9α-fluoro-11β,17α-dihydroxy-20β,21-iso-propy-lidenedioxy-1,4-pregnadien-3-one	0.25	260(306) 308(143)	285(86)	116
			2	260(306) 308(143)	285(86)	116
			20	259(297) 307(135)	284(76)	116
321	$C_{26}H_{42}O_6NNa$	Sodium 3α,7α-dihy-droxy-5β-cholanyl-glycinate (sodium glycochenodesoxy-cholate)	2	308(180) 388(69) 446(30)	250(41) 381(64) 428(28)	44
322	$C_{26}H_{43}O_4N$	5β-Cholanylglycine (glycocholanic acid)	2	315(32)	250(7)	44
323	$C_{26}H_{43}O_5N$	3α-Hydroxy-5β-cholanylglycine (glycolithocholic acid)	2	315(95)	250(25)	44
324	$C_{26}H_{43}O_6N$	3α,12α-Dihydroxy-5β-cholanylglycine (glycodesoxycholic acid)	2	313(206)	252(62)	44
325	$C_{26}H_{43}O_7N$	3α,7α,12α-Trihydroxy-5β-cholanylglycine (glycocholic acid)	2	303(96) 389(637) 479(62)	255(37) 332(72) 433(36)	44
326	$C_{26}H_{44}O_5NSNa$	Sodium 5β-cholanyl-taurinate(sodium taurocholanate)	2	315(22)	250(13)	44

TABLE X—*continued*

No.	Empirical Formula	Compound	Time, hours	λ_{max} in mμ ($E_{1\,cm}^{1\%}$)	λ_{min} in mμ ($E_{1\,cm}^{1\%}$)	Reference
327	$C_{26}H_{44}O_7NSNa$	Sodium 3α,7α-dihydroxy-5β-cholanyltaurinate(sodium taurochenodesoxycholate)	2	308(150) 384(87) 450(30)	252(43) 380(81) 430(27)	44
328	$C_{26}H_{44}O_7NSNa$	Sodium 3α,12α-dihydroxy-5β-cholanyltaurinate(sodium taurodesoxycholanate)	2	315(174)	252(60)	44
329	$C_{26}H_{45}O_6NS$	3α-Hydroxy-5β-cholanyltaurine (taurolithocholic acid)	2	312(95)	250(19)	44
330	$C_{26}H_{45}O_8NS$	3α,7α,21α-Trihydroxy-5β-cholanyltaurine (taurocholic acid)	2	303(81) 389(546) 480(54)	255(39) 333(61) 436(29)	44

TABLE XI. ABSORPTION SPECTRA OF C_{27} STEROIDS.

No.	Empirical Formula	Compound	Time, hours	λ_{max} in mμ ($E^{1\%}_{1\,cm}$)	λ_{min} in mμ ($E^{1\%}_{1\,cm}$)	Reference
331	$C_{27}H_{33}O_9F$	11β,16α,21-Triacetoxy-9α-fluoro-17α-hydroxy-1,4-pregna-diene-3,20-dione	0.25	261(260) 308(114)	—	48
			2	260(266) 308(117)	—	48
			20	260(275) 308(156)	—	48
332	$C_{27}H_{34}O_6$	3β-Acetoxy-5,7-pregnadien-20-one maleic anhydride adduct	2	240(328) 261(175) I 309(81) 403(31)	295(75) 356(22)	13
333	$C_{27}H_{35}O_9F$	16α,20β,21-Triacetoxy-9α-fluoro-11β,17α-dihydroxy-1,4-pregnadien-3-one	0.25	259(242) 309(111)	284(63)	116
			2	259(243) 309(111)	284(66)	116
			20	259(238) 308(114)	283(63)	116
334	$C_{27}H_{37}O_6F$	9α-Fluoro-11β-hydroxy-16α,17α; 20β,21-bis-isopropylidenedioxy-1,4-pregnadien-3-one	0.25	258(262) 308(134)	285(94)	116
			2	258(262) 308(134)	285(94)	116
			20	258(258) 308(132)	285(88)	116
335	$C_{27}H_{37}O_9F$	16α,20β,21-Triacetoxy-9α-fluoro-11β,17α-dihydroxy-4-pregnen-3-one	0.25	281(344)	none	116
			2	281(337)	none	116
			20	281(317)	none	116
336	$C_{27}H_{38}O_3$	22a-Spirosta-4,7-dien-3-one	2	287(403) 403(66) 468(55)	236(121) 343(41) 431(48)	13
337	$C_{27}H_{38}O_7$	21-Acetoxy-3,20-bis-ethylenedioxy-5,7-pregnadien-17α-ol	2	238(252) I 292(309) 380(152) I 392(170) 476(215)	251(215) 352(112) 412(124)	13
338	$C_{27}H_{40}O_3$	22a-Spirost-4-en-3-one	2	292(397)	239(83)	13
339	$C_{27}H_{40}O_7$	21-Acetoxy-3,20-bis-ethylenedioxy-5-pregnen-17α-ol	2	239(294) 296(397) 339(188) 496(94) I 543(159) 569(162)	252(174) 327(177) 397(35) 553(153)	13
340	$C_{27}H_{42}O$	3,5-Cholestadien-7-one	—	356	—	36

TABLE XI—*continued*

No.	Empirical Formula	Compound	Time, hours	λ_{max} in mμ ($E^{1\%}_{1\,cm}$)	λ_{min} in mμ ($E^{1\%}_{1\,cm}$)	Reference
341	$C_{27}H_{42}O_4$	3β-Hydroxy-5α,22a-spirostan-11-one	2	280(57) 320(67) 401(110)	259(52) 360(37)	13
342	$C_{27}H_{44}O$	4-Cholesten-3-one	2	292(437)	232(89)	13
343	$C_{27}H_{44}O$	7-Cholesten-3-one	2	240(86) 317(189)	228(179) 263(68)	13
344	$C_{27}H_{44}O_3$	5β,22b-Spirostan-3β-ol	2	317(123) 330(123) 401(47)	260(47) 324(120) 378(37)	13
345	$C_{27}H_{46}O$	5α-Cholestan-3-one	2	312(152)	255(52)	13
346	$C_{27}H_{46}O$	5β-Cholestan-3-one	2	235(91) I 316(146) 477(12)	263(66) 430(10)	13
347	$C_{27}H_{46}O$	5-Cholesten-3β-ol (Cholesterol)	2	242(69) 319(196) 415(61) 489(22) I	226(63) 258(61) 393(56)	13
348	$C_{27}H_{48}O$	5β-Cholestan-3β-ol (coprosterol)	2	240(54) 320(117) 410(27) I	224(48) 260(43)	13
349	$C_{27}H_{48}O_3$	5β-Cholestane-3α,7α,12α-triol	2	322(177) 390(334) 484(126)	257(67) 347(153) 439(93)	43

TABLE XII. ABSORPTION SPECTRA OF C_{28} STEROIDS.

No.	Empirical Formula	Compound	Time, hours	λ_{max} in mμ ($E^{1\%}_{1\,cm}$)	λ_{min} in mμ ($E^{1\%}_{1\,cm}$)	Reference
350	$C_{28}H_{40}O$	4,7,9(11),22-Ergosta-tetraen-3-one	2	240(189) I 292(496) 400(86) 455(61) I	228(172) 378(75)	13
351	$C_{28}H_{42}O$	5,7,9(11),22-Ergosta-tetraen-3β-ol (dehydroergosterol)	2	249(269) I 278(355) 332(179) I 373(221) 433(314) 517(104) I	230(245) 344(166) 384(210)	13
352	$C_{28}H_{42}O$	4,7,22-Ergostatrien-3-one	2	294(504) 444(29)	233(111) 396(18)	13
353	$C_{28}H_{44}O$	7,22-Ergostadien-3-one	2	328(103) 312(272)	225(97) 258(90)	13
354	$C_{28}H_{44}O$	5,7,22-Ergostatrien-3β-ol (ergosterol)	2	231(146) I 309(289) 416(168) 436(143) I 490(93) I	255(111) 379(129)	13
355	$C_{28}H_{44}O_7$	3α,7α-Diacetoxy-12α-hydroxy-5β-cholanic acid	2	316(208) 390(224) 500(78)	253(55) 342(75) 460(54)	43
356	$C_{28}H_{46}O$	5,24(28)-Ergostadien-3β-ol(24-methylene-cholesterol, chalinasterol)	2	240(117) 314(221) 421(117) 440(107) I 499(69)	229(114) 255(103) 387(97) 483(66)	13
357	$C_{28}H_{46}O$	7,22-Ergostadien-3β-ol	2	238(93) 319(224) 419(81) 441(66) I 469(48) I	229(90) 256(79) 400(76)	13
358	$C_{28}H_{48}O$	5α-Ergostan-3-one	2	240(46) 313(125)	230(45) 257(41)	13
359	$C_{28}H_{48}O$	24a-Ergost-5-en-3β-ol (campesterol)	2	242(80) 318(220) 415(71) 500(29) I	226(71) 258(68) 387(59)	13
360	$C_{28}H_{48}O$	5α,24a-Ergost-22-en-3β-ol (neospongo-sterol)	2	240(76) 319(204) 393(64) I 423(72) 446(62) I 478(45) I	228(72) 256(66) 383(60)	13
361	$C_{28}H_{48}O$	5α,24a-Ergost-8(14)-en-3β-ol (α-stellastenol)	2	240(107) I 316(207) 420(90) 441(67) I 504(31) I	258(93) 388(83)	13

TABLE XII—*continued*

No.	Empirical Formula	Compound	Time, hours	λ_{max} in mμ ($E^{1\%}_{1\,cm}$)	λ_{min} in mμ ($E^{1\%}_{1\,cm}$)	Reference
362	$C_{28}H_{48}O$	5α,24a-Ergost-14-en-3β-ol (β-stellastenol)	2	239(97) 319(217) 394(76) I 423(79) 440(67) I 489(41) I	229(93) 257(83) 402(72)	13
363	$C_{28}H_{48}O_2$	14,15-Epoxy-5α-ergostan-3β-ol	2	237(121) I 308(311) 340(189) I 368(125) I 415(98) 448(70) I 497(54) I	256(96) 398(86)	13
364	$C_{28}H_{50}O$	5α,24a-Ergostan-3β-ol (stellastanol)	2	240(72) 320(171) 415(33) I 478(17) I	227(66) 259(62)	13
365	$C_{28}H_{50}O$	5α-Ergostan-3α-ol	2	321(162) 416(27) I 473(12) I	254(54)	13
366	$C_{28}H_{50}O$	5α-Ergostan-3β-ol	2	321(165) 406(31) I 470(15) I	254(55)	13
			2	321(164) 410(29) I 480(14) I	255(54)	13

TABLE XIII. ABSORPTION SPECTRA OF C_{29} STEROIDS.

No.	Empirical Formula	Compound	Time, hours	λ_{max} in mμ ($E^{1\%}_{1\,cm}$)	λ_{min} in mμ ($E^{1\%}_{1\,cm}$)	Reference
367	$C_{29}H_{40}O_4$	22a-Spirosta-5,7,9(11)-trien-3β-ol acetate	2	245(244) I 347(359) 409(81) 474(50)	279(100) 383(59) 458(47)	13
368	$C_{29}H_{42}O_4$	5α,22a-Spirosta-7,9(11)-dien-3β-ol-acetate	2	236(197) I 286(195) 409(325) 469(300)	256(136) 343(88) 437(230)	13
369	$C_{29}H_{42}O_4$	22a-Spirosta-5,7-dien-3β-ol acetate	2	240(272) 285(156) 327(94) I 406(238) 471(153)	226(247) 269(141) 346(84) 440(122)	13
370	$C_{29}H_{44}O_4$	3,5,7-Cholestatrien-3β-ol acetate	2	291(336) 373(81) I 460(106)	230(126) 390(47)	13
371	$C_{29}H_{44}O_4$	5,7,9(11)-Cholestatrien-3β-ol acetate	2	279(210) 368(377) 438(92)	251(161) 319(126) 407(77)	13
372	$C_{29}H_{44}O_4$	22a-Spirost-5-en-3β-ol acetate	2	320(94) 339(86) I 412(319) 490(28)	265(44) 358(78) 458(25)	13
373	$C_{29}H_{44}O_4$	5α,22a-Spirost-7-en-3β-ol acetate	2	239(109) I 325(105) I 409(397) 469(44) 500(26) I 537(5) I	270(71) 458(41)	13
374	$C_{29}H_{45}O_2N$	5-Solaniden-3β-ol acetate	2	241(81) 320(160) 346(142) 413(242)	227(74) 270(58) 334(135) 376(106)	13
375	$C_{29}H_{46}O_2$	5,7-Cholestadien-3β-ol acetate	2	235(108) I 312(393) 406(56) I 486(50) I	254(97)	13
376	$C_{29}H_{46}O_2$	5α-Cholesta-8(9),24-dien-3β-ol acetate	2	239(116) I 312(218) 391(97) I 414(90) 500(39) I	253(113) 405(89)	13
377	$C_{29}H_{46}O_3$	2α-Acetoxy-4-cholesten-3-one	0.25	296(295)	none	115
			2	297(308)	234(121)	115
			20	289(266) 349(297) 430(125)	248(174) 313(274) 382(106)	115

TABLE XIII—*continued*

No.	Empirical Formula	Compound	Time, hours	λ_{max} in mμ ($E^{1\%}_{1\ cm}$)	λ_{min} in mμ ($E^{1\%}_{1\ cm}$)	Reference
378	$C_{29}H_{46}O_3$	3β-Acetoxy-5-cholesten-7-one	2	285(107) I 355(419) 411(23) I 484(13) I	241(58)	13
379	$C_{29}H_{46}O_7$	Methyl 3α,7α-diacetoxy-12α-hydroxy-5β-cholanate	2	317(199) 390(232) 505(78)	255(52) 344(78) 460(62)	43
380	$C_{29}H_{48}O$	24a-Stigmasta-5,22-dien-3β-ol (poriferasterol)	2	240(107) 315(257) 428(127) 498(63)	229(103) 259(97) 387(82) 486(60)	13
381	$C_{29}H_{48}O$	24a-Stigmasta-7,22-dien-3β-ol (chondrillasterol)	2	238(103) 313(271) 440(100) 494(45) I	230(102) 255(91) 390(79)	13
382	$C_{29}H_{48}O$	5,22-Stigmastadien-3β-ol	2	233(117) I 314(259) 425(115) 498(48) I	255(97) 385(76)	13
383	$C_{29}H_{48}O$	5,24(28)-Stigmastadien-3β-ol(fucosterol)	2	234(113) I 317(200) 431(177) 500(97)	258(93) 388(107) 488(92)	13
			2	238(113) I 318(187) 431(198) 500(103)	260(93) 389(112) 486(97)	13
384	$C_{29}H_{48}O$	7,22-Stigmastadien-3β-ol	2	235(93) I 314(260) 446(114) 496(55) I	256(83) 390(79)	13
385	$C_{29}H_{48}OS$	5-Cholestene-3β-thiol acetate	2	246(52) 320(148) 338(121) I 407(13) I	228(42) 264(45)	13
386	$C_{29}H_{48}O_2$	5-Cholesten-3β-ol acetate(cholesteryl acetate)	2	315(200) 415(73) 494(27) I	255(73) 389(62)	13
387	$C_{29}H_{48}O_2$	5α-Cholest-6-en-3β-ol acetate	2	239(84) I 319(226) 418(80) 441(66) I 480(40) I	257(76) 385(70)	13
388	$C_{29}H_{48}O_2$	5α-Cholest-7-en-3β-ol acetate	2	238(60) I 318(200) 418(87) 482(45) I	253(55) 383(73)	13

TABLE XIII—*continued*

No.	Empirical Formula	Compound	Time, hours	λ_{max} in mμ ($E^{1\%}_{1\ cm}$)	λ_{min} in mμ ($E^{1\%}_{1\ cm}$)	Reference
389	$C_{29}H_{48}O_2$	5α-Cholest-8(14)-en-3β-ol acetate	2	239(83) I 316(207) 395(73) I 422(78) 494(32) I	253(75) 383(70)	13
390	$C_{29}H_{48}O_3$	3β-Acetoxy-5α-cholestan-7-one	2	305(189) 402(42) 475(9) I	243(63) 370(31)	13
391	$C_{29}H_{50}O$	Palysterol	2	242(100) 318(248) 421(103) 440(90) I 500(48)	228(97) 258(88) 388(76) 486(47)	13
392	$C_{29}H_{50}O$	5-Stigmasten-3β-ol	2	233(77) I 317(190) 416(60) 500(22) I	253(67) 390(50)	13

TABLE XIV. ABSORPTION SPECTRA OF C_{30} STEROIDS.

No.	Empirical Formula	Compound	Time, hours	λ_{max} in mμ ($E^{1\%}_{1\,cm}$)	λ_{min} in mμ ($E^{1\%}_{1\,cm}$)	Reference
393	$C_{30}H_{46}O_8$	3α,7α,12α-Triacetoxy-5β-cholanic acid	2	310(192)	252(56)	43
394	$C_{30}H_{48}O_2$	5α-Ergosta-7,22-dien-3β-ol acetate	2	311(265) 395(79) I 418(84)	252(76) 382(76)	13
395	$C_{30}H_{48}O_2$	5α-Ergosta-8(9),14-dien-3β-ol acetate	2	229(106) I 310(323) 377(77) I 415(74)	252(87) 401(73)	13
396	$C_{30}H_{50}O_2$	5α-Ergost-7-en-3β-ol acetate	2	234(79) I 318(216) 395(84) I 413(87) 470(53) I	254(63) 382(76)	13
397	$C_{30}H_{50}O_2$	5α-Ergost-8(14)-en-3β-ol acetate	2	319(213) 399(81) I 416(84) 472(52) I	253(60) 381(71)	13
398	$C_{30}H_{50}O_2$	5α-Ergost-14-en-3β-ol acetate	2	318(223) 392(82) I 418(87) 478(53) I	252(61) 381(74)	13
399	$C_{30}H_{52}O_2$	5α-Ergostan-3α-ol acetate	2	320(150) 402(55) 475(18) I	257(41) 386(50)	13
400	$C_{30}H_{52}O_2$	5α-Ergostan-3β-ol acetate	2	320(156) 400(32) I	258(52)	13

TABLE XV. ABSORPTION SPECTRA OF C_{31} STEROIDS.

No.	Empirical Formula	Compound	Time, hours	λ_{max} in mμ ($E^{1\%}_{1\,cm}$)	λ_{min} in mμ ($E^{1\%}_{1\,cm}$)	Reference
401	$C_{31}H_{52}O_2$	24a-Stigmast-5-en-3β-ol acetate (clionasterol acetate)	2	241(76) 318(194) 415(73) 440(49) I 497(27) I	228(70) 255(67) 386(58)	13
402	$C_{31}H_{54}O_2$	5α-Stigmastan-3β-ol acetate	2	233(61) I 320(161) 402(48) 474(19) I	255(52) 389(45)	13

TABLE XVI. ABSORPTION SPECTRA OF C_{34} STEROIDS.

No.	Empirical Formula	Compound	Time, hours	λ_{max} in mμ ($E^{1\%}_{1\,cm}$)	λ_{min} in mμ ($E^{1\%}_{1\,cm}$)	Reference
403	$C_{34}H_{50}O_2$	5-Cholesten-3β-ol benzoate	2	262(429) 312(212) 414(56) 440(40) I 495(19) I	284(147) 391(47)	13

Note added in proof

Significant use of spectra in concentrated sulfuric acid of cardiac glycosides and aglycones has been published since this review was written. See:

(1) BROWN, B. T. and WRIGHT, S. E., *J. Amer. Pharm. Assoc.*, **49**, 777 (1960).

(2) REPKE, K. and KLESCZEWSKI, S., *Arch. Exptl. Pathol. Pharmakol.*, **239**, 131 (1960).

(3) BROWN, B. T. and WRIGHT, S. E., *J. Pharm. Pharmacol.*, **13**, 262 (1961).

Acknowledgement—The authors wish to acknowledge the assistance of Miss Phyllis Ablondi and Mr. Walter Hearn in preparing the many spectral curves presented.

VII. REFERENCES

[1] ANTONUCCI, R., BERNSTEIN, S., HELLER, M., LENHARD, R., LITTELL, R. and WILLIAMS, J. H., *J. Org. Chem.* **18**, 70 (1953).
[2] ARROYAVE, G. and AXELROD, L. R., *J. Biol. Chem.* **208**, 579 (1954).
[3] AXELROD, L. R., *J. Amer. Chem. Soc.* **75**, 6301 (1953).
[4] AXELROD, L. R., *J. Biol. Chem.* **201**, 59 (1953).
[5] AXELROD, L. R., *J. Biol. Chem.* **205**, 173 (1953).
[6] AXELROD, L. R. and ARROYAVE, G., *J. Amer. Chem. Soc.* **75**, 5729 (1953).
[7] AXELROD, L. R. and MILLER, L. L., *Arch. Biochem. Biophys.* **49**, 248 (1954).
[8] AXELROD, L. R., MILLER, L. L. and HERLING, F., *J. Biol. Chem.* **219**, 455 (1956).
[9] BACCHUS, H., *Amer. J. Physiol.* **188**, 297 (1957).
[10] BALFOUR, W. E., COMLINE, R. S. and SHORT, R. V., *Nature, Lond.* **183**, 467 (1959).
[11] BERLINER, D. L., JONES, J. E. and SALHANICK, H. A., *J. Biol. Chem.* **223**, 1043 (1956).

[12] Bernstein, S., Allen, W. S., Heller, M., Lenhard, R. H., Feldman, L. I. and Blank, R. H., *J. Org. Chem.* **24**, 286 (1959).
[13] Bernstein, S. and Lenhard, R. H., *J. Org. Chem.* **18**, 1146 (1953).
[14] Bernstein, S. and Lenhard, R. H., *J. Org. Chem.* **19**, 1269 (1954).
[15] Bernstein, S. and Lenhard, R. H., *J. Org. Chem.* **25**, 1405 (1960).
[16] Bernstein, S. and Lenhard, R. H., unpublished studies.
[17] Bernstein, S., Lenhard, R. H. and Allen, W. S., U.S. Patent No. 2,789,118, April 16 (1957).
[18] Bernstein, S., Lenhard, R. H. and Williams, J. H., *J. Org. Chem.* **18**, 1166 (1953).
[19] Bianchini, P. and Osima, B., *Boll. Soc. Ital. Biol. Sper.* **34**, 1791 (1958).
[20] Birmingham, M. K. and Kurlents, E., *Canad. J. Biochem. and Physiol.* **37**, 510 (1959).
[21] Bitman, J., Rosselet, J.-P., De Reddy, A. M. and Lieberman, S., *J. Biol. Chem.* **225**, 39 (1957).
[22] Bongiovanni, A. M. and Clayton, G. W., Jr., *Johns Hopk. Hosp. Bull.* **94**, 180 (1954).
[23] Bongiovanni, A. M. and Eberlein, W. R., *Analyt. Chem.* **30**, 388 (1958).
[24] Burstein, S., *J. Amer. Chem. Soc.* **78**, 1769 (1956).
[25] Burstein, S. and Dorfman, R. I., *J. Amer. Chem. Soc.* **77**, 4668 (1955).
[26] Burstein, S. and Dorfman, R. I., *J. Biol. Chem.* **213**, 581 (1955).
[27] Burstein, S., Dorfman, R. I. and Nadel, E. M., *J. Biol. Chem.* **213**, 597 (1955).
[28] Burton, R. B., Keutmann, E. H. and Waterhouse, C., *J. Clin. Endocrin. Met.* **13**, 48 (1953).
[29] Bush, I. E., *Recent Progr. Hormone Res.* **9**, 321 (1954).
[30] Bush, I. E., *Ciba Foundation Colloquia on Endocrinology* **11**, 200 (1958).
[31] Carstensen, H., Burgers, A. C. J. and Li, C. H., *J. Amer. Chem. Soc.* **81**, 4109 (1959).
[32] Carstensen, H., Oertel, G. W. and Eik-Nes, K. B., *J. Biol. Chem.* **234**, 2570 (1959).
[33] Caspi, E. and Bergen, J. R., *Arch. Biochem. Biophys.* **59**, 207 (1955).
[34] Caspi, E. and Pechet, M. M., *J. Biol. Chem.* **230**, 843 (1958).
[35] Clark, I., *Nature, Lond.* **175**, 123 (1955).
[36] Cunningham, N. F. and Morton, R. A., *Biochem. J.* **72**, 92 (1959).
[37] Diaz, G., Zaffaroni, A., Rosenkranz, G. and Djerassi, C., *J. Org. Chem.* **17**, 747 (1952).
[38] Dohan, F. C., Touchstone, J. C. and Richardson, E. M., *J. Clin. Invest.* **34**, 485 (1955).
[39] Dorfman, L., *Chem. Rev.* **53**, 47 (1953).
[40] Dyrenfurth, I., Sybulski, S., Notchev, V., Beck, J. C. and Venning, E. H., *J. Clin. Endocrin. Met.* **18**, 391 (1958).
[41] Eberlein, W. R. and Bongiovanni, A. M., *J. Biol. Chem.* **223**, 85 (1956).
[42] Eisenstein, A. B., *Proc. Soc. Exptl. Biol., N.Y.* **91**, 657 (1956).
[43] Eriksson, S. and Sjövall, J., *Ark. Kemi* **8**, 303 (1955).
[44] Eriksson, S. and Sjövall, J., *Ark. Kemi* **8**, 311 (1955).
[45] Farrell, G. L., Royce, P. C., Rauschkolb, E. W. and Hirschman, H., *Proc. Soc. Exptl. Biol. N.Y.* **87**, 141 (1954).
[46] Fish, C. A., Hayano, M. and Pincus, G., *Arch. Biochem. Biophys.* **42**, 480 (1953).
[47] Fotherby, K., *Biochem. J.* **71**, 209 (1959).
[48] Fox, S. M., Origoni, V. E. and Smith, L. L., *J. Amer. Chem. Soc.* **82**, 2580 (1960).
[49] Ganis, F. M., Axelrod, L. R. and Miller, L. L., *J. Biol. Chem.* **218**, 841 (1956).
[50] Gillam, A. E. and Stern, E. S., *An Introduction to Electronic Absorption Spectroscopy in Organic Chemistry* pp. 47–51. Arnold, London (1954).
[51] Gillespie, R. J. and Leisten, J. A., *Quart. Rev. Chem. Soc., Lond.* **8**, 40 (1954).
[52] Göbel, P., Heni, F. and D'Addabbo, A., *Hoppe-Seyl. Z.* **311**, 201 (1958).
[53] Goldberg, H. F. and Linford, J. H., *Canad. J. Biochem. Physiol.* **36**, 1221 (1958).
[54] Gornall, A. G. and Gwilliam, C., *Canad. J. Biochem. Physiol.* **35**, 71 (1957).
[55] Graff, M. M., *J. Biol. Chem.* **197**, 741 (1952).
[56] Gray, C. H., Green, M. A. S., Holness, N. J. and Lunnon, J. B., *J. Endocrin.* **14**, 146 (1956).
[57] Hagopian, M., Pincus, G., Carlo, J. and Romanoff, E. B., *Endocrinology* **58**, 387 (1956).
[58] Harman, R. E., Ham, E. A., DeYoung, J. J., Brink, N. G. and Sarett, L. H., *J. Amer. Chem. Soc.* **76**, 5035 (1954).
[59] Haynes, R. C., Jr., Koritz, S. B., Péron, F. G. and Robidoux, W. F., *J. Biol. Chem.* **234**, 1421 (1959).
[60] Heard, R. D. H. and O'Donnell, V. J., *Endocrinology* **54**, 209 (1954).
[61] Hirschmann, R. F., Miller, R., Beyler, R. E., Sarett, L. H. and Tishler, M., *J. Amer. Chem. Soc.* **77**, 3166 (1955).
[62] Holness, N. J., *Lancet* **2**, 952 (1957).
[63] Holness, N. J. and Gray, C. H., *J. Endocrin.* **17**, 237 (1958).
[64] Holness, N. J., Lunnon, J. B. and Gray, C. H., *J. Endocrin.* **14**, 138 (1956).
[65] Hudson, P. B. and Lombardo, M. E., *J. Clin. Endocrin. Met.* **15**, 324 (1955).
[66] Idler, D. R., Ronald, A. P. and Schmidt, P. J., *J. Amer. Chem. Soc.* **81**, 1260 (1959).
[67] Jensen, C. C., *Acta Endocr.* **30**, 222 (1959).

[68] KALANT, H., *Biochem. J.* **63**, 10P (1956).
[69] KALANT, H., *Biochem. J.* **69**, 79 (1958).
[70] KLOPPER, A. I. and MACNAUGHTON, M. C., *J. Endocrin.* **18**, 319 (1959).
[71] LEVINE, V. E. and TAO, A. H., *Federation Proc.* **12**, 238 (1953).
[72] LEVY, H. R. and TALALAY, P., *J. Biol. Chem.* **234**, 2009 (1959).
[73] LINFORD, J. H., *Canad. J. Med. Sci.* **30**, 199 (1952).
[74] LINFORD, J. H., *Canad. J. Biochem. and Physiol.* **35**, 299 (1957).
[75] LINFORD, J. H. and FLEMING, O. J., *Canad. J. Med. Sci.* **31**, 182 (1953).
[76] LINFORD, J. H. and PAULSON, O. B., *Canad. J. Med. Sci.* **30**, 213 (1952).
[77] LITTELL, R. and BERNSTEIN, S., *J. Amer. Chem. Soc.* **78**, 984 (1956).
[78] LOKE, K. H., MARRIAN, G. F. and WATSON, E. J. D., *Biochem. J.* **71**, 43 (1959).
[79] LOMBARDO, M. E. and HUDSON, P. B., *J. Biol. Chem.* **229**, 181 (1957).
[80] LOMBARDO, M. E. and HUDSON, P. B., *Endocrinology* **65**, 417 (1959).
[81] LOMBARDO, M. E., HUDSON, P. B. and YANDEL, F., Jr., *J. Biol. Chem.* **220**, 699 (1956).
[82] LOMBARDO, M. E., MCMORRIS, C. and HUDSON, P. B., *Endocrinology* **65**, 426 (1959).
[83] LOMBARDO, M. E., ROITMAN, E. and HUDSON, P. B., *J. Clin. Endocrin. Met.* **16**, 1283 (1956).
[84] MARRIAN, G. F., LOKE, K. H., WATSON, E. J. D. and PANATTONI, M., *Biochem. J.* **66**, 60 (1957).
[85] MATTOX, V. R., MASON, H. L., ALBERT, A. and CODE, C. F., *J. Amer. Chem. Soc.* **75**, 4869 (1953).
[86] MCALEER, W. J., private communication.
[87] MILLER, L. L. and AXELROD, L. R., *Metabolism* **3**, 438 (1954).
[88] NADEL, E. M., YOUNG, B. G., HILGAR, A. C. and BURSTEIN, S., *Acta Endocr.* **28**, 283 (1958).
[89] NORMAN, A. and SJÖVALL, J., *J. Biol. Chem.* **233**, 872 (1958).
[90] NOWACZYNSKI, W., KOIW, E. and GENEST, J., *Canad. J. Biochem. and Physiol.* **35**, 425 (1957).
[91] NOWACZYNSKI, W., SANDOR, T., KOIW, E., JONES, R. N. and GENEST, J., *Canad. J. Biochem. and Physiol.* **36**, 869 (1958).
[92] NOWACZYNSKI, W. J. and STEYERMARK, P. R., *Arch. Biochem. Biophys.* **58**, 453 (1955).
[93] NOWACZYNSKI, W. J. and STEYERMARK, P. R., *Canad. J. Biochem. and Physiol.* **34**, 592 (1956).
[94] NOWACZYNSKI, W. J., STEYERMARK, P. R., KOIW, E., GENEST, J. and JONES, R. N., *Canad. J. Biochem. and Physiol.* **34**, 1023 (1956).
[95] OERTEL, G. W. and EIK-NES, K. B., *Analyt. Chem.* **31**, 98 (1959).
[96] OERTEL, G. W. and EIK-NES, K. B., *Endocrinology* **65**, 766 (1959).
[97] PÉRON, F. G. and DORFMAN, R. I., *J. Biol. Chem.* **223**, 877 (1956).
[98] PETERSON, R. E., *J. Biol. Chem.* **225**, 25 (1957).
[99] PETERSON, R. E., PIERCE, C. E. and KLIMAN, B., *Arch. Biochem. Biophys.* **70**, 614 (1957).
[100] PETERSON, R. E. and WYNGAARDEN, J. B., *J. Clin. Invest.* **35**, 552 (1956).
[101] PONTIUS, D., BECKMANN, I. and VOIGT, K. D., *Acta Endocr.* **20**, 19 (1955).
[102] REICH, H., NELSON, D. H. and ZAFFARONI, A., *J. Biol. Chem.* **187**, 411 (1950).
[103] REIF, A. E. and LONGWELL, B. B., *Endocrinology* **62**, 573 (1958).
[104] RICHARDSON, E. M., BULASCHENKO, H. and DOHAN, F. C., *J. Clin. Endocrin. Met.* **18**, 666 (1958).
[105] RICHARDSON, E. M., TOUCHSTONE, J. C. and DOHAN, F. C., *J. Clin. Invest.* **34**, 285 (1955).
[106] RICHARDSON, E. M., BULASCHENKO, H. and DOHAN, F. C., *J. Clin. Endocrin. Met.* **18**, 1399 (1958).
[107] ROMANOFF, L. P., SEELYE, J., RODRIGUEZ, R. and PINCUS, G., *J. Clin. Endocrin. Met.* **17**, 434 (1957).
[108] ROMO, J., ZAFFARONI, A., HENDRICHS, J., ROSENKRANZ, G., DJERASSI, C. and SONDHEIMER, F. *Chem. & Ind.* 783 (1952)
[109] SALHANICK, H. A. and BERLINER, D. L., *J. Biol. Chem.* **227**, 583 (1957).
[110] SCHNEIDER, J. J., *J. Biol. Chem.* **194**, 337 (1952).
[111] SIMPSON, S. A., TAIT, J. F., WETTSTEIN, A., NEHER, R., VON EUW, J., SCHINDLER, O. and REICHSTEIN, T., *Helv. Chim. Acta* **37**, 1163 (1954).
[112] SJÖVALL, J., *Ark. Kemi* **8**, 317 (1955).
[113] SLAUNWHITE, W. R., ENGEL, L. L., SCOTT, J. F. and HAM, C. L., *J. Biol. Chem.* **201**, 615 (1953).
[114] SLAUNWHITE, W. R. and SANDBERG, A. A., *J. Clin. Endocrin. Met.* **17**, 395 (1957).
[115] SMITH, L. L., unpublished results.
[116] SMITH, L. L., GARBARINI, J. J., GOODMAN, J. J., MARX, M. and MENDELSOHN, H., *J. Amer. Chem. Soc.* **82**, 1437 (1960).
[117] SMITH, L. L. and HALWER, M., *J. Amer. Pharm. Assoc.* **48**, 348 (1959).
[118] SMITH, L. L., MARX, M., GARBARINI, J. J., FOELL, T., ORIGONI, V. E. and GOODMAN, J. J., *J. Amer. Chem. Soc.*, **82**, 4616 (1960).
[119] SMITH, L. L. and MULLER, W. H., *J. Org. Chem.* **23**, 960 (1958).
[120] SOMMERVILLE, I. F. and DESHPANDE, G. N., *J. Clin. Endocrin. Met.* **18**, 1223 (1958).

[121] SOUTHCOTT, C. M., BANDY, H. E., NEWSOM, S. E. and DARRACH, M., *Canad. J. Biochem. Physiol.* **34**, 913 (1956).
[122] SOUTHCOTT, C. M., GANDOSSI, S. K., BARKER, A. D., BANDY, H. E., MCINTOSH, H. and DARRACH, M., *Canad. J. Biochem. and Physiol.* **34**, 146 (1956).
[123] SOUTHCOTT, C. M., SPROULE, V. A., MCINTOSH, H. and DARRACH, M., *Canad. J. Biochem. and Physiol.* **36**, 819 (1958).
[124] STEYERMARK, P. R. and NOWACZYNSKI, W. J., *Arch. Biochem. Biophys.* **59**, 1 (1955).
[125] STOUDT, T. H., MCALEER, W. J., CHEMERDA, J. M., KOZLOWSKI, M. A., HIRSCHMANN, R. F., MARLATT, V. and MILLER, R., *Arch. Biochem. Biophys.* **59**, 304 (1955).
[126] TAUBER, H., *Analyt. Chem.* **24**, 1494 (1952).
[127] TELLER, W. and STAIB, W., *Acta Endocr.* **32**, 209 (1959).
[128] TOUCHSTONE, J. C., BULASCHENKO, H. and DOHAN, F. C., *J. Clin. Endocrin. Met.* **15**, 760 (1955).
[129] TOUCHSTONE, J. C., COOPER, D. Y., KASPAROW, M. and BLAKEMORE, W. S., *J. Clin. Endocrin. Met.* **19**, 487 (1959).
[130] TOUCHSTONE, J. C., GLAZIER, L., COOPER, D. Y. and ROBERTS, J. M., *J. Clin. Endocrin. Met.* **15**, 382 (1955).
[131] TOUCHSTONE, J. C., KEISMAN, R. A., MARCANTONIO, A. F. and GREENE, J. W., Jr., *Analyt. Chem.* **30**, 1707 (1958).
[132] VAN ZEELST, A. M. C., SCHWARZ, F. and FAST, A. K., *Lancet* **2**, 896 (1957).
[133] VERMEULEN, A., *J. Endocrin.* **18**, 278 (1959).
[134] WALENS, H. A., TURNER, A. and WALL, M. E., *Analyt. Chem.* **26**, 325 (1954).
[135] WILSON, H., BORRIS, J. J. and BAHN, R. C., *Endocrinology* **62**, 135 (1958).
[136] WILSON, H., FAIRBANKS, R., SCIALABBA, D., MCEWEN, C. and ZIFF, M., *J. Clin. Endocrin. Met.* **16**, 86 (1956).
[137] ZAFFARONI, A., *J. Amer. Chem. Soc.* **72**, 3828 (1950).
[138] ZAFFARONI, A., *Recent Progr. Hormone Res.* **8**, 51 (1953).
[139] ZAFFARONI, A. and BURTON, R. B., *J. Biol. Chem.* **193**, 749 (1951).
[140] ZAFFARONI, A. and BURTON, R. B., *Arch. Biochem. Biophys.* **42**, 1 (1953).
[141] ZAFFARONI, A., RINGOLD, H. J., ROSENKRANZ, G., SONDHEIMER, F., THOMAS, G. H. and DJERASSI, C., *J. Amer. Chem. Soc.* **80**, 6110 (1958).

INDEX

As the compounds listed in the index are not all named according to the IUPAC system, the following suggestions are given :

If the steroid sought is not filed where expected, look it up according to other systems of nomenclature, bearing also in mind that there is considerable variation about which substituent group will be named first.

Compounds are filed alphabetically for the most part. In the case of a series of steroids all with the same general name, i.e. "Hydroxypregnendiones," the position of ring double bonds is the next determinant of ordering (lower to higher numbers). Within these groups of similar unsaturation, the steroid with a lower numbered carbon bearing the first type of substituent mentioned comes before a steroid having this group at a carbon higher number. 11β-Hydroxy-4-pregnene-3,20-dione comes before : 17α-Hydroxy-4-pregnene-3,20-dione which is filed before : 11β-Hydroxy-5-pregnene-3,20-dione, then : 17α-Hydroxy-5-pregnene-3,20-dione.

Some acetates are filed under "Acetoxy," or "Diacetoxy," etc., as well as being listed as acetates under the parent compound. All derivatives are filed under the parent compound.

If a compound contains halogen or nitrogen, this is *usually* indicated in the first prefix of its name.

Steroids may also be filed under : Bis, carboxy, epoxy, ethinyl, ethoxy, di, homo, iso, methoxy, nor, seco.

Not affecting alphabetical position are the following : ring letter designations, *N*, (for nitrogen substituents), *cis*, *trans*, *d*, *l*, Greek letters, or any numbers (except as mentioned in paragraph three).

Where the hydrogen atom at the A/B ring juncture is α, the following terms may be used : 5α, androst-, allopregn-, cholest-.

When the hydrogen is in the β configuration, terms 5β, etiochol-, pregn-, coprost-, may be used.

When the configuration at a ring juncture is given for a steroid with unsaturation in the steroid nucleus, the IUPAC system is used in the index as : 3α-Hydroxy-5β-pregna-6,9(11)-dien-20-one. This does not affect the alphabetical position, of course, but is done for reasons of clarity in the reading of the names.

The Editor wishes to express his deep appreciation to Miss Priscilla Carter and Mrs. George Wein for the patience, care and skill they devoted to the preparation of the index.

INDEX